Linda Meeks
The Ohio State University

Philip Heit
The Ohio State University

Randy Page
University of Idaho

Meeks Heit

Health and Wellness

Meeks Heit Publishing Company
Editorial, Sales, and Customer Service
P.O. Box 121
Blacklick, OH 43004
(614) 759-7780

Contributing Author

Candace Purdy, M.S.
Health Education Consultant

Director of Editorial: Julie DeVillers
Managing Editor: Myra Immell
Art Direction and Design: Mary Geer
Director of Art and Design: Jim Brower
Production: Elizabeth Kim
Photography: Lew Lause, Roman Sapecki, Chas Krider
Illustration: Deborah Rubenstein
Editorial Assistant: Tamre Edwards

Unit 10 outlines emergency care procedures that reflect the standard of knowledge and accepted practices in the United States at the time this book was published. It is the teacher's responsibility to stay informed of changes in emergency care procedures in order to teach current accepted practices. The teacher also may recommend that students gain complete, comprehensive training from courses offered by the American Red Cross.

Printed in the United States of America

2 3 4 5 6 7 8 9 10   99 98

Library of Congress Catalog Number: 97-093756

ISBN: 1-886693-14-5

About Meeks Heit Publishing Company

Professor Linda Meeks   **Dr. Philip Heit**

Linda Meeks and Philip Heit are professors emeriti at The Ohio State University. Linda and Philip held joint appointments as faculty members in Health Education in the College of Education and Allied Medicine in the College of Medicine. They have collaborated for more than 20 years, co-authoring more than 150 health books that are used by millions of students preschool through college. Together, they have helped state departments of education as well as thousands of school districts develop comprehensive school health education curricula. Their books and curricula are used throughout the United States as well as in Canada, Japan, Mexico, England, Puerto Rico, Spain, Egypt, Jordan, Saudi Arabia, Bermuda, and the Virgin Islands. Linda and Philip train professors as well as educators in state departments of education and school districts. Their book, *Comprehensive School Health Education: Totally Awesome® Strategies for Teaching Health,* is the most widely used book for teacher training in colleges, universities, and school districts. Thousands of teachers throughout the world have participated in their Totally Awesome® Teacher Training Workshops. Linda and Philip have been the keynote speakers for many teacher institutes and wellness conferences. They are personally and professionally committed to the health and well-being of youth.

Advisory Board

iv

Medical Reviewer

Donna Bacchi, M.D., M.Ph.
Medical Directory of Community
  and Neighborhood Health Services
Austin/Travis County Health
  Department
Austin, Texas

Reviewers

Kymm Ballard, M.A.
Physical Education, Athletics, and
  Sports Medicine Consultant
North Carolina Department of
  Public Instruction
Raleigh, North Carolina

Kay Bridges
Health Educator
Gaston County Public School
Gaston, North Carolina

Reba Bullock, M.Ed.
Health Education Curriculum
  Specialist
Baltimore City Public Schools
Baltimore, Maryland

Anthony S. Catalano, Ph.D.
K–12 Health Coordinator
Melrose Public Schools
Melrose, Massachusetts

Galen Cole, Ph.D.
Division of Health
  Communication
Office of the Director
Centers for Disease Control
  and Prevention
Atlanta, Georgia

Brian Colwell, Ph.D.
Professor
Texas A&M
Department of HLKN
College Station, Texas

Sylvia Douglas, M.S.
Supervisor of Physical Education
Mobile County Schools
Mobile, Alabama

Tommy Fleming, Ph.D.
Director of Health and
  Physical Education
Texas Education Agency
Austin, Texas

Denyce Ford, M.Ed., Ph.D.
Coordinator, Comprehensive
  School Health Education District
  of Columbia Public Schools
Washington, D.C.

Joanne Frasier, Ed.D.
Education Associate
Comprehensive Health and HIV,
  Office of Technical Assistance
South Carolina Department
  of Education
Columbia, South Carolina

Elizabeth Gallun, M.A.
Supervisor of Drug Programs
Prince George's County Public
  Schools
Upper Marlboro, Maryland

Linda Harrill-Rudisill, M.A.
Chairperson of Health Education
York Chester Junior High School
Gastonia, North Carolina

Janet Henke
Middle School Team Leader
Baltimore County Public Schools
Baltimore, Maryland

Russell Henke
Coordinator of Health
Montgomery County Public
  Schools
Rockville, Maryland

Larry Herrold, M.S.
Supervisor, Office of Health
  and Physical Education K–12
Baltimore County Schools
Baltimore, Maryland

Susan Jackson, B.S., M.A.
Health Promotion Specialist
Healthworks, Wake Medical
  Center
Raleigh, North Carolina

Linda Johnson, M.Ed.
HIV/AIDS Education
  Coordinator
Department of Public Instruction
Bismarck, North Dakota

Joe Leake, CHES
Curriculum Specialist
Baltimore City Public Schools
Baltimore, Maryland

Debra Ogden, M.A.
Coordinator of Health, Physical
  Education, Driver Education and
  Safe and Drug-Free Program
Collier County Public Schools
Naples, Florida

Diane S. Scalise, R.N., M.S.
Coordinator, Health Education
  Services
The School Board of Broward
  County
Fort Lauderdale, Florida

Michael Schaffer, M.A.
Supervisor of Health
  Education K–12
Prince George's County
  Public Schools
Upper Marlboro, Maryland

**Sharon Vassiere, M.S., M.A.T.,
  CHES**
Health and Physical Education
  Curriculum Coordinator
Anchorage School District
Anchorage, Alaska

George Walker, M.A.
Health Instructor
Murphy High School
Mobile, Alabama

Linda Wright, M.A.
Project Director
HIV/AIDS Education Program
Washington, D.C.

Unit 1
Page 2

Mental and Emotional Health

Unit 2
Page 86

Family and Social Health

Unit 3
Page 174

Growth and Development

Unit 4
Page 254

Nutrition

Unit 5
Page 326

Personal Health and Physical Activity

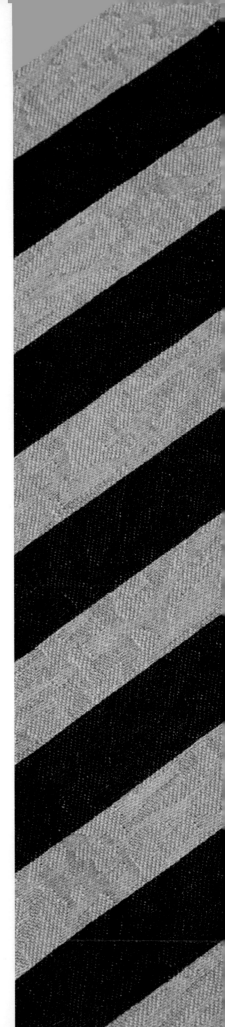

Unit 6
Page 400

Alcohol, Tobacco, and Other Drugs

Unit 7
Page 478

Communicable and Chronic Diseases

Unit 8
Page 542

Consumer and Community Health

Unit 9
Page 596

Environmental Health

Unit 10
Page 648

Injury Prevention and Safety

Unit 1

Mental and Emotional Health

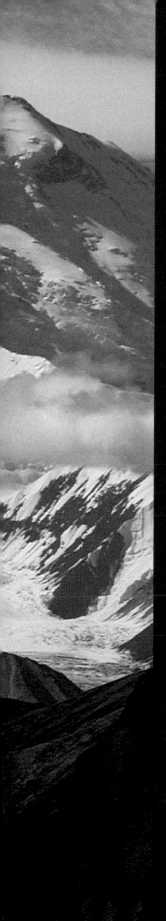

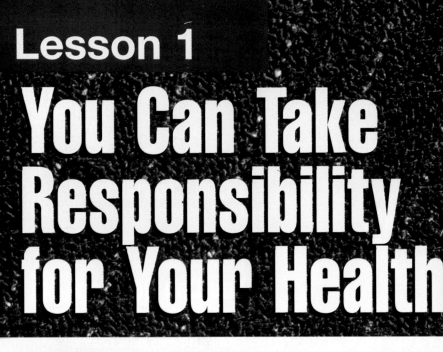

Lesson 1

You Can Take Responsibility for Your Health

Life Skill **I will take responsibility for my health.**

Who is responsible for the quality of your health? Your parents or guardian? Your family? You? Certainly your parents or guardian and your family contribute to your health. However, it may surprise you to learn that you control many of the factors that influence your health. To a great extent, you are in the driver's seat. This lesson will discuss what you should know about health status. You will learn ten factors that influence your health status. This lesson will explain how you can take responsibility for your health. You will learn how you can become a health literate person.

The Lesson Outline

What to Know About Health Status

How to Take Responsibility for Your Health

How to Be a Health Literate Person

Objectives

1. List and briefly discuss ten factors that affect health status. **pages 5–8**

2. Use The Wellness Scale to explain how to take responsibility for your health status. **page 9**

3. List and explain the four skills needed to be a health literate person. **page 10**

Vocabulary Words

health status
heredity
protective factor
risk factor
environment
random event
health care
healthful behavior
risk behavior
healthful situation
risk situation
healthful relationship
harmful relationship
responsible decision
wrong decision
resistance skills
risk
calculated risk
unnecessary risk
resiliency
quality of life
wellness
The Wellness Scale
health literate person
health advocate

What to Know About
Health Status

Health status is the condition of a person's body, mind, emotions, and relationships. There are ten factors that affect a person's health status. They are as follows.

1. A person's **heredity**
2. The quality of the **environment** in which a person lives
3. The **random events** that occur in a person's life
4. The **health care** a person receives
5. The **behaviors** and **situations** a person chooses
6. The quality of the **relationships** a person has
7. The **decisions** a person makes
8. A person's ability to use **resistance skills**
9. The kinds of **risks** a person takes
10. The degree to which a person is **resilient**

Studies in Europe, Canada, and the United States show that being poor and having an income in the lowest 20 percent of the people in your country shortens life spans by an average of seven to ten years.
Are We Scaring Ourselves to Death? ABC News, Show #ABC-53, April 21, 1994.

How Heredity Affects Health Status

Heredity is the passing of characteristics from biological parents to their children. Inherited characteristics may be protective factors or risk factors. A **protective factor** is something that increases the likelihood of a positive outcome. Characteristics passed on to you from your parents may promote your health status. Suppose your biological parents enjoy good health into their eighties or nineties. Your life expectancy would be greater than someone whose parents died from heart disease in their fifties. Of course, you could offset this protective factor if you chose harmful habits, such as smoking cigarettes.

Inherited characteristics can be a risk factor for some diseases. A **risk factor** is something that increases the likelihood of a negative outcome. Having a biological parent with premature heart disease is a risk factor for heart disease. Knowing the risk factors you may have inherited is valuable. Suppose you are at risk for heart disease because of your heredity. You can make choices to offset this risk factor. You can choose to eat a healthful diet, to exercise regularly, and to learn to manage your stress.

How Environment Affects Health Status

The **environment** is everything around a person. Your environment includes the air you breathe, the water you drink, and the place in which you live. Some people have better living conditions than others. Their environment is a protective factor and promotes their health status. Other people live in crowded and poor environments. Their environment is a risk factor and compromises their health status. They are sick more often and have shorter life spans.

How Random Events Affect Health Status

A **random event** is an event over which a person has little or no control. You often hear about random events on the news. For example, a person may be in a hotel during a fire and suffer from smoke inhalation. A person may be injured by falling debris in an earthquake. A person may be walking in a crosswalk and be struck by a car because the car's brakes failed. These people had little or no control over the random events that changed their health status.

How Health Care Affects Health Status

Health care is the professional medical and dental help that promotes a person's health. The kind of health care available to you and the way you use it affects your health status. For example, to maintain or improve health status, you need regular medical and dental checkups. If you experience signs and symptoms of a disease, you need prompt medical care. When treatment is recommended, it must be available to you.

How Behaviors and Situations Affect Health Status

Your behavior choices affect your health status. A **healthful behavior** is an action a person chooses that:

- promotes health;
- prevents injury, illness, and premature death;
- improves the quality of the environment.

Examples of healthful behaviors are wearing a safety belt, exercising regularly, eating healthful foods, and getting sufficient rest and sleep. When you choose healthful behaviors, you protect your health status.

A **risk behavior** is an action a person chooses that:

- threatens health;
- can cause injury, illness, and premature death;
- destroys the environment.

Examples of risk behaviors are rollerblading without safety equipment, smoking cigarettes, and joining a gang. If you choose risk behaviors, you may harm your health status.

Different situations also affect your health status. A **healthful situation** is a circumstance that:

- promotes health;
- prevents injury, illness, and premature death;
- improves the quality of the environment.

Examples of healthful situations are attending drug-free parties, sitting in non-smoking sections of restaurants, and being a passenger in a car driven by someone who obeys safety rules.

A **risk situation** is a circumstance that:

- threatens health;
- can cause injury, illness, and premature death;
- destroys the environment.

Examples of risk situations include being in another country without having had the recommended immunizations, being in a room where people are smoking cigarettes, and riding in a car driven by a person who has been using alcohol or other drugs.

Six Categories of Risk Behaviors in Teens

1. **Behaviors that result in unintentional and intentional injuries**

2. **Tobacco use**

3. **Alcohol and other drug use**

4. **Sexual behaviors that result in HIV infection or other sexually transmitted diseases and in unintended pregnancies**

5. **Diet choices that contribute to disease**

6. **Lack of physical activity**

Source: Centers for Disease Control and Prevention

How Relationships Affect Health Status

Did you know that the quality of your relationships may affect your health status? A **healthful relationship** is a relationship that:

◆ promotes self-respect,

◆ encourages productivity and health,

◆ is free of violence and/or drug misuse and abuse.

Examples of healthful relationships include those in which people identify strengths in each other, encourage each other to study, support each other's exercise plans, and motivate each other to avoid risk behaviors.

A **harmful relationship** is a relationship that:

◆ harms self-respect,

◆ interferes with productivity and health,

◆ includes violence and/or drug misuse and abuse.

Examples of harmful relationships include those in which one or both people criticize each other, interrupt each other's work, encourage each other to engage in risk behaviors, or drain each other of energy.

How Decisions Affect Health Status

The decisions you make result in actions that affect your health status. A **responsible decision** is a choice that leads to actions that:

◆ promote health,

◆ protect safety,

◆ follow laws,

◆ show respect for self and others,

◆ follow the guidelines of parents and other responsible adults,

◆ demonstrate good character.

A **wrong decision** is a choice that leads to actions that:

◆ harm health,

◆ are unsafe,

◆ are illegal,

◆ show disrespect for self and others,

◆ disregard the guidelines of parents and other responsible adults,

◆ lack good character.

When you make a wrong decision, you threaten your health status. ●●●●●●●●●●●●➤

How Resistance Skills Affect Health Status

Knowing that responsible decisions are the best decisions is not enough. To promote health status, you need to know how to make responsible decisions when others pressure you to make wrong decisions. **Resistance skills** are skills that help a person say NO to an action or to leave a situation.

Suppose someone pressures you to smoke a cigarette. You know that cigarette smoking harms health. But, you are unable to say NO. You give in to pressure and smoke. Your inability to say NO leads to an action that threatens your health status.

Suppose you know how to deal with pressure. You are able to say NO when others pressure you to make wrong decisions. You use resistance skills when someone pressures you to smoke. You do not give in and smoke. Your ability to use resistance skills helps you protect your health.

How Risk-Taking Affects Health Status

A **risk** is a chance that a person takes that has an unknown outcome. Taking risks can have a positive or negative effect on your health status. A **calculated risk** is a chance that a person takes after careful consideration of the possible outcomes. For example, you may consider the possible outcomes of trying out for an athletic team. If you make the team, you will be involved in regular physical activity and competition. If you do not make the team, you might feel disappointed. You decide that the risk is worth taking. You decide to try out for the team.

An **unnecessary risk** is a chance that is not worth taking after the possible outcomes are considered. For example, you have a choice of ways to walk to school. The shorter route takes you through gang turf. But, you would chance being injured if you take the shorter route. You take the longer route after considering the risk to your safety. To protect your health status, you must avoid taking unnecessary risks.

Are you a calculated risk-taker? Do you consider the possible outcomes before you act? Or do you take unnecessary risks?

How Resiliency Affects Health Status

Throughout life, everyone experiences difficult times. However, difficult times may not affect your health status as much as how you respond to them.

Suppose you experience difficult times. You do not make adjustments that help you bounce back and recover from what has happened. You choose harmful behaviors instead. Perhaps you start a fight at school or drink alcohol to forget your troubles. These actions harm health status and make difficult times worse.

Suppose you experience difficult times but quickly make adjustments. **Resiliency** (ri·ZIL·yuhn·see) is the ability to adjust, recover, bounce back, and learn from difficult times. You might reach out for the help and support of others. You stay optimistic and do not let tough times interfere with your goals and dreams. You examine what has happened and try to learn and grow. Being resilient helps you protect your health status.

How to
Take Responsibility for Your Health

Quality of life is the degree to which a person lives life to the fullest capacity. **Wellness** is the quality of life that results from a person's health status. **The Wellness Scale** is a scale that shows the ranges in quality of life. Quality of life can range from optimal wellness to premature death. High-level wellness, average wellness, minor illness or injury, and major illness or injury fall in between.

There are ten factors that affect your health status and wellness. A factor that has a positive effect promotes optimal wellness. A factor that has a negative effect increases your risk of illness, injury, and premature death. Take responsibility for your health and wellness. Examine the ten factors listed on The Wellness Scale. Which of the factors are under your control?

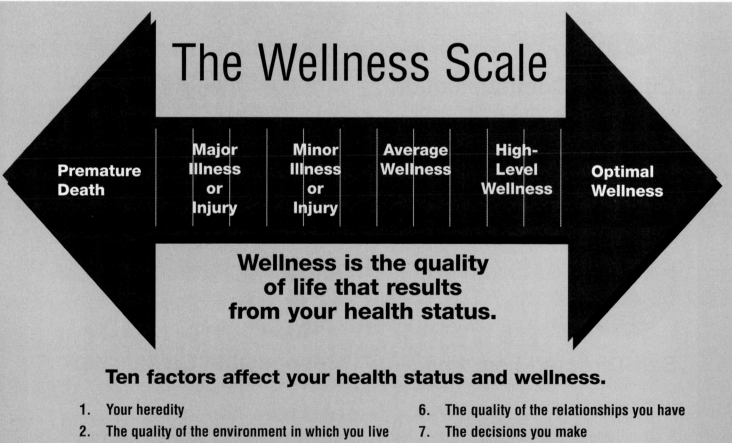

The Wellness Scale

| Premature Death | Major Illness or Injury | Minor Illness or Injury | Average Wellness | High-Level Wellness | Optimal Wellness |

Wellness is the quality of life that results from your health status.

Ten factors affect your health status and wellness.

1. Your heredity
2. The quality of the environment in which you live
3. The random events that occur in your life
4. The health care you receive
5. The behaviors and situations you choose
6. The quality of the relationships you have
7. The decisions you make
8. Your ability to use resistance skills
9. The kinds of risks you take
10. The degree to which you are resilient

How to Be a
Health Literate Person

Health literacy includes skills that help you take responsibility for your health. A **health literate person** is a person skilled in:

- effective communication,
- self-directed learning,
- critical thinking (problem solving),
- responsible citizenship.

The four skills needed for health literacy are described in more detail below. There is a symbol to represent each skill. You will see these four symbols repeated in each of the Lesson Reviews in this book. As you complete each Lesson Review, you will be practicing the skills you need to become health literate.

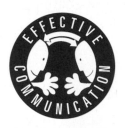

Effective Communication

involves expressing your health knowledge, beliefs, and ideas. To become an effective communicator, practice expressing yourself in different ways. Have conversations with others about health. Write, design art, make graphs, and use technology to express your health knowledge, beliefs, and ideas.

Critical Thinking

involves evaluating the facts and examining possible outcomes before making decisions. To become a critical thinker, practice using The Responsible Decision-Making Model outlined in Lesson 4. This model includes six questions you can use to evaluate the possible consequences of a decision.

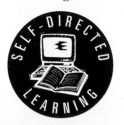

Self-Directed Learning

involves gathering and using health-related information. To become a self-directed learner, set aside time to stay informed about health-related matters. Read magazines and books, watch videos, listen to books on tape, access health-related information on a computer, watch up-to-date programs on television, and attend talks.

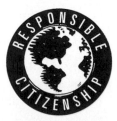

Responsible Citizenship

involves behaving in ways that make your home, school, community, nation, and world a better place. To be a responsible citizen, always choose responsible behavior. Listen to the advice of responsible adults. Practice being a health advocate. A **health advocate** is a person who promotes health.

Lesson 1

Review

Vocabulary Words

Write a separate sentence using each of the vocabulary words listed on page 4.

Objectives

1. What are ten factors that affect health status? **Objective 1**
2. What are six categories of risk behaviors in teens? **Objective 1**
3. What is the difference between taking calculated risks and taking unnecessary risks? **Objective 1**
4. How would you rate your health status using The Wellness Scale? **Objective 2**
5. What are the four skills needed to be a health literate person? **Objective 3**

Responsible Decision-Making

Your friend is trying to decide whether (s)he should attend a party where there will be drinking. Some classmates encourage him/her to go, while others do not. Your friend does not know what to do. Write a response to this situation.

1. Describe the situation that requires your friend to make a decision.
2. List possible decisions your friend might make.
3. Name two responsible adults with whom your friend might discuss his/her decisions.
4. Evaluate the possible consequences of your friend's decisions. Determine if each decision will lead to actions that:
   - promote health,
   - protect safety,
   - follow laws,
   - show respect for your friend and others,
   - follow the guidelines of your friend's parents and of other responsible adults,
   - demonstrate good character.
5. Decide which decision is most responsible and appropriate for your friend.
6. Tell two results your friend can expect if (s)he makes this decision.

 Effective Communication

Prepare a three-minute story for the evening newscast on the ten factors that affect health status. Make a written or printed copy of your story. Rehearse the story. Present it to classmates.

 Self-Directed Learning

Check the library or Internet for information on one of the six categories of risk behaviors in teens. Make a written or printed copy of this information.

 Critical Thinking

Evaluate your risk-taking behavior. What type of risk-taker are you? Are you a calculated risk-taker? Do you consider the possible outcomes before acting? Or do you take unnecessary risks? Would you try something that you know is harmful?

 Responsible Citizenship

Write a ten-line pledge about taking responsibility for your health. Sign and date the pledge. Share the pledge with family members and classmates.

Lesson 2

You Can Practice Life Skills for Health

Life Skill **I will practice life skills for health.**

Perhaps you have artistic or musical skills. Perhaps you have athletic skills. Whatever your skills are, you have learned to become more proficient in them due to practice. What about your skills to improve the quality of your health? Do you discipline yourself to practice these skills? This lesson will explain what you should know about life skills for health. You will learn 100 life skills you can practice to promote your health. This lesson includes a health behavior inventory. A health behavior inventory is a checklist you complete to learn if you practice life skills for health. You will learn how to make a health behavior contract to practice life skills.

Vocabulary Words
life skill
health behavior inventory
health behavior contract

The Lesson Outline
What to Know About Life Skills
How to Complete a Health Behavior Inventory
How to Make a Health Behavior Contract

Objectives
1. Explain why it is important to practice life skills. **page 13**
2. Discuss the purpose of a health behavior inventory. **page 13**
3. List the five parts of a health behavior contract. **page 16**

What to Know About
Life Skills

Your quality of life is improved when you have optimal wellness. Optimal wellness is achieved by practicing life skills. A **life skill** is a healthful action that is learned and practiced for a lifetime. The Health Behavior Inventory of 100 Life Skills for Health on pages 14 and 15 identifies 100 life skills you can practice for optimal wellness. Each of the 100 lessons in this book focuses on one of these skills and contains practical suggestions for practicing the skill. The suggestions help you put your knowledge into action.

How to Complete a
Health Behavior Inventory

What do you do on a regular basis to promote your health? You can check on yourself by using The Health Behavior Inventory of 100 Life Skills for Health. A **health behavior inventory** is a checklist a person completes to learn if (s)he is practicing life skills for health. When you have completed the health behavior inventory, you will be more aware of what you are doing or not doing to promote your health status.

The life skills listed in a health behavior inventory are not of equal value. For example, consider these two life skills: "I will avoid tobacco use and secondhand smoke." "I will investigate health careers." Both of these life skills contribute to quality of life. However, if you practiced these two life skills, they would not have an equal effect on your health status. Choosing to avoid tobacco use and secondhand smoke helps prevent heart disease and cancer.

Investigating health careers helps you plan for your future. You benefit from practicing both of these life skills. However, your health status is protected more by choosing not to use tobacco products than by investigating health careers.

An example of a health behavior inventory appears on the next two pages. Read and respond to each life skill listed on the inventory. Answer "YES" if you practice the life skill, "NO" if you do not. Review your responses after you finish. YES responses indicate life skills you practice to promote your health status. Continue to practice these life skills. NO responses indicate life skills you do not practice. Plan to begin practicing these life skills. Determine which life skills to begin practicing first. The next part of this lesson will explain how to make a plan to develop the habit of practicing a life skill.

The Health Behavior Inventory

Directions: Number from 1 to 100 on a sheet of paper. Read each life skill carefully. Write YES or NO next to the same number on your paper. Each YES response indicates a life skill you practice to promote your health status. Each NO response indicates a life skill you do not practice. Plan to begin practicing these life skills.

Growth and Development

21. I will keep my body systems healthy.
22. I will recognize habits that protect female reproductive health.
23. I will recognize habits that protect male reproductive health.
24. I will learn about pregnancy and childbirth.
25. I will practice abstinence to avoid the risks of teen pregnancy and parenthood.
26. I will provide responsible care for infants and children.
27. I will achieve the developmental tasks of adolescence.
28. I will develop my learning style.
29. I will develop habits that promote healthful aging.
30. I will share with my family my feelings about dying and death.

Mental and Emotional Health

1. I will take responsibility for my health.
2. I will practice life skills for health.
3. I will gain health knowledge.
4. I will make responsible decisions.
5. I will use resistance skills when appropriate.
6. I will develop good character.
7. I will choose behaviors to promote a healthy mind.
8. I will express emotions in healthful ways.
9. I will follow a plan to manage stress.
10. I will be resilient during difficult times.

Nutrition

31. I will select foods that contain nutrients.
32. I will eat the recommended number of servings from the Food Guide Pyramid.
33. I will follow the Dietary Guidelines.
34. I will plan a healthful diet that reduces the risk of disease.
35. I will evaluate food labels.
36. I will develop healthful eating habits.
37. I will follow the Dietary Guidelines when I go out to eat.
38. I will protect myself from food-borne illnesses.
39. I will maintain a desirable weight and body composition.
40. I will develop skills to prevent eating disorders.

Family and Social Health

11. I will develop healthful family relationships.
12. I will work to improve difficult family relationships.
13. I will use conflict resolution skills.
14. I will develop healthful friendships.
15. I will develop dating skills.
16. I will practice abstinence.
17. I will recognize harmful relationships.
18. I will develop skills to prepare for marriage.
19. I will develop skills to prepare for parenthood.
20. I will make healthful adjustments to family changes.

Personal Health and Physical Activity

41. I will have regular examinations.
42. I will follow a dental health plan.
43. I will be well-groomed.
44. I will get adequate rest and sleep.
45. I will participate in regular physical activity.
46. I will develop and maintain health-related fitness.
47. I will develop and maintain skill-related fitness.
48. I will prevent physical activity-related injuries and illnesses.
49. I will follow a physical fitness plan.
50. I will be a responsible spectator and participant in sports.

of 100 Life Skills for Health

Alcohol, Tobacco, and Other Drugs

51. I will follow guidelines for the safe use of prescription and OTC drugs.
52. I will not misuse or abuse drugs.
53. I will avoid risk factors and practice protective factors for drug misuse and abuse.
54. I will use resistance skills if I am pressured to misuse or abuse drugs.
55. I will not drink alcohol.
56. I will avoid tobacco use and secondhand smoke.
57. I will not be involved in illegal drug use.
58. I will choose a drug-free lifestyle to reduce the risk of HIV infection and unwanted pregnancy.
59. I will choose a drug-free lifestyle to reduce the risk of violence and accidents.
60. I will be aware of resources for the treatment of drug misuse and abuse.

Consumer and Community Health

71. I will choose sources of health information wisely.
72. I will recognize my rights as a consumer.
73. I will take action if my consumer rights are violated.
74. I will evaluate advertisements.
75. I will make a plan to manage time and money.
76. I will choose healthful entertainment.
77. I will make responsible choices about health care providers and facilities.
78. I will evaluate ways to pay for health care.
79. I will be a health advocate by being a volunteer.
80. I will investigate health careers.

Environmental Health

81. I will stay informed about environmental issues.
82. I will help keep the air clean.
83. I will help keep the water safe.
84. I will help keep noise at a safe level.
85. I will precycle, recycle, and dispose of waste properly.
86. I will help conserve energy and natural resources.
87. I will protect the natural environment.
88. I will help improve my visual environment.
89. I will take actions to improve my social-emotional environment.
90. I will be a health advocate for the environment.

Communicable and Chronic Diseases

61. I will choose behaviors to reduce my risk of infection with communicable diseases.
62. I will choose behaviors to reduce my risk of infection with respiratory diseases.
63. I will choose behaviors to reduce my risk of infection with sexually transmitted diseases.
64. I will choose behaviors to reduce my risk of HIV infection.
65. I will choose behaviors to reduce my risk of cardiovascular diseases.
66. I will choose behaviors to reduce my risk of diabetes.
67. I will choose behaviors to reduce my risk of cancer.
68. I will recognize ways to manage asthma and allergies.
69. I will recognize ways to manage chronic health conditions.
70. I will keep a personal health record.

Injury Prevention and Safety

91. I will follow safety guidelines to reduce the risk of unintentional injuries.
92. I will follow safety guidelines for severe weather and natural disasters.
93. I will follow guidelines for motor vehicle safety.
94. I will practice protective factors to reduce the risk of violence.
95. I will respect authority and obey laws.
96. I will practice self-protection strategies.
97. I will stay away from gangs.
98. I will not carry a weapon.
99. I will participate in victim recovery if I am harmed by violence.
100. I will be skilled in first aid procedures.

How to Make a
Health Behavior Contract

A **health behavior contract** is a written plan to develop the habit of practicing a life skill. A health behavior contract includes the following five items.

1. Your name and the date (this shows your commitment to the contract);
2. The life skill that needs to become a new habit;
3. A few statements describing how the life skill will improve your health status;
4. A specific plan for recording your progress;
5. An evaluation of how the plan worked for you.

Health Behavior Contract

1. **Name**_____**Date**_____

2. **Life Skill:** I will plan a healthful diet that reduces the risk of disease.

3. **Effects on Health Status:** The American Cancer Society (ACS) suggests eating cruciferous vegetables to reduce the risk of colon cancer. Cruciferous vegetables are vegetables that belong to the cabbage family. Cruciferous vegetables include broccoli, cauliflower, and brussels sprouts. The ACS also recommends eating a diet high in fiber to reduce colon cancer. Foods high in fiber include whole-wheat bread, cereals containing grains, and fruits and vegetables.

4. **Plan and Method to Record Progress:** I will eat three servings of vegetables each day. At least one serving will be a cruciferous vegetable. I will eat at least two servings of fruit each day. For breakfast, I will have a bowl of cereal and whole-wheat toast. I will keep a food diary for one week and then evaluate my food selections.

My Calendar

M	T	W	Th	F	S	S
cereal	cereal	oops!	cereal	cereal	oops!	oops!
toast	toast	toast	toast	toast	oops!	oops!
peas	corn	squash	okra	lettuce	cabbage	broccoli
spinach	lima beans	peas	sprouts	peas	corn	peppers
radishes	broccoli	broccoli	cabbage	broccoli	lettuce	lettuce
orange juice	orange juice	orange juice	orange juice	orange juice	pear	apple
raspberries	grapes	grapes	apple	grapes	pineapple	grapes
strawberries	pear	plum	plum	watermelon	plum	plum

5. **Evaluation:** I was rushed on the weekend and didn't always eat cereal. I could eat another serving of whole-wheat bread to get my fiber. I felt stuffed eating all those vegetables, but I am getting used to it. I enjoyed eating the fruits for snacks. They gave me quick energy.

Lesson 2

Review

Vocabulary Words

Write a separate sentence using each of the vocabulary words listed on page 12.

Objectives

1. Why is it important to practice life skills? **Objective 1**

2. How long should you practice a life skill? **Objective 1**

3. What is the purpose of a health behavior inventory? **Objective 2**

4. Why do the life skills listed in a health behavior inventory have unequal effects on your health status? **Objective 2**

5. What are the five parts of a health behavior contract? **Objective 3**

Responsible Decision-Making

In health class, you have just read about 100 life skills for health. After class, the student next to you tells you (s)he belongs to a gang. (S)he was surprised to read the life skill, "I will stay away from gangs." (S)he asks you if (s)he made a wrong decision when (s)he joined a gang. Write a response to this situation.

1. Describe the situation that requires your classmate to make a decision.
2. List possible decisions your classmate might make.
3. Name two responsible adults with whom your classmate might discuss his/her decisions.
4. Evaluate the possible consequences of your classmate's decisions. Determine if each decision will lead to actions that:
   - promote health,
   - protect safety,
   - follow laws,
   - show respect for yourself and others,
   - follow the guidelines of your parents and of other responsible adults,
   - demonstrate good character.
5. Decide which decision is most responsible and appropriate for your classmate.
6. Tell two results you expect if your classmate makes this decision.

 Effective Communication

Select a life skill from The Health Behavior Inventory of 100 Life Skills for Health. Design a poster to motivate young people to practice this life skill. Find a place in your community to display your poster.

 Self-Directed Learning

Check the library or Internet for American Heart Association materials. Locate a health behavior inventory that focuses on risk factors for heart disease.

Critical Thinking

A friend from another school notices your health book. The friend opens the book to The Health Behavior Inventory of 100 Life Skills for Health. After completing the inventory, the friend says, "I scored really well. I practice several life skills." However, you notice that your friend does not practice these life skills: "I will not drink alcohol." "I will avoid tobacco use and secondhand smoke." Write a response to your friend's statement, "I scored really well."

 Responsible Citizenship

A responsible citizen obeys laws. Review the life skills listed on The Health Behavior Inventory of 100 Life Skills for Health. List five life skills that require you to obey laws.

Lesson 3

You Can Acquire Health Knowledge

Life Skill **I will gain health knowledge.**

Why are certain foods recommended for optimal health? Why do you need to sit in the nonsmoking section of a restaurant? Why do you need to wear a safety belt when riding in an automobile? The questions you have about your health and the health of others are very important. The answers to these questions might affect the quality of your health—and your life. This lesson examines ways you can acquire health knowledge. You will learn the ten areas into which health knowledge is organized. This lesson will explain how you can use technology to locate health-related information. You will learn ways to locate information on television, videos, laser discs, and computers. This lesson also will include ways to locate health-related information in printed materials.

The Lesson Outline

How Health Knowledge Is Organized

How to Use Technology

How to Use Printed Materials

Objectives

1. Name the ten areas of health into which health knowledge is organized. **page 19**

2. List and explain different types of technology you can use to access health-related information. **pages 20–21**

3. List and explain different types of printed materials you can use to gain health-related information. **page 22**

Vocabulary Words

health knowledge

infomercial

video

laser disc

computer

CD-ROM

on-line

modem

electronic mail (e-mail)

Internet

World Wide Web (WWW)

web site

database

pamphlet

periodical

reference materials

card catalog

plagiarism

How Health Knowledge Is Organized

Health knowledge is the information and understanding a person has about health. In this book, information about health is organized into ten content areas. Ten life skills are suggested for each of the ten areas of health. As you study the ten areas of health, you will gain knowledge about each area. As a result, you will benefit in at least two ways:

1. **Health knowledge will help you make a plan to practice life skills.**

2. **Health knowledge will help you learn to make responsible decisions about your health.**

The Ten Areas of Health

1. **Mental and Emotional Health**
2. **Family and Social Health**
3. **Growth and Development**
4. **Nutrition**
5. **Personal Health and Physical Activity**
6. **Alcohol, Tobacco, and Other Drugs**
7. **Communicable and Chronic Diseases**
8. **Consumer and Community Health**
9. **Environmental Health**
10. **Injury Prevention and Safety**

Media are the various forms of mass communication. You can acquire health knowledge through the media. Media literacy is the ability to recognize and evaluate the messages in media.

Questions to Evaluate Media Messages™

1. What is the purpose of the message?
2. Who is the target audience for the message?
3. Who will profit if members of the target audience are influenced by the message?
4. Does the message encourage members of the target audience to choose responsible behavior? How?
5. What techniques are used to make the message appealing to the target audience? Why?
6. What information is missing from the message? Why?
7. Is this message consistent with messages found in other media on the same subject? How?

How to Use
Technology

Technology, such as television, videos, laser discs, and computers, can help you find health-related information.

Television

Many programs on network and cable TV focus on health-related issues. These programs can be identified by exploring TV channels or by reading TV listings. Local hospitals, universities, and health organizations can provide the names of specific health-related programs available in your broadcast area.

When health-related information is presented on TV, the purpose may be to inform, to sell, or to entertain. If a program is produced by the medical staff at the local hospital, the purpose is to inform. The health-related information should be reliable.

Some TV programs are produced by advertisers who represent companies that want to sell health-related products. An **infomercial** is a TV program meant to sell products or services. The purpose of infomercials is to influence what you buy, not to provide reliable health-related information.

Other TV programs are produced for entertainment. You probably have watched weekly shows focusing on emergency room settings or on doctors at a hospital. The purpose of these shows is to create a high level of interest, not to provide reliable health-related information.

Videos

A **video** is a tape of video images and sound that is recorded and played using a videocassette recorder and a TV. Many videos focus on health-related issues. Check for these videos in the education or health section of your local video store. Many health organizations and community agencies produce videos on health-related topics that you can borrow. You also can borrow videos from your local public or school library. As with TV programs, you should always check the source of the information that appears in videos.

Laser discs

A **laser disc** is a hard, plastic disc used to record, store, and retrieve video images and sound. Laser discs are played on a laser disc player that displays the information from the disc onto a TV screen or computer monitor. You can use a remote control to immediately access any frame on a laser disc. Laser discs are available at many retail stores. Laser discs also may be available at your local public library.

Computers

A **computer** is an electronic device used to process, translate, and transmit information. In addition to home and school computers, computers also are available at libraries. Pay-per-use locations, such as copy centers or cyber-cafés that have on-line access, let you use their computers for a small fee. Pay-per-use locations usually have access to the latest computer technology.

CD-ROMs

A CD-ROM is a small, plastic disc used to store and retrieve still and video images, sound, and text. A CD-ROM is played on a computer that has a special CD-ROM drive. You can use CD-ROMs to access large information sources. An entire encyclopedia or several years of a magazine can fit on one CD-ROM. Check in the local public library, in school, and in the education section of a computer store for health-related information on CD-ROM. Several health magazines, journals, and texts also are available on CD-ROM.

Modems

Going on-line is another source of health-related information. **On-line** is the interactive use of computers using telecommunication technology. To go on-line, you need a computer, a modem, communications software, and a telephone line. A **modem** is an electronic device that allows computers to send, receive, and retrieve information over telephone lines. Modems are used with on-line systems such as the Internet and services such as electronic mail to send information from one computer to another.

Electronic mail (e-mail) is a message sent instantly from one computer to another. You can access health-related information through e-mail by sending messages to health organizations and to people who are knowledgeable about health. You can send e-mail to a teacher, an author, a politician, and health care professionals.

The **Internet** is an on-line telecommunications system that connects computer networks from around the world. On the Internet, you can find health-related information by searching for health topics on the World Wide Web. The **World Wide Web (WWW)** is a graphic system on the Internet made up of a huge collection of documents. It is easy to use and offers a vast amount of information. For example, if you want to find the latest information on HIV/AIDS, attempt a search using the words "HIV" and "AIDS." A menu of topics and subtopics should appear, along with the addresses of several health-related web sites. A **web site** is the specific location where information is found.

Databases

A database is a collection of related information organized for quick access to specific items of information. For example, if you are specifically looking for information on breast cancer, you might use the CANCERLIT database. You can access databases through the Internet, at your local public library, or by using CD-ROMs.

How to Check Sources

How do you know if a source is reliable? Reliable information is based on research. It does not try to influence your decisions to buy something. It does not make false claims. Consider the following questions when you evaluate health-related information:

1. **What is the source of the information?** Reliable sources include government agencies, community organizations, professional organizations, and the medical staff at universities.

2. **Is the information based on research and scientific evidence?** You should be able to obtain copies of the research. Other sources should be provided upon request.

3. **Do physicians, dentists, and other health care professionals believe the information?** Local health care professionals should confirm the information.

Health-Related Agencies You Can Find on the World Wide Web

- The Centers for Disease Control and Prevention (CDC)
- The American Red Cross
- The Environmental Protection Agency (EPA)
- The National Institute of Health (NIH)
- The United States Department of Health and Human Services (HHS)
- The United States Department of Education
- The American Cancer Society (ACS)
- The American Heart Association (AHA)
- The Food and Drug Administration (FDA)
- The United States Department of Agriculture (USDA)
- The National Institute of Drug Abuse (NIDA)

How to Use
Printed Materials

Printed materials, such as magazines, journals, pamphlets, periodicals, and books, can be reliable sources of health-related information. Many health organizations and private agencies distribute printed materials. For example, the American Heart Association distributes pamphlets and information sheets about cardiovascular diseases. Other health organizations publish pamphlets about other health concerns, such as cancer, diabetes, and arthritis. A **pamphlet** is a short publication that generally focuses on a specific topic.

You can find in-depth health-related information in periodicals, such as journals, newspapers, and magazines. A **periodical** is a publication that is distributed at regular intervals of time. Local and national newspapers sometimes have entire sections dedicated to health. Journals and magazines often contain articles that include up-to-date health-related information. For example, if you are looking for information on current cancer research, you might check a medical journal. If you are interested in fitness, you might check a fitness magazine. Newspapers, journals, and magazines can be purchased or obtained from stores, private organizations, and public agencies. You also can find periodicals at the library.

Local public libraries and school libraries are good sources of printed materials. Besides magazines, journals, and newspapers, libraries contain books and reference materials. **Reference materials** are publications that contain facts and information and are used for consultation. As you read this health book, you may find a topic you want to study further. You can check an encyclopedia or a health reference guide for more information on the topic.

To locate books and reference materials at the library, check the card catalog or the computer database. A **card catalog** is a collection of note cards that lists information about all the books and many of the other materials available in the library. The cards are organized in the numerical system used by the library. Many libraries now use computer databases in place of card catalogs.

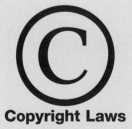

Copyright Laws

Suppose you have a report due tomorrow for health class. You find an entry in the encyclopedia on your topic. You consider copying the entry word for word. No harm will be done, right? Wrong! **Plagiarism** (PLAY·juh·riz·uhm) is copying and passing off the ideas or words of another person or persons as one's own. Copyright laws protect people's original work. Plagiarism violates copyright laws. Examples of plagiarism include copying:

- **paragraphs from a book,**
- **a newspaper article,**
- **information on the Internet,**
- **another student's paper.**

It is not wrong to use some information from a source. However, if you do, you should identify the source. Write the name of the source, the author, and the copyright date after the information you have used. This shows that the information is not your original work. Always follow the correct bibliographical form when listing sources.

Lesson 3
Review

Vocabulary Words

Write a separate sentence using each of the vocabulary words listed on page 18.

Objectives

1. What are the ten areas of health into which health knowledge is organized? **Objective 1**

2. What are different types of technology you can use to access health-related information? **Objective 2**

3. What are 11 examples of health-related agencies you can find on the World Wide Web? **Objective 2**

4. What are different types of printed materials you can use to gain health-related information? **Objective 3**

5. What are four examples of plagiarism? **Objective 3**

Responsible Decision-Making

Suppose you use a computer away from home to access the Internet. As you search, you find a web site with obscene pictures and stories. You know that on your family's computer this web site is blocked. Write a response to this situation.

1. **Describe the situation that requires you to make a decision.**
2. **List possible decisions you might make.**
3. **Name two responsible adults with whom you might discuss your decisions.**
4. **Evaluate the possible consequences of your decisions. Determine if each decision will lead to actions that:**
   - **promote health,**
   - **protect safety,**
   - **follow laws,**
   - **show respect for yourself and others,**
   - **follow the guidelines of your parents and of other responsible adults,**
   - **demonstrate good character.**
5. **Decide which decision is most responsible and appropriate.**
6. **Tell two results you expect if you make this decision.**

Effective Communication

Write a letter to a health agency or a person who is knowledgeable in health, such as a professor, a teacher, a physician, or a nurse. Ask for information concerning a health-related issue or topic that is of particular interest to you. If you have access to e-mail, send an electronic message.

Self-Directed Learning

Go to your school or public library and learn how to use the card catalog or computer to find health-related sources. Find three health-related sources and write them in correct bibliographical form on notebook paper.

Critical Thinking

Suppose you have to do a research project for your health class. You have put off doing the project until the night before it is due. A classmate finds a short report on the Internet on the topic you have selected. (S)he suggests that you copy it. (S)he says the odds are that your teacher will think it is your original work. Why is it wrong to copy the report from the Internet?

Responsible Citizenship

Investigate the rules and laws that govern on-line communication. Make a list of these regulations. Share the list with your family members and classmates.

Lesson 4

You Can Make Responsible Decisions

Life Skill I will make responsible decisions.

How do you make decisions? Do you weigh information carefully and consider the consequences before you make a decision? Do you make decisions based on what your friends are doing? Do you discuss important decisions with your parents or guardian? What do you do if you make a wrong decision? This lesson helps you to evaluate your decision-making style. You will learn whether or not your decision-making style promotes health status. This lesson includes The Responsible Decision-Making Model. You will learn how to make responsible decisions. This lesson also outlines steps you can take if you make a wrong decision.

The Lesson Outline

How to Evaluate Your Decision-Making Style

How to Use The Responsible Decision-Making Model

What to Do If You Make a Wrong Decision

Objectives

1. Describe the three decision-making styles. **page 25**
2. Outline the six steps in The Responsible Decision-Making Model.
   page 26
3. List and explain four steps to take if you make a wrong decision.
   page 28

Vocabulary Words

inactive decision-making style

procrastinate

reactive decision-making style

proactive decision-making style

empowered

The Responsible
Decision-Making Model

wrong decision

restitution

How to Evaluate Your
Decision-Making Style

Y ou may have one of three possible styles of making decisions.

An **inactive decision-making style** is a habit in which a person fails to make choices, and this failure determines the outcome. Teens who use the inactive decision-making style:

- often procrastinate (To **procrastinate** is to postpone something until a future time.);
- have little control over the direction their lives take;
- have difficulty gaining the self-confidence that would result if they took responsibility for making decisions when they should.

A **reactive decision-making style** is a habit in which a person allows others to make his/her decisions. Teens who use the reactive decision-making style:

- are easily influenced by what others think, do, or suggest;
- lack self-confidence and have a great need to be liked by others;
- give control of the direction of their lives to others.

A **proactive decision-making style** is a habit in which a person describes the situation that requires a decision, identifies and evaluates possible decisions, and makes a decision and takes responsibility for the consequences. Teens who use the proactive decision-making style:

- are not driven by circumstances and conditions;
- are not easily influenced by peers;
- have principles, such as integrity, honesty, and dignity, that guide their decisions and behavior; and are empowered. To be **empowered** is to be energized because a person has some control over his/her decisions and behavior.

How to Use
The Responsible Decision-Making Model

The Responsible Decision-Making Model is a series of steps to follow to assure that the decisions a person makes result in actions that:

1. promote health,
2. protect safety,
3. follow laws,
4. show respect for self and others,
5. follow the guidelines of parents and of other responsible adults,
6. demonstrate good character.

The Responsible Decision-Making Model

Step 1. Describe the situation that requires a decision.
Describe the situation in writing if no immediate decision is necessary. Describe the situation out loud or to yourself in a few sentences if an immediate decision is necessary. Being able to describe the situation in your own words helps you see it more clearly.

Step 2. List possible decisions you might make.
List all the possible decisions you can think of in writing, if no immediate decision is necessary. If you must decide right away, review the possible decisions out loud or to yourself.

Step 3. Share the list of possible decisions with a parent, guardian, or other responsible adult.
Share possible decisions with a responsible adult, when no immediate decision is necessary. If possible, delay making a decision. An adult may think of other possibilities. (S)he may help you evaluate the possible consequences of each decision. Consider your options seriously.

Step 4. Use six questions to evaluate the possible consequences of each decision.

1. Will this decision result in actions that promote health?
2. Will this decision result in actions that protect safety?
3. Will this decision result in actions that follow laws?
4. Will this decision result in actions that show respect for myself and others?
5. Will this decision result in actions that follow the guidelines of my parents and of other responsible adults?
6. Will this decision result in actions that demonstrate good character?

Step 5. Decide which decision is most responsible and appropriate.
Rely on the six questions in Step 4 as you compare the decisions.

Step 6. Act on your decision and evaluate the results.
Follow through with your decision with confidence. You will be confident if you pay attention to the six questions in Step 4.

Activity

Using The Responsible Decision-Making Model

Life Skill: I will make responsible decisions.

Materials: paper, pen or pencil

Directions: Follow the steps listed below to practice using The Responsible Decision-Making Model. Think about the situation and complete Steps 4 and 5 on a separate sheet of paper. Due to the fictional nature of the activity, do not complete Step 6. DO NOT WRITE IN THIS BOOK.

 Describe the situation that requires a decision. Tonight is the big game between my school and its biggest rival. My friends are going to the game together. One friend says, "Remember the sign just outside their stadium? I've got a can of spray paint. Why don't we get there early and paint a score in BIG numbers on that sign!" My friends think the idea is a blast. I am not so sure.

 List possible decisions I might make. A. Help my friends spray paint a make-believe score on the sign outside the stadium. B. Tell my friends I will not spray paint the other school's sign.

 Share the list of possible decisions with a parent, guardian, or other responsible adult. I could call my parent or guardian or my older sibling, say I am being pressured to spray paint the sign, and discuss my decisions with them.

Use six questions to evaluate the possible consequences of each decision. Suppose I decide to help spray paint the sign. Will my decision lead to actions that:

1. promote health?
2. protect safety?
3. follow laws?
4. show respect for myself and others?
5. follow the guidelines of my parents and of other responsible adults?
6. demonstrate good character?

Suppose I decide not to help spray paint the sign. Will my decision lead to actions that:

1. promote health?
2. protect safety?
3. follow laws?
4. show respect for myself and others?
5. follow the guidelines of my parents and of other responsible adults?
6. demonstrate good character?

Decide which decision is most responsible and appropriate.

Act on your decision and evaluate the results.

What to Do If You Make a
Wrong Decision

A **wrong decision** is a choice that leads to actions that:

1. **harm health,**
2. **are unsafe,**
3. **are illegal,**
4. **show disrespect for self and others,**
5. **disregard the guidelines of parents and of other responsible adults,**
6. **lack good character.**

If you make a wrong decision, do something about it. Don't just hope that no one will find out that you have done something wrong.

Four Steps

You Can Take When You Have Made a Wrong Decision

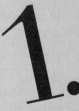

1. **Take responsibility and admit you have made a wrong decision.** Wrong is wrong! Do not make excuses if you make a wrong decision. Do not try to cover up what you have done.

Do not continue actions based on wrong decisions. The very moment you recognize you have made a wrong decision, examine what actions you have taken based on your wrong decision. Begin to make corrections.

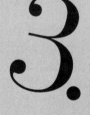

3. **Discuss the wrong decision with a parent, guardian, or other responsible adult.** Your parents or guardian are responsible for guiding the decisions you make. Suppose you make a wrong decision. Your parents or guardian need to know. They can help you correct what you have done.

4. **Make restitution for harm done to others.** **Restitution** is making good for any loss or damage. It is making up for any harm you have caused. An apology is not always enough to correct the harm done. Suppose you borrowed a friend's jacket without asking and lost it. You should apologize and make restitution. You need to pay to replace the jacket.

Lesson 4

Review

Vocabulary Words

Write a separate sentence using each of the vocabulary words listed on page 24.

Objectives

1. What are the three decision-making styles? **Objective 1**

2. What are the benefits associated with using a proactive decision-making style? **Objective 1**

3. What are the six steps in The Responsible Decision-Making Model? **Objective 2**

4. When is a decision a wrong decision? **Objective 3**

5. What are four steps you can take if you make a wrong decision? **Objective 3**

Responsible Decision-Making

Some classmates want you to try chewing tobacco. They pressure you by giving you reasons why you should chew, such as "everyone is doing it," "your parents will never know you tried it," and "you'll look cool if you chew." Write a response to this situation.

1. Describe the situation that requires you to make a decision.

2. List possible decisions you might make.

3. Name two responsible adults with whom you might discuss your decisions.

4. Evaluate the possible consequences of your decisions. Determine if each decision will lead to actions that:
   - promote health,
   - protect safety,
   - follow laws,
   - show respect for yourself and others,
   - follow the guidelines of your parents and of other responsible adults,
   - demonstrate good character.

5. Decide which decision is most responsible and appropriate.

6. Tell two results you expect if you make this decision.

Effective Communication

Develop a slogan to remind teens to correct wrong decisions. An example of a slogan might be "Just Correct It."

Self-Directed Learning

Read a copy of your local newspaper. Study the crime reports and the traffic accidents. Find three examples of harm done by a person who has made a wrong decision.

Critical Thinking

Evaluate your own decision-making skills. What decision-making styles do you use? When do you use each style and why? How might you improve your ability to make responsible decisions?

Responsible Citizenship

Make a poster of the steps in The Responsible Decision-Making Model. Include an example for each step. Obtain permission from a school administrator to hang the poster in a prominent place in the school.

Lesson 5

You Can Resist Negative Peer Pressure

Life Skill **I will use resistance skills when appropriate.**

Have you ever been pressured to do something you did not want to do? Of course you have! The real question is, "How did you respond?" Did you resist the pressure? Or, did you give in? Often your peers are the ones who pressure you. A **peer** is a person of similar age or status. This lesson focuses on ways to resist negative peer pressure. You will learn how to recognize negative peer pressure and resistance skills. You will learn steps to take to be self-confident and assertive. This lesson also teaches you five actions you can take if you have given in to negative peer pressure.

The Lesson Outline

How to Recognize Peer Pressure

How to Use Resistance Skills

How to Be Self-Confident and Assertive

What to Do If You Give in to Negative Peer Pressure

Objectives

1. Identify ten pressure statements peers might use to pressure you to make a wrong decision. **page 31**

2. List and explain eight resistance skills to resist negative peer pressure. **page 32**

3. Explain three steps you can take to be assertive and demonstrate self-confidence. **page 33**

4. Identify ten possible negative outcomes that might result if you give in to negative peer pressure. **page 35**

5. Discuss five actions you can take if you have given in to negative peer pressure. **page 36**

Vocabulary Words

peer

peer pressure

positive peer pressure

negative peer pressure

resistance skills

The Model for Using Resistance Skills

broken-record technique

nonverbal behavior

self-confidence

assertive behavior

passive behavior

aggressive behavior

How to Recognize
Peer Pressure

Peer pressure is influence that people of similar age or status place on others to behave in a certain way. Peer pressure can be either positive or negative. Suppose a test is scheduled tomorrow. Tonight, a teen calls a friend in class to go to a movie. The friend says "no" and convinces the teen to study for the test instead. Or, suppose a teen tries to convince a friend to see an R-rated movie. The friend says "no" and instead encourages the teen to see a movie that is rated PG. These situations are examples of positive peer pressure. **Positive peer pressure** is influence from peers to behave in a responsible way.

Peers can pressure in negative ways, too. Suppose a teen is pressured to go to a party where there will be drugs. It is dangerous and illegal for teens to use alcohol and other harmful drugs, such as marijuana. Several classmates going to the party pressure this teen to go, too. Or, suppose a classmate wants to copy a friend's homework instead of doing it himself/herself. (S)he keeps pressuring the friend for his/her notebook. These situations are examples of negative peer pressure. **Negative peer pressure** is influence from peers to behave in a way that is not responsible.

People who are mature, responsible, and caring want the best for others. They are careful not to exert negative peer pressure. People who exert negative peer pressure on you do not have your best interest in mind. For example, peers who want you to attend a party where there is drinking are not considering what is best for you. They want you to drink because they want you to support their wrong action. Remember the following advice about peer pressure:

Peers who pressure you to make wrong decisions often want support for their wrong actions. They do not consider the possible negative outcomes you may experience as a result.

Ten Negative Peer Pressure Statements

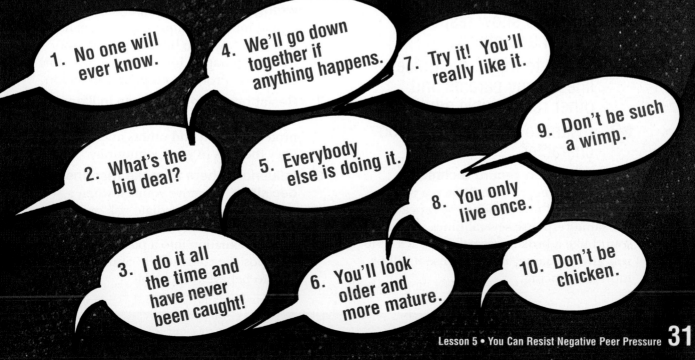

1. No one will ever know.

2. What's the big deal?

3. I do it all the time and have never been caught!

4. We'll go down together if anything happens.

5. Everybody else is doing it.

6. You'll look older and more mature.

7. Try it! You'll really like it.

8. You only live once.

9. Don't be such a wimp.

10. Don't be chicken.

How to Use
Resistance Skills

Resistance skills are skills that help a person say "no" to an action or to leave a situation. Resistance skills are sometimes called refusal skills and can be used to resist negative peer pressure.

The Model for Using Resistance Skills below is a list of suggested ways to resist negative peer pressure.

The Model for Using Resistance Skills

Say No!

1. **Say NO with self-confidence.** Look directly at the person or persons to whom you are speaking. Express yourself clearly.

2. **Give reasons for saying NO.** Use the six guidelines for making responsible decisions as your reasons for saying NO.

   NO. I want to promote my health.

   NO. I want to protect my safety.

   NO. I want to follow laws.

   NO. I want to show respect for myself and others.

   NO. I want to follow the guidelines of my parents and other responsible adults.

   NO. I want to demonstrate good character.

3. **Use the broken-record technique.** The **broken-record technique** is a way to strengthen a "no" response by repeating the same response several times. You will sound like a broken record, but each time you give the same "no" response it will be more convincing.

4. **Use nonverbal behavior to match verbal behavior.** Nonverbal behavior is the use of actions to express emotions and thoughts. Shaking your head "no" is an example of nonverbal behavior. Your verbal "no" should not be confused by a nonverbal behavior that is misleading.

5. **Avoid being in situations in which there will be pressure to make wrong decisions.** Think ahead. Avoid situations that might be tempting. For example, do not spend time at a peer's house when his/her parents or guardians are not home.

6. **Avoid being with people who make wrong decisions.** Remember that your reputation is the impression others have of you. Choose to be with people who have a reputation for making responsible decisions. Protect your good reputation.

7. **Resist pressure to engage in illegal behavior.** You have a responsibility to protect yourself and others and to obey the laws in your community.

8. **Influence others to make responsible decisions.** Remove yourself when a situation poses immediate risk or danger. If there is no immediate risk, try to turn a negative situation into a positive situation. Be a positive role model. Show others how to behave responsibly.

How to Be
Self-Confident and Assertive

How do you feel when you tell others about a decision you have made? Do you feel secure and confident when you express your ideas and feelings? Or do you get a knot in your stomach?

Self-confidence is belief in oneself. When you are self-confident, you believe in your ideas, feelings, and decisions. You convey confidence when you express yourself to others. Your behavior is assertive rather than passive or aggressive.

Assertive behavior is the honest expression of ideas, feelings, and decisions without worrying or feeling threatened. When your behavior is assertive, you show others that you are in control of yourself. You look directly at the person or persons to whom you are speaking. You clearly state your feelings or decisions and do not back down.

Assertive behavior differs from passive behavior and aggressive behavior. **Passive behavior** is the holding back of ideas, feelings, and decisions. Teens with passive behavior do not stand up for themselves. They make excuses for their behavior. They might look away or laugh when sharing feelings or making decisions. They may be unwilling to share their feelings. They lack self-confidence.

Aggressive behavior is the use of words or actions that are disrespectful toward others. Teens with aggressive behavior might interrupt others or monopolize a conversation. They might call others cruel names or make loud, sarcastic remarks. They might glare at someone or make threatening hand gestures. They threaten others because they lack self-confidence.

Steps to Be Self-Confident and Assertive

Step 1. Always use the six questions in The Responsible Decision-Making Model to evaluate the possible consequences of your decisions.

- Will this decision result in actions that promote health?

- Will this decision result in actions that protect safety?

- Will this decision result in actions that follow laws?

- Will this decision result in actions that show respect for myself and others?

- Will this decision result in actions that follow the guidelines of my parents and of other responsible adults?

- Will this decision result in actions that demonstrate good character?

A positive response to each of the six questions helps guarantee that a decision is responsible. The more often you make responsible decisions, the more self-confidence you gain. You become more assertive and more confident when expressing yourself.

Step 2. Imagine a shield of protection in front of you when peers pressure you to make wrong decisions. If peers make negative pressure statements, imagine the statements bouncing off your shield. The statements don't get through to you.

Step 3. When you doubt yourself, talk with a parent, guardian, or other responsible adult. Your parents or guardian can give you a morale boost and help you resist negative peer pressure. Teens who are self-confident and assertive appreciate and rely on their parents or guardians who support and encourage them.

Activity

Recognizing Peer Pressure

Life Skill: I will use resistance skills when appropriate.

Materials: note card, paper, pen or pencil

Directions: Practice recognizing peer pressure. Form groups and plan two short skits that examine peer pressure situations. Skits are brief sketches or dramatic performances. Complete the activity by following the six steps listed below.

 Following your teacher's instructions, form groups of three or four people.

 Make a list of possible peer pressure situations. In your groups, brainstorm a list of possible peer pressure situations to use in skits. You have to do two skits. One skit should concentrate on positive peer pressure. The other skit should concentrate on negative peer pressure. Choose two situations from your list to use in the skits.

 Plan your skit. As you plan your two skits, think about everything you have learned in Lesson 5. Include at least two phrases from the list of negative peer pressure statements on page 31, and demonstrate at least two of the ways to resist peer pressure suggested in The Model for Using Resistance Skills. The two skits should be no longer than a total of five minutes.

 Write the scripts for your two skits. You do not have to write the scripts word for word. Each person in your group should have a note card with an outline of his/her part in the two skits.

 Perform the two skits on the day specified by your teacher.

 Ask classmates to use the information from the lesson to analyze and evaluate the two skits. Classmates should:

1. Briefly describe the peer pressure situations portrayed in the two skits.

2. Tell which words or phrases from page 31 the group used.

3. List five additional words or phrases that peers might use to pressure each other.

4. Tell which suggestions from The Model for Using Resistance Skills the group used and say which suggestions were most effective.

What to Do If You Give in to
Negative Peer Pressure

**Suppose you give in to negative peer pressure.
There is often a price to pay. Consider ten
possible negative outcomes that might result
if you give in to negative peer pressure.**

1. **Giving in to negative peer pressure may harm health.** Suppose you give in to pressure to smoke cigarettes. The nicotine in tobacco would increase your heart rate and blood pressure. You would increase your risk of heart disease.

2. **Giving in to negative peer pressure may threaten your safety.** Suppose you give in to pressure to ride in a motor vehicle driven by someone who has been drinking beer. You would risk being injured—or killed—in a traffic accident.

3. **Giving in to negative peer pressure may cause you to break laws.** Suppose you give in to pressure to drink alcohol. It is against the law for minors to drink alcoholic beverages. You would risk being in trouble with law enforcement officers.

4. **Giving in to negative peer pressure may cause you to show disrespect for yourself and others.** Suppose you give in to pressure to call a classmate a cruel name. You would risk offending or hurting the feelings of your classmate.

5. **Giving in to negative peer pressure may cause you to disregard the guidelines of your parents and other responsible adults.** Suppose you give in to pressure to break curfew. Curfew is a fixed time when a person is to be at home. You would risk your parents' or guardian's anger and punishment for breaking curfew.

6. **Giving in to negative peer pressure does not demonstrate good character.** Suppose you give in to pressure to spray paint a wall of the school building. You would risk being caught and disciplined by school officials. You would risk getting a reputation as a troublemaker.

7. **Giving in to negative peer pressure may cause you to feel disappointed in yourself.** Suppose you give in to pressure and do something you do not want to do. You would risk being disappointed in yourself and regret not being able to stand up for yourself under pressure.

8. **Giving in to negative peer pressure may cause you to feel resentment toward peers**. Suppose you give in to pressure and make a wrong decision that results in injury to yourself. You would resent your peers as you deal with your injury.

9. **Giving in to negative peer pressure may harm your self-confidence.** Suppose you give in to pressure and change your mind about doing what you know is best. Deep down inside you would know that you were not in control of yourself or of the situation. You would risk destroying your self-confidence.

10. **Giving in to negative peer pressure may cause you to feel guilty and ashamed.** Suppose you give in to negative peer pressure and another person is harmed because of your actions. You would feel guilty and ashamed that you were responsible for what happened.

Five Actions to Take if You Have Given in to Negative Peer Pressure

1. **Take responsibility for any decisions, actions, or judgments that result from having given in to negative peer pressure.** Be honest and do not blame others for your actions.

2. **Consider ways to deal with the negative outcomes.** You already have learned about restitution. Restitution is making good for any loss or damage. Remember, you must make things right. Responsible adults can help you decide how to correct any harm you have done to others.

3. **Examine the reasons why you have given in to negative peer pressure.** Think about the situation and about the peers who pressured you. Were there specific pressure statements that caused you to change your mind? Why? Did some peers influence you more than others? Why?

4. **Make a plan to handle similar situations in the future.** Learn from your mistakes and be better prepared in the future. Be ready for pressure statements that influence you. Bolster your self-confidence so the approval of peers is not necessary.

5. **Ask a parent, guardian, or other responsible adult to help you review situations in which you have given in to negative peer pressure.**

Lesson 5
Review

Vocabulary Words

Write a separate sentence using each of the vocabulary words listed on page 30.

Objectives

1. What are ten pressure statements peers might use to pressure you to make a wrong decision? **Objective 1**

2. What are eight resistance skills you can use to resist negative peer pressure? **Objective 2**

3. What are three steps you can take to be assertive and demonstrate self-confidence? **Objective 3**

4. What are ten possible negative outcomes that might result if you give in to negative peer pressure? **Objective 4**

5. What are five actions you can take if you have given in to negative peer pressure? **Objective 5**

Responsible Decision-Making

Some of your friends have stolen the master key to your school and plan to break in over the weekend. They have decided that "trashing" the principal's office would be a great practical joke. They have invited you to join them. Write a response to this situation.

1. Describe the situation that requires you to make a decision.
2. List possible decisions you might make.
3. Name two responsible adults with whom you might discuss your decisions.
4. Evaluate the possible consequences of your decisions. Determine if each decision will lead to actions that:
   • promote health,
   • protect safety,
   • follow laws,
   • show respect for yourself and others,
   • follow the guidelines of your parents and of other responsible adults,
   • demonstrate good character.
5. Decide which decision is most responsible and appropriate.
6. Tell two results you expect if you make this decision.

Effective Communication

Recall a situation in which you were influenced by positive peer pressure. Write a letter to the person who influenced you in a positive way. Explain how you benefited from his/her positive peer pressure.

Self-Directed Learning

Interview an adult. Ask this adult to share a situation in which (s)he was pressured by peers. Share The Model for Using Resistance Skills with this adult, and ask him/her which resistance skills (s)he finds most effective.

Critical Thinking

Suppose that you are usually self-confident and assertive. But, around one particular person you become shy and exhibit passive behavior. What might cause you to be passive around this person? What can you do to be more assertive around this person?

Responsible Citizenship

After you review The Model for Using Resistance Skills, share it with a family member, neighbor, or friend. Explain the model in your own words. Be sure to give at least two examples of when and how to use the model.

Lesson 6

You Can Develop Good Character

Life Skill **I will develop good character.**

You are preparing for the responsibilities of adulthood. Your preparation should include an evaluation of your actions. If your actions are responsible, you develop self-respect. **Self-respect** is a high regard for oneself because one behaves in responsible ways. Self-respect should not be confused with conceit. **Conceit** is excessive appreciation of one's worth. Confusion exists about the notion of feeling good about oneself. Some people might lead you to believe that you should always feel good about yourself. But you should not feel good about yourself when you choose wrong actions. You should forgive yourself only after correcting wrong actions. This lesson explains how to develop good character and improve self-esteem. You will learn why having good character should be the basis for having good feelings about yourself.

The Lesson Outline

What to Know About Character

What to Know About Self-Esteem

How to Develop Good Character and Improve Self-Esteem

Objectives

1. Discuss the use of self-control and delayed gratification in building good character. **page 39**

2. List and discuss six reasons why it is important to develop positive self-esteem based on responsible actions. **page 40**

3. List and discuss three steps to take to develop good character and improve self-esteem. **page 42**

4. List and discuss ten ways to improve self-respect. **page 43**

Vocabulary Words

self-respect

conceit

value

family value

character

self-control

moderation

delayed gratification

self-esteem

positive self-esteem

negative self-esteem

beta-endorphins

What to Know About
Character

How would you describe yourself?

Are you honest?
Fair?
Trustworthy?
Patient?
Compassionate?
Health-conscious?

What are your values? A **value** is a standard or belief. An example of a value that ought to be important to you is to always tell the truth. Think about the values you hold. A **family value** is a standard that is held and copied by members of a family. You learn family values from your parents or guardian and other adults. For example, your family may value education. They encourage you to learn new ideas and new skills and to do your best in school. Think about your family's values. How have those values influenced you? Your values will determine your character.

Character is a person's use of self-control to act on responsible values. **Self-control** is the degree to which a person regulates his/her own behavior. For example, suppose you value honesty. At the drugstore, you give the clerk a $10 bill for a magazine you want to purchase. The clerk gives you change for a $20 bill. Would you tell the clerk (s)he gave you too much change? If you have good character, you would use self-control and avoid the temptation to keep the extra change.

Suppose you value your health. As you pass through a food line at a restaurant, you make food selections. Self-control helps keep you from taking too much food. Self-control helps you practice moderation. **Moderation** is placing limits to avoid excess. Although the food looks delicious, you practice moderation and do not pig out.

When you have good character, self-control helps you delay gratification when it is appropriate. **Delayed gratification** is voluntarily postponing an immediate reward in order to complete a task before enjoying a reward. For example, suppose you value your education. Tomorrow you have a test for which you need to study. But, tonight is opening night of a movie you want to see. A friend tries to persuade you to see the movie tonight. You use self-control and choose to study and see the movie another night.

When you have good character, you set limits for yourself. Your behavior reflects responsible values. You practice delayed gratification when it is appropriate.

What to Know About
Self-Esteem

Self-esteem is a person's belief about his/her worth. **Positive self-esteem** is a person's belief that (s)he is worthy and deserves respect. **Negative self-esteem** is a person's belief that (s)he is not worthy and does not deserve respect. A person's belief about himself/herself should be based on the appropriateness of his/her actions.

Six Reasons Why It Is Important to Develop Positive Self-Esteem Based on Responsible Actions

1.

You are more likely to practice life skills. You take responsibility for your health. You keep your body, mind, and relationships in top condition.

2.

You are more likely to make responsible decisions. When you understand that you are special, you do not have to go along with the crowd to feel accepted. You rely on your own judgment and make responsible decisions.

3.

You appreciate your uniqueness. To be unique is to be one of a kind. You are confident and do not give in to pressure to be like everyone else. For example, you select your clothing and hairstyle with confidence.

4.

You have a firm foundation for difficult times. You understand that everyone experiences difficult times. You know difficult times will pass and you do not give up because you believe in yourself.

5.

You are more likely to take calculated risks to mature. When you believe in yourself, you do not worry about failing. If you try something new, you may not be satisfied with the results. That does not wipe you out because you know you are capable. You try again or try another task. You are willing to take a calculated risk again.

6.

You expect others to treat you with respect. If your actions are worthy, you have self-respect. Your good feelings about yourself are based on self-respect. Other people notice your responsible behavior and your respect for yourself. They, in turn, treat you with the respect you deserve.

Activity

Your Internal Tapes—Evaluate Your Beliefs

Life Skill: I will develop good character.

Materials: paper, pen or pencil

Directions: Evaluate your beliefs. Pretend you have an internal tape recorder that plays a tape of statements that are repeated over and over. Read the ten statements below. Each statement represents a belief. What beliefs do you hear most often as you listen to your internal tape? YOUR TEACHER WILL NOT ASK YOU TO SHARE ANY OF THESE BELIEFS WITH HIM/HER OR WITH CLASSMATES.

1. It is important to always tell the truth.

2. Sometimes it is best to lie.

3. It is important to consider others before acting.

4. I must look out only for number one.

5. It is important to always obey laws.

6. Laws were made to be broken.

7. It is important to respect authority.

8. No one can tell me what to do.

9. It is important to play by the rules.

10. I must do what I need to do to win at all costs.

Evaluation: What are the beliefs that you allow to play in your mind? The odd-numbered statements are beliefs your internal tape plays that motivate you to behave in responsible ways. If these statements describe you, your actions can help you develop positive self-esteem. The even-numbered statements are beliefs your internal tape plays that motivate you to behave in wrong ways. If these statements describe you, you must change your behavior.

How to
Develop Good Character and Improve Self-Esteem

To possess good character, your actions must reflect responsible values. To improve self-esteem, your belief statements must be responsible. The following three steps can be used to develop good character and improve self-esteem:

1. **Make a character check to determine if your actions reflect responsible values.**

2. **Control the belief statements that motivate you.**

3. **Give yourself a dose of self-respect.**

How to Make a Character Check

Are you proud of your actions?

Do your actions reflect responsible values?

Character is your use of self-control to act on responsible values. If you behave in ways that contradict responsible values, you should not have positive beliefs about yourself. For example, if you have good character, you would not feel good about yourself if you lied to others or cheated someone. Behaving in these ways would not build character. If you lied and cheated and did not feel bad, you would have bad character.

Throughout life, you must make checks of your character. List responsible values. Ask yourself if your actions reflect these values. Ask responsible adults who have good character for feedback. Suppose your actions do not reflect the values that you listed. Then you should change your actions to reflect these values.

Control the Belief Statements That Motivate You

Suppose your actions reflect responsible values and you have good character. Why might you have negative self-esteem? Negative belief statements, such as "I am worthless" or "I will fail no matter how hard I try," have different origins. Parents, guardians, or other responsible adults and trained counselors can help teens change negative belief statements. Remember, you will want to control the belief statements that play in your mind. You must have a set of belief statements that motivate you to behave in responsible ways. Then you will feel good about yourself. This is the key to healthful, positive self-esteem.

Give Yourself a Dose of Self-Respect

Do you respect yourself?

Do you expect others to respect you?

There is truth to the saying, "Actions speak louder than words." If you say you have self-respect, you must treat yourself in special ways. Other people will notice your behavior. They will respect you.

1. **Pay attention to your appearance.** Being well-groomed is one of the first indicators of self-respect. When you carefully choose what you will wear or you brush your hair, you put your best foot forward. You will feel more self-confident when you look your best.

2. **Make a list of your responsible actions and review the list often.** Knowing your actions are responsible helps keep you from getting down on yourself. Give yourself credit for behaving in responsible ways. Change behavior that is not responsible.

3. **Be a friend to yourself by enjoying activities, such as hobbies, by yourself.** Being by yourself allows quiet time to get in touch with your thoughts and feelings. You also can develop a talent or hobby that helps you feel unique.

4. **Write your feelings in a journal.** Writing about feelings is a good way to examine what is happening in your life. Writing about feelings also is a way to vent feelings such as anger, resentment, and disappointment. Review what you have written to gain self-knowledge.

5. **Make spending time with members of your family a priority.** If you have a loving, supportive family, members of your family believe you are special. They build you up and encourage you. When you are down on yourself, they help you change your attitude.

6. **Care for other people in the way you would like them to care for you.** For example, suppose you want to receive cards and notes. Send cards and notes to friends and relatives.

7. **Let other people know what helps you feel special.** For example, suppose you would like your birthday to be a big deal. Don't take it for granted that others know how you feel. Be honest and tell others you want them to help you celebrate your birthday.

8. **Support the interests of family members and friends and ask them to support your interests.** For example, suppose your sister plays on the volleyball team. Go to her games and support her efforts. Ask her to attend the activities in which you participate.

9. **Ask family members and friends to tell you examples of your actions that show you have character.** Listen carefully to their feedback. Thank them for recognizing your effort to use self-control to act responsible.

10. **Get plenty of exercise to generate feelings of well-being.** After vigorous exercise, beta-endorphins are released in the bloodstream. **Beta-endorphins** (BAY·tuh·en·DOR·finz) are substances produced in the brain that create a feeling of well-being.

Activity

Create a Tape of Belief Statements to Motivate You

Life Skill: I will develop good character.

Materials: tape recorder and blank tape (optional*), paper, pen or pencil

Directions: Complete the activity by following the ten steps below.

 Read through the belief statements listed on page 41. On a sheet of paper, list any even-numbered belief statements that play in your mind. Now list other belief statements that play in your mind and motivate you to behave in wrong ways. YOUR TEACHER WILL NOT ASK YOU TO SHARE THIS LIST.

 Place the tape in a recorder and record the even-numbered state-ments that you checked previously. Record any other belief statements that motivate you to behave in wrong ways. Listen to these belief statements one last time.

 You may choose to share this tape with a parent, guardian, other responsible adult, or trained coun-selor who is helping you develop character and improve self-esteem.

 Refer back to the paper on which you listed any even-numbered statements. Cross off each belief statement that motivates you to behave in wrong ways. Replace it with a posi-tive belief statement. For example, if you wrote "No one can tell me what to do," replace it with "I must respect authority." Add other positive belief statements.

 Place your tape of negative belief statements in the tape recorder. Erase the tape so the negative beliefs are gone. The tape is now blank and you have the opportunity to record other beliefs on it.

 Record the list of positive belief statements on the blank tape.

 Listen to the tape of positive belief statements several times.

 Listen to the tape whenever you begin to focus on negative belief statements.

 Discuss your negative belief statements with your parents, guardian, other responsible adults, or a trained coun-selor. Then share your tape of positive belief statements. Ask for suggestions for other positive belief statements.

 On a sheet of paper, list an action you can take to match each of your positive belief statements. For example, you might list an action to match the positive belief statement "I must always obey laws." You might write "I will wear my safety belt when riding in an automobile."

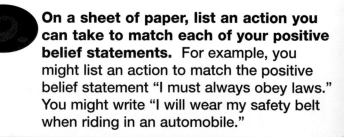
* If you do not have a tape recorder and tape, use two sheets of paper and a pen or pencil. On the first paper, write the negative beliefs you have about yourself. Review the list. As you read each negative belief, cross it out and, on the second sheet of paper, write a positive belief to replace it. When you have finished, tear up the sheet of paper with the negative beliefs written on it. Keep the second sheet of paper that has the list of positive beliefs. Review this list often.

Lesson 6

Review

Vocabulary Words

Write a separate sentence using each of the vocabulary words listed on page 38.

Objectives

1. Why does a person with good character need to have self-control? **Objective 1**

2. When does a person with good character practice delayed gratification? **Objective 1**

3. What are six reasons why it is important to develop positive self-esteem based on responsible actions? **Objective 2**

4. What are three steps to take to develop good character and improve self-esteem? **Objective 3**

5. What are ten ways to improve self-respect? **Objective 4**

Responsible Decision-Making

You are with a friend outside the movie theater. Your friend has left his/her wallet at home. You do not have enough money for both of you to see the movie. (S)he suggests, "Pay and go into the movie. Open the exit door and I'll sneak in for free." Write a response to this situation.

1. Describe the situation that requires you to make a decision.
2. List possible decisions you might make.
3. Name two responsible adults with whom you might discuss your decisions.
4. Evaluate the possible consequences of your decisions. Determine if each decision will lead to actions that:
   • promote health,
   • protect safety,
   • follow laws,
   • show respect for yourself and others,
   • follow the guidelines of your parents and of other responsible adults,
   • demonstrate good character.
5. Decide which decision is most responsible and appropriate.
6. Tell two results you expect if you make this decision.

 ### Effective Communication

Design a "Top Ten List of Ways to Demonstrate Good Character." Create your list using computer graphics or some other artistic form.

 ### Self-Directed Learning

Find a definition for the word "character" in two different sources. Copy each definition and its source on a sheet of paper. Use the two definitions to create your own definition of character.

 ### Critical Thinking

Self-control helps a person practice moderation. Moderation is placing limits to avoid excess. Name two health problems that are a result of doing something in excess.

 ### Responsible Citizenship

Suggest to the appropriate community leader or local newspaper that your community have a Responsible Citizen Award. Write a brief statement (fewer than 200 words) that explains the criteria for the award. Suggest a person to nominate for the award. Discuss three of his/her actions that demonstrate that (s)he has good character and is a responsible citizen.

You Can Develop a Healthy Mind

Life Skill **I will choose behaviors to promote a healthy mind.**

You will face many challenges in your life. Some challenges will be more difficult for you than others. The way you respond to challenges in your life is important. Every challenge is an opportunity to learn about yourself and to develop your potential. This lesson explains how you can develop a healthy mind. You will learn about personality characteristics that can keep you afloat when life becomes difficult. You will learn how and why you should avoid addictions. You also will learn what teens can do if they have addictive behavior or codependence. This lesson outlines different mental disorders. You will learn how mental disorders can affect health status.

The Lesson Outline

What to Know About Personality

What to Know About Addictions

What to Know About Codependence

What to Know About Mental Disorders

Objectives

1. Identify 25 personality characteristics that promote health status. **page 47**

2. List and discuss 11 addictions that some teens develop. **pages 50–51**

3. Identify five signs of addiction and three ways to avoid addictions. **page 52**

4. Discuss the characteristics of and treatment for codependence. **page 53**

5. Outline six categories of mental disorders. **pages 54–55**

Vocabulary Words

personality
addiction
drug addiction
eating disorder
exercise addiction
gambling addiction
nicotine addiction
nicotine
perfectionism
relationship addiction
shopping addiction
television addiction
thrill-seeking addiction
workaholism
formal intervention
relapse
codependence
codependent
enabler
honest talk
support group
mental disorder
affective disorder
anxiety disorder
dissociative disorder
personality disorder
somatoform disorder
schizophrenia

What to Know About
Personality

Personality is an individual's unique pattern of characteristics. Characteristics often are used to describe a person. Certain personality characteristics promote health status. When you possess these characteristics, you are more likely to take responsibility for your health.

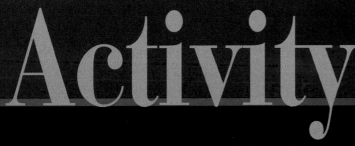

Activity
Your Personality Checkup

Life Skill: I will choose behaviors to promote a healthy mind.

Materials: paper, pen or pencil

Directions: Read the following list of personality characteristics. Select the ten characteristics you find most desirable. On a separate sheet of paper, make a "Top Ten List of Personality Characteristics."

ambitious: showing a strong desire to achieve a particular goal

compassionate: showing concern and a desire to be helpful

confident: having a belief in one's own abilities

cooperative: willing to work with others for a common benefit

courageous: having mental or moral strength to go on when there is danger, fear, or difficulty

dedicated: being devoted to a cause, ideal, or purpose

enthusiastic: being filled with strong excitement

faithful: being loyal and dedicated

generous: willing to give or share

honest: being truthful and fair

hopeful: believing that what is wanted will happen

loyal: being supportive and faithful

optimistic: tending to expect a positive outcome

patient: waiting or enduring difficulty without complaining

perceptive: having insight or understanding

persistent: continuing a course of action

reliable: being trustworthy and dependable

resilient: being able to adjust, recover, bounce back, and learn from difficulties

resolute: being firm in one's decisions

respectful: showing high regard for something or somebody

responsible: being accountable for one's behavior

secure: having no doubt in opinions or expectations

self-determined: acting in a certain manner without outside influence

self-disciplined: following through on what one intends or promises to do

sincere: being honest and trustworthy

What to Know About
Addictions

What do you do when you feel anxious and tense? How do you cope with difficult situations? Are you able to acknowledge a problem and deal with it? Some teens do not deal with their problems. They use drugs or rely on harmful behaviors as a way of coping. They develop addictions. An **addiction** is a compelling need to take a drug or engage in a specific behavior.

You may be familiar with drug addiction. Some teens drink alcohol to avoid dealing with problems. They feel a compelling need or urge to drink alcohol whenever they feel bored, lonely, or frustrated. They depend on alcohol to avoid their problems and change their mood. Some teens depend on other drugs to avoid their problems and change their mood. They depend on drugs such as cocaine, crack, and marijuana. Drug addiction also is referred to as chemical dependence and drug dependence.

Even a healthful behavior that is carried to extremes can become an addictive behavior. For example, many teens enjoy shopping. However, teens who feel compelled to shop when they are unhappy may cross the line from shopping to shopping addiction. Many teens enjoy exercise. However, teens who exercise to extremes to avoid facing problems have an addiction. A Teen's Guide to Addictions on pages 50 and 51 reviews 11 addictions teens may have.

Characteristics of Teens Who Are at Risk for Developing Addictions

⟶

Teens who are at risk for developing addictions:

1. are depressed,
2. have negative self-esteem,
3. have many unmet needs,
4. do not know how to have fun,
5. feel guilty and ashamed,
6. live in a fantasy world,
7. have had traumatic childhoods,
8. feel tense and anxious,
9. have difficulty expressing feelings,
10. have trouble with anger,
11. blame others when things go wrong,
12. constantly seek approval,
13. want to control others,
14. have poor coping skills,
15. have difficulty with authority figures,
16. feel empty inside,
17. are bored,
18. are unable to delay gratification,
19. are lonely,
20. deny personal problems.

How Addictions Affect Health Status

Addictions can harm health status in several ways:

◆ **An addiction can harm physical health.**
Using drugs, such as nicotine, alcohol, crack, cocaine, or marijuana, harms body organs. Exercising to extremes can cause injuries.

◆ **An addiction can jeopardize safety.**
Using drugs, such as alcohol, crack, cocaine, or marijuana, changes the way a person thinks. Teens who use drugs may choose unsafe actions and have accidents. Use of drugs can lead to fights that result in injuries. Drug use is a major cause of motor vehicle accidents that result in injury or death. Teens with thrill-seeking addiction take unnecessary risks that can result in injury or death. Thrill-seeking addiction is discussed further on page 51.

◆ **An addiction can harm relationships.**
Teens with addictions focus most of their attention on a drug or a behavior. They neglect their relationships. They deny their addiction(s) and begin to lie or be secretive. They are unable to share feelings in healthful ways. As a result, their relationships with family and friends suffer.

◆ **An addiction can cause legal problems.**
The use of crack, cocaine, marijuana, and other drugs is illegal. Drinking alcohol and gambling, including the purchase of lottery tickets, is illegal for minors. Teens can get busted for these addictions. They may be suspended from school, be arrested, or go to jail.

◆ **An addiction can cause financial problems.** Teens with shopping addiction often overspend. They may borrow credit cards or steal to pay for purchases. They get into financial difficulty and may even break the law in order to continue their addiction. Teens with drug addiction may spend large amounts of money on drugs. Teens with gambling addiction may continue betting when they do not have money.

Activity

How to Recognize an Addiction

Life Skill: I will choose behaviors to promote a healthy mind.

Materials: paper, pen or pencil

Directions: Below is a list of addictions and a series of incomplete statements with blanks. Fill in any of the behaviors that describe you. If any do describe you, share them with a parent, guardian, or other responsible adult. DO NOT WRITE IN THIS BOOK.

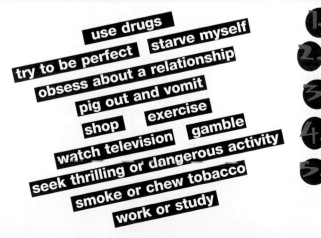

use drugs
try to be perfect   starve myself
obsess about a relationship
pig out and vomit
shop   exercise
watch television   gamble
seek thrilling or dangerous activity
smoke or chew tobacco
work or study

1. I frequently feel the need to _____.

2. I _____ instead of dealing with my feelings of depression, loneliness, boredom, or anxiety.

3. Sometimes I feel bad about myself after I _____.

4. I continue to _____ even when there are negative consequences.

5. I promise myself and others that I will not _____, but I cannot seem to stop.

A Teen's Guide to

Addictions

Drug Addiction (Chemical Dependence, Drug Dependence)

Drug addiction is the compelling need for a drug even though it harms the body, mind, or relationships. Teens with drug addiction feel the need for drugs when they are anxious, bored, or depressed. They depend on drugs to change their moods. They use drugs to avoid facing problems. They usually deny that they use drugs for these reasons.

> **Lesson 52 will include more information on drug addiction.**

Eating Disorders

An **eating disorder** is a mental disorder in which a person has a compelling need to starve, to binge, or to binge and purge. To purge is to rid the body of food by vomiting or by using laxatives or diuretics. Teens with eating disorders usually have negative self-esteem. They often do not feel good about their appearance. They want more control over their lives. They substitute harmful eating habits for the control they think they are lacking.

> **Lesson 40 will include more information on eating disorders.**

Exercise Addiction

Exercise addiction is the compelling need to exercise. Teens with exercise addiction make exercise the focus of their lives. They exercise to relieve tension and to feel in control of their lives. They put their exercise routine ahead of family, friends, studying, and other responsibilities. They may push themselves to the limit and injure themselves. If they do not exercise, they are depressed, anxious, and unhappy and have difficulty sleeping.

Gambling Addiction

Gambling addiction is the compelling need to bet money or something else. Teens with gambling addiction often are bored and restless. They get a "high" when they place bets. Gambling addiction often begins in childhood with shooting marbles and flipping baseball cards and progresses to pinball machines and video games and then to bets on sports events and card games. There is no cure. Teens who develop gambling addiction will struggle to control the urge to gamble for the rest of their lives. More than one-third of teens with gambling addiction have other addictions as well.

Nicotine Addiction (Nicotine Dependence)

Nicotine addiction or nicotine dependence is the compelling need for nicotine. **Nicotine** is a stimulant drug found in tobacco products, including cigarettes and chewing tobacco. Teens addicted to nicotine develop their schedule around smoking or chewing tobacco. They may rely on nicotine to wake up in the morning. They may smoke or chew to relieve tension or boredom.

> **Lesson 56 will include more information on nicotine addiction.**

Perfectionism

Perfectionism is the compelling need to be accurate. Teens who are perfectionists often repeat the same task because they are never satisfied with their performance. They are overly critical of themselves and of others. Nothing is ever good enough for them. Perfectionism is the result of feeling inadequate and insecure. Some teens become perfectionists because adults had unrealistic expectations of them during their childhood.

A Teen's Guide to

Addictions

Relationship Addiction

Relationship addiction is the compelling need to be connected to another person. Teens with relationship addiction use relationships like they would drugs. When they feel depressed or insecure, contact with a specific person gives them a quick fix. But they feel better only for a brief time. They need the other person to "fill up" their emptiness. They feel a constant need to be with this other person. Teens with relationship addiction are often described as being needy. The person with whom they have a relationship feels suffocated and drained of energy.

Lesson 17 will include more information on relationship addiction.

Shopping Addiction

Shopping addiction is the compelling need to purchase things. Teens with shopping addiction may describe themselves as "born to shop" and may "shop 'til they drop." These teens are insecure. Shopping gives them a quick fix for depressed feelings. Salespeople may give them special attention. They feel in control and powerful when they make purchases. They feel better, but not for long. After a shopping spree, they often feel guilty. Shopping addiction can lead to severe emotional and financial problems.

Television Addiction

Television addiction is the compelling need to watch television. Teens with television addiction plan their schedules around the television programs they watch. They may watch six to seven hours of TV a day. When these teens become anxious or bored, they turn on the TV. They get a quick fix from watching TV. They are unable to manage their time and get other things done. As a result, they have no time to be involved in school activities. These teens usually do not get good grades. They usually are not physically fit.

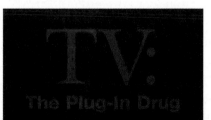

The number of teens with television addiction has increased dramatically. In 1985, a book describing television as "The Plug-In Drug" was published.

Marie Winn. *The Plug-In Drug.* Penguin Books, 1985.

Thrill-Seeking Addiction

Thrill-seeking addiction is the compelling need to take unnecessary risks. Teens with thrill-seeking addiction enjoy scary situations. They are willing to take dangerous dares. During risky experiences, there are biochemical changes in the brain. Some teens get hooked and constantly seek these changes. Thrill-seeking becomes a quick fix. Teens with this addiction may take unnecessary risks and injure themselves.

Workaholism

Workaholism is the compelling need to work to fill an emptiness. Teens who are workaholics may feel the need to work whenever they are not in school. This may include excessive studying. This does not mean that all teens who study and get good grades are workaholics. It is healthy to set goals and work hard to reach them. Workaholics do not enjoy themselves when they are not working or studying. Working long hours keeps them from dealing with other aspects of their lives, such as emotions and relationships. They need the constant praise they may get from work. They get a high from work that helps them overcome feelings of depression and are anxious, tense, and upset when they not working.

What to Do About Addictions

Five Signs of Addiction

1. Having a compelling need to take a drug or engage in a behavior

2. Taking a drug or engaging in a behavior instead of dealing with feelings of anxiety, depression, boredom, or loneliness

3. Feeling bad about oneself after taking a drug or engaging in a behavior

4. Taking a drug or engaging in a behavior even when there are negative consequences

5. Trying to stop taking a drug or engaging in a behavior, but being unable to do so

Having one or more addictions is a serious threat to a person's health. Be on the lookout for signs of addictions in yourself and in others. The following suggestions will help you avoid addictions:

1. **Stay informed.** Review up-to-date information about addictions often.

2. **Make a self-check to learn if you have any of the characteristics of teens who are at risk for developing addictions.** Refer to the list on page 48 of the characteristics of teens who are at risk for developing addictions. Talk to a parent, guardian, or other responsible adult if you have any of the characteristics listed.

3. **Make a self-check to determine if you have an addiction.** Complete the activity on page 49, How to Recognize an Addiction. If you complete the blanks with a drug or specific behavior that interferes with healthful living, talk to your parent, guardian, or other responsible adult about getting help for an addiction.

Teens often deny addictions and refuse to get help. They may need to be confronted by parents, guardians or other caring people. A **formal intervention** is an action by people, such as family members, who want a person to get treatment. The people involved in a formal intervention prepare ahead of time. They review what the teen has said and done. They review how the teen's addiction affects them. A trained counselor can help them prepare. During a formal intervention, these people confront the teen with the addiction. The counselor can be present. They are very specific as they tell the teen what they have observed. They explain why treatment is needed.

There are different approaches to treatment for addictions. Individual therapy is treatment that involves a trained professional and the person with an addiction. Group therapy involves a trained professional who works with more than one person at a time. Family therapy involves a trained professional who works with the person and his/her family members. Some teens who have addictions must be hospitalized. Treatment for physical health problems may be needed.

Teens who have been treated for an addiction may have a relapse. A **relapse** is a return to a previous behavior or condition. These teens return to their addiction when they feel depressed, anxious, or lonely. To avoid relapse, teens must stick to their plan for recovery. Part of any recovery plan for teens with addictions is to have a support network. The purpose of the support network is to allow the teens to feel secure enough to share their feelings and needs. People in the support network also provide encouragement.

What to Know About
Codependence

People sometimes become very involved with other people who have an addiction. They want to rescue people with an addiction and fix their problems. **Codependence** is a mental disorder in which a person denies feelings and begins to cope in harmful ways. A **codependent** is a person who wants to rescue and control another person. People with codependence have characteristics in common.

People with codependence are enablers. An **enabler** is a person who supports the harmful behavior of others. For example, an enabler might lend money to someone with a gambling addiction or make excuses for a friend who uses drugs. An enabler might praise someone who exercises to extremes for being in condition. These responses encourage people with addictions to continue their addiction. People with codependence are unable to participate in honest talk. **Honest talk** is the straightforward sharing of feelings.

People with codependence may benefit from individual, group, or family therapy. They also may benefit from being in a support group. A **support group** is a group of people who help one another recover from an addiction, a particular disease, or a difficult situation. Various lessons in this book include information about different available support groups.

People with codependence:

- deny their feelings,
- focus on fixing other people's problems,
- try to control other people,
- feel responsible for what other people say or do,
- seek the approval of others,
- have difficulty having fun,
- have difficulty allowing others to care for them,
- try to protect others from the harmful consequences of their behavior,
- do not meet their own needs,
- avoid living their own lives by concentrating on other people.

Lessons 12 and 17 will include more information on codependence.

Recovery from codependence involves:

- **developing a better sense of self,**
- **learning to share feelings,**
- **learning to stay focused on solving one's own problems,**
- **allowing other people to be responsible for their own lives,**
- **using honest talk to confront people with problems.**

What to Know About
Mental Disorders

A **mental disorder** is a mental or emotional condition that makes it difficult for a person to live in a normal way. The causes of mental disorders can be organic or functional. Organic mental disorders are caused by physical injuries and illnesses that affect the brain. Some causes include strokes, brain tumors, automobile accidents, alcoholism, sexually transmitted diseases, and meningitis. Functional mental disorders have causes that are not physical. Some causes include environmental conditions, stress, traumatic experiences, and poor coping skills.

A Guide to Mental Disorders

The American Psychiatric Association classifies mental disorders according to their common patterns of behaviors.

Affective Disorders

An **affective disorder** is a disorder involving moods that are extreme. The exact causes of affective disorders are not known, but they are more common in some families.

Clinical depression is long-lasting feelings of hopelessness, sadness, or helplessness. People are considered to have clinical depression if they have not had a recent trauma and still experience five of nine general symptoms for two weeks or more. General symptoms include deep sadness, apathy, fatigue, agitation, sleep disturbances, weight or appetite change, lack of concentration, feelings of worthlessness, and morbid thoughts.

Bipolar disorder or **manic-depressive disorder** is a disorder in which a person's moods vary from extreme happiness to depression. During the manic phase, the person experiences great joy for no reason and is very talkative and restless. (S)he may have outbursts of anger that turn into violence. During the depressive phase, the person is in a passive mood, has little energy, and may think of suicide. This phase ends when the person's mood swings back to the manic phase.

Seasonal affective disorder is a type of depression that occurs when a person has reduced exposure to sunlight. People with this disorder usually experience symptoms during the months when there is reduced sunlight. Symptoms include increased appetite, decreased physical activity, irritability, and general depression. The change in mood may be due to the absence of sunlight. Special light therapy for short periods daily will relieve many of these symptoms.

Anxiety Disorders

An **anxiety disorder** is a disorder in which real or imagined fears prevent a person from enjoying life. People who have an anxiety disorder may have panic attacks. A panic attack is a period of intense fear and anxiety that is accompanied by body changes. Body changes may include increased heart rate, sweating, shaking, shortness of breath, discomfort, nausea, loss of control, chills, hot flashes, and fear of dying.

General anxiety disorder is a recurring state of anxiety, fear, and tenseness. People with this disorder feel anxious most of the time. No specific object or situation produces the fear.

Phobia is an excessive fear of certain objects, situations, or people. The fear is very real to the person even though it is not realistic. A panic attack may occur when the object, situation, or person is near. Mental health professionals link phobias with past experiences. For example, an adult who was locked in a small space as a child may fear closed spaces.

Some common phobias are:

- aerophobia: fear of flying
- agoraphobia: fear of being in open spaces
- algophobia: fear of pain
- arachnophobia: fear of spiders
- claustrophobia: fear of closed spaces
- hematophobia: fear of the sight of blood
- hydrophobia: fear of water
- nyctophobia: fear of darkness
- pyrophobia: fear of fire
- xenophobia: fear of strangers

Obsessive-compulsive disorder is the urgent need to repeat a thought or an action. People with this disorder may not be able to clear a thought from their mind. They may repeat an action so often that they cannot attend to other responsibilities.

Post-traumatic stress disorder (PTSD) is a condition in which the after-effects of a past event keep a person from living in a normal way. People who suffer from PTSD may have been in military combat or sexually abused. They may have recurring dreams or nightmares of what took place. They may have difficulty concentrating and sleeping.

Dissociative Disorders

A **dissociative** (di·SOH·shee·ay·tiv) **disorder** is a disorder in which a person has memory loss, confused identity, or more than one identity.

Amnesia is the inability to recall past experiences. Amnesia is the result of aging, illness, or injury, not intentional forgetting. A person might not recall who (s)he is and assume a different identity. Usually, amnesia lasts a short time and is not as dramatic as portrayed in movies or on television.

Multiple personality is a rare mental disorder in which two or more personalities coexist within the same person. The person may shift from one personality to another. Each personality is unaware of the other personality's thoughts and actions.

Personality Disorders

A **personality disorder** is a disorder in which a person's patterns of thinking, feeling, and acting interfere with daily living.

Antisocial personality disorder is a disorder in which a person's patterns of behavior are in conflict with society. People who are antisocial are often hateful, aggressive, and irritable. They may be indifferent to the needs of others. They may break the law and place others in danger.

Avoidant personality disorder is a disorder in which a person avoids all social contact. People with this disorder have negative self-esteem and fear rejection from other people.

Dependent personality disorder is a disorder in which a person cannot function without the advice and help of others. People with this disorder are afraid of making decisions or doing anything without help because they fear rejection.

Histrionic personality disorder is a disorder in which a person has emotional outbursts and constantly draws attention to himself/herself.

Narcissistic personality disorder is a disorder in which a person is boastful, conceited, and inconsiderate of others. People with this disorder believe they are better than others. They are preoccupied with their own wants and needs.

Passive-aggressive personality disorder is a disorder in which a person switches back and forth from being forceful with people and events and being frightened of them.

Somatoform Disorders

A **somatoform** (soh·MA·toh·form) **disorder** is a disorder in which a person has symptoms of disease but no physical cause can be found.

Hypochondria (hy·puh·KAHN·dree·uh) is a disorder in which a person is constantly worried about illness. Such a person is called a hypochondriac. A hypochondriac constantly feels aches and pains and worries about developing some illnesse or disease.

Conversion disorder is disorder in which a person experiences sudden health changes as a result of an emotional state. Health changes that might occur include sudden loss of vision or hearing, loss of sensation in the skin, or paralysis of a body part.

Schizophrenia

Schizophrenia (skitz·oh·FREN·ee·uh) is a disorder in which there is a split or breakdown in logical thought processes. The split results in unusual behaviors. Actions, words, and emotions are confused and usually are inappropriate. A person with this disorder may appear desperate and withdraw into an inner world of fantasy.

Paranoid schizophrenia is a type of schizophrenia in which a person has delusions of either persecution or grandeur. Delusions of persecution are feelings that other people are trying to harm you. Delusions of grandeur are feelings that you are unusually great.

How Can People with Mental Disorders Be Helped?

People with mental disorders can be helped in the following ways:

Formal intervention. A formal intervention may be needed to help people who deny their condition and refuse to get help.

Evaluations. People with mental disorders may need both a medical evaluation and a psychological evaluation.

Medications. Some people with mental disorders need medication that must be prescribed by a physician.

Therapy. Most people with mental disorders benefit from individual, group, or family therapy in which a trained mental health professional helps them make adjustments to daily living.

Support groups. People with mental disorders may benefit from sharing their feelings and needs. Family members also may benefit from being in support groups.

Recovery plan. People with mental disorders must have a long-range recovery plan. They must continue their therapy and/or medication when recommended to prevent a relapse.

Activity

Mental Health Owner's Manual

Life Skill: I will choose behaviors to promote a healthy mind.

Materials: computer and printer (optional), paper, colored pens and pencils

Directions: A car owner's manual tells the owner how to get the best performance from the car. It includes important operating, maintenance, and service information. A Mental Health Owner's Manual tells a person how to maintain a healthy mind. Follow the steps below to design a Mental Health Owner's Manual.

 Design a clever cover for your owner's manual. Create your own logo to depict positive mental health.

 Create a Table of Contents page that includes the following: Chapter 1. Special Features of this Model, Chapter 2. Maintenance Problems, Chapter 3. Service Warranty.

 Create information for Chapter 1. Describe your personality. Refer to the personality characteristics listed on page 47. Include the personality characteristics you "own" and would like to "own."

 Create information for Chapter 2. Maintenance Problems are things that could go wrong with the owner's mental health. Include information from this chapter on addictions and mental disorders.

Create information for Chapter 3. This chapter should explain where and how to get service. Use the information you have learned about how people with mental disorders can be helped.

Lesson 7

Review

Vocabulary Words

Write a separate sentence using each of the vocabulary words listed on page 46.

Objectives

1. What are 25 personality characteristics that promote health status? **Objective 1**

2. What are 11 addictions that some teens develop? **Objective 2**

3. What are five signs of addiction and three ways to avoid addictions? **Objective 3**

4. What are the characteristics of and treatment for codependence? **Objective 4**

5. What are six categories of mental disorders? **Objective 5**

Responsible Decision-Making

You are visiting a teen in a community that has a lottery that has grown to over $25 million. Your friend encourages you to buy several tickets for yourself. You are not at the legal age. The teen has a friend who will purchase the tickets for you. Write a response to this situation.

1. Describe the situation that requires you to make a decision.
2. List possible decisions you might make.
3. Name two responsible adults with whom you might discuss your decisions.
4. Evaluate the possible consequences of your decisions. Determine if each decision will lead to actions that:
   • promote health,
   • protect safety,
   • follow laws,
   • show respect for yourself and others,
   • follow the guidelines of your parents and of other responsible adults,
   • demonstrate good character.
5. Decide which decision is most responsible and appropriate.
6. Tell two results you expect if you make this decision.

Effective Communication

Design an ad that can be placed in the catalog of your favorite store to warn about the dangers of shopping addiction.

Self-Directed Learning

Write a short report on seasonal affective disorder. Locate information in three magazines or journals. Cite your sources.

Critical Thinking

One of your friends seems very "needy." This friend calls you several times every evening and wants to be with you all the time. You feel like you need space. What kind of an addiction might your friend have? How might you use honest talk to help your friend?

Responsible Citizenship

Select one of the addictions discussed in A Teen's Guide to Addictions. Write an editorial for the school newspaper discussing how this addiction might lead to illegal behaviors.

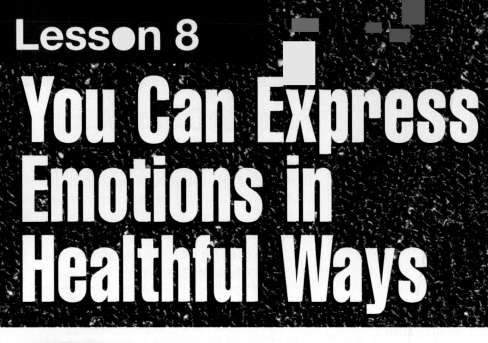

Lesson 8

You Can Express Emotions in Healthful Ways

Life Skill **I will express emotions in healthful ways.**

You express your emotions in a number of different ways—with spoken words, written or printed words, sign language, or actions. This lesson discusses the influence emotions have on your health status. You will learn about the mind-body connection. This lesson provides guidelines for expressing emotions in healthful ways. You will learn how to use I-messages and active listening. This lesson also discusses how to express anger in healthful ways. You will learn how to use anger management skills.

The Lesson Outline

How Emotions Affect Your Mind and Body

How to Express Emotions in Healthful Ways

How to Use I-Messages and Active Listening

How to Use Anger Management Skills

Objectives

1. Explain how emotions affect the mind-body connection. **page 59**
2. Outline the five guidelines for expressing emotions in healthful ways. **page 60**
3. Write an example of an I-message, a you-message, and active listening. **page 61**
4. Discuss hidden anger and anger cues. **page 62**
5. List and discuss ten anger management skills to help a teen manage anger. **page 63**

Vocabulary Words

communication

emotion

mind-body connection

psychosomatic disease

nonverbal behavior

mixed message

I-message

you-message

active listening

anger

anger trigger

anger cue

hidden anger

hostility syndrome

serotonin

projection

displacement

anger management skills

self-statements

How Emotions Affect Your Mind and Body

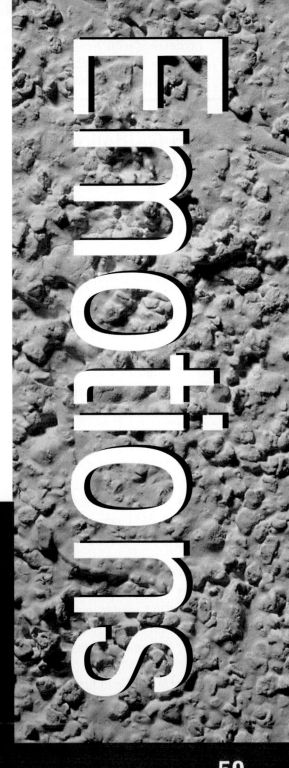

Communication is the sharing of emotions, thoughts, and information with another person. An **emotion** is a specific feeling. The listing below names many different emotions you may have experienced.

Your response to an emotion is mental as well as physical. The **mind-body connection** is the close relationship between mental and physical responses. Suppose you have a test tomorrow and you respond by worrying. Your response affects your mind and your body. It may become difficult for you to concentrate (mental response). Your heart rate and blood pressure may increase (physical response). Knowing how to express your emotions in healthful ways helps keep your mind and body healthy.

Being unable to express emotions in healthful ways can harm your body. A **psychosomatic disease** is a physical disorder caused or aggravated by emotional responses. Suppose a teen does not know how to handle an argument with friends. (S)he may get a stomachache or a headache— an emotional response caused a physical disorder.

Suppose a teen has asthma. Asthma is a chronic condition in which breathing becomes difficult. This teen may worry about a test in school and have difficulty breathing—an emotional response aggravated a physical disorder.

Remember that your health status includes the condition of your body, mind, emotions, and relationships. To promote your health status, you must pay attention to your mind-body connection. Expressing emotions in healthful ways is essential to having healthful relationships.

Types of Emotions

Have you ever felt:

depressed	afraid	resentful	guilty
optimistic	lonely	excited	stressed
disgusted	angry	sad	happy
rejected	loving	frustrated	surprised
envious	anxious	shy	jealous
	nervous		thrilled

How to Express Emotions in Healthful Ways

How well do you express your emotions? When you express your emotions, are your actions responsible? Do you think about protecting your health when you experience an intense emotional response? Review the five guidelines that appear below for expressing emotions in healthful ways.

Five Guidelines for Expressing Emotions in Healthful Ways

1. **Identify the emotion.**
   - What emotion am I experiencing?

2. **Identify the source of the emotion.**
   - Why do I feel this way?

3. **Decide whether or not you need to respond right away.**
   - Should I talk to a parent, guardian, or other responsible adult about the emotions I am experiencing?
   - Should I try to sort out my emotions by myself?
   - Do I need more information before I respond?
   - Do I need to rehearse what I will say before I respond?

4. **Choose a responsible and healthful response.**
   - What I-message might I use? (I-messages are explained on the next page.)
   - Would it be helpful to express my emotions by writing in a journal?
   - Could I write a poem, sculpt clay, or draw a picture to express my emotions?

5. **Protect your health.**
   - Do I need extra sleep?
   - Do I need to work off my strong emotions with vigorous exercise?
   - Am I aware of any physical disorders that might be connected to the emotional response I am experiencing? If so, I may need to see a physician.
   - Am I able to function in daily activities? If not, I may need to ask my parent(s) or guardian about counseling.

Nonverbal Communications and Mixed Messages

Did you know that your actions also express how you feel? **Nonverbal behavior** is the use of actions to express emotions and thoughts. For example, twisting your hair might express anxiety. Tapping your foot might express impatience. Smiling usually indicates pleasure. These are examples of actions that send a message to anyone who is observing you.

Avoid sending mixed messages when you express your feelings. A **mixed message** is a message that gives out two different meanings. For example, the words you use and the tone of your voice when you speak may send different meanings. Suppose a friend apologizes for something that (s)he has done to you. If you accept the apology with a smirk on your face, your words and actions give a mixed message.

How to Use
I-Messages and Active Listening

When You Speak

Using I-messages is a healthful way to express feelings. An **I-message** is a statement that contains a specific behavior or event, the effect of the behavior or event on a person, and the emotions that result. You can become skilled at using I-messages to share your feelings. Examine the box at the bottom of the page for an example of an I-message. When you use an I-message, you express your emotions without blaming or shaming another person. You do not attack another person or put the person on the defensive. When you use an I-message, you give the other person a chance to respond.

Using you-messages results in the opposite response. A **you-message** is a statement that blames or shames another person. A you-message puts down another person for what (s)he has said or done. When a you-message is used, emotions are not shared in a healthful way. A you-message brings out a different response from another person.

Compare the I-message and the you-message in the box below.

When You Listen

Active listening is a way of responding to show that a person hears and understands. An active listener might respond in four different ways to let the other person know that (s)he is really hearing and understanding. The listener may:

1. ask for more information (clarifying response),
2. repeat in his/her own words what the speaker said (restating response),
3. summarize the main ideas (summarizing response),
4. acknowledge and show appreciation for the speaker's feelings (confirming response).

If You Don't Listen

Have you ever stopped listening to someone because:

...you were thinking of something or someone else?

...you could not hear the speaker?

...you were tired and dozing off?

...you were thinking about what you were going to say next?

...you were distracted by other noise?

...you thought you knew what the speaker was going to say next?

When you tune out someone who is speaking to you, the person may feel unimportant. You risk harming your relationship with the person.

Situation: Your younger sister picks up the phone several times while you are trying to work out a disagreement with a friend. You are very irritated with the interruptions. You tell your friend that you will call him/her back in a few minutes. You go into your sister's room and say...

What Would You Say?

I-message:

When I was interrupted on the phone (event) I couldn't talk with my friend (effect) and I am irritated (emotions).

You-message:

You are rude and selfish to pick up the phone when I am trying to have a conversation.

How to Use
Anger Management Skills

What causes you to feel angry? **Anger** is the feeling of being irritated or annoyed. Anger is usually a response to being hurt, frustrated, insulted, or rejected. An **anger trigger** is a thought or event that causes a person to become angry. An **anger cue** is a body change that occurs when a person is angry. Anger cues are part of your response to anger. Response to anger is often called the fight-or-flight response because your body changes to prepare you for an emergency. You are prepared to take quick action or to run away to protect yourself.

Hidden anger is anger that is not recognized and is expressed in an inappropriate way. The following types of behavior may be signs of hidden anger: being negative, making cruel remarks to others, being sarcastic, procrastinating, blowing up easily, having very little interest in anything, being bored, sighing frequently, being depressed. If you have hidden anger, your health will be affected. You

may experience tense facial muscles, stiff or sore neck and shoulder muscles, ulcers, headaches, high blood pressure, some types of cancer, and weight loss or gain.

Some teens are always angry. They have a chip on their shoulder and seem ready to blow up. Imagine what is going on inside their bodies! They exhibit hostility syndrome. **Hostility syndrome** is a physical state in which the body is in the fight-or-flight state at all times. In other words, the person's body always feels that there is an emergency about to happen. The person's body is on overdrive and gets very little rest. The person's immune system, the body system that fights disease, does not work well.

Teens who have hostility syndrome have lowered brain serotonin levels. **Serotonin** is a chemical in the body that helps regulate primitive drives and emotions. Teens with lowered brain serotonin levels can become very aggressive.

Teens with hidden anger may express their anger in harmful ways. They may express their anger with projection. **Projection** is blaming others for actions or events for which they are not responsible. For example, a teen who scores poorly on a test may say the test was unfair and blame a teacher. Teens with hidden anger may express anger with displacement. **Displacement** is the releasing of anger on someone or something other than the cause of the anger. For example, a teen angry about a family situation might destroy school property. Some teens do not know they have hidden anger.

It is not harmful to feel angry. Feeling angry is a normal and healthful response to many situations. However, it is essential that you learn to control your anger and to express anger in appropriate ways. **Anger management skills** are healthful ways to control and express anger. Review the anger management skills on the facing page.

Anger Cues

- Rapid breathing
- Increase in heart rate
- Rise in blood pressure
- Increased sweating from sweat glands in the face
- Sweaty palms
- Dryness of the mouth
- Increased alertness
- Decreased sensitivity to pain
- Increased muscle strength as a result of increased availability of blood sugar to the muscles
- Tensed eyebrows
- Pursed lips
- Reddening of the face

Anger Management Skills

1. **Keep an Anger Self-Inventory.** An Anger Self-Inventory helps you examine your anger. Use the questions in the inventory when you recognize that you are experiencing anger cues. Decide if you are overreacting to a situation or person. Determine if a situation or person is worth your attention. If your anger is justified, examine ways to respond.

Anger Self-Inventory

- What am I feeling?
- What is causing me to feel this way?
- Is my anger justified?
- Am I still angry? (If yes, continue.)
- What are healthful ways I can express my anger?

2. **Use self-statements to control anger.** **Self-statements** are words a person can say to himself/herself when (s)he experiences anger triggers and cues.

- I can manage this situation.
- I will take a few deep breaths before I say anything.
- I'll just count to ten. One, two, three....
- I am in control as long as I keep cool.
- I am not going to explode over this.

3. **Use I-messages instead of you-messages.** An I-message can be used to express your anger about the behavior of another person. Using I-messages keeps communication lines open. The other person can respond without feeling threatened.

4. **Write a letter.** Writing a letter provides a safe way to express anger. You can express your reasons for being angry without being interrupted. You can read your letter and make changes before sending it. You can hold the letter until you cool down. You may even decide not to send the letter after you have written it.

5. **Write in a journal.** Writing in a journal can help you vent your anger. Write answers to the questions in the Anger Self-Inventory. Review your answers to learn more about your anger.

6. **Reduce the effects of anger cues with physical activity.** Vigorous physical activity can relieve anger cues. Try activities such as dancing, jogging, swimming, martial arts, weightlifting, or rollerblading.

7. **Use safe physical actions to blow off steam.** Express anger in a physical way that will not have harmful consequences to yourself or to others:

- Stomp on the floor.
- Scream into a pillow.
- Hit a pillow.
- Squeeze a tennis ball.
- Throw a fluff ball.

8. **Keep a sense of humor.** Telling a joke or poking fun at a situation or yourself (in a good-spirited way that does not attack others) can lighten up a situation. Laughing helps reduce the effects of anger cues.

9. **Rehearse what to do in situations that you know are your anger triggers.** Think of situations that make you angry. Imagine what you would say and do in these situations to control your anger. Rehearse in front of a mirror or with a friend, parent, or counselor.

10. **Talk with a parent or mentor.** Responsible adults can help you recognize anger triggers and cues. They can help you choose healthful actions.

Activity

Filled with Hostility

Life Skill: I will express emotions in healthful ways.
Materials: two water glasses, one clear and the other colored; a pitcher of water
Directions: Follow the steps below to learn about the hostility syndrome.

 Three student volunteers are needed for this activity. One volunteer will hold the colored glass. One volunteer will hold the clear glass. One volunteer will hold the pitcher of water.

 A classmate will name an anger trigger—something that makes him/her angry. The student volunteer holding the pitcher of water will pour a small amount of water into both the clear glass and the colored glass. The water poured into the glasses represents anger.

 The student holding the clear glass will state an appropriate anger management skill and pour the water from the glass back into the pitcher. This student has expressed his/her anger and gotten rid of it.

 The student holding the colored glass does nothing. Because the glass is colored, you cannot see the water. But, you know there is anger inside.

 Repeat the same sequence. Another classmate will name an anger trigger—something that makes him/her angry. The student volunteer holding the pitcher of water will pour water into the two glasses.

 The student holding the clear glass will state an appropriate anger management skill and pour the water from the glass back into the pitcher. This student has expressed and gotten rid of his/her anger.

 The student holding the colored glass does nothing. Although the anger (water) is hidden, you know there is even more anger (water) in this glass.

 Repeat the same sequence several times.

 Examine the contents of the clear glass. The student holding the clear glass used appropriate anger management skills. What skills did (s)he use? What happens when you use anger management skills?

 Examine the contents of the colored glass. The student holding the colored glass did not express anger. What happens when you do not express anger?

Lesson 8

Review

Vocabulary Words

Write a separate sentence using each of the vocabulary words listed on page 58.

Objectives

1. How do emotions affect the mind-body connection? **Objective 1**
2. What are five guidelines for expressing emotions in healthful ways? **Objective 2**
3. What examples can you give of an I-message, a you-message, and active listening? **Objective 3**
4. What is hidden anger and what are 12 examples of anger cues? **Objective 4**
5. What are ten anger management skills to help a teen manage anger? **Objective 5**

Responsible Decision-Making

Some classmates toilet paper your friend's house. Your friend is furious and wants revenge. (S)he gets some rotten eggs and asks you to help splatter them on your classmates' houses. Write a response to this situation.

1. Describe the situation that requires you to make a decision.
2. List possible decisions you might make.
3. Name two responsible adults with whom you might discuss your decisions.
4. Evaluate the possible consequences of your decisions. Determine if each decision will lead to actions that:
   - promote health,
   - protect safety,
   - follow laws,
   - show respect for yourself and others,
   - follow the guidelines of your parents and of other responsible adults,
   - demonstrate good character.
5. Decide which decision is most responsible and appropriate.
6. Tell two results you expect if you make this decision.

Effective Communication

Refer to the self-statements to control anger listed on page 63. Make your own list of five self-statements that you can use when you experience anger triggers and cues.

Self-Directed Learning

Check the library or Internet for an article containing information on the hostility syndrome or anger management skills. Write a one-page summary of the article. Include the complete bibliographical reference for the article.

Critical Thinking

A friend uses you-messages when (s)he is angry with you. (S)he blames and shames you when you do something (s)he doesn't like. You feel put down and on the defensive when this happens. How might you change the way you and your friend communicate with each other?

Responsible Citizenship

You decide to run for a class office. A group of friends helps you with your campaign. After much effort, you lose by only a few votes. However, you are very grateful for your friends' time and effort. Write a note to the group that contains at least one I-message expressing your feelings of gratitude.

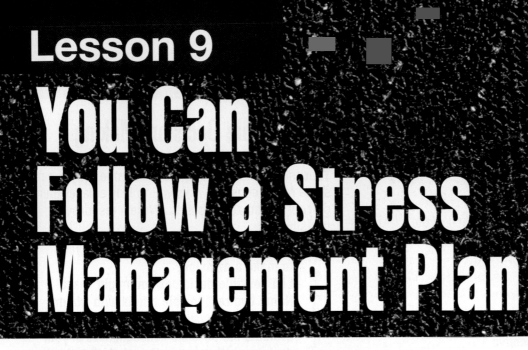

Lesson 9

You Can Follow a Stress Management Plan

Life Skill I will follow a plan to manage stress.

Have you ever felt "stressed out?" **Stress** is the response of the body to the demands of daily living. A **stressor** is a source or cause of stress. Stressors may be physical, mental, social, or environmental. Exercising until you are exhausted is a physical stressor. Preparing for a difficult test is a mental stressor. Being introduced to someone new is a social stressor. Being in a room filled with cigarette smoke is an environmental stressor. This lesson explains what you need to know about stress and stressors. You will learn about the three stages of stress. You will learn ways prolonged stress can affect your health status. This lesson also includes stress management skills. You will learn how to prevent and deal with stressful situations. You will learn how to protect your health if life changes occur.

The Lesson Outline

What to Know About Stress

How Stress Affects Your Health Status

How to Use Stress Management Skills

Objectives

1. List and discuss the three stages of the general adaptation syndrome. **page 67**

2. Explain ways prolonged stress can affect each of the ten areas of health. **pages 68–69**

3. List and discuss ten stress management skills that can be used to prevent and control stress. **pages 70–71**

4. Give the top five life changes that are most stressful for teens. **page 72**

Vocabulary Words

stress

stressor

general adaptation syndrome (GAS)

alarm stage

adrenaline

resistance stage

exhaustion stage

psychosomatic disease

caffeine

pollutants

stress management skills

time management plan

budget

beta-endorphins

helper T cell

life change

What to Know About
Stress

One thing is certain. You cannot avoid stressors in your life. When you experience stressors, changes occur in your body. The **general adaptation syndrome (GAS)** is a series of body changes that result from stress. The GAS occurs in three stages: the alarm stage, the resistance stage, and the exhaustion stage.

The **alarm stage** is the first stage of the GAS in which the body gets ready for quick action. During this stage, adrenaline is secreted into the bloodstream. **Adrenaline** is a hormone that prepares the body to react during times of stress or in an emergency. Your heart rate and blood pressure increase, digestion slows, muscles contract, respiration and sweating increase, and mental activity increases. Your pupils dilate so you can see more sharply, and your hearing sharpens as well. You experience a burst of quick energy. Sometimes the alarm stage is called the fight-or-flight response because the GAS gets you ready to take action or to run away to protect yourself.

The **resistance stage** is the second stage of the GAS in which the body attempts to regain internal balance. The body no longer is in the emergency state. Adrenaline no longer is secreted. Heart rate and blood pressure decrease and digestion begins again. Muscles relax, respiration returns to normal, and sweating stops.

The first two stages of the GAS are normal and healthful. When you experience a stressor, the alarm stage helps you respond. After your initial response, the resistance stage occurs and your body regains internal balance.

However, some people are not able to manage stress. As a result, their bodies are in the alarm stage for long periods of time. People who do not know positive actions to take when stress occurs force their bodies to stay ready for an emergency. The body becomes exhausted, and a third stage occurs. The **exhaustion stage** is the third stage of the GAS in which wear and tear on the body increases the risk of injury, illness, and premature death.

General Adaptation Syndrome (GAS)

During the ALARM STAGE, the sympathetic nervous system prepares to meet the demand of the stressor.

During the RESISTANCE STAGE, the parasympathetic nervous system attempts to return the body to a state of homeostasis.

ALARM STAGE	RESISTANCE STAGE
Pupils dilate	Pupils constrict
Hearing sharpens	Hearing is normal
Saliva decreases	Saliva increases
Heart rate increases	Heart rate decreases
Blood pressure increases	Blood pressure decreases
Bronchioles dilate	Bronchioles constrict
Digestion slows	Intestinal secretions increase to normal
Blood flow to muscles increases	Blood flow to muscles decreases
Muscles tighten	Muscles relax

How Stress Affects
Your Health Status

Stress has a holistic effect. This means a stressor in any of the ten areas of health may affect one or more of the other areas. Suppose a teen's parents get divorced. The teen may find it difficult to study (Mental and Emotional Health), to eat (Nutrition), and to sleep (Personal Health and Physical Activity). The original stressor, the divorce, creates other stressors that affect the teen's health status. Since your health status involves every aspect of your life, consider how stress can affect the ten areas of your health.

Stress and Mental and Emotional Health

Prolonged stress makes it difficult for you to think clearly and concentrate. This may affect your grades. You may feel edgy and express emotions in inappropriate ways. You are more likely to experience psychosomatic diseases. A **psychosomatic disease** is a physical disorder caused or aggravated by emotional responses. Physical disorders, such as headaches, stomach-aches, and ulcers are common examples of psychosomatic diseases. Other physical disorders, such as asthma and chronic fatigue syndrome, also can be aggravated by stress.

Stress and Family and Social Health

Have you ever heard someone say, "(S)he makes me sick." There is some truth to this saying. Suppose you are in a stressful relationship. When prolonged stress occurs in a relationship, changes may take place inside your body. The number of white blood cells that fight disease may decrease. The likelihood that you will become ill increases.

Stress and Growth and Development

During puberty, hormones cause body changes. For example, growth hormones may cause you to experience a growth spurt. It is not uncommon for teens to grow four inches taller in one year. Other hormones cause secondary sex characteristics to develop. Teens who cannot adjust to these changes may choose harmful ways of coping. For example, eating disorders are more common in teens who are uncomfortable with their body changes.

Stress and Nutrition

When you are stressed, your body secretes adrenaline. This causes the body to use up its supply of vitamins B and C. Additional vitamins B and C are needed. Suppose you drink caffeine. **Caffeine** is a stimulant found in chocolate, coffee, tea, some soda pops, and some prescription and over-the-counter drugs. When you consume 250 to 300 milligrams of caffeine within a two-hour period, the alarm stage of the GAS begins. A 12-ounce (336-gram) cola contains about 50 milligrams of caffeine, a one-ounce (28-gram) chocolate bar contains 20 milligrams, and a cup of coffee contains about 100 milligrams.

Suppose you eat salty foods when you feel stress. When you eat salty foods or add salt to your food, your body retains fluids. This could increase your blood pressure. High blood pressure is a contributing factor to heart disease. Suppose you respond to stress by pigging out on sweets. High concentrations of refined sugar may cause your body to increase the production of insulin, a hormone that helps your body use sugar in the blood. Too much insulin results in low blood sugar and will cause you to lose energy.

Stress and Personal Health and Physical Activity

Recall that your body uses up vitamin C during stressful periods. Without enough vitamin C, you may notice that your gums bleed. Suppose you exercise to exhaustion when you are stressed. Too much exercise can affect your immune system, the body system that helps fight disease. You may become fatigued and run down.

Stress and Alcohol, Tobacco, and Other Drugs

The use of drugs, such as tobacco, marijuana, cocaine, alcohol, or tranquilizers, may decrease your ability to cope with stress. Using tobacco, marijuana, or cocaine may actually cause a person to experience the alarm stage of the GAS. Alcohol and tranquilizers depress the part of the brain responsible for reasoning and judgment. Your decision-making skills may be affected.

Stress and Communicable and Chronic Diseases

Periods of being overwhelmed and frustrated may cause the body's immune system to be suppressed. This results in lowered resistance to disease. You would become more susceptible to communicable diseases, such as flu and the common cold. Prolonged stress might affect a person's risk of cancer. Cancer cells are more likely to develop, multiply, and spread. Being stressed keeps the body in the alarm stage of the GAS. Heart rate and blood pressure remain high. This affects the heart and blood vessels. Cardio-vascular diseases are more likely to occur.

Stress and Consumer and Community Health

Boredom is a stressor. Boredom results from a lack of challenge. People who are bored with their lives may turn to harmful behavior. Shopping addiction, television addiction, video game addiction, and gambling addiction are more common in people who are stressed from boredom.

Stress and Environmental Health

The environment includes everything around you. **Pollutants** are harmful substances in the environment. Pollutants may be in the air you breathe, the water you drink, or the food you eat. Pollutants activate the GAS. Loud noise, such as from rock music and concerts, heavy traffic, and airports, also initiates the alarm stage of GAS. Suppose you are exposed to loud noises. You are more likely to make mistakes and have accidents. For example, teens typing on a computer make more mistakes when loud music is playing. Teens who smoke or who listen to loud music while driving have more accidents.

Stress and Injury Prevention and Safety

Stress is a major contributing factor in almost all kinds of accidents. Motor vehicle accidents are the leading cause of death in the 15-to-24 age group. In his book *Psychology and the Road*, David Shinar explains that "people drive as they live." People whose lifestyles are filled with caution, tolerance, thrift, loyalty, foresight, and consideration usually have safe driving records. People who are frustrated, aggressive, and angry because of stress in their lives may not be able to concentrate on safe driving. These people have higher accident rates.

How to Use
Stress Management Skills

Throughout life, you will experience many stressors. you may not be able to control all of these stressors. However, you can control your response to them. **Stress management skills** are techniques to:

1. prevent and deal with stressors,
2. protect one's health from the harmful effects produced by the stress response.

How to Prevent and Deal with Stressful Situations

Use Responsible Decision-Making Skills. When a situation is difficult and requires a decision, you will be less stressed if you approach the situation in a logical way. The Responsible Decision-Making Model provides steps to follow when you are stressed out, but need to think clearly. Always use the six questions to evaluate the possible consequences of each decision.

- Will this decision result in actions that promote health?
- Will this decision result in actions that protect safety?
- Will this decision result in actions that follow laws?
- Will this decision result in actions that show respect for myself and others?
- Will this decision result in actions that follow the guidelines of my parents and of other responsible adults?
- Will this decision result in actions that demonstrate good character?

Keep a time management plan. A **time management plan** is a plan that shows how a person will spend time. Having a time management plan helps keep you from being overwhelmed. Poor time management is a major stressor.

> Lesson 75 will include more information on time management plans.

Keep a budget. A **budget** is a plan for spending and saving money. Spending more money than you have is a major stressor. Knowing your income and expenses keeps you from spending money and regretting it later.

> Lesson 75 will include more information on budgets.

Talk with parents, a guardian, or other responsible adults. You can benefit from the wisdom of adults. They can help you explore ways to deal with stressors. They can help you evaluate decisions you must make. They can provide support, encouragement, and suggestions.

Have a support network of friends. Friends can listen and offer suggestions. They can share healthful ways they dealt with similar experiences. When you have a support network of friends, you do not feel alone. You know others care about you and will be there for you during difficult times.

How to Protect Yourself During Stressful Periods

Participate in physical activity. During the alarm stage of the GAS, adrenaline and sugar are released into the bloodstream. These body changes prepare you for quick action. But, suppose these body changes occur for a long time. These changes will cause wear and tear on the body. Regular physical activity helps the body regain internal balance during times of stress. Physical activity uses up the extra adrenaline and sugar. Participate in physical activity often. Take a walk or choose other activities when you feel stressed. Physical activity up to 24 hours after the onset of stress is beneficial. Consider the other benefits of physical activity. If you are physically active for at least 25 minutes three times a week for seven to ten weeks, your body will release beta-endorphins for up to 90 minutes after your workout. **Beta-endorphins** are substances produced in the brain that create a feeling of well-being. Regular physical activity will help you become physically fit. When you are physically fit, the stress response is not as great, your body regains internal balance more easily, and you have improved resistance to disease.

Write in a journal. Writing in a journal can help you organize your thoughts and feelings. You can review how a stressor is affecting you and learn more about how you cope. Writing in a journal has been shown to elevate the number of helper T cells. A **helper T cell** is a white blood cell that signals B cells to produce antibodies. Blood samples were taken from teens who had experienced major life changes. Their helper T cell count was down. This increased their risk of disease. They were asked to write their feelings about the major life changes in a journal each day. More blood samples were taken. After writing in a journal for a period of time, their helper T cell count increased. This was because their bodies were regaining internal balance.

Use breathing techniques. When you experience a stressor, your body begins the alarm stage of the GAS. Breathing techniques help to relax you and restore internal balance. Breathe in deeply through your nose keeping your mouth shut. Then, slowly blow the air out through your mouth. This breathing technique will calm you and help stop the alarm stage of the GAS.

Eat a healthful diet. You may have seen vitamins that are sold as "stress vitamins." These vitamins contain extra doses of vitamins B and C. Vitamin B is needed for a healthy nervous system. Vitamin C helps the immune system function. When you are stressed out, your body uses up an extra supply of these two vitamins. It is very important for you to replenish these vitamins by choosing foods that are good sources. Vitamin B is found in foods such as whole-grain cereals, rice, legumes, and breads. Vitamin C is found in foods such as oranges, grapefruit, tomatoes, limes, lemons, and broccoli. You can make other changes in your diet. Reduce your intake of caffeine. Caffeine is found in coffee, tea, some soda pops, and chocolate. Caffeine is a stimulant drug that will increase the effects of the alarm stage of the GAS. Decrease your intake of sugar. During the alarm stage of the GAS, extra sugar is already in your bloodstream. Too much sugar will stress you out even more.

Get plenty of rest and sleep. When you are stressed out, your body is working extra hard. Your heart rate, breathing rate, and blood pressure are increased. Your muscles are tense. Getting rest and sleep keeps you from becoming too tired. When you are resting or sleeping, your blood pressure lowers, breathing rate decreases, and heart rate slows. Your muscles relax, and your body has a chance to rest. Rest and sleep help you feel refreshed. You will have more energy to deal with the stressor.

Activity

Calculate Your Life-Change Units

Life Skill: I will follow a plan to manage stress.

Materials: paper, pen, or pencil

Directions: A **life change** is an event or situation that requires a person to make a readjustment. Life changes are stressors. Read through the following list of life changes in teens. Calculate your life-change units for the past 12 months. A score less than 150 indicates that you have experienced little change. A score between 150 and 300 indicates moderate change. If your score is over 300, your life has changed significantly. You may not be able to control life changes. But you can control your response to life changes.

Life Change	Life-Change Units
Getting married	101
Being pregnant and unmarried	92
Experiencing the death of a parent	87
Acquiring a visible deformity	81
Experiencing divorce of parents	77
Becoming an unmarried father	77
Becoming involved with drugs	76
Having a parent sentenced to jail for a year or more	75
Having parents who are separated	69
Experiencing the death of a brother or sister	68
Experiencing a change in being accepted by peers	67
Having a teenage sister who is unmarried and pregnant	64
Learning that you are adopted	64
Having a parent remarry	63
Experiencing the death of a close friend	62
Having a visible congenital deformity	62
Having a serious illness requiring hospitalization	58
Moving to a new school district	56
Failing a grade in school	56
Not making a desired extracurricular activity	55
Having a parent who has a serious illness	55

Life Change	Life-Change Units
Breaking up with a boyfriend or girlfriend	53
Having a parent sentenced to jail for 30 or fewer days	53
Beginning to date	51
Being suspended from school	50
Having a newborn sister or brother	47
Having an outstanding personal achievement	46
Observing more arguments between parents	46
Having a parent who loses his/her job	46
Experiencing a change in the financial status of parents	45
Being accepted at the college of your choice	43
Beginning high school	42
Having a brother or sister who has a serious illness	41
Having a parent who is at home less because of his/her occupation	38
Having a brother or sister who moves out to live somewhere else	37
Experiencing the death of a grandparent	36
Having a third adult begin to live with the family	34
Becoming a full member of a religion	31
Observing fewer arguments between parents	26
Having a parent who begins to work	26

Lesson 9

Review

Vocabulary Words

Write a separate sentence using each of the vocabulary words listed on page 66.

Objectives

1. What happens during each of the three stages of the general adaptation syndrome? **Objective 1**

2. How can prolonged stress affect each of the ten areas of health? **Objective 2**

3. What are two purposes of stress management skills? **Objective 3**

4. What are ten stress management skills that can be used to prevent and control stress? **Objective 3**

5. What are the top five life changes that are most stressful for teens? **Objective 4**

Responsible Decision-Making

You are stressed about a test tomorrow in your most difficult subject. You call a friend who is in your class. She says she is staying up all night to study. She suggests that you make a pot of strong coffee. She says the coffee helps her stay awake. Write a response to this situation.

1. Describe the situation that requires you to make a decision.
2. List possible decisions you might make.
3. Name two responsible adults with whom you might discuss your decisions.
4. Evaluate the possible consequences of your decisions. Determine if each decision will lead to actions that:
   • promote health,
   • protect safety,
   • follow laws,
   • show respect for yourself and others,
   • follow the guidelines of your parents and of other responsible adults,
   • demonstrate good character.
5. Decide which decision is most responsible and appropriate.
6. Tell two results you expect if you make this decision.

Effective Communication

Illustrate the three stages of the general adaptation syndrome. Use posterboard and markers to create a visual, or use a computer to create a graphic.

Self-Directed Learning

Obtain a brochure from the American Heart Association, a local hospital or clinic, or a physician that focuses on heart disease. Find out the risk factors for heart disease. How does stress rank as a risk factor? Summarize your findings.

Critical Thinking

Last night, your friend decided to go to a party. The weather was stormy, so you decided not to go. This morning you get a call from your friend's mother. Your friend was in a serious accident on the way home from the party and is in a coma. You are very stressed. How can you protect your health during this stressful period?

Responsible Citizenship

Contact a person in the business community. Ask if you can prepare a pamphlet on stress management to be given to employees. Your pamphlet should discuss stress, describe stress management skills, and include a sample health behavior contract.

Lesson 10

You Can Be Resilient

Life Skill **I will be resilient during difficult times.**

Are you familiar with these sayings? "When the going gets tough, the tough get going." "Tough times never last, but tough people do." There are ups and downs in everyone's life. And, some people seem to have more difficult times than other people. But, difficult times do not have to last. People who hang in are resilient. To be **resilient** is to be able to adjust, recover, bounce back, and learn from difficult times. This lesson discusses what to do if life seems difficult. You will learn what to do if anger or depression lasts. You will learn how to prevent suicide. This lesson also describes how to be resilient. You will learn eight steps you can take to be resilient.

The Lesson Outline

If Life Seems Difficult

If Anger or Depression Lasts

How to Prevent Suicide

How to Be Resilient

Objectives

1. List and discuss five emotional responses used to cope with life crises. **page 75**

2. Discuss four causes of long-lasting anger and depression. **page 76**

3. Identify 14 warning signs that a teen may be considering a suicide attempt. **page 78**

4. Identify seven suicide prevention strategies. **page 79**

5. Discuss eight steps teens can take to be resilient. **page 80**

Vocabulary Words

resilient

life crisis

clinical depression

serotonin

suicide

parasuicide

suicide prevention strategies

mentor

support group

If Life Seems Difficult

Sometimes life seems to be a bummer. Events happen over which you have no control —a loved one dies; a parent loses a job; an earthquake, fire, or tornado destroys your property; you are in a car accident. You may have disappointments—you don't make an athletic team, your parents argue, your boyfriend or girlfriend dumps you.

A **life crisis** is an experience that causes a high level of stress. Most people respond to life crises by working through a series of five emotional responses. The five responses are listed below. A person has worked through a life crisis when (s)he accepts what has happened, adjusts, and bounces back. This does not mean that (s)he likes what has happened.

The following example illustrates how a teen might work through a life crisis. Suppose a teen's parents tell him/her they are getting divorced. The teen convinces himself/herself that the divorce will never happen. This is a form of denial. Then the father moves away from home. The teen no longer can deny that his/her parents are having problems. The teen responds with anger. (S)he asks, "Why does this have to happen to me?" (S)he is angry at both parents and copes by bargaining. (S)he tries to change the parents' decision. If the family is having financial difficulties, the teen may offer to get a part-time job. (S)he may promise to get better grades. The promises often are motivated by guilt. The teen may believe (s)he is at fault for the divorce. But (s)he is not responsible, and the bargaining does not save the marriage.

The teen realizes his/her efforts are hopeless. Nothing (s)he can do will change the outcome. The parents will get divorced, and things will change. Now, depression begins. The teen is very sad about the divorce. This period of sadness is necessary. Sadness allows the teen to feel the pain and experience the loss of change. In the end, this teen accepts the fact that his/her parents are divorced. (S)he begins to adjust to the new family situation.

This is only one example of a life crisis. But, the feelings the teen experienced are the same feelings teens experience in other life crises. People of all ages experience these feelings as they try to cope with life crises. When you experience a life crisis, you need to work through your feelings. Learning to work through your feelings during difficult times helps you become emotionally mature.

Five Emotional Responses Used to Cope with Life Crises

People respond to life crises by working through the following emotional responses.

1. **Denying** or refusing to believe what is happening.

2. **Being angry** about what is happening.

3. **Bargaining** or making promises hoping it will change what is happening.

4. **Being depressed** when you recognize the outcome is unlikely to change.

5. **Accepting** what is happening, adjusting, and bouncing back.

These five stages have been adapted from Dr. Elisabeth Kübler-Ross' work on death and dying.

If Anger or Depression Lasts

It is a normal reaction to feel angry or depressed while trying to adjust to a life crisis. For example, suppose a classmate was killed in a motor vehicle accident. You might feel angry about the accident. Later, you might feel sad and depressed because you will not see your friend again. Or, suppose a boyfriend or girlfriend dumps you for someone else. You might feel angry and betrayed. Then you might feel depressed and lonely. Suppose you share your feelings with a parent or close friend. This is a healthful way to express feelings. Eventually, you work through your anger and depression. You bounce back and are ready to move forward.

Some people do not know how to work through anger and depression. Have you ever known anyone who stayed angry and bitter? This person may have continued to be angry long after the crisis had passed. This person is stuck and cannot get on with his/her life. A person whose anger is long-lasting needs help. A person who is depressed for two weeks or more is experiencing clinical depression. **Clinical depression** is long-lasting feelings of hopelessness, sadness, or helplessness.

Four Causes of Long-Lasting Anger and Depression

1. **Inability to cope with a life crisis.** Some people are unable to get through life crises. For example, teens who have been physically or sexually abused may not know how to deal with their feelings. They remain depressed unless they get help. Other life crises may not be as severe—loss of a boyfriend or girlfriend, failing to make an athletic team, being bullied—but teens still cannot get through them. These may be everyday situations for some teens but difficult for others. Counseling may help teens learn to cope with life crises.

2. **Illness.** Do you remember the mind-body connection? The mind-body connection is the close relationship between mental and physical responses. When a person has a physical illness, mental and emotional health is affected. For example, a person who has flu or a severe cold may feel depressed. People with serious illnesses, such as AIDS, cancer, or heart disease, often feel depressed. Physicians who help with a person's physical illness can make recommendations for how to relieve depression.

3. **Family history.** Some people have a family history of depression. Depression may be due to lowered brain serotonin levels. **Serotonin** is a chemical in the body that helps regulate primitive drives and emotions. Fortunately, there are medications that affect serotonin levels and relieve biochemical depression. These medications must be prescribed and monitored by a physician. A physician may recommend counseling, support groups, diet changes, and regular exercise as part of treatment.

4. **Alcohol and other drug use.** People who abuse drugs have much higher rates of depression than people who do not abuse drugs. Alcohol and other depressant drugs change a person's mood. People who drink and abuse other depressant drugs are more at risk for harming themselves and others.

CAUTION

Drinking alcohol interferes with a person's ability to cope with life crises. Alcohol intensifies feelings of anger and depression. People with a family history of depression become even more depressed when they drink. Remember, drinking alcohol to relieve problems does not work. It creates more problems. People who drink when they are depressed are more at risk for harming themselves and others.

How to Prevent
Suicide

Symptoms of Depression

A person is diagnosed as being clinically depressed if (s)he has at least five of nine general symptoms for a duration of two weeks. Mild depression is diagnosed with two to four symptoms for a duration of at least two weeks.

- Deep sadness
- Apathy
- Fatigue
- Agitation
- Sleep disturbances
- Weight or appetite change
- Lack of concentration
- Feelings of worthlessness
- Morbid thoughts

The philosopher Joseph Addison once said, "The three grand essentials to happiness in life are something to do, someone to love, and something to hope for." Think about his message for a moment. Having something to do and doing it well gives you a feeling of accomplishment. Having people to love gives you the opportunity to share your feelings, hopes, dreams, and disappointments. Having something to hope for gives you a reason to live. When you have something to hope for, you look forward to your future. Teens who do not have things to do, people to love, and something to hope for are more at risk for suicide than are other teens.

Suicide is the intentional taking of one's own life. Some teens view suicide as a way to escape problems. Other teens view suicide as a way to gain attention. Still others view suicide as a way to get even with those who have rejected them. Suicide cannot be undone. There is always a better choice than suicide.

What to Know About Suicide Attempts

Parasuicide is a suicide attempt in which a person does not intend to die. Parasuicide is a cry for help. Teens who make a suicide attempt are depressed, discouraged, and lack hope. They want others to know that they are in a lot of pain. Without help, teens who have attempted suicide once may attempt suicide again. For this reason, a suicide attempt or talk of a suicide attempt must always be taken seriously. Some teens who make a suicide attempt and do not intend to die are not discovered. Their cries for help end in tragic death. Each of us must do everything possible to prevent suicides.

- Never make a suicide attempt, even as a way to get attention.
- A suicide attempt is a risky way of trying to get help.
- If you are depressed or discouraged, ask a parent, a guardian, or other responsible adult for help. Do not give up hope.

What to Know About Suicidal Tendencies

Teens who are at risk for attempting suicide may have one or more of the following characteristics:

- **Aggressive behavior**
- **Perfectionistic behavior**
- **Feelings of hopelessness**
- **Low self-esteem**
- **Inadequate social skills**
- **Mental disorders**
- **Depression**
- **Hidden anger**

Teens who attempt suicide may have had a difficult life experience, such as a breakup of a relationship, an unwanted pregnancy, or failure at school. Teens are more likely to attempt suicide if they:

- **abuse alcohol and other drugs;**
- **have experienced the death of a parent, parental separation, or parental divorce;**
- **feel alienated from family and friends;**
- **are teased or rejected by peers;**
- **have difficulty coping with body changes and sexuality.**

How to Recognize Signs of Suicide

Teens who are thinking about making a suicide attempt often provide warning signs. By trying to warn others, they are crying out for help and hoping someone will step in and help them. Signs that a teen may be considering a suicide attempt include:

- **making a direct statement about killing oneself, such as "I wish I was never born;"**
- **making an indirect statement about killing oneself, such as, "I wonder where I can get a gun;"**
- **having a change in personality;**
- **withdrawing from family and friends;**
- **losing interest in personal appearance;**
- **having a preoccupation with death and dying;**
- **making frequent complaints about physical symptoms related to emotions, such as stomachaches;**
- **using alcohol and other drugs;**
- **losing interest in schoolwork;**
- **giving away possessions;**
- **talking about getting even with others;**
- **failing to recover from a disappointment or a loss;**
- **running away from home;**
- **having a close friend or relative who has committed suicide.**

How to Practice Suicide Prevention Strategies

Suicide prevention strategies are techniques that can be used to help prevent a person from thinking about, attempting, and completing suicide. If you are concerned about a teen:

- **Look for warning signs when a teen is depressed.**
- **Listen without giving advice.**
- **Take a suicide threat seriously.**

- **Ask if the teen has a specific plan and means to follow through.**
- **Do not be sworn to secrecy.**
- **Call a parent, a guardian, or other responsible adult immediately.**
- **Stay with the teen until professional help arrives.**

Activity

Staying Connected

Life Skill: I will be resilient during difficult times.

Materials: ball of yarn

Directions: Follow the six steps below to learn more about having a support network.

 Sit or kneel in a circle with classmates.

 Think of two people who provide you support or to whom you would go for support if you needed it. You need to have a support network of responsible adults and friends who will give you encouragement and support during difficult times.

 One classmate will begin. This classmate will take the ball of yarn and wrap a small piece around his/her finger. (S)he will name the two people who provide him/her support. Then this classmate will roll the ball of yarn to another classmate.

 This classmate will take the ball of yarn and wrap a small piece around his/her finger. (S)he will name the two people who provide him/her support. Then this classmate will roll the ball of yarn to another classmate.

 Repeat until each classmate has had the ball of yarn and shared the names of two people who provide him/her support.

 Notice that all your classmates are connected by the yarn. Staying connected to other people improves health. It helps you to be resilient. Write a one-page essay on "ways you can stay connected to your support network."

How to Be
Resilient

Do you remember these sayings? "When the going gets tough, the tough get going." "Tough times never last, but tough people do." These sayings are about people who are resilient. To be resilient is to be able to adjust, recover, bounce back, and learn from difficult times. Some teens are more resilient than others. They are prepared for life crises and respond in healthful ways should they occur. Do you want to be more resilient? Do you want to be prepared to deal with difficult situations? There are steps you can take.

You can bounce back from difficult times.

Take Steps to Be Resilient

Step 1: Work on your relationships with members of your family. You are working on skills to gain independence from your parents or guardian. Yet at the same time, you need to remain close. Feeling connected to family members gives you added strength during tough times. Do not wait for tough times to happen. Spend time talking to your parents or guardian and other family members every day. Share what is happening in your life—both good and bad.

Step 2: Develop a close relationship with a mentor. A **mentor** is a responsible person who guides another person. A coach, member of the clergy, teacher, counselor, principal, guardian, aunt, uncle, grandparent, or other responsible adult can be a mentor. Spend time with the person you choose as a mentor. Discuss difficult situations with your mentor. Get suggestions on ways to handle life crises.

Step 3: Choose friends who are supportive and who have responsible behavior. Select your friends wisely. Friends who choose responsible behavior will encourage you to make wise choices during difficult times. They will listen to your feelings and respond. Stay away from teens who behave in harmful ways.

Step 4: Do not put off dealing with difficult situations. At first, you may respond to a difficult situation by denying what is happening. Do not get stuck in this stage of working through your feelings. Remember—tough times do not go away by pretending nothing is wrong. Face up to what is happening.

Step 5: Avoid choosing harmful behaviors as a way of coping with tough times. You cannot adjust and bounce back from tough times by choosing harmful behavior. Choosing to drink, smoke, gamble, starve yourself, steal, or lie will make tough times worse.

Step 6: Ask for support when you need it. Reach out and ask for help during tough times. If the first person you ask for help is not supportive, don't go into your shell. Reach out again. Being willing to ask for help is a key ingredient in being resilient.

Step 7: Discuss available support groups with a parent, guardian, or other responsible adult. A **support group** is a group of people who help one another recover from an addiction, a particular disease, or a difficult situation. Sometimes it is helpful to be in a group with other teens who have experienced the same life crisis. You will not feel like you are the only one who has ever felt the way you do.

Step 8: Be involved in school and community activities. Being involved is an important way to feel connected to others. Being a member of a school team or participating in an activity gives you a sense of belonging. Volunteering to help others helps you feel needed.

Lesson 10

Review

Vocabulary Words

Write a separate sentence using each of the vocabulary words listed on page 74.

Objectives

1. What are five emotional responses used to cope with life crises? **Objective 1**

2. What are four causes of long-lasting anger and depression? **Objective 2**

3. What are 14 warning signs that a teen may be considering a suicide attempt? **Objective 3**

4. What are seven suicide prevention strategies? **Objective 4**

5. What are eight steps teens can take to be resilient? **Objective 5**

Responsible Decision-Making

Your boyfriend or girlfriend has dumped you for someone else. You are feeling down and lonely. You wonder if you are interesting and attractive. Your best friend suggests that you drown your sorrows with a six-pack of beer. (S)he says drinking helps people forget their problems and get on with life. Write a response to this situation.

1. Describe the situation that requires you to make a decision.

2. List possible decisions you might make.

3. Name two responsible adults with whom you might discuss your decisions.

4. Evaluate the possible consequences of your decisions. Determine if each decision will lead to actions that:
   - promote health,
   - protect safety,
   - follow laws,
   - show respect for yourself and others,
   - follow the guidelines of your parents and of other responsible adults,
   - demonstrate good character.

5. Decide which decision is most responsible and appropriate.

6. Tell two results you expect if you make this decision.

Effective Communication

Two sayings appear in this lesson. "When the going gets tough, the tough get going." "Tough times never last, but tough people do." Create your own saying to get across the same message.

Self-Directed Learning

Find out what support groups are especially helpful for teens. List the groups and their purposes. Discuss the list with your parents or guardian. After your discussion, list the three support groups that you believe may be most helpful. Give the purpose of each group and the dates, meeting times, and place the group meets.

Critical Thinking

A natural disaster (flood, earthquake, hurricane, tornado) has destroyed your friend's belongings. Your friend is very angry. What other feelings might you expect your friend to experience? How can your friend be resilient?

Responsible Citizenship

Younger people need mentors to provide encouragement and support. Think of a younger person in your community for whom you could be a mentor. Suppose you were to spend an hour a week with this person for six weeks. On a sheet of paper, describe what you might do. Share your plan with your parents or guardian and consider acting upon it.

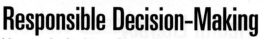

Responsible Decision-Making

You are invited to a Super Bowl party. When you arrive, you are asked to contribute $3 to a football pool. Some of the teens at this party borrow money so that they will have more than one chance to win. They seem psyched when they sign up for the football pool. The person having the party says to you, "Bet everything you've got. You can win big!" Write a response to this situation.

1. Describe the situation that requires you to make a decision.
2. List possible decisions you might make.
3. Name two responsible adults with whom you might discuss your decisions.
4. Evaluate the possible consequences of your decisions. Determine if each decision will lead to actions that:
   - promote health,
   - protect safety,
   - follow laws,
   - show respect for yourself and others,
   - follow the guidelines of your parents and of other responsible adults,
   - demonstrate good character.
5. Decide which decision is most responsible and appropriate.
6. Tell two results you expect if you make this decision.

Health Behavior Inventory of Life Skills

Number from 1 to 10 on a sheet of paper. Read each life skill carefully. Write YES or NO next to the same number on your paper. Each YES response indicates a life skill you practice to promote your health status. Each NO response indicates a life skill you do not practice. Plan to begin practicing these life skills.

1. I will take responsibility for my health.
2. I will practice life skills for health.
3. I will gain health knowledge.
4. I will make responsible decisions.
5. I will use resistance skills when appropriate.
6. I will develop good character.
7. I will choose behaviors to promote a healthy mind.
8. I will express emotions in healthful ways.
9. I will follow a plan to manage stress.
10. I will be resilient during difficult times.

Multicultural Health

You can find health-related information on the Internet and at your local library. The information you locate may be designed for specific cultures. Locate information about heart disease for two cultures other than your own.

Family Involvement

Many programs on network and cable TV stations focus on health-related issues. These programs can be identified by exploring available TV channels or by reading TV listings. Local hospitals, universities, and health organizations can provide the names of specific health-related programs in your broadcast area. Select a program to watch with members of your family. After viewing the program, ask each family member what (s)he learned. Write a summary.

Health Behavior Contract

Copy and complete the following health behavior contract. Evaluate your progress.
Share the results with your family.

Health Behavior Contract

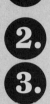

1. Name_____ Date_____

2. **Life Skill:** I will follow a plan to manage stress.

3. **Effects on Health Status:** Stress management skills are techniques to prevent and deal with stressors and to protect my health from the harmful effects produced by the stress response. When I practice these skills, I am less likely to develop psychosomatic diseases. I will be less likely to develop communicable and chronic diseases. I will be less likely to make mistakes in my schoolwork or have accidents. I will sleep better and enjoy my leisure time.

4. **Plan and Method to Record Progress:** I will practice at least two stress management skills each day. I will choose from the following list:

1. Use responsible decision-making skills
2. Keep a time management plan
3. Keep a budget
4. Talk with parents, a guardian, or other responsible adults
5. Have a support network of friends
6. Participate in physical activity
7. Write in a journal
8. Use breathing techniques
9. Eat a healthful diet
10. Get plenty of rest and sleep

My Calendar

M	T	W	Th	F	S	S

5. **Evaluation:** _____
_____
_____

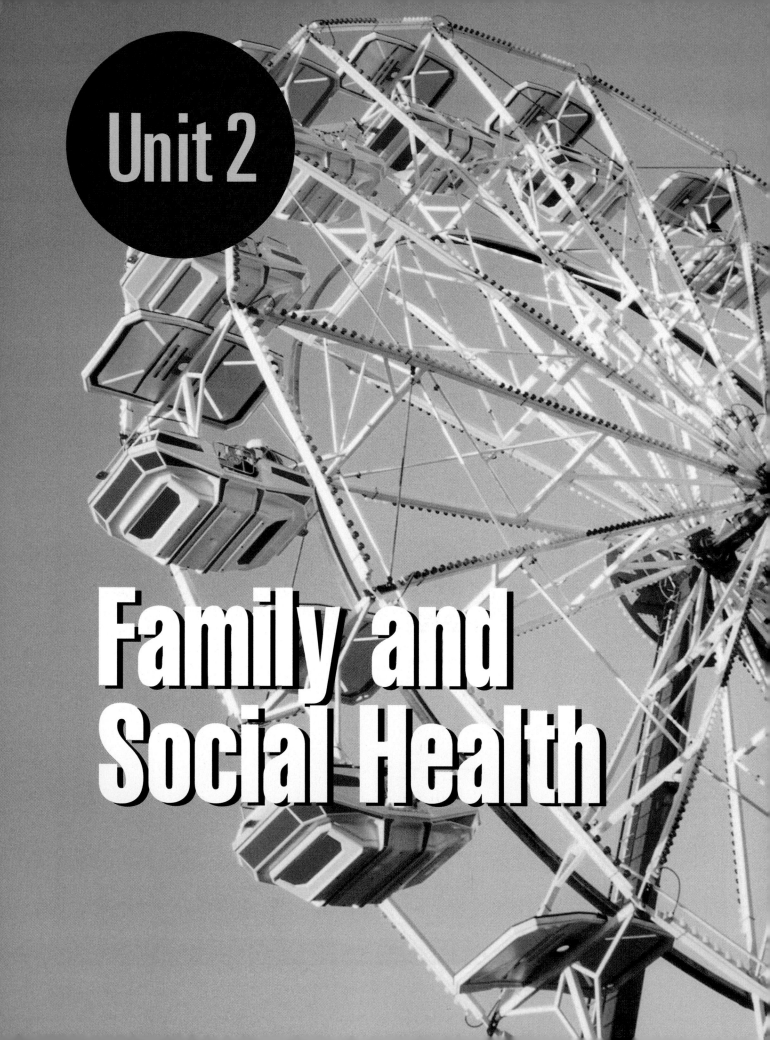

Unit 2

Family and Social Health

Lesson 11

You Can Be a Loving Family Member

Life Skill **I will develop healthful family relationships.**

A **family** is a group of people who are related by blood, adoption, or marriage. Your family relationships influence you and your behavior. The parents or adults who raised you have the greatest influence on you. Parents or other adults who "parent" you are your role models for relationships. This lesson discusses family relationships. You will examine skills that are learned in an ideal family. You will learn how to be a loving family member.

The Lesson Outline

What to Know About Families

What Skills Are Learned in an Ideal Family

How to Be a Loving Family Member

Objectives

1. Contrast the ideal family with the dysfunctional family using The Family Continuum. **page 89**

2. List and explain 12 skills parents in an ideal family teach their children about loving, responsible relationships. **pages 90–93**

3. Identify three ways to be a loving family member. **page 94**

Vocabulary Words

family
ideal family
dysfunctional family
self-respecting behavior
self-centered behavior
sexuality
sex role
communication
value
conflict
delayed gratification
affection
work ethic
authority
curfew

What to Know About
Families

Everyone belongs to a family. Each family is different, but all families share certain characteristics with other families. The Family Continuum shows two extremes of family life. Studying these two extremes of family life—the ideal family and the dysfunctional family—is an important way to learn about relationships.

An **ideal family** is a family that has all the skills needed for loving, responsible relationships. A **dysfunctional family** is a family that lacks the skills to be successful and function in healthful ways. In this lesson, you will learn about the ideal family.

Lesson 12 will include more information on the dysfunctional family.

The Family Continuum

The Family Continuum indicates the degree to which a family promotes skills needed for loving, responsible relationships.

Dysfunctional Family

Ideal Family

The majority of families, eight out of ten to be exact, rank in the middle of the continuum. They are not ideal, but neither are they completely dysfunctional.

What Skills Are Learned in an Ideal Family

Perhaps you have watched a television sitcom about a family. The family members in this sitcom may have seemed to relate well to each other. They may have seemed almost perfect to you. In reality, most families are not perfect. After all, families are made up of family members who are human. And to be human is to have strengths as well as weaknesses. Many families possess various characteristics of an ideal family, but no family is perfect all the time. What are the skills needed for loving, responsible relationships that are taught in ideal families?

In an ideal family, parents teach their children:

1. Self-respecting behavior
2. Healthful attitudes toward sexuality
3. Effective communication
4. A clear sense of values
5. Responsible decision-making
6. Ways to resolve conflict
7. Effective coping skills
8. Ways to delay gratification
9. Ways to express affection and integrate love and sexuality
10. How to give and receive acts of kindness
11. A work ethic
12. Respect for authority

How You Learn Self-Respecting Behavior

Self-respecting behavior is treating oneself in healthful and responsible ways. It is an outgrowth of the ways you were treated by the adults who raised you from birth. If you received love and felt accepted, then you began to feel good about yourself. If you were well-cared for, you learned how to take care of yourself. As a result, you learned how to treat yourself in healthful and kind ways. You learned to choose behaviors that would not harm you. Teens raised in an ideal family also learn the difference between self-respecting and self-centered behavior. **Self-centered behavior** is actions that fulfill personal needs with little regard for the needs of others. Self-centered behavior does not contribute to healthful family relationships.

How You Learn Healthful Attitudes Toward Sexuality

Sexuality is the feelings and attitudes a person has about his/her body, sex role, and relationships. Your sexuality is influenced from birth, when you are born either male or female. Your parents or guardians talk to you about your body and shape your attitudes about being male or female. They influence your sex role. A **sex role** is a way a person acts and the feelings and attitudes (s)he has about being male or female. Sex roles also include the expectations people have for other males or females. Your parents or guardians helped you learn about sex roles. For example, you may have learned that it is acceptable for males as well as females to cry and share feelings. You may have learned that males and females differ but deserve equal respect. In an ideal family, parents or guardians discuss puberty with their teens. They explain the changes in feelings and emotions that accompany puberty. Their openness and sensitivity help teens learn how to accept their sexuality.

How You Learn Effective Communication

Communication is the sharing of emotions, thoughts, and information with another person. You first learn to communicate in your family. Suppose your parents or guardians use I-messages to express feelings and listen carefully when you speak. Then, as you begin to copy their way of communicating, you develop skills in communicating with others. Suppose your parents or guardians know how to express anger, sadness, and disappointment in healthful ways. Then you learn healthful ways to express these emotions. In an ideal family, you feel secure practicing communication skills. You use these communication skills in other relationships.

How You Learn a Clear Sense of Values

A **value** is a standard or belief. In an ideal family, parents or guardians teach their children values. For example, your parents or guardians may value hard work, honesty, and close family relationships. They behave in ways consistent with these values. They work hard, are honest in their dealings with others, and spend time with members of their family. They discuss these values with you. You listen to what they say, and their behavior confirms what they say. You observe their everyday behavior. You internalize their values and behave in similar ways. When you relate to others, you remember these family values. They become the standard for what you think and believe. You will have a clear sense of values for the rest of your life.

How You Learn to Make Responsible Decisions

In an ideal family, parents or guardians serve as role models for decision-making. You observe your parents or guardians using the decision-making process. They carefully evaluate options before deciding what to do. They weigh the consequences of possible actions. They make responsible decisions and teach you to do the same. In an ideal family, parents or guardians expect responsible behavior from their children. They set guidelines and make expectations clear. There are consequences for breaking family guidelines. You learn that there always are consequences for wrong behavior. This helps you when you are pressured by peers. You think about consequences and say NO to wrong behaviors. When you have difficulty saying NO, you turn to your parents or guardians for support. If you make a mistake, your parents or guardians help you learn from it.

How You Learn to Resolve Conflicts

A **conflict** is a disagreement between two or more people or between two or more choices. In every relationship, there are conflicts. In an ideal family, parents or guardians teach their children to resolve conflicts in healthful ways. They listen to both sides of a disagreement and work to find an acceptable solution. In an ideal family, conflicts are resolved without violence. You learn healthful ways to resolve conflicts. You have skills to resolve conflicts in other relationships.

Lesson 13 will include more information on conflict resolution.

How You Learn Effective Coping Skills

In Lesson 10 you learned the five emotional responses that people use to cope with a life crisis. They are: 1. denying or refusing to believe what is happening; 2. being angry about what is happening; 3. bargaining or making promises hoping it will change what is happening; 4. being depressed when you recognize the outcome is unlikely to change; 5. accepting what is happening, adjusting, and bouncing back. In an ideal family, parents or guardians want their children to develop emotional strength. They understand and recognize ways people deal with a life crisis. Suppose your parents or guardians encourage you to share your feelings during a life crisis. You will learn how to cope during difficult times you may experience later in your life.

How You Learn to Delay Gratification

In an ideal family, parents or guardians teach their children the importance of delayed gratification. **Delayed gratification** is voluntarily postponing an immediate reward in order to complete a task before enjoying a reward. If you have learned to delay gratification, you are patient. You are not tempted to choose something you want right now rather than wait until a more appropriate time. Being able to delay gratification is especially important in relationships. During your teen years, you may experience sexual feelings. But, it is not appropriate for you to be sexually active. Waiting until marriage to express intimate sexual feelings protects your health and follows family guidelines.

How You Learn to Express Affection and Integrate Love and Sexuality

Affection is a fond or tender feeling that a person has toward another person. In an ideal family, parents or guardians teach their children how to express affection. For example, your parents or guardians may hug you, kiss you good night or good-bye, or hold you when you are sad. Their expressions of warm feelings help you feel loved. They also teach you appropriate ways to express affection. You learn who has the right to touch you, when, and how. For example, you may allow a doctor to touch certain parts of your body during a physical examination. However, you learn when it is not appropriate for someone to touch your body. In an ideal family, parents or guardians teach their children that sex and love belong together in a committed marriage. You learn that sex belongs in marriage, and you practice delayed gratification.

How You Learn to Give and Receive Acts of Kindness

In an ideal family, parents or guardians demonstrate acts of kindness and express thankfulness. They do kind things for family members and for other people in the community. They accept and are grateful for acts of kindness from others. As you observe your parents or guardians giving and receiving, you learn to act in similar ways. You are willing to give to others and express thankfulness. You are able to receive kind acts from others. Giving and receiving are both needed to sustain healthful relationships.

How You Learn a Work Ethic

A **work ethic** is an attitude of discipline, motivation, and commitment toward tasks. In an ideal family, parents or guardians teach their children a work ethic. Parents and guardians work hard and serve as role models for their children. As you observe your parents or guardians, you learn to do your best and not give up when work is challenging. You learn the rewards that result from hard work. You learn to demonstrate a work ethic by completing schoolwork, doing household chores, participating in athletics, holding a part-time job, or doing volunteer work.

How You Learn to Respect Authority

In a healthful family, children learn to respect authority. **Authority** is the power and right to apply laws and rules. Authority is first learned within the family. In an ideal family, children respect the authority of their parents or guardians. Parents or guardians set and enforce guidelines for behavior. For example, your parents or guardians may set a curfew. A **curfew** is a fixed time when a person is to be at home. You respect your parents or guardians and do not break the curfew. You recognize that if you break the curfew, there will be consequences. Your parents or guardians will then use appropriate discipline, such as taking away certain privileges. In an ideal family, parents or guardians also serve as role models for their children. They, too, respect authority by obeying laws and rules. As you observe their behavior, you learn to obey laws and rules set by authority figures such as teachers, principals, and police officers.

How to Be a
Loving Family Member

In this lesson, you have learned about an ideal or "perfect" family. As you learned about an ideal family, you may have thought to yourself, "This point describes my family." At other times, you may have thought, "My family certainly could improve in this area." All humans have strengths and weaknesses. Your parents or guardians are human. They may try hard but fall short. This is the reason that family relationships will not be perfect and family life will not be ideal. Yet, the struggle to have the best family life possible is worth the effort. Your task is to be the very best family member you can be. Remember the life skill for this lesson: I will develop healthful family relationships. Consider the following acronym: **ACT.**

Action: Choose actions that promote healthful family relationships.
Commitment: Make a promise to be a loving family member.
Time: Spend time with your family.

Activity

Family Sitcom Ratings

Life Skill: I will develop healthful family relationships.

Materials: pencil, paper, television guide, newspaper, computer (optional)

Directions: Review the listing of programs in the television guide or newspaper to find descriptions of family sitcoms. Then complete this activity.

 Select two family sitcoms to investigate further. Ask your parent or guardian if it is appropriate to view these sitcoms.

 Make a list of the ten characteristics of an ideal family.

 As you view each sitcom, refer to the list you have made. Take notes about how each sitcom family functions.

 Draw The Family Continuum. Rate the family shown in each sitcom and show where you would place it on the continuum. Write several reasons to defend your rating. Title your continuum Family Sitcom Ratings.

 Share your Family Sitcom Ratings with classmates.

Lesson 11

Review

Vocabulary Words

Write a separate sentence using each of the vocabulary words listed on page 88.

Objectives

1. How does the ideal family contrast with the dysfunctional family on The Family Continuum? **Objective 1**

2. What are 12 skills that children in an ideal family are taught by their parents or guardians? **Objective 2**

3. What is the difference between self-respecting behavior and self-centered behavior? **Objective 2**

4. Why is it important to be able to delay gratification? **Objective 2**

5. What are three ways to be a loving family member? **Objective 3**

Responsible Decision-Making

A friend of yours is trying to decide whether (s)he should attend a party at which there will be drinking. Some classmates encourage the friend to go, while others do not. Your friend does not know how to make up his/her mind. Write a response to this situation.

1. Describe the situation that requires your friend to make a decision.
2. List possible decisions your friend might make.
3. Name two responsible adults with whom your friend might discuss his/her decisions.
4. Evaluate the possible consequences of your friend's decisions. Determine if each decision will lead to actions that:
   - promote health,
   - protect safety,
   - follow laws,
   - show respect for your friend and others,
   - follow the guidelines of your friend's parents and of other responsible adults,
   - demonstrate good character.
5. Decide which decision is most responsible and appropriate for your friend.
6. Tell two results your friend can expect if (s)he makes this decision.

 Effective Communication

Write a paragraph describing the ideal family. Work with a friend or family member who knows more than one language or use a foreign language dictionary. Translate your paragraph into another language.

 Self-Directed Learning

Interview a parent or another adult who helped raise you. Ask this person to identify three values important to your family. Write these three values on one side of an index card. On the opposite side of the card, write three values that are important to you. Share what you have written with your parent or with another adult.

 Critical Thinking

Describe a situation that requires that you practice delayed gratification. Identify the immediate reward that you must postpone. Explain why it would be best for you to be patient and wait.

Responsible Citizenship

In a balanced relationship, you give and receive acts of kindness. Consider people in your community who would benefit from an act of kindness from you. Plan to "give" an act of kindness to someone each day this week.

You Can Recognize Ways to Improve Family Relationships

Life Skill **I will work to improve difficult family relationships.**

An **ideal family** is a family that has all the skills needed for loving, responsible relationships. The ideal family is the family that you visualize as being perfect. Although few families are perfect, it is important to recognize what is ideal. Then you have a model toward which you can work. Lesson 11 focused on the ideal family. This lesson focuses on the dysfunctional family. A **dysfunctional family** is a family that lacks the skills to be successful and function in healthful ways. You will learn what skills are lacking in dysfunctional families so you will know how to avoid behaviors that break down the family. You will learn about codependent relationships. You also will learn how to improve dysfunctional family relationships.

The Lesson Outline

What to Know About the Dysfunctional Family

What to Know About Codependent Relationships

How to Improve Dysfunctional Family Relationships

Objectives

1. Discuss ten causes of dysfunctional family relationships.
   pages 97–99

2. List and discuss ten feelings and behaviors that describe people who are codependent. **page 100**

3. Outline ways to improve dysfunctional family relationships.
   page 102

Vocabulary Words

ideal family
dysfunctional family
chemical dependence
codependence
addiction
perfectionism
violence
domestic violence
juvenile offender
abuse
child abuse
spouse abuse
parent abuse
elder abuse
physical abuse
emotional abuse
neglect
sexual abuse
abandonment
mental disorder
intimacy
enmeshment
interdependence
recovery program
Alcoholics Anonymous (AA)
Al-Anon
Al-Ateen

What to Know About the
Dysfunctional Family

The term dysfunctional family was first used to describe families in which there was alcoholism. The family member with alcoholism did not function in healthful ways. The family members who lived with alcoholism also began to function in ways that were harmful. The term dysfunctional family is now applied to all families in which members relate to one another in destructive and irresponsible ways.

Causes of Dysfunctional Families

- **Chemical dependence**
- **Other addictions**
- **Perfectionism**
- **Violence**
- **Physical abuse**
- **Emotional abuse**
- **Neglect**
- **Sexual abuse**
- **Abandonment**
- **Mental disorders**

Chemical Dependence in the Family

Chemical dependence is the compelling need to take a drug even though it harms the body, mind, or relationships. Chemical dependence also is called drug addiction and drug dependence. The lives of family members who are drug-dependent become dominated by the need to obtain and use drugs. The drugs, in turn, cause changes in thinking and behaving. There is more violence in families in which there is drug dependence. There also is more sexual abuse. Teens who are raised in a family in which there is chemical dependence are at risk for being harmed by violence. They may use drugs to cope with difficult situations.

There is evidence that chemical dependence may be inherited. Teens with a family history of chemical dependence who experiment with alcohol and other drugs have an increased risk of developing chemical dependence. Teens and other family members may develop codependence. **Codependence** is a mental disorder in which a person denies feelings and begins to cope in harmful ways. Codependence will be discussed in greater detail later in this lesson.

Other Addictions in the Family

An **addiction** is a compelling need to take a drug or engage in a specific behavior. Besides chemical dependence, the following addictions contribute to dysfunctional family life: eating disorders, exercise addiction, perfectionism, gambling addiction, nicotine addiction, relationship addiction, shopping addiction, television addiction, thrill-seeking addiction, and workaholism.

A family member with an addiction becomes obsessed with his/her addiction. The addiction becomes a top priority. Family life is neglected. Teens who live with a family member who has an addiction may develop codependence. They may develop the same or other addictions as ways of coping.

> **Lesson 7 will include more information about addictions.**

Perfectionism in the Family

Perfectionism is the compelling need to be accurate. Perfectionism is an addiction that is becoming more common. It can affect other family members. Parents or guardians who are perfectionists are overly critical of themselves and of their children. Teens who live with a perfectionistic parent or guardian may feel inadequate and insecure. These teens also may become perfectionists. They may criticize others and never be satisfied with anything. They may be overly critical of themselves. Their behavior is self-destructive and harms their relationships with others.

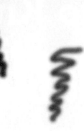

Violence in the Family

Violence is the use of physical force to injure, damage, or destroy oneself, others, or property. **Domestic violence** is violence that occurs within a family. Domestic violence includes physical abuse and sexual abuse. The family member who is violent usually is very controlling. Often, the violent family member abuses drugs. Other family members try to keep peace by avoiding disagreements. They may blame themselves when the family member has violent outbursts. Between acts of violence, the family member who is violent may be kind, gentle, and apologetic. But, the cycle of drug use and violent outbursts continues.

Teens who live in homes with domestic violence are at risk. They may be injured by the violent family member. They may copy the behavior of the violent family member and become controlling and violent. These teens are at risk for becoming juvenile offenders. A **juvenile offender** is a legal minor who commits a criminal act. Teens who are sexually abused are at risk for becoming pregnant or infected with HIV and other STDs.

Abuse in the Family

Abuse is the harmful treatment of another person. **Child abuse** is the harmful treatment of a minor. **Spouse abuse** is the harmful treatment of a husband or wife. **Parent abuse** is the harmful treatment of a parent. **Elder abuse** is the harmful treatment of an aged family member.

Four Kinds of Abuse

- **Physical abuse** is harmful treatment that results in physical injury to the victim.
- **Emotional abuse** is "putting down" another person and making the person feel worthless.
- **Neglect** is failure to provide proper care and guidance.
- **Sexual abuse** is sexual contact that is forced on a person.

An abusive family member is controlling and moody. Often, abusive family members are drug-dependent. Their need for control and their moodiness increase when they are under the influence of drugs. Teens who live with an abusive family member may be afraid and confused. They cannot understand why an abusive family member can be loving at one moment and abusive the next. They want to believe they are loved. For this reason, they deny their feelings and cover up what is happening. They may blame themselves and believe they deserve to be abused.

Abandonment in the Family

Abandonment is removing oneself from those whose care is one's responsibility. Parents who abandon their children are not available for them. Their absence from their children's lives may cause their children pain, suffering, and confusion. For example, a married couple may separate and divorce. Later, one parent may no longer see the children. The children feel a great loss. They may begin to feel unlovable, worthless, or guilty. They may think, "Why doesn't my parent want to be part of my life? What did I do wrong? I must not be lovable." They may experience the same feelings in other relationships. Abandoned teens have difficulty getting close to others. They may feel that if they get close to someone, that person too may abandon them. Abandoned teens may push away others. Or, they may be very needy. They may demand the attention of others to fulfill childhood needs that were not met.

Mental Disorders in the Family

A **mental disorder** is a mental or emotional condition that makes it difficult for a person to live in a normal way. Families in which one or more family members have a mental disorder have special stressors. Suppose a family member suffers from clinical depression. Other family members might respond in a healthful way. They might recognize that this family member has a mental disorder that requires treatment. They are sensitive to this but do not let this person's depression dominate their lives. In a dysfunctional family, family members do not respond in a healthful way. They may feel responsible for the family member's depression and feel guilty. They may try to "fix" the family member's depression and attempt to cheer up him/her. When the family member remains depressed, they feel personally responsible. They may allow the family member's depression to dominate family life.

What to Know About
Codependent Relationships

Family members living in a dysfunctional family may develop codependence. Codependence is a mental disorder in which a person denies feelings and begins to cope in harmful ways. People who have codependence are called codependent.

The Tree of Codependence illustrates how dysfunctional family life can lead to codependence. The roots are labeled with behaviors that occur in dysfunctional families. The branches are labeled with feelings and behaviors that describe people who are codependent.

Try to fix others' problems

Fear abandonment

Resist authority figures

Are very controlling

Have low self-esteem

Are people pleasers

Withdraw for protection

Are overly responsible

Hide anger

Deny feelings

Chemical dependency

Other addictions

Perfectionism

Violence

Neglect

Emotional abuse

Physical abuse

Sexual abuse

Mental disorders

Abandonment

People who are codependent struggle in their relationships. They cannot develop intimacy. **Intimacy** is a deep and meaningful kind of sharing between two people. People with codependence avoid intimacy by choosing one extreme or another:

1. **They focus on trying to please another person or people and deny their own needs.**

    or

2. **They avoid being close to another person or people to keep from being hurt.**

The two sides of codependence—obsessing about others and avoiding others—are at the root of much unhappiness. Suppose you obsess about another person. You constantly want to please the person. The person's needs become so important that you overlook your own. Eventually you lose your identity. This is enmeshment. **Enmeshment** is a condition in which a person becomes obsessed with the needs of another person and no longer can recognize his/her own needs.

In a healthy relationship, there is interdependence. **Interdependence** is a condition in which two people depend upon one another, yet each has a separate identity. Both are aware of their own and the other person's needs and feelings

People with codependence may avoid intimacy by choosing relationships that offer little or no chance for closeness. Teens with codependence are more comfortable with someone with problems. This is because teens from dysfunctional families choose relationships similar to the family relationships they have had.

Activity

Self-Check: Can You Recognize Codependence?

Life Skill: I will work to improve difficult family relationships.

Materials: paper, pen or pencil

Directions: Healthy people have some of the behaviors and feelings that describe people who are codependent but do not rely on them excessively. Number a sheet of paper from one to ten. Make a check next to a number if it describes a feeling or behavior you experience often and/or intensely. Discuss your responses with a parent or other responsible adult. YOU WILL NOT BE ASKED TO SHARE YOUR ANSWERS WITH YOUR TEACHER OR CLASSMATES.

 1. Do you try to hide your anger? Hidden anger is anger that is not recognized and is expressed in an inappropriate way.

2. Are you a people pleaser? People pleasing is needing the approval of others to feel good about yourself.

3. Are you a caretaker? You are a caretaker if you assume responsibility for the problems of others so they will need you.

4. Are you a controlling person? You are controlling if you want others to do as you say so you can feel secure.

5. Do you fear abandonment? If you fear abandonment, you are worried that something will be taken away from you.

6. Do you fear authority figures? If you were constantly criticized by parents or other adult family members, you may fear authority figures.

 7. Do you have frozen feelings? If your feelings were met with disapproval, anger, or rejection, you may have stopped recognizing them.

 8. Do you lack self-confidence? You lack self-confidence if you always worry that you will make a mistake or fail.

 9. Are you overly responsible? If you are overly responsible, you take on too much and do tasks that others should do themselves.

 10. Do you isolate yourself? If you isolate yourself, you withdraw when you are uncomfortable.

Recognizing codependent behaviors and feelings is the first step toward improving family relationships. Review any items you checked. Discuss your responses with a responsible adult.

How to Improve Dysfunctional Family Relationships

Suppose you are raised in a dysfunctional family and are codependent. Is there any hope for your recovery from codependence? Can family members learn how to relate in responsible and healthful ways? It is important to recognize that parents, guardians, and family members may choose behaviors that are harmful and are not responsible. Their actions and behaviors may be wrong. But, it is still important to give them your love and respect as much as possible. Recognize that you may be copying your parent's or guardian's behavior, and change your responses. Remember, you are responsible for your own actions.

Individual and group therapy can help ensure recovery from codependence. In individual therapy, a skilled therapist works one-on-one with the codependent. (S)he assists the codependent in discovering how much of what (s)he feels and believes was shaped by the dysfunctional family. Then the therapist helps the codependent learn healthier ways to express feelings and relate to others.

In group therapy, a skilled therapist works with a group of people to help them learn healthful ways to express feelings and relate to others. The group members practice new ways of relating within the safety of the group. These new ways of relating are transferred into real-life situations.

Recovery programs help people bounce back from codependence. A **recovery program** is a group that supports members as they change their behavior to be responsible. One of the first recovery programs was Alcoholics Anonymous. **Alcoholics Anonymous (AA)** is a recovery program for people who have alcoholism.

Then, recovery programs were developed for family members of people with alcoholism. **Al-Anon** is a recovery program for people who have friends or family members with alcoholism. **Al-Ateen** is a recovery program for teens who have a family member or friend with alcoholism.

Today, there are many different recovery programs. There are recovery programs for codependence, gambling, workaholism, and many other addictions.

Lesson 12
Review

Vocabulary Words

Write a separate sentence using each of the vocabulary words listed on page 96.

Objectives

1. What are ten causes of dysfunctional family relationships? **Objective 1**

2. What are ten feelings and behaviors that describe people who are codependent? **Objective 2**

3. What are two ways people who are codependent block intimacy with other people? **Objective 2**

4. What are three ways to improve dysfunctional family relationships? **Objective 3**

5. What is the purpose of a recovery program? **Objective 3**

Responsible Decision-Making

You spend the evening at a friend's home. Your friend's brother has cocaine in his room. Your friend tells you their parents do not know. Your friend has to make excuses for his brother when he does not show up at school or at his part-time job. Your friend's brother makes threats if the topic of drug use comes up. Your friend is embarrassed about his brother's behavior and asks you to keep it a secret. Write a response to this situation.

1. Describe the situation that requires you to make a decision.

2. List possible decisions you might make.

3. Name two responsible adults with whom you might discuss your decisions.

4. Evaluate the possible consequences of your decisions. Determine if each decision will lead to actions that:
   - promote health,
   - protect safety,
   - follow laws,
   - show respect for yourself and others,
   - follow the guidelines of your parents and of other responsible adults,
   - demonstrate good character.

5. Decide which decision is most responsible and appropriate.

6. Tell two results you expect if you make this decision.

 ## Effective Communication

Develop a "Top Ten List of Ways to Stop Codependence." Refer to the behaviors and feelings on page 100 that describe people who are codependent.

 ## Self-Directed Learning

Check the card catalog at the library for books on family life. Select one book of interest to you. Write a book report summarizing what you learn from reading the book.

 ## Critical Thinking

You plan to attend college or vocational school when you graduate from high school. So now you must study and get the best grades possible. How might you recognize the difference between hard work and perfectionism?

 ## Responsible Citizenship

One form of elder abuse is neglect. Some senior citizens are abandoned by their families. They do not receive cards, letters, or visits. Ask your parents or guardian to consider a way you might stay in touch with a senior citizen who is lonely.

Lesson 13

You Can Use Conflict Resolution Skills

Life Skill **I will use conflict resolution skills.**

Conflicts occur everyday. Conflicts occur within relationships—in a family, in a school, and in a community. They occur between strangers. They also may occur within yourself and center on your needs and values. Conflict often involves strong emotions. These emotions might serve as motivators to help you resolve a conflict in a responsible manner. At other times, emotions might cloud your judgment and you might resolve the conflict in a way you will regret later. This lesson focuses on types of conflict and conflict response styles. You will learn how to use conflict resolution skills and mediation. You also will learn how to avoid behaviors that discriminate against others.

The Lesson Outline

What to Know About Conflict

How to Use Conflict Resolution Skills

How to Use Mediation

How to Avoid Discriminatory Behavior

Objectives

1. Explain four types of conflict and three conflict response styles. **page 105**
2. Outline conflict resolution skills. **pages 106–107**
3. Outline the eight steps in mediation. **page 108**
4. Discuss ways to avoid discriminatory behavior. **page 109**

Vocabulary Words

conflict

intrapersonal conflict

interpersonal conflict

intragroup conflict

intergroup conflict

conflict response style

conflict avoidance

conflict confrontation

conflict resolution

conflict resolution skills

mediation

mediator

discriminate

prejudice

hate crime

stereotype

synergy

diversity

empathy

What to Know About Conflict

A **conflict** is a disagreement between two or more people or between two or more choices. There are four types of conflict and three conflict response styles.

1. An **intrapersonal conflict** is a conflict that occurs within a person. For example, you may say to yourself, "I would like to watch television after dinner." You also may think, "I should study for the test I have tomorrow." You are involved in intrapersonal conflict.

2. An **interpersonal conflict** is a conflict that occurs between two or more people. Suppose you and a sibling alternate doing the dinner dishes. Your sibling was sick yesterday so you did the dishes two days in a row. You believe your sibling should do dishes for the next two days. Your sibling disagrees. You and your sibling are involved in interpersonal conflict.

3. An **intragroup conflict** is a conflict that occurs between people that identify themselves as belonging to the same group. Suppose your group of friends has been pranked by another group of teens. Some of your friends want to get even by "egging" the other group's school. You and your friend do not want to take part. You and your friend are involved in an intragroup conflict.

4. An **intergroup conflict** is a conflict that occurs between two or more groups of people. The conflict may involve different neighborhoods, schools, gangs, racial groups, religious groups, or nations. For example, you may be on an athletic team that is playing another school. A player on your school's team bumps into a player on the other team. The team members of the other school believe the action was intended to harm their team member. Players from your school and players from the other school are involved in an intergroup conflict.

What Is Your Conflict Response Style?

A **conflict response style** is a pattern of behavior a person demonstrates when a conflict arises. The person may demonstrate one or a combination of the following conflict response styles.

- **Conflict avoidance** is a conflict response style in which a person avoids disagreements at all costs. If you have this style, you do not tell others when you disagree with them. You may be so concerned that others will not like you that you are not willing to challenge their behavior. Rather than disagree with someone, you sit back and allow others to solve problems in a method of their choosing.

- **Conflict confrontation** is a conflict response style in which a person attempts to settle a disagreement in a hostile, defiant, and aggressive way. If you use conflict confrontation, you like to confront others. As a confronter, you want to win or be right at all costs. You view conflict as a win-lose proposition. You believe your side of the story is the only one worth considering.

- **Conflict resolution** is a conflict response style in which a person uses conflict resolution skills to resolve a disagreement. **Conflict resolution skills** are steps that can be taken to settle a disagreement in a responsible way. If you use these skills, you remain rational and in control when you have disagreements with others. You listen to the other person's side of the story. You see the potential for a win-win solution in situations and relationships in which there is conflict.

How to Use
Conflict Resolution Skills

A guiding principal of conflict resolution is the concept of win-win. When those involved in a conflict feel that they have won, it is a win-win situation. When only one side in a conflict feels it has won, the situation is a win-lose. It is important to realize that there does not have to be a loser in every conflict. To repeat the definition, conflict resolution skills are steps that can be taken to settle a disagreement in a responsible way. The following list identifies the ten steps necessary to resolve conflict in a responsible way.

1. Remain calm.

Ralph Waldo Emerson, a nineteenth-century philosopher, once said, "We boil at different degrees." Make a personal assessment of your boiling point. Try to increase your patience so that you lower your boiling point. For some people, counting to ten is helpful. For others, a few deep breaths help. Still others need a time out before trying to resolve a conflict.

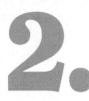

2. Set the tone.

Reassure the other person that you want to play fair and find a mutually acceptable solution. Practice positive communication skills: avoid blaming, avoid interrupting, affirm others, be sincere, avoid put-downs, reserve judgment, avoid threats, separate the person from the problem, help others save face, and use positive nonverbal responses.

3. Define the conflict.

Define the conflict in writing. The description of what you are in conflict about should be short and to the point. If the conflict is between you and another person or other persons, each of you should describe the conflict. In describing the conflict, it is important to continue to follow the rules for setting the tone. The focus should be on describing the conflict, not on describing the people involved in the conflict.

4. Take responsibility for personal actions.

Think about your personal actions that may have led to the conflict. Recognize what part you have played. Apologize if any of your actions were questionable or wrong.

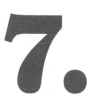

5. Use I-messages to express needs and feelings.

The needs and feelings of people involved in a conflict are important in finding a successful solution. A win-win solution usually recognizes the feelings and needs of each person who is involved. When you use I-messages, you take responsibility for your feelings. You do not blame and shame others and put them on the defensive.

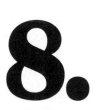

6. Listen to the needs and feelings of others.

Take time to allow other people to share their needs and feelings. Do not interrupt or judge. Listening to people shows that you sincerely want to resolve a conflict in a manner that will be win-win if possible.

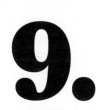

7. List and evaluate possible solutions.

This step involves brainstorming as many solutions as possible for the conflict. Identify all possible solutions before you discuss each one. When discussing each solution, predict the outcome. Will the solution result in actions that are healthful, safe, legal, respectful of all people involved, and nonviolent?

8. Agree on a solution.

To avoid future conflicts, restate or summarize what each of you will do to honor the agreement reached. Sometimes it is helpful to put the agreement in writing so that the agreement may be reviewed at a later time. Remember that the solution should be healthful, safe, legal, respectful of all people involved, and nonviolent.

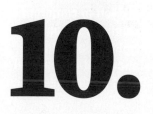

9. Keep your word and follow the agreement.

You should always intend to do what you say you will do. Sometimes, people need help keeping their word and following the agreement that has been reached. If this is the case, people need to share the difficulty that they expect to have and examine ways they can be helped. Trust is very important in conflict resolution.

10. Ask for the assistance of a trusted adult if the conflict cannot be resolved.

Sometimes people in conflict need the help of a trusted adult to reach a solution. Conflict resolution does not mean compromising your values or the guidelines of your parents or guardian. The agreement should involve a solution that is healthful, safe, legal, respectful of all people involved, and nonviolent.

How to Use
Mediation

Mediation is a process in which an outside person helps people in conflict reach a solution. A **mediator** is a person who helps people in conflict reach a solution. Mediation involves eight steps.

1. **A mediator is agreed upon.** The purpose of a mediator is to help the people involved in the conflict find an acceptable solution. The mediator should be objective. The only bias the mediator should have is for the solution to be healthful, safe, legal, respectful of all people involved, and nonviolent.

2. **Set ground rules.** Appropriate ground rules include: tell the truth; commit to resolve the conflict; avoid blaming; avoid put-downs; avoid threats; avoid sneering; avoid pushing; avoid hitting; reserve judgment; and listen without interruption.

3. **Define the conflict.** The people involved need to begin by describing the conflict. They need to agree about what has taken place.

4. **Identify solutions to the conflict.** The people involved brainstorm ways to resolve the conflict. The mediator also can suggest ways to resolve the conflict.

5. **Evaluate suggested solutions.** When evaluating each solution, predict the probable outcome. Will the solution result in actions that are healthful, safe, legal, respectful of all people involved, and nonviolent?

6. **Negotiate a solution.** The mediator helps the people involved negotiate a solution. The mediator may suggest making tradeoffs in order for all people involved to feel that they are in a win-win situation. In some situations, all people meet together; in others, only one side meets with the mediator at a time.

7. **Write and sign an agreement.** The people involved should enter into the agreement in an entirely voluntary manner. After they agree to do so, an agreement should be written. Time should be allowed for those involved to review the agreement and to ask questions. The people involved and the mediator should sign and date the agreement and keep a copy. The agreement can be used as a reference point should questions or further conflicts arise.

8. **Schedule a follow-up meeting.** The mediator and people involved can agree to the desired length of time that might pass before a follow-up meeting. They might even determine the agenda for the meeting. The purpose of the meeting is to review how well the agreement is working.

A mediator will not ask you to compromise your values or the guidelines of your parents or guardian. The negotiated agreement should involve a solution that is healthful, safe, legal, respectful of all people involved, and nonviolent.

How to Avoid Discriminatory Behavior

To **discriminate** is to treat some people or groups of people differently from others. **Prejudice** is suspicion, intolerance, or irrational hatred directed at an individual or group of people. Prejudice motivates hate crimes. A **hate crime** is a crime motivated by prejudice. Discriminatory behavior and prejudice divide people. Those who are targets of discriminatory behavior and prejudice are angry because they are treated unfairly.

It is important to show respect for all people. When you show respect for others, you increase the likelihood that they will be at their best and contribute to society. You increase the likelihood that people will be able to live together, be productive, and behave in nonviolent ways. To avoid discriminatory behavior, you must recognize this kind of behavior, and you yourself must not do it. You also must challenge others who choose to behave in a discriminatory manner.

1. Challenge stereotypes. A **stereotype** is a prejudiced attitude that assigns a specific quality or characteristic to all people who belong to a particular group. Stereotypes imply that an individual is the same as every other member in the group with which (s)he is identified. It is unfair to make generalizations about people based on stereotypes. People who belong to a specific racial, religious, ethnic, or gender group have their race, religion, ethnicity, or gender in common. However, they are different in other ways. You must avoid believing that all people belonging to the same group have the same problems.

2. Create synergy through diversity. **Synergy** is a positive outcome that occurs when different people cooperate and respect one another and create more energy for all. **Diversity** is the quality of being different or varied. When there is synergy, people with different backgrounds, talents, and skills work together to produce better solutions than would be possible if everyone were exactly alike.

3. Show empathy for all people. **Empathy** is the ability to share in another person's emotions or feelings. When you have empathy, you understand what the person is feeling and express that understanding. You might express it with words or actions.

4. Avoid discriminatory comments. Words often cause emotional wounds more difficult to heal than physical wounds. Always think before you speak. Avoid making jokes or snide remarks about other people. Avoid laughing or affirming others when they make jokes or snide remarks about other people.

5. Ask others to stop discriminatory behavior. One way to support discriminatory behavior is to say or do nothing when people around you behave in a discriminatory way. Instead, state your disapproval when someone makes a snide remark or tells a joke about a person belonging to a specific group. Tell the person making the remark or telling the joke that (s)he may have meant no harm but that this behavior is hurtful to other people.

6. Learn about people who are different from you. As you learn more about others, you appreciate their talents. You are more likely to develop empathy for the pain they may feel. You are better able to see how people who are different might live and work together. There are many ways to learn about people different from you. Study a foreign language. Read about other races or cultures. Get to know a student in your school or community who is different from you.

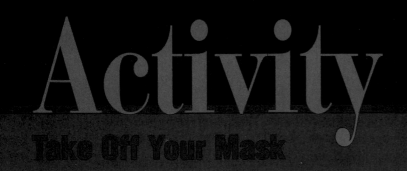

Activity
Take Off Your Mask

Life Skill: I will use conflict resolution skills.

Materials: construction paper, scissors, markers; newspaper cut into strips, wire, and papier-mâché, paints (optional); paper and pencil

Directions: Follow the steps below to practice conflict resolution skills with your teacher or classmates.

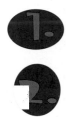 **1.** Allow classmates to select one of the following conflict response styles: conflict avoidance or conflict confrontation.

2. Each classmate is to make a mask of a face expressing the feelings of the conflict response style (s)he selected. Classmates who have selected conflict avoidance will make a mask of a face without expression or fearful. Classmates who have selected conflict confrontation will make a mask of a face that appears hostile, angry, or aggressive. The masks may be made from construction paper, paper, or papier-mâché. To make the mask from papier-mâché, begin by molding a face from flexible wire. Dip the newspaper strips into the papier-mâché and cover the wire. Paint the face to add expression to the eyes and mouth. To make the mask from construction paper, draw an outline of a face with eyes and mouth. Cut out the face, eyes, and mouth. Add expression to the face by drawing on it with markers.

 3. Divide the class into four groups to write a short scenario in which there is conflict. Each group should brainstorm ideas for the scenario. The group can begin by asking group members to identify situations they believe make teens angry. For example, a teen may be angry if (s)he is waiting in line at a movie theatre and someone cuts in ahead of him/her. Have one member in the group write the scenario on a sheet of paper.

 4. A spokesperson from one of the groups should read the short scenario written by his/her group.

 5. A volunteer with a mask of a face expressing conflict avoidance should show the class his/her mask and explain how (s)he would respond using conflict avoidance.

 6. The same volunteer should then put down or "take off the mask" and say how (s)he might respond using conflict resolution.

 7. A volunteer with a mask of a face expressing conflict confrontation should show the class his/her mask and explain how (s)he would respond using conflict confrontation.

 8. The same volunteer should then put down or "take off the mask" and say how (s)he might respond using conflict resolution.

 9. The spokespersons from the other three groups should take turns reading the short scenarios from their groups, and steps five through eight should be repeated.

10. Have classmates share what they have discovered about the three conflict response styles by completing this activity.

Lesson 13

Review

Vocabulary Words

Write a separate sentence using each of the vocabulary words listed on page 104.

Objectives

1. What are four types of conflict a person might have? **Objective 1**

2. What are three conflict response styles? **Objective 1**

3. What are the ten steps in conflict resolution? **Objective 2**

4. What are the eight steps in mediation? **Objective 3**

5. What are six ways to avoid discriminatory behavior? **Objective 4**

Responsible Decision-Making

One of your classmates has just moved here from a different country. Some students make fun of this student. They make snide remarks and have made up a list of cruel nicknames. Two students carry this behavior a step further. They decide to call your classmate's house and make cruel remarks or leave threatening messages. They ask you to participate in their "fun." Write a response to this situation.

1. Describe the situation that requires you to make a decision.
2. List possible decisions you might make.
3. Name two responsible adults with whom you might discuss your decisions.
4. Evaluate the possible consequences of your decisions. Determine if each decision will lead to actions that:
   • promote health,
   • protect safety,
   • follow laws,
   • show respect for yourself and others,
   • follow the guidelines of your parents and of other responsible adults,
   • demonstrate good character.
5. Decide which decision is most responsible and appropriate.
6. Tell two results you expect if you make this decision.

 Effective Communication

Divide a piece of paper into three columns. At the top of each column, write one of the conflict response styles: conflict avoidance, conflict confrontation, conflict resolution. List five words under each head. Each word should describe the conflict response style under which it is written. Which of the three columns best describes you?

 Self-Directed Learning

Locate a newspaper or magazine article about a teen who was injured during a fight. Write a short report in which you summarize what happened and explain how conflict resolution and mediation would have been helpful.

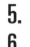 **Critical Thinking**

A classmate frequently tells jokes about people of a specific ethnic group. Your classmate expects you to join in and laugh. Write a paragraph in which you explain to your friend the harmful effects of his/her behavior.

 Responsible Citizenship

Set aside time to discuss mediation with a parent or guardian. Explain what you have learned about the mediation process. Emphasize that mediation should never compromise your values or the guidelines of your parent or guardian. Together, make a list of three adults who would be responsible mediators for teens in your community.

Lesson 14

You Can Develop Healthful Friendships

Life Skill **I will develop healthful friendships.**

A **healthful friendship** is a balanced relationship that promotes mutual respect and healthful behavior. Having healthful friendships improves the quality of your life. Friends take a personal interest in you. They support you when you are successful. They encourage you during difficult times. You can participate in social activities with friends. This lesson will explain how to initiate friendships. You will learn how to handle rejection. This lesson explains how to maintain balanced friendships. You will learn the difference between a one-sided friendship and a balanced friendship. You also will learn why some teens are people pleasers.

Vocabulary Words
healthful friendship
conversation
rejection
balanced friendship
one-sided friendship
people pleaser

The Lesson Outline
How to Initiate Friendships
How to Maintain Balanced Friendships

Objectives
1. Explain how to initiate friendships. **page 113**
2. Explain how to maintain balanced friendships. **page 114**

How to
Initiate Friendships

Have you ever watched two people play a game of chess? Each person gets ready to play by placing his/her chess pieces on the board. Then one of the players makes an opening move. Friendships begin the same way. First, two people must want to initiate, or begin, the friendship. Then one of them must make an opening move.

Opening Moves

Suppose you want to make a new friend. Before making an opening move, it is smart to make a background check. There are questions you should ask yourself about anyone who might become a friend.

- **What do I know about this person?**
- **Does this person have good character?**
- **Do my parents or guardian know this person?**
- **Will my parents or guardian approve of my spending time with this person?**

Pursue the friendship only if the person has good character and your parents or guardians approve. Now you are ready to make an opening move. There always is an element of risk involved. After all, you may not be certain that a person whom you want as a friend wants to pursue a friendship with you. Consider the possible opening moves you might make. You might wait in the hall after class and begin a conversation or call a person on the telephone. Each of these opening moves involves risk as well as the possibility of reward. You risk being rejected, but you may be rewarded with the opportunity to develop a new friendship.

Conversation Tips ....

Suppose your opening move was a success. Where do you go now? Your success in developing new friendships often depends on your ability to carry on a conversation. A **conversation** is a verbal exchange of feelings, thoughts, ideas, and opinions. How skilled are you at having conversations? The Conversation Keepers and Conversation Killers are do's and don'ts for having conversations.

How to Handle Rejection

Everyone experiences rejection at times. **Rejection** is the feeling of being unwelcome or unwanted. You may approach a person and speak, and (s)he may blow you off. A friend, or at least someone you thought was a friend, may not include you in plans for the weekend. How do you respond to rejection? Do you become angry and try to get even? Or, do you bury your feelings and pretend not to care? These responses destroy relationships. Express your hurt, anger, or disappointment in a healthful way.

- **Use I-messages to share your feelings with the person who rejected you.** You might respond to the example stated above by saying, "When I wasn't included in plans for the weekend, and you went out without me, I was disappointed."

- **Share your feelings with a trusted adult if you cannot share them with the person who rejected you.**

- **Remember that you are worthwhile even when a person does not want to be your friend or a friend does not include you.**

Conversation Keepers	Conversation Killers
Asking questions	Talking about yourself
Showing interest in what someone else is saying	Appearing disinterested in what someone else is saying
Listening carefully	Interrupting someone
Responding to others	Changing the topic
Considering other ideas	Being a know-it-all
Using correct grammar	Using slang words
Encouraging another person	Bragging
Being positive	Complaining
Sharing your ideas and feelings	Talking about others
Encouraging someone to talk	Dominating the conversation
Making eye contact	Avoiding eye contact

What to Know About
Dating Skills

Being Ready for Steady

Q. Suppose you are dating only one person. Your parents discourage this steady relationship. They want you to go out with different people and spend more time with your friends. What are the advantages of dating several people versus going steady?

A. Going steady provides a comfort zone. You feel secure when you always have someone there for you. This person can help you feel accepted. But, staying in the comfort zone has disadvantages too. During your teen years, you have the opportunity to practice your dating skills. You can take risks and ask out different people and accept other invitations. You can learn to handle rejection when someone does not want to go out with you. Different dating experiences help you meet new people and gain self-confidence.

Getting Up Courage

Q. Suppose there is someone in math class whom you think is "hot." You'd like to ask this person to a party your friend is having. But, you get tongue-tied whenever you begin to speak. What can you do?

A. To calm your nerves, do a practice run first. Rehearse with a family member, trusted friend, or in front of a mirror how you will ask this person out. Be honest and share your feelings. It's OK to be up front and tell a person you wish to date that you are nervous. It will ease the tension. Then, take a deep breath, smile, and ask for the date. Now consider your dating attitude. If you ask someone for a date, do not consider yourself a success or failure based on the person's acceptance or rejection of your invitation. Instead, give yourself credit for doing the asking. Always remember: If a person turns down a date with you, it does not mean you are a loser.

Being Up Front

Q. Suppose someone you have been dying to go out with asks you out. The plans involve going out with people who have a reputation for drinking. Should you accept the date?

A. Ask questions and get the facts before you accept the date. Explain that you do not drink and that you do not hang out with people who do. You need to know if there will be any drinking before you can accept. Your potential date may reassure you that there will be no alcohol. You need to make it clear that if there is drinking, you will leave immediately. You also may suggest going out with other people who do not drink. However, suppose your potential date does not reassure you that there will be no drinking. Turn down the date and do not be too disappointed. Remember, dating situations that include drinking lead to trouble.

How to Turn Down a Date

Q. A friend told me someone in my English class is going to ask me out. I know the person, and there is NO WAY I want to go. How can I keep from hurting this person's feelings?

A. Tune into your social graces and handle the situation with class. Thank the person for asking you. Say directly, but gently, that you are not interested in going out. Avoid dishonesty. For example, do not say you are busy when you are not.

Making a Fast Exit

Q. Suppose you are at a party where teens are drinking alcohol or experimenting with other drugs. You tell your date you want to leave. Your date suggests staying another hour. Should you stay or make a fast exit?

A. Easy decision...MAKE A FAST EXIT. The faster you leave, the better. There can be serious consequences if you stay. Suppose someone calls the police to report alcohol and other drug use at the party. The police arrive and find teens drinking and using other drugs. You will appear guilty even though you did not drink or use drugs. People who hear about the party will believe you were drinking because you were at the party. Remember, your parents or guardian gave you the privilege to date. They believe that you are trustworthy and responsible. Now, what should you do if your date will not leave? Make a fast exit yourself. Call your parents, or guardians, or another responsible adult to pick you up.

It's OK Not to Go Out

Q. My friends talk about going out all the time. I feel like something is wrong with me because I am not interested in going out. Should I go out anyhow to keep up my image?

A. Going out, or dating, should be a choice. You may not be ready or you may not be interested right now. Do not doubt yourself because you are not interested in going out right now. Do not date because you feel pressured to do so.

Loan or Gift?

Q. I gave my steady a family ring to wear. After we broke up, I asked for the ring back. My former steady likes the ring and wants to keep it. Who should have the ring?

A. A gift is something that is voluntarily given with no strings attached. Usually, a gift becomes the property of the person to whom it was given. When you gave your steady the ring, you intended your steady to wear it as long as you were together. Now you realize that you should have made this clear. You each view the giving of the ring differently. Apologize for not being clear as to your intentions. Explain that the ring has special meaning to you.

When Someone Better Asks You Out

Q. Suppose you have plans to go on a date with someone this Saturday. Then you run into another person you like better. The second person asks if you have plans Saturday. Should you try to get out of your other plans?

A. Character is essential when dating. You must always treat people with respect. How would you feel if someone cancelled plans with you for someone (s)he liked better? Always keep the commitments that you make to others. Set a date with the second person for a different night.

Dating Skills Checklist

Rate your dating skills. Pat yourself on the back for each of the following statements that describes your behavior.

1. I do not base my self-worth on my ability to get a date.
2. I ask questions and get the facts before I accept a date.
3. I decline a date when there will be pressure to drink or be sexually active.
4. I honor my dating commitments and do not change plans if someone better comes along.
5. I recognize the advantages of dating different people rather than going steady.
6. I would make a fast exit from a date instead of being or staying in a situation that is against my parents' or guardian's guidelines.
7. I would not hesitate to call my parents or guardian if I were on a date and needed help.
8. I am comfortable staying home when I do not want to date.
9. I am clear as to my expectations when I give or receive a gift in a dating situation.
10. I am honest and kind when I turn down someone for a date.

What to Know About
Date Rape

In social situations, you must be concerned about your safety and the safety of others. **Rape** is the threatened or actual use of physical force to get someone to have sex without giving consent. Rape usually is motivated by a combination of power, anger, and sexual desire. When rape is committed by a person unknown to the person being raped, power and anger are usually the motivating factors. However, the majority of rape cases involve a form of rape known as acquaintance rape. **Acquaintance rape** is rape in which the rapist is known to the person who is raped. **Date rape** is rape that occurs in a dating situation. The motivation for date rape is often sexual desire. In some cases it is the desire to control. Date rape is more likely to be an impulsive act rather than a planned activity. Acquaintance rape and date rape are forms of violence.

Why You Need the Facts About Date Rape

Surveys of high school students indicate that teens are sometimes confused about date rape. They may believe that sex without consent is OK in some situations. Sex without consent is NEVER OK.

FACT: Sex without consent is rape. Circumstances do not change this definition of unlawful behavior.

- Suppose a female puts herself in a risk situation. Perhaps she goes into a male's bedroom when no adults are home. Do her actions indicate consent to have sex even if she says "no?" NO. If a male forces a female to have sex when she is in a risk situation, he has committed rape. Caution to females: Do not put yourself in risk situations. If you do, it can be very difficult to defend yourself. No one will hear your call for help should sexual advances occur. If date rape occurs, others may believe that you said "yes" even if you did not.

- Suppose a female wears sexy clothes, such as a very short skirt, a tight sweater, or a low-cut dress. Is she "asking for it" because she dresses in this way? NO. If a male assumes she wants to have sex and forces her to do so, he has committed rape. Caution to females: Dress in an appropriate way to avoid sending mixed messages. Remember, the way you dress affects your reputation.

- Suppose a male believes the male role is to be the aggressor and the female role is to be the resister. He may believe his sex role includes making forceful sexual advances. In addition, he may believe that when a female says "no" she really means "maybe," and when she says "maybe" she really means "yes." As a result, he ignores messages of nonconsent and forces the female to have sex, especially if he encounters little physical resistance. He is guilty of committing rape. Caution to females: Be consistent. Say "no" clearly. Do not encourage sexual advances.

- Suppose a male misinterprets signs of affection. He may believe that cuddling or kissing indicate a desire to have sex. He may interpret a female's "no" as token resistance. He may believe she does not want to appear too easy and that he needs to be more forceful. As a result, he ignores her resistance and forces sex. He is guilty of committing rape. Caution to females: Keep your limits clear when you express affection. If a male becomes more forceful, offer more than token resistance. Say "no" firmly and yell, scream, or run away if necessary.

Why Alcohol and Other Drug Use Increases the Risk of Date Rape

Most cases of date rape involve the use of alcohol and other drugs because of the following reasons:

1. **Drinking alcohol or using other drugs increases the likelihood that you might be in a risk situation.** Suppose a female has been drinking alcohol or smoking marijuana. As a result, she is not thinking clearly. She is in a risk situation in which she normally would not be. For example, she might leave a party with a male she doesn't know. She might go to a male's home when no adults are there and listen to music in his bedroom. She is now in a risk situation. It may be difficult for her to defend herself from sexual advances or rape.

2. **Drinking alcohol or using other drugs interferes with judgment.** Suppose a male has a strong sexual desire for a female he is dating. The female tries to make her limits for expressing affection clear to him. She says NO. However, the male has been drinking or using other drugs. He is unable to think clearly and to respond in an appropriate way. He does not respect his female companion's NO response. He rapes her because his judgment is impaired.

3. **Drinking alcohol and using other drugs intensifies feelings and the need for control.** Date rape is an act of violence. A male who is a rapist often has an increased need to control a female companion. He also is more likely to act upon that need after using alcohol or other drugs. Indeed, many rapes are reported after alcohol or other drug use has occurred.

Know About Laws Concerning Date Rape

- A female who is under the influence of alcohol or other drugs cannot give legal consent to have sex. In other words, having sex with a female who has been drinking or using drugs can be considered date rape in a court of law, even if the woman did not say "no."

- Drunkeness or being high on drugs is not a legal defense against date rape. In other words, if a man has been drinking alcohol or using drugs before he commits a rape, this is not a legal excuse. He still has committed rape.

What to Know About the Date Rape Drugs

Flunitrazepam (floo·nuh·TRAZ·i·pam) is an odorless, colorless sedative drug. On the street, the drug is known as "roofies," "rope," "the forget pill," and "roach." This drug is ten times stronger than valium, which is a tranquilizer. Like alcohol, it makes some users fearless and aggressive. It is referred to as "the date-rape drug" because it can cause blackouts, with complete or partial loss of memory. A male can slip a "roofie" into a female's drink and commit date rape after she blacks out. Other effects include aggressiveness and fearlessness. It can cause breathing irregularities and can be fatal. Law enforcement officers are particularly concerned about the increasing number of rapes associated with "roofies." There also is concern about the potential for addiction to flunitrazepam and overdosing on the drug.

Other date rape drugs include GHB and MDMA (ecstasy).

Why Practicing Abstinence Is a Responsible Decision

Throughout your life, you will have many important decisions to make. The quality of your life will be determined by your decisions. Lesson 4 included information on how to make responsible decisions. A **responsible decision** is a choice that leads to actions that:

- **promote health,**
- **protect safety,**
- **follow laws,**
- **show respect for self and others,**
- **follow the guidelines of parents and of other responsible adults,**
- **demonstrate good character.**

Practicing abstinence until marriage is a responsible decision.

Practicing Abstinence Promotes Health

You reduce the risk of becoming infected with HIV and developing AIDS. The number of AIDS cases among teens and young adults increased more than 75 percent in the last few years. Many more teens are likely to be HIV-infected; millions more are at risk because a person infected with HIV may not know it or may not tell a partner. To date, there is no effective cure for AIDS. When you practice abstinence, you help protect yourself from HIV infection and AIDS.

You reduce the risk of becoming infected with sexually transmitted diseases (STDs). To date, there is treatment but no cure for genital herpes and genital warts. Teens infected with either of these STDs can have recurrences the rest of their lives. There is an increase in the number of cases of pelvic inflammatory disease (PID) in teen females. PID can lead to permanent scarring of the Fallopian tubes. This can result in sterility. When you practice abstinence, you protect yourself from infection with STDs.

You will not become a teenage parent. More than three out of ten teenage females become pregnant before age 20; many become pregnant more than once as teens. Of those who become pregnant before age 15, 60 percent will become pregnant more than once as teens. Most teen females who have babies are not married. They do not have the emotional support of a loving husband. Their babies do not live with a father who can love and nurture them. Teens who marry have a lower continuing financial status than they would have if they had married and had children in their twenties. When you practice abstinence, you do not risk becoming pregnant or getting someone pregnant.

Practicing Abstinence Protects Safety

You reduce the risk of violence that is associated with teen parenthood.

- The suicide rate of teen mothers is ten times that of the general population.
- The number of teen parents who abuse and neglect their children because of frustration is extremely high.

When you practice abstinence, you reduce the risk of being a teen parent who is stressed out and more at risk for being violent.

Practicing Abstinence Follows Laws

You avoid being in situations in which you can be prosecuted for having sex with a minor. In most states, having sex with a person before the legal age of consent is considered corruption of a minor. The **legal age of consent** is that age when a person is legally able to give permission. A person who is mentally disabled may not understand what it means to give permission even if (s)he is not a minor. A person can be prosecuted for having sex with a minor or with someone who is mentally disabled.

You avoid sexual behavior for which you can be prosecuted for date rape. When you practice abstinence, you will not be guilty of having sex with an unwilling partner. You will not be accused of date rape.

Practicing Abstinence Shows Respect for Self and Others

You maintain a good reputation because you are responsible. Self-respect is a high regard for oneself because one behaves in responsible ways. Practicing abstinence is a responsible behavior. When you practice abstinence, you maintain self-respect. You show respect for others when you support their decision to be responsible by practicing abstinence. Other teens will respect you when you behave in responsible ways. Other teens will be comfortable and confident dating you because you do not pressure them to be sexually active. You will maintain your good reputation.

Practicing Abstinence Follows the Guidelines of Parents and of Other Responsible Adults

You avoid having conflicts with your parents or guardian because you follow their guidelines. Several surveys conducted by various groups indicate that as many as 97 percent of parents and guardians of teens want them to practice abstinence. Your parents or guardian want you to live a quality life. They set high standards for your behavior because they know you will benefit. They know the serious consequences that can occur from being sexually active. They want to protect you.

Practicing Abstinence Demonstrates Good Character

You are self-disciplined and can delay gratification in order to uphold your values. A **value** is a standard or belief. **Character** is a person's use of self-control to act on his/her values. When you have good character, you uphold family values and practice abstinence. You recognize the importance of delayed gratification. You postpone sexual intercourse until marriage. As a result, you do not feel guilty or anxious about your behavior. You can concentrate on other aspects of your life, including dating relationships.

How to Set Limits for Expressing Physical Affection

Each of us has a need to be liked, especially by those who are important to us. Liking includes both affection and respect. **Affection** is a fond or tender feeling that a person has toward another person. It is experienced as emotional warmth, or closeness.

Affection is expressed in different ways. Words such as "I like you" express affection. Physical touch also expresses affection.

Respect is high regard for someone or something. Respect for another person is high regard for this person's admirable characteristics and responsible and caring actions. In a relationship, there may be affection, respect, neither, or both.

Knowing how to set limits for expressing affection helps you maintain self-respect and the respect of a dating partner.

Setting limits helps you keep your sexual feelings under control. **Sexual feelings** are feelings that result from a strong physical and emotional attraction to another person. Sexual feelings may occur when you see a certain person, kiss or touch that person, look at a picture, or read certain material. Sexual feelings may occur when you have certain thoughts.

It is important for you to know how sexual feelings intensify when you express physical affection. When two people are attracted to each other, they may express physical affection by kissing or hugging. These ways of expressing physical affection are enjoyable. Kissing and hugging, in turn, may result in sexual feelings.

The couple's expressions of affection may not stop with a hug or a casual kiss. They may continue to prolonged kissing. Prolonged kissing further intensifies sexual feelings. Caressing or touching also strengthens sexual feelings. Intimate expressions of physical affection cause physical changes to occur in the body. There is increased blood flow to the reproductive organs. In the male, the penis fills with blood and becomes erect. This intensifies sexual feelings in the male. In the female, there is increased blood flow to the vagina, creating a warm feeling.

These physical changes prepare the body for sex even if the couple previously had decided to abstain from sex. Each of their bodies now says, "YES, I am ready for sex" even though their brains say, "NO, I do not want to be sexually active."

There is an important reason why you need to set limits on expressing affection in a physical manner. If you become too involved, your body's message "YES, I am ready to have sex," may attempt to override your brain's message "NO, I do not want to be sexually active." You need to keep your brain's message in charge in order to practice abstinence.

1. Limit your expressions of affection to hand holding, hugging, and casual kissing to keep your brain in control of your decisions and actions.

2. Tell a person your limits before expressing affection.

3. Do not date someone who does not respect your limits.

4. Avoid drinking alcohol and using other drugs that dull your brain and interfere with wise judgment.

5. Do not date someone who drinks alcohol or uses other drugs that dull his/her brain and interfere with his/her wise judgment.

How to Say NO If You Are Pressured to Be Sexually Active

Peer pressure exists in many situations throughout your life. However, peer pressure is most powerful during your teen years. As a teen you are searching for identity and discovering who you are. You are examining your values and learning ways to act on them. Your peers may challenge what you believe and how you behave. Unless you are very self-confident, you may weaken when you are challenged. You may weaken because you want to be liked and accepted. But, giving in to peers will not get you what you really need to be happy. Happiness is more a result of being respected for your values than being liked because you went along with the crowd. Consider this quote:

> The only way to be is me, then those who like me, like me.
>
> Hugh Prather, *Notes to Myself*

Do you understand what the quote means? The quote explains why you need to be yourself and act on your values. Unless you show others who you really are and what you really believe, they cannot really like you because they do not really know you. Do not be swayed to change your values.

Stick to your values so you can be at peace with yourself. Suppose you are challenged by your peers to be sexually active. They may try to convince you that all teens are sexually active. They may try to convince you that you will be more liked or accepted if you are sexually active. But, remember, you have to live with yourself. Giving in to peer pressure will not give you self-respect. And, peers usually lose respect for those who give in to them. Equip yourself with resistance skills.

Resistance skills are skills that help a person say NO to an action or to leave a situation. The next two pages contain a list of eight suggested ways to resist negative peer pressure to be sexually active.

Hold On... to What You've Got

Some teens feel empty inside. They may not feel loved and appreciated. They may not feel close to members of their families. For example, some teens have little or no contact with their fathers if their parents have divorced. These teens are at risk for becoming sexually active. They may believe that having sex will help them hold on to a boyfriend or girlfriend. They may believe that sex is a substitute for being loved and appreciated. But, having sex with a boyfriend or girlfriend does not stop empty feelings. AND, it does not help a teen hold on to a boyfriend or girlfriend. Hold on to what is really important—self-respect. If you feel empty...if you do not feel close to anyone...if a parent has abandoned you..., talk to your other parent, a counselor, or a teacher. These adults can help you deal with your empty feelings.

Turn the page to learn how to resist negative peer pressure to be sexually active.

How to Use Resistance Skills If You Are Pressured to Be Sexually Active

1. **Be confident and say "NO, I do not want to be sexually active."**

Look directly at the person to whom you are speaking. State your limits for expressing physical affection.

2. **Give reasons why you practice abstinence.**

Use the six questions from The Responsible Decision-Making Model to develop your reasons for saying "NO, I do not want to be sexually active."

I practice abstinence to promote my health.

- I do not want to become infected with HIV and develop AIDS.
- I do not want to become infected with other STDs, such as genital herpes and genital warts.
- I do not want to become a teenage parent.

I practice abstinence to protect the safety of others.

- I do not want to risk being a stressed teen parent who neglects or abuses a child.

I practice abstinence to follow laws.

- I do not want my partner or myself to be prosecuted for having sex with a minor.
- I do not want to be accused of date rape.

I practice abstinence to show respect for myself and others.

- I want to protect my good reputation and the reputation of others.
- I want to uphold my personal values.
- I want to protect my health and the health of others.

I practice abstinence to follow the guidelines of my parents and other responsible adults.

- I want to practice family values.
- I do not want to disappoint or disobey my parents or guardian.

I want to demonstrate good character.

- I want to have a good reputation.
- I do not want to feel guilty or anxious.
- I want to postpone sexual intercourse until marriage.

3. Use the broken record technique and repeat several times the same reason you practice abstinence.

For example, you might say, "NO, I do not want to be sexually active. I practice abstinence to promote my health. I do not want to become infected with HIV and develop AIDS." If you continue to get pressure, repeat this response several times. You will sound like a broken record. But, each time you give the same response you will be more convincing.

4. Use nonverbal behavior to support your message that you do not want to be sexually active.

Do not lead someone on or "go too far" when you express affection. These behaviors do not match the limits you have set.

5. Avoid being in situations in which you may be pressured to be sexually active.

Do not spend time in situations in which you might be vulnerable, such as being in someone's bedroom. Do not go to parties at which teens will be drinking alcohol or using other drugs. Avoid watching movies, videos, and television shows that imply teen sex is OK. Avoid reading books and magazines that are filled with pictures and stories that encourage teen sex.

6. Avoid being with anyone who pressures you to be sexually active.

Expect someone whom you are dating to respect your limits and do not date this person if (s)he pressures you to have sex. Avoid being with teens who brag about "scoring" or having "sexual conquests." Date people your own age. Older people may exert additional sexual pressure. Pay attention to what your parents or guardian say when they advise against being with certain teens.

7. Know the laws regarding sex that protect you and follow them.

Tell a parent or guardian if an adult makes sexual advances toward you. Tell a parent or guardian if you suspect date rape.

8. Influence your friends to practice abstinence.

Be confident and share with friends your decision to practice abstinence. Encourage a friend who is sexually active to practice abstinence.

How Teens Who Have Been Sexually Active Can Change Their Behavior

Wisdom is good judgment and intelligence in knowing what is responsible and appropriate. People gain wisdom as they gain more knowledge and experience. Some teens who have been sexually active in the past learn from their experience. They gain knowledge as they experience the negative consequences of their activity. They begin to recognize that being sexually active was not the best choice. They understand the benefits of sexual abstinence. They may feel guilty or anxious about their behavior. They may take another look at the facts—the risk of HIV infection, the risk of other STDs, unwanted parenthood. These teens may regret that they have not followed family guidelines. They may have given in to pressure to have sex and now they regret having done so. If you practice abstinence, you can be proud of your behavior. If you are sexually active, you must change your behavior.

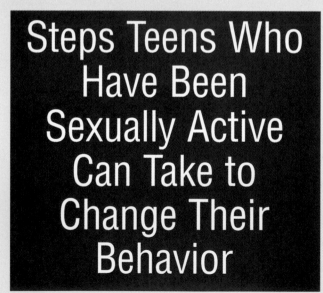

Steps Teens Who Have Been Sexually Active Can Take to Change Their Behavior

1. **Make a written list of your reasons for choosing abstinence.** Review this list often. The list will keep you aware of the risks you take when you are sexually active. It will serve as a constant reminder of why you should practice abstinence. For example, you may list "I do not want to become infected with HIV" or "I do not want to be pregnant or get someone pregnant."

2. **Talk to a trusted adult about your behavior and your decision to practice abstinence.** Your parents or guardian may be angry when they learn that you have been sexually active. However, they will support your decision to change your behavior. Remember, their role is to guide you. They can offer suggestions to strengthen you as you make changes. They can help you with the relationship in which you are involved. They can help you set new guidelines for expressing affection.

3. **Consider the health consequences that may have occurred from being sexually involved.** You and any sexual partners you have had may have become infected with HIV or another STD. You or your partner may be pregnant. With your parents or guardian, discuss appropriate examinations that may be needed.

4. **Set new guidelines for expressing affection.** Obviously, your old guidelines did not work. Be honest with yourself in order to avoid temptation. Remember, your parents or guardian can help you.

5. **Have a frank discussion with the partner with whom you were sexually involved.** Explain that you regret having been sexually active. Share your reasons for making a renewed commitment to practice abstinence.

6. **Get reassurance from your partner that (s)he will practice abstinence.** In a healthful relationship, two people acknowledge mistakes and work together to correct them. They help each other avoid temptation. They look at ways to improve the quality of their lives.

7. **Break off a relationship with a partner who will not agree to practice abstinence.** Remember, you have examined your values and beliefs and you know your decision is the right one. Any partner who continues to pressure you at this point does not really respect you.

8. **Reevaluate the influence of the group of friends with whom you associate.** Most people are drawn to friends who support what they are doing. This often is the case with people who are doing something wrong. They are most comfortable with friends who say it is OK to do whatever they are doing. In fact, these friends also may be choosing wrong actions. When you gain wisdom and want to change, these friends may want you to continue wrong actions. After all, if you change, they may have to think more about what they are doing. Any time you need to change your behavior, it is best to look at the role your friends play. If they support wrong behavior, they may be enablers. An **enabler** is a person who supports the harmful behavior of others. Avoid being with friends who are enablers. Instead, select friends who challenge you to be at your best. Select friends who pressure you to change wrong behavior.

9. **Be honest and direct about your commitment to practice abstinence in new relationships.** Get off to the right start when you begin new relationships. Set standards for expressing affection with dating partners. Stick to these standards.

10. **Avoid behaviors, such as using alcohol or other drugs and being in tempting situations, that impair your wise judgment.** You may have the best intentions and say you will practice abstinence. But, certain behaviors may affect your ability to stick to what you say you will do. Most teens who have been sexually active were under the influence of alcohol, placed themselves in tempting situations, or continued to "go too far" without setting limits.

Activity

Hook, Line, and Sinker

Life Skill: I will practice abstinence.

Materials: paper, pen or pencil

Directions: A line is a short statement that may have a "hook" to it. A line may be intended to "hook" you and "reel" you into doing something you should not do. Below are ten lines designed to hook you into being sexually active. Do not get reeled in if someone tries to hook you by using one of these lines. Respond by giving your reason for practicing abstinence. Refer to step 2 of How to Use Resistance Skills If You Are Pressured to Be Sexually Active on page 130. Consider how you would respond to each of the ten lines listed below using resistance skills. Number a sheet of paper from one to ten. Write a response to each line next to the corresponding number on your paper.

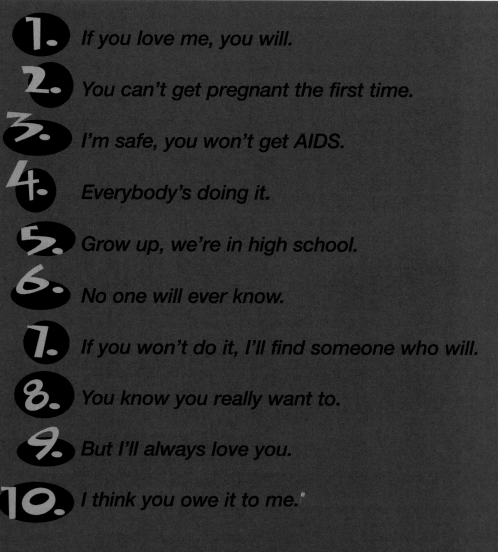

1. *If you love me, you will.*

2. *You can't get pregnant the first time.*

3. *I'm safe, you won't get AIDS.*

4. *Everybody's doing it.*

5. *Grow up, we're in high school.*

6. *No one will ever know.*

7. *If you won't do it, I'll find someone who will.*

8. *You know you really want to.*

9. *But I'll always love you.*

10. *I think you owe it to me.*

Lesson 16

Review

Vocabulary Words

Write a separate sentence using each of the vocabulary words listed on page 124.

Objectives

1. What are five reasons to wait until marriage to have sex? **Objective 1**

2. Why is it a responsible decision to practice abstinence? **Objective 2**

3. How can you set limits on expressing physical affection? **Objective 3**

4. What resistance skills can you use to say NO if you are pressured to be sexually active? **Objective 4**

5. What are ten steps teens who have been sexually active can take to change their behavior? **Objective 5**

Responsible Decision-Making

You really like one of your classmates. So far, you have spent time with this person only in a group with friends. Now you are finally alone with this person. (S)he holds your hand and you feel something really special. (S)he says (s)he is really turned on and begins to touch you. You do not want to go too far. Write a response to this situation.

1. Describe the situation that requires you to make a decision.
2. List possible decisions you might make.
3. Name two responsible adults with whom you might discuss your decisions.
4. Evaluate the possible consequences of your decisions. Determine if each decision will lead to actions that:
   • promote health,
   • protect safety,
   • follow laws,
   • show respect for yourself and others,
   • follow the guidelines of your parents and of other responsible adults,
   • demonstrate good character.
5. Decide which decision is most responsible and appropriate.
6. Tell two results you expect if you make this decision.

 ### Effective Communication

Pretend you are an advice columnist for a teen magazine. A teen who is sexually active writes you. This teen wants to change his/her behavior and practice abstinence but does not want to lose his/her boyfriend or girlfriend. Write a response addressing this teen's concerns.

 ### Self-Directed Learning

In this lesson, you learned that the number of AIDS cases in teens and young adults increased more than 75 percent in the last few years. Check the library or Internet for additional statistics that support the importance of choosing abstinence. Make a written or printed copy of the statistics you locate to share with your classmates.

 ### Critical Thinking

You and a friend are discussing sex. Your friend says, "I like to go a little bit farther each time I date. I can always stop if things get too heated." Your friend has ignored how the body and mind work when a person has sexual feelings for someone. Write a paragraph explaining why your friend needs to set limits for expressing physical affection.

 ### Responsible Citizenship

Be an abstinence advocate. Evaluate social activities in which teens in your community can participate. Develop a list of healthful activities in which teens can participate on a date.

You Can Recognize Harmful Relationships

Life Skill **I will recognize harmful relationships.**

A **relationship** is a connection a person has with another person. Your health status is affected by the quality of the relationships you have with others. You may have different kinds of relationships. In general, relationships are usually healthful or harmful. A **healthful relationship** is a relationship that promotes self-respect, encourages productivity and health, and is free of violence and/or drug misuse and abuse. A **harmful relationship** is a relationship that harms self-respect, interferes with productivity and health, and includes violence and/or drug misuse and abuse. This lesson describes how and why people relate to each other in harmful ways. You will learn why people get involved in harmful relationships. You will learn what you can do if any of your relationships are harmful.

Vocabulary Words

relationship

healthful relationship

harmful relationship

people pleaser

enabler

clinger

fixer

distancer

controller

center

abuser

liar

promise breaker

The Lesson Outline

How People Relate in Harmful Ways

Why People Get Involved in Harmful Relationships

What to Do About Harmful Relationships

Objectives

1. Identify behaviors associated with the Ten Profiles of People Who Relate in Harmful Ways. **pages 137–139**

2. Explain why people get involved in harmful relationships. **pages 140–141**

3. Outline what to do about harmful relationships. **page 142**

How People Relate in Harmful Ways

Some people lack self-respect. They are not interested in the health of others. They do not encourage others to be productive and to do their best. They relate with others in harmful ways.

Ten Profiles of People Who Relate in Harmful Ways

1. The People Pleaser

The **people pleaser** is a person who constantly seeks the approval of others. A people pleaser will do almost anything to be liked. This may include harmful behavior, such as using alcohol or other drugs. Other people describe a people pleaser as a "doormat" because they can walk all over the people pleaser with no consequences. The people pleaser sabotages the chance to have healthful relationships because others do not respect him/her.

The People Pleaser:

- Seeks the approval of others
- Will do anything to be liked
- Is a "doormat"

2. The Enabler

The **enabler** is a person who supports the harmful behavior of others. The enabler may deny what another person does. For example, the enabler may overlook another person's drinking, gambling, or cheating. The enabler may make excuses or cover up for another person. The enabler also may contribute to another person's harmful behavior. For example, the enabler may place a bet for a friend who has a gambling problem or drink with a person who is a problem drinker. The enabler sabotages the chance to have healthful relationships when (s)he does not expect other people to behave in responsible ways. As a result, the enabler cannot get his/her own needs for attention, affection, and support met.

The Enabler:

- Supports the harmful behavior of others
- Makes excuses for the wrong behavior of others
- Denies his/her feelings

3. The Clinger

The **clinger** is a person who is needy and dependent. The clinger feels empty inside and constantly turns to another person to feel better. When the clinger has this person's attention or affection, the clinger feels better. But, no amount of attention or affection keeps the clinger fulfilled. The clinger keeps demanding more and eventually "suffocates" the other person because the clinger wants all of the other person's time or attention. The clinger sabotages the chance to have healthful relationships by not giving other people space. When people pull away, the clinger is threatened and clings even more.

The Clinger:
- Is needy and dependent
- Chases and clings to others
- Suffocates others

4. The Fixer

The **fixer** is a person who tries to fix other people's problems. The fixer takes on problems that are not his/her responsibility but are the responsibility of another person. The fixer is quick to give advice. (S)he will identify different possible solutions to the other person's problems and try them for the person. In the process of getting involved with someone else's problems, the fixer avoids his/her own feelings and problems. The fixer sabotages the chance to have healthful relationships because healthy people do not want others to solve their problems. Healthy people solve their own problems with the support of others. They do not want others to "take over."

The Fixer:
- Tries to fix other people's problems
- Is quick to give advice
- Takes over other people's responsibilities

5. The Distancer

The **distancer** is a person who is emotionally unavailable to others. There are a number of ways that the distancer keeps other people from getting too close. The distancer may be too busy to spend time with other people. The distancer may avoid sharing feelings. The distancer keeps others at a distance so (s)he will not get hurt. The distancer sabotages the chance to have healthful relationships by not risking emotional involvement.

The Distancer:
- Is emotionally unavailable
- Avoids sharing feelings
- Keeps people at arm's length

6. The Controller

The **controller** is a person who is possessive, jealous, and domineering. The controller seeks power. The controller may tell another person what to do, what to wear, and what to believe. The controller does not like to share the object of his/her attention with anyone else. The controller may monopolize a boyfriend's or girlfriend's time. The controller sabotages the chance to have healthful relationships by not respecting the interests or opinions of others. Healthy people want to participate in the decisions made in a relationship. A person may be fearful of a controller, and with good reason. You may have seen media coverage of teens who harmed their boyfriend or girlfriend. In many instances, the teen causing the harm was a controller. There may have been signs of jealous and possessive behavior before the harm occurred, but they were not recognized or dealt with. Trust your feelings if ever you feel someone is being too jealous or possessive of you. Talk to a trusted adult.

The Controller:
- Is possessive, jealous, and domineering
- Does not respect the will of others
- Demands his/her own way

7. The Center

The **center** is a person who is self-centered. It is almost as if the center is wearing a badge that says, "ME, ME, ME." Talk to the center on the telephone, and the center will do most of the talking. But the center will not show much interest in what you have to say. The center wants to do what the center wants to do, when the center wants to do it. And, the center is not too concerned about what other people want to do or how other people feel. The center sabotages the chance to have healthful relationships by being so focused on being the center of attention that the needs of others are ignored.

The Center:

- Is self-centered
- Does the talking but not the listening
- Ignores the needs of others

8. The Abuser

The **abuser** is a person who is abusive. The abuser may constantly put down others or cause others personal harm. The abuser may threaten others, begin fights, and act in violent ways. The abuser may force someone to have sex. Other people find the abuser's behavior confusing. This is because the abuser may follow acts of abuse with periods of gentleness. However, the abusive behavior returns. An abuser may miss the chance to have healthful relationships by threatening and harming others. Stay away from a person you suspect may be an abuser. This person can cause you physical or emotional harm.

The Abuser:

- Is abusive
- Puts down others
- Threatens and harms others

9. The Liar

The **liar** is a person who does not tell the truth. Honesty is a foundation in any healthful relationship. People base their responses on what you tell them in your conversations and actions. When a liar does not tell the truth, other people make responses based on false information. Other people say and do things they might not have said or done had they known the truth. This is exactly what the liar wants. The liar may lie about himself/herself to try to look good. For example, the liar may pretend to be something (s)he is not, in order to impress others. His/her relationships are based on lies. The liar avoids the truth to manipulate others into the responses the liar wants. The liar sabotages the chance to have healthful relationships by lying to others to get the response (s)he wants.

The Liar:

- Does not tell the truth
- Builds relationships based on lies
- Manipulates others into the responses (s)he wants

10. The Promise Breaker

The **promise breaker** is a person who is not reliable. The promise breaker will make plans with another person and be a "no show." The promise breaker often makes plans with another person and changes them if something better comes along. The promise breaker may agree to change annoying behaviors but does not make the changes. The promise breaker sabotages the chance to have healthful relationships by not keeping his/her word. Other people doubt the promise breaker's sincerity and commitment.

The Promise Breaker:

- Is unreliable
- Makes plans and cancels them
- Agrees to change behavior and does not do so

Why People Get Involved in
Harmful Relationships

You need to understand the interaction in harmful relationships. People who relate in harmful ways often are drawn to each other. They have a magnetic attraction toward being in a relationship together. Being together helps each of them play out his/her profile as a people pleaser, enabler, clinger, fixer, distancer, controller, center, abuser, liar, or promise breaker. The following examples can help you understand why some people end up in harmful relationships.

Match-Up:

A Promise Breaker and a People Pleaser

The promise breaker makes plans to go to a movie with a people pleaser. When the promise breaker gets another more interesting invitation, (s)he cancels the plans. The people pleaser is angry but keeps the anger inside. The people pleaser accommodates the promise breaker and agrees to go to the movie at a later date.

Suppose you are a friend of the promise breaker. (S)he mentions (s)he cancelled plans with someone to do something more interesting. Would you approve of what the promise breaker did? You do not know the other person in that relationship is a people pleaser, so you do not recognize that (s)he too is relating in a harmful way. But, if you knew the interaction of the two people in the relationship, you would have known that both people relate in harmful ways. The promise breaker needs to learn to keep commitments. The people pleaser must set limits and share his/her feelings.

Match-Up:

A Controller and an Enabler

The controller is a very jealous teen male who demands all of his girlfriend's attention. He objects when she spends time with her girlfriends. He has angry outbursts if a male classmate speaks to her. The controller is very suspicious and accuses his girlfriend of seeing other guys. She is an enabler and makes excuses for him. She convinces herself "He loves me so much that he wants me with him all the time." She gives up her friends to spend all her time with him. She supports his wrong behavior.

Suppose the female is your friend and she tells you about her boyfriend's love for her. From what she says, you might think she is in a very loving relationship. You might not recognize that this is a harmful relationship and that both of them relate in harmful ways. The boyfriend must respect his girlfriend's right to have friends and encourage her to run her own life. The girlfriend must take responsibility for her life and not deny her own feelings and needs.

Match-Up:

A Clinger and a Distancer

The clinger is a female who was raised in a divorced family. Her father abandoned the family when she was ten years old, and she rarely speaks with him. She was very hurt and feels the loss of her father's presence in the home. Deep down inside, she fears that she will be abandoned again. As a result, she is afraid to be vulnerable and close. She becomes attracted to a distancer. The distancer is the perfect match because he is emotionally unavailable.

Both the clinger and the distancer are afraid to be close. They protect themselves in different ways. The clinger chases someone who cannot be close. The distancer runs away from relationships and does not get emotionally involved with the clinger. He spends some time with her and then backs off. She then chases harder. They continue to play into each other's game. Both the clinger and the distancer must change to have healthful relationships. The clinger must address the emptiness (s)he feels and develop greater self-confidence. The distancer must address his/her fears of sharing feelings and becoming close to others.

Changing Profiles in Different Relationships

There are many match-ups of people who relate in harmful ways, such as a center and a fixer, and a people pleaser and an abuser. It is important to know that a person can be described one way in one relationship and a different way in another relationship. For example, suppose a female has several close friends but is an enabler only when she is with her boyfriend. She needs to examine what it is about this relationship that causes her to relate in harmful ways.

What to Do About
Harmful Relationships

1. **Evaluate each of your relationships on a regular basis.**

   - List ways you relate to others that concern you.
   - List ways another person relates to you that concern you.
   - Ask a parent, guardian, or other trusted adult to review the lists with you. This adult may recognize behaviors in one of your relationships that you do not recognize.

2. **Recognize when you must end a harmful relationship rather than work to change it.**

   - End a relationship with anyone who chooses illegal behavior.
   - End a relationship with anyone who threatens your health or safety.
   - End a relationship when your parents or guardian ask you to do so.
   - Get help from a trusted adult if the harmful relationship is with a family member.

3. **Identify changes in behavior that must occur in any existing harmful relationship that you would like to continue.**

   - List changes you expect in yourself. For example, you might write, "I will not make plans and cancel them because I have something better to do."
   - List changes you expect the other person to make. For example, you might write, "I expect (person's name) to tell the truth at all times."

4. **Talk to a parent, guardian, or other trusted adult about the changes you expect in the relationship.**

   - Share your concerns about the relationship.
   - Share the behaviors you expect to change.
   - Share the behaviors you expect the other person to change.
   - Discuss whether your expectations are realistic.
   - Discuss whether or not it is wise to continue the relationship.
   - Discuss your other relationships. Do you notice any similarities?
   - Discuss ways to improve your relationship skills.

5. **Have a frank discussion with the other person in the relationship in which you share your concerns and expectations.**

   - Identify your concerns and your expectations.
   - Ask the other person to identify his/her concerns and expectations.
   - Discuss whether or not the relationship should be continued.
   - Make a plan to work on the relationship if you want to continue together.

6. **Set a future date in which you will evaluate the relationship again.**

   - Identify a realistic time frame for making the necessary changes.
   - Evaluate whether or not your expectations have been fulfilled.

Lesson 17

Review

Vocabulary Words

Write a separate sentence using each of the vocabulary words listed on page 136.

Objectives

1. What are three behaviors that describe each of the following people: people pleaser, enabler, clinger, fixer, distancer, controller, center, abuser, liar, promise breaker? **Objective 1**

2. Why do people get involved in harmful relationships? **Objective 2**

3. Why might a controller match up with an enabler? **Objective 2**

4. Why might a teen have several healthful friendships but relate to a boyfriend or girlfriend in harmful ways? **Objective 2**

5. What might a teen do about harmful relationships? **Objective 3**

Responsible Decision-Making

Your friend always complains about her boyfriend: "My boyfriend doesn't treat me well." "He spends more time with his friends than he spends with me." "He always is looking at other girls." "The only time we spend together is when he doesn't have anything better to do." Your friend often says that she wants to break up with her boyfriend, but she continues to date him. Write a response to this situation.

1. Describe the situation that requires your friend to make a decision.

2. List possible decisions your friend might make.

3. Name two responsible adults with whom your friend might discuss his/her decisions.

4. Evaluate the possible consequences of your friend's decisions. Determine if each decision will lead to actions that:
   • promote health,
   • protect safety,
   • follow laws,
   • show respect for your friend and others,
   • follow the guidelines of your friend's parents and of other responsible adults,
   • demonstrate good character.

5. Decide which decision is most responsible and appropriate for your friend.

6. Tell two results your friend can expect if (s)he makes this decision.

 Effective Communication

This lesson included different examples of relationship match-ups. Select a match-up that was not discussed in the lesson. Write a paragraph to explain why the two people you have selected get involved in a match-up and what the consequences would be.

 Self-Directed Learning

Select an adult you trust, such as your parent or guardian. Ask this person to review one of your relationships with you. Refer to the six steps on page 142.

 Critical Thinking

Suppose you have many healthful relationships. However, with a certain friend you are a people pleaser. This friend is a controller. Why might you be a people pleaser with this friend? What steps can you take to change the relationship?

 Responsible Citizenship

Share with a friend or family member the information you have learned about harmful relationships. Explain how the friend or family member can use the information to evaluate his/her relationships.

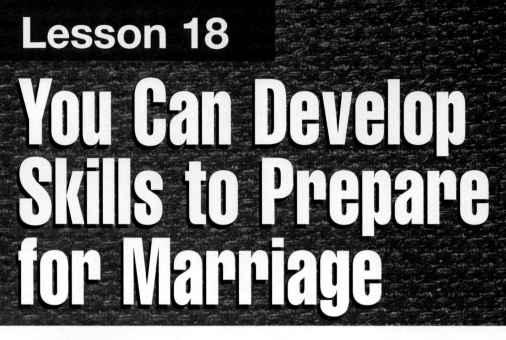

You Can Develop Skills to Prepare for Marriage

Life Skill I will develop skills to prepare for marriage.

A **traditional marriage** is an emotional, spiritual, and legal commitment a man and woman make to one another. Most people marry at least once and have high expectations for their marriage. Marriage provides intimacy and companionship as well as feelings of well-being. Marriage provides a framework for sustaining the family unit and having and raising children. Although you are not ready for marriage right now, you can learn information that will help you make decisions in the future. This lesson will include information on the marriage relationship. You will learn factors that help predict success in marriage. You will learn about the marriage commitment. This lesson also will focus on why teen marriage is risky.

The Lesson Outline

What to Know About the Marriage Relationship

How to Predict Success in Marriage

What to Know About the Marriage Commitment

Why Teen Marriage Is Risky

Objectives

1. Explain the four kinds of intimacy in marriage. **page 145**

2. Identify ten factors used to predict success in marriage. **page 146**

3. Explain two important ways marriage partners can ensure that their marriage will last. **page 147**

4. Explain how teen marriage interferes with mastery of the eight developmental tasks of adolescence. **pages 149–150**

Vocabulary Words

traditional marriage

intimacy

philosophical intimacy

psychological intimacy

creative intimacy

physical intimacy

developmental stages of marriage

developmental task

puberty

What to Know About the
Marriage Relationship

You are not ready for marriage right now. However, your high school education is helping you prepare for your future. You are gaining information and skills to use as an adult. You already have learned something about marriage by observing your parents, guardian, and other adults who are married or have been married. From them, you may have learned something about intimacy.

Intimacy is a deep and meaningful kind of sharing between two people. There are many kinds of intimacy but, for a marriage to be sustained over the years, four kinds of intimacy are of particular importance. The four kinds of intimacy are: philosophical, psychological, creative, and physical.

Philosophical intimacy is the sharing of beliefs and values. Marriage partners share how their beliefs influence their decisions. Marriage partners share the values that determine their day-to-day priorities. For example, one partner might value his/her relationship with parents. As a result, spending holidays with parents is a priority to this partner. The other partner recognizes and respects this priority even though this particular value may not be as important to him/her.

Psychological intimacy is the sharing of needs, emotions, weaknesses, and strengths. Marriage partners share their needs, such as the need for a hug or the need to have someone who will listen. Marriage partners share and rejoice in their individual successes. They ask one another for support when a disappointment occurs. When they share weaknesses, they feel accepted rather than rejected. Psychological intimacy deepens through the years.

Creative intimacy is the sharing of efforts to accomplish tasks and projects. This kind of sharing goes beyond discussion and emotional responses. Marriage partners engage in many cooperative efforts. For example, they may work together to make their apartment or house a home. They may choose furniture together, plant a garden, and select wallpaper. Marriage partners may plan a vacation together. They may take lessons to learn a sport they can enjoy together. Raising children also involves creative intimacy. Marriage partners plan activities in which they can participate with their children. They share child-raising responsibilities, such as discipline. For marriage partners to have creative intimacy, each partner must do his/her share of the work with a willing attitude. Marriage partners must agree on expectations and on who does what.

Physical intimacy is the sharing of physical affection. Physical intimacy includes a wide range of behaviors that express warmth and closeness. Marriage partners show physical affection when they touch, caress, hold hands, and kiss. Marriage partners express physical affection when they have sexual intercourse. To be physically intimate, marriage partners should be sexually attracted to one another. Each marriage partner should have a healthful attitude about sex. Each marriage partner needs the commitment and security of marriage. The commitment that the marriage partners make to each other provides a real sense of security to each partner. This enhances physical intimacy.

Potential marriage partners can assess the warmth and closeness that each partner feels for the other without having sexual intercourse. **FACT: Sex before marriage DOES NOT predict sexual satisfaction during marriage. Remember, it is a responsible decision to wait until marriage to have sex. Sex before marriage does not involve a commitment. So, there is no feeling of security. Real intimacy is not involved.**

How to Predict Success in Marriage

There are factors that help predict whether or not a marriage will be a success. These factors appear in the chart Ten Factors Used to Predict Success in Marriage.

Ten Factors Used to Predict Success in Marriage

1. **Age.** Couples who marry during their teen years have a high divorce rate. Couples who marry when they are in their twenties or older usually enjoy more success. Marriage partners who are similar in age have greater success in marriage than marriage partners with large age differences because they are at similar stages of development.

2. **Reasons for marriage.** Couples who marry to love and nurture one another and to share intimacy are more likely to succeed at marriage than those who marry to escape a difficult and unhappy family situation, to get even with parents, or to escape loneliness.

3. **Length of the relationship and engagement.** Longer relationships and engagements provide the opportunity for couples to examine their relationship and to develop intimacy. Longer relationships are usually associated with success in marriage.

4. **Similar attitudes about children and child-raising.** Discussing attitudes toward having and raising children contributes to a successful marriage. Couples should discuss these issues before they are married: if and when they want children, how many children they want, how they intend to raise their children. Couples should work through any disagreement on these issues before they are married.

5. **Similar interests.** Although marriages can sustain differences in interests, the old saying "opposites attract" may not apply when predicting success at marriage. Differences provide stressors that must be worked out. Studies report that couples who are similar with regard to race, ethnic background, religious beliefs, socioeconomic status, education, and intelligence are more likely to succeed at marriage.

6. **Commitment to sexual fidelity.** Physical intimacy in marriage provides a closeness and a feeling of security. Sexual fidelity is important in establishing trust. Couples who honor a commitment to sexual fidelity and who trust each other are more likely to succeed at marriage.

7. **Good character.** People who have good character make responsible decisions. They are self-disciplined. They are aware that their actions will affect the quality of their marriage.

8. **Parents' success at marriage.** People whose parents are divorced are more likely to get divorced themselves. This may be because they have not lived in a family in which parents resolved conflicts and maintained their marriage.

9. **Parental attitudes toward the potential marriage partner.** A marriage is more likely to succeed when a person's parents approve of the future husband or wife.

10. **Careful selection of marriage partner.** A marriage is more likely to succeed when people are cautious when selecting a mate. This includes using the factors that contribute to successful marriage when considering a partner.

What to Know About the
Marriage Commitment

Today, because of rising divorce rates, it seems wise to examine two important ways marriage partners can help ensure that their marriage will last.

1. **Marriage partners must be committed to actions that honor their wedding vows.**

2. **Marriage partners must work together to master the developmental stages of marriage.**

Marriage partners must be committed to actions that honor their wedding vows. When two people marry, they take vows, or make promises. This is what commitment is. Yet, there are two ways partners can view marriage. One view of marriage is commitment-motivated: "I will behave in my marriage in the ways I have promised." Another view of marriage is feelings-motivated: "I will behave in my marriage according to how I feel about my marriage at the moment."

Examine the difference between these two views of marriage and the potential consequences. A partner who is commitment-motivated behaves as (s)he says (s)he will rather than as (s)he happens to "feel" at the time. Suppose this partner does not "feel" like being supportive of the other person's needs but uses discipline to do so to honor the marriage commitment. Suppose this partner does not "feel" like being sexually faithful, but uses discipline to say, "NO" to tempting situations. When a partner acts in these ways without feeling resentment, (s)he indicates that the marriage commitment is a priority. These kinds of actions reinforce the marriage commitment.

Now examine the opposite type of marriage. Suppose a partner believes in a feelings-motivated marriage. This partner believes how (s)he feels at any given moment determines whether or not (s)he should keep the vows that were made. When this partner "feels" like loving the other partner at times during the marriage, the marriage thrives. But suppose, at times, the partner does not "feel" like being loving or being loved. The partner may not "feel" like being supportive or listening or being faithful. The partner decides to honor these "feelings" rather than the promises made in the wedding vows. Habits that interfere with the marriage commitment begin to creep into the marriage. This partner acts on these feelings and is not supportive, doesn't listen and is not sexually faithful. The consequences are loss of trust, loss of security, and loss of commitment.

Responsible actions cause good "feelings;" however, "feelings" may or may not cause responsible actions. A commitment involves responsible actions. No one can promise how (s)he will feel for a lifetime; however, (s)he can promise how (s)he will act.

Marriage partners must work together to master the developmental stages of marriage. The **developmental stages of marriage** are five stages of marriage during which couples must master certain tasks in order to develop and maintain intimacy. The five stages and the tasks to be mastered in each stage are identified on the next page in The Major Tasks of the Five Stages of Marriage. The appropriateness of the tasks within each stage depends on the ages of the married partners and the length of the marriage. The tasks are designed for people who marry in their twenties and stay married to the same person. People who marry much younger or much older may experience other stressors that affect the tasks. They may need to master tasks from different stages at the same time. These people may be working on tasks that are different from those of their peers who married in their twenties and stayed married.

The Major Tasks of the Five Stages of Marriage

The First Stage:

The First Two Years

The newly married couple overcome their idealistic notions of marriage and begin to form a family. The partners strive to:

- maintain individual identity at the same time as they form a family;
- develop cooperation and reduce the need to control the other;
- develop a sexual bond with the other that leads to deeper intimacy;
- develop an effective decision-making style;
- recognize the difficulties in their parents' marriages and anticipate how those difficulties might affect their marriage.

The Second Stage:

The Third Through the Tenth Year

The couple gain a realistic view of their marriage and of one another and must settle into dealing with their individual weaknesses and make an effort to avoid dysfunctional behaviors. Their goals are to:

- recognize and confront the weaknesses of both partners;
- examine relationships and avoid dysfunctional behaviors;
- reaffirm commitment to sexual intimacy, including sexual fidelity;
- examine the influence of children on marriage and to agree upon child-raising methods.

The Third Stage:

The Eleventh Through the Twenty-fifth Year

The couple establish and maintain individual identity and deal with issues of forgiveness, aging, adolescent children, and intimacy. They recognize the need to:

- reexamine and maintain individual identity and develop mutual dependence;
- recognize that one another will not be perfect;
- forgive one another for shortcomings and mistakes;
- confront the crises of middle age, including aging, sexuality, and job and financial security; they struggle for individuality;
- reevaluate and make a plan for maintaining and developing intimacy.

The Fourth Stage:

The Twenty-sixth Through the Thirty-fifth Year

The couple must master tasks from the first three stages that were not previously mastered, confront changes in sexuality, and grieve over their losses. They determine to:

- reevaluate the tasks from the previous stages and determine if they have been successfully mastered;
- recognize the physical changes that accompany aging and affect sexuality and to rekindle romance;
- grieve over losses such as the death of parents and children leaving home.

The Fifth Stage:

The Thirty-sixth Year and On

The couple find new reasons for existing after the major life tasks of achieving financial security and nurturing their family have been completed; partners confront their feelings about death. They agree to:

- prepare for retirement;
- renew intimacy and develop ways to continue sexual intimacy;
- prepare for death and for the death of the marriage partner;
- accept death as a stage of life.

Adapted from *Passages of Marriage*, Appendix, Thomas Nelson Publishers, 1991.

Why Teen Marriage Is Risky

One way to reduce the number of separations and divorces is to reduce the number of teen marriages. More than 75 percent of teen marriages end in divorce. There are many reasons why teen marriages do not succeed. Teens need to master the developmental tasks of adolescence before tackling the tasks that are appropriate for the stages of marriage. Robert Havinghurst, a sociologist, identified eight developmental tasks of adolescence. A **developmental task** is an achievement that needs to be mastered to reach the next level of maturity. The following discussion explains why teen marriage interferes with reaching the next level of maturity necessary for a successful marriage.

> Teens who marry do not have enough time to work on the developmental tasks of adolescence. Instead, married teens must work on the tasks of the early stages of marriage.

Task 1:
Teen marriage does not give you enough time to...
Develop healthful friendships with members of both sexes.

During adolescence, you need to have friendships with members of both sexes. You need to learn how to communicate and how to develop friendships. You need to be selective and learn to evaluate your friendships. To do this, you must identify characteristics of people you admire. Examining issues such as trust, honesty, and loyalty is important. Having friendships with members of both sexes helps you learn more about yourself, which is an important aspect of forming personal identity. You need to gain a sense of who you are. Teen marriage cuts short the time you need to develop friendships with members of both sexes. Teens who marry are less likely to have a support network of mature friends who will be helpful during the stressful first years of marriage.

Task 2:
Teen marriage does not give you enough time to...
Become comfortable with your maleness or femaleness.

Dating helps you learn to respond to people of the opposite sex. Having the opportunity to date different people is very beneficial. You can test ways of interacting you have learned from your role models. You may become aware of harmful patterns in your behavior and the need for change. Teens who marry are robbed of the time they need to become comfortable with their maleness or femaleness. They pass up much of the fun that their peers have participating in social activities.

Task 3:
Teen marriage does not give you enough time to...
Become comfortable with your body.

Your body is still growing and developing. Hormonal changes that accompany puberty cause new feelings as well as body changes. **Puberty** is the stage of growth and development when both the male and female body become capable of producing offspring. You may notice that your moods change. You need time to adjust to these changes in your emotions. You need time to be comfortable with changes in your body. Teens who marry may do so because they have a strong sexual attraction to one another. They may lack the skills needed to tell the difference between love and sexual attraction. As a result, they make mistakes in selecting a marriage partner.

Task 4:
Teen marriage does not give you enough time to...
Become emotionally independent from adults.

One of the reasons teens are described as rebellious is that they challenge their parents or guardian. You may have challenged your parents or guardian as a way to show your independence. At times you still may want to be dependent on your parents or guardian, while at other times you want to break away from their influence. This is normal. After all, you are learning to be an adult and preparing to run your own life. During your teen years, you need the safety and security your parents or guardians provide. They help you test your ways of becoming independent. Teens who marry are faced with adulthood without the safety and security of being parented themselves when they really need it. If they marry and live with parents or guardians who continue in the parent role, the teens are unable to master one of the primary tasks of the first stage of marriage—to mold into one family with their partner.

Task 5:
Teen marriage does not give you enough time to...
Learn skills you will need later for a successful marriage and parenthood.

As teens mature and complete different developmental tasks, they acquire skills they can use later when they marry and become parents. Teens need to develop effective communication skills to help them achieve intimacy in adulthood. Intimacy is a deep and meaningful kind of sharing between two people. Teens also need to develop conflict resolution skills to learn how to settle disagreements when they are married and become parents. Teens who marry do not have time to fully develop these and other skills necessary for marriage and parenthood.

Task 6:
Teen marriage does not give you enough time to...
Prepare for a career.

During adolescence, you are gaining skills and knowledge about yourself to help you prepare for a career. Your education should be a top priority. Your goal is to have the skills needed to get a job, support yourself, and be financially independent. Teens who marry usually have difficulty completing their education. When they try to get a job, they have difficulty competing with their skilled peers who stayed in school. As a result, they earn less money. If they rely on parents or a guardian for financial support, they are not able to achieve their own financial independence. Living with very limited income places stress on marriage.

Task 7:
Teen marriage does not give you enough time to...
Have a clear set of values to guide your behavior.

A value is a standard or belief. Your parents or guardians have taught you many values that have helped to guide your choices and behavior. As an adolescent, you are beginning to achieve emotional independence from your parents or guardian. As a result, you have time to take a second look at the values you have learned from your parents or guardian. You gain confidence when you move from "these are my parents' or guardian's values" to "these are my values." Teens who marry may do so before they are certain of their own values. They may marry someone who has different values.

Task 8:
Teen marriage does not give you enough time to...
Understand and achieve socially responsible behavior.

Adolescence has been described as the "me" stage. During early and middle adolescence, you may focus on your needs. You may spend much time thinking about your appearance, your social life, and your friends. In the next few years, this focus will change. You will look at the world around you and identify ways to be helpful. Teens who marry do not have the time to get involved in their community and help others. The demands of a teen marriage take up all of their time.

Lesson 18

Review

Vocabulary Words

Write a separate sentence using each of the vocabulary words listed on page 144.

Objectives

1. What are four kinds of intimacy in marriage? **Objective 1**

2. What are ten factors used to predict success in marriage? **Objective 2**

3. What are two important ways marriage partners can ensure that their marriage will last? **Objective 3**

4. What are the five stages of marriage and what are examples of tasks to master in each stage? **Objective 3**

5. How does teen marriage interfere with the mastery of the eight developmental tasks of adolescence? **Objective 4**

Responsible Decision-Making

Suppose you have a classmate who is considering getting married. Her boyfriend proposed to her, but she still has not given an answer. Your classmate has plans to go to college and follow a career. However, she is seriously considering the proposal. Write a response to this situation.

1. Describe the situation that requires your classmate to make a decision.

2. List possible decisions your classmate might make.

3. Name two responsible adults with whom your classmate might discuss his/her decisions.

4. Evaluate the possible consequences of your classmate's decisions. Determine if each decision will lead to actions that:
   • promote health,
   • protect safety,
   • follow laws,
   • show respect for your classmate and others,
   • follow the guidelines of your classmate's parents and of other responsible adults,
   • demonstrate good character.

5. Decide which decision is most responsible and appropriate for your classmate.

6. Tell two results your classmate can expect if (s)he makes this decision.

 Effective Communication

Design a symbol to represent a committed marriage. Explain to classmates the meaning of your symbol.

 Self-Directed Learning

Interview a parent, guardian, or other responsible adult who is or has been married. Ask this person about the elements of a successful marriage. What factors have made his/her marriage successful or unsuccessful? Write a summary of the interview. Be prepared to share your findings with your classmates.

 Critical Thinking

The sixth developmental task of adolescence is to prepare for a career. Suppose you marry as a teen. Will you have enough time to finish school and prepare for a career? How might teen marriage affect your plans for a career?

 Responsible Citizenship

Part of being a responsible citizen is following laws. Check the library or Internet for information regarding teen marriage. What laws govern teen marriage? Do different states have different laws concerning teen marriage? Share the information with your classmates.

Lesson 19

You Can Develop Skills to Prepare for Parenthood

Life Skill **I will develop skills to prepare for parenthood.**

Someday you may choose to be a parent. If you make this choice, you will need certain knowledge and skills. Even if you do not become a parent, it is important to know about parenthood. This lesson will discuss the factors that should be considered before becoming a parent and the responsibilities that parents must be willing to assume. You will examine different discipline techniques. This lesson will discuss four kinds of child abuse. You will learn the difference between discipline and child abuse. You also will learn the importance of breaking the cycle of child abuse.

The Lesson Outline

Before Becoming a Parent
How to Be a Responsible Parent
What to Know About Child Abuse

Objectives

1. Explain the three "Rs" (Reasons, Resources, Responsibilities) to consider before becoming a parent. **pages 153–154**
2. Explain what it means to be a responsible parent. **pages 155–156**
3. Discuss child abuse and how to break the cycle of abuse. **pages 157–158**

Vocabulary Words

parent
philosophical intimacy
psychological intimacy
creative intimacy
physical intimacy
discipline
preventive discipline
behavior modification
logical consequences discipline
physical punishment
abuse
physical abuse
emotional abuse
neglect
sexual abuse
incest
cycle of abuse

Before Becoming a Parent

Most teens look forward to having their driver's license. Do you look forward to having yours or do you already have it? To get a driver's license, you must pass a written test and a test that demonstrates your skills. To prepare for the written test you must read a manual that contains the motor vehicle laws for your state. You also prepare by practicing your driving skills. In most states, a temporary license is issued and you practice driving while accompanied by a licensed driver. You may take a driver's training course in school or in your community. Your driver's license indicates that you have the required knowledge and skills needed to be a responsible driver. This protects not only you but others as well. No one who does not have a license should drive a car. Now, think about being a parent. There is no license that is required before becoming a parent. There is no written test and no test of parenting skills. Yet, being a parent is one of the most important tasks in our society.

Most teens who are parents did not want to be parents at the time they learned of the pregnancy. Some teens do want to be parents, but their reasons for wanting a baby usually are not appropriate—to get even with parents, to keep a boyfriend, to have someone to love. This lesson will discuss being a responsible adult and a parent.

When you are a responsible adult, your marital status and the quality of your marriage are important if you are considering parenthood. Children benefit from living with a loving father and mother who are married and respect one another. Many children do not live with both their parents. Perhaps a parent died. Perhaps their parents are divorced. The parent with whom they live may be very loving and have parenting skills. Some children live with both parents, but only one is loving and the other is abusive. These kinds of situations change the structure of a family. The ideal situation is for children to live with two loving, married parents.

Lesson 24 will include more information on teen pregnancy and parenthood.

There are three "Rs" to consider before becoming a parent:

R: The REASONS you want to have a child.

R: The RESOURCES you will need to raise a child.

R: The RESPONSIBILITIES you will have as a parent.

Reasons for Becoming a Parent

The reasons for having children can be grouped into four categories. These four categories and examples from each appear in the chart Reasons People Want to Become Parents. Suppose someone chooses one or more of the first three reasons in the chart. They focus more on the person's needs than on the child's. Being ready for parenthood means being ready to focus on someone else's needs in addition to your own. The fourth reason, the desire to love and guide a child, is the best reason to have a child.

Reasons People Want to Become Parents

1. **To build up one's ego**
   - To have a child who looks like me
   - To have a child who will carry on the family name
   - To have a child who will inherit the family business, money, or property
2. **To compensate for something that is missing in one's life**
   - To save one's marriage
   - To make up for one's unhappy childhood
   - To help one feel more secure as a male or female
3. **To conform to what peers are doing or what others expect**
   - To please one's parents or guardian
   - To do what one's peers are doing
   - To keep from being criticized for being childless
4. **To love and guide someone**
   - To have the satisfaction of loving a child
   - To help a child grow and develop
   - To teach a child how to be responsible

Adapted from Peck and Granzig. *The Parent Test,* 1978.

Resources Needed for Parenthood

Suppose a married couple wants to purchase a car. The cost of the car and of various options for the car would be considered. If the purchase could not be financed, the decision to buy the car would have to be delayed. Financial resources also must be evaluated when a couple considers having a child. Some of the costs a couple might expect are:

- health and hospitalization insurance;
- prenatal care for the mother-to-be;
- maternity clothes for the mother-to-be;
- delivery and postpartum care for the mother and baby in a hospital or a birth center or at home;
- hospitalization for the baby;
- pediatrician's hospital visits, regular well-baby checkups, required immunizations, sick visits, medications;
- nursery furnishings: bassinet, crib, bedding, linens, bathtub, stroller, highchair, chest, car seat, infant carrier, toys;
- clothing for the baby;
- diapers and/or diaper service;
- formula, food, and vitamins for the baby;
- baby supplies: bottles, swabs, baby wipes, diaper rash ointment, tissues, powder, baby soap and shampoo, oil;
- the possible need for child care or day care.

For many families, there is the additional cost of lost income during the mother's maternity leave. One of the parents may cut back to part-time work or stop working altogether after the birth of a baby. The first year of childrearing is very expensive. These financial considerations are a must when deciding if and when to become parents.

Responsibilities of Parenthood

When people become parents, they take responsibility for raising a child. Whether the child is newborn or adopted, there are certain promises parents should make. These ten promises are listed below in The Parent Pledge to a Child.

The Parent Pledge to a Child

1. I will set aside a quantity of time as well as quality time to spend with you.
2. I will learn about your age-appropriate development so that I can have realistic expectations for you.
3. I will teach you rules to ensure your health and safety.
4. I will give you love and affection.
5. I will teach you with a positive attitude, avoiding criticism.
6. I will teach you my moral and ethical values.
7. I will teach you self-discipline and self-control with effective discipline, not child abuse.
8. I will provide economic security for you.
9. I will recognize that you have rights, and I will respect those rights.
10. I will raise you in a stable, secure family that is free from substance abuse (free from the abuse of alcohol, marijuana, and other drugs).

How to Be a
Responsible Parent

Parenting involves having more than loving feelings for a child. To **parent** is to guide a child to responsible adulthood. Being a responsible and caring parent is not an easy task. It involves developing intimacy with a child, caring for a child as (s)he grows and develops, and helping a child develop self-discipline and self-control.

Developing intimacy with a child. This lesson has focused on the reasons for becoming a parent, the resources needed, and the responsibilities involved. Developing intimacy with a child is one of the responsibilities of parenting. The early lessons a child learns from parents with regard to intimacy influence his/her ability to become intimate with others.

Philosophical intimacy is the sharing of beliefs and values. Responsible parents teach their children beliefs and values. They discipline their children when they act in wrong ways. This helps children know how to behave. It helps them develop good character.

Psychological intimacy is the sharing of needs, emotions, weaknesses, and strengths. Responsible parents are trustworthy and accepting. Their children can talk to them about sensitive topics. Responsible parents encourage and support their children when their children have disappointments.

Creative intimacy is the sharing of efforts to accomplish tasks and projects. Responsible parents give their children their first feelings of teamwork. They ask their children to help with tasks in the home. They share fun projects.

Physical intimacy is the sharing of physical affection. Responsible parents express physical affection for children in appropriate ways. Babies who receive soft touches, are spoken to, held, and looked at frequently by the mother and father in the first few days of life cry less and smile and laugh more than babies who are not treated in these ways. Children who are loved learn to feel secure in ways of expressing affection. They are able to receive affection from others.

Caring for a child as (s)he grows and develops. Responsible parents help their children develop emotional, social, verbal, intellectual, and motor skills. They understand that age-appropriate skills help keep their children safe from harm. They understand emotional development and reassure their children if they are fearful or anxious. They obtain medical help for their children when needed.

Helping a child develop self-discipline and self-control. Responsible parents discipline their children. **Discipline** is training that develops self-discipline and self-control. **Preventive discipline** is training in which a parent explains correct behavior and the consequences of wrong behavior. Suppose a child gets a new bicycle for his/her birthday. The parent explains his/her expectations. For example, the parent says (s)he expects the child to put away the bicycle after riding it. The parent further explains that if the bicycle is not put away, the child will not permitted to ride the bicycle for three days.

Behavior modification is a disciplinary technique in which positive rewards are used to encourage desirable behavior and negative consequences are used to stop undesirable behavior. For example, a parent might praise a child for remembering to put away his/her bicycle. The parent might plan a special reward. On the other hand, the parent wants to change undesirable behavior. The child who leaves the bicycle in an unsafe place may not be permitted to ride the bicycle for three days.

Logical consequences discipline is a disciplinary technique in which the child is allowed the opportunity to experience the results of undesirable behavior so that (s)he will want to change the undesirable behavior. An example might be a child who frequently forgets to take his/her packed lunch to school. The child calls the parent and asks the parent to bring the forgotten lunch to school. The parent disciplines the child by refusing to take the forgotten lunch to school. The child experiences the consequences—no lunch. As a result, the child is not as forgetful in the future.

Physical punishment is a disciplinary technique in which an act is used to teach a child not to repeat undesirable behavior. Slapping and spanking are examples of physical punishment. Slapping and spanking appear to be helpful in only two instances. First, when a child is young, a parent might slap the child's hand to prevent a behavior that might harm the child. For example, the parent might slap the child's hand if (s)he tries to put a fork in an electrical outlet. Second, a parent might use a very light slap on the young child's buttocks or hand to get the child's attention. The slap should not be severe enough to hurt or injure the child.

Spanking is usually ineffective in teaching long-range discipline and self-control. For example, consider the two examples—the child who did not put away his/her bicycle, and the child who forgot to take his/her packed lunch to school. If a child is spanked for either of these behaviors, the discipline creates fear rather than changing undesirable behavior. The other approaches to discipline that were discussed are more effective than physical punishment in teaching the desired behavior. Spanking usually creates hostility and anxiety in children. In many cases, physical punishment is physical abuse. Physical abuse is discussed later in this lesson.

The parents who are most effective in helping their children learn self-discipline and self-control are those who:

1. set limits for their children,
2. are consistent in their actions,
3. are neither too strict nor too permissive,
4. discuss acceptable behavior with their children,
5. listen to their children and pay attention to their feelings.

What to Know About
Child Abuse

Abuse is the harmful treatment of another person. You learned earlier that abuse is one cause of dysfunctional families. Now you will look more closely at how and why parents, stepparents, or guardians might abuse their children.

Recall the four kinds of abuse: physical, emotional, neglect, and sexual. **Physical abuse** is harmful treatment that results in physical injury to the victim. **Emotional abuse** is "putting down" another person and making the person feel worthless. **Neglect** is failure to provide proper care and guidance. **Sexual abuse** is sexual contact that is forced on a person.

Physical abuse is not the same as discipline. Physical abuse is harmful. Discipline is training. Suppose a parent, stepparent, or guardian kicks a child and says, "I'll teach you to follow my rules." Actions such as this are not appropriate forms of discipline. They are acts of violence. Physical abuse includes actions such as striking a child with a belt buckle, rope, or other object to inflict harm. Burning, bruising, cutting, or breaking bones on purpose also are forms of physical abuse. They are not methods of discipline. They do not develop self-control and self-discipline.

Emotional abuse may be difficult to recognize. Suppose a parent, stepparent, or guardian puts down a child. Perhaps the parent, stepparent, or guardian makes comments such as: "You are worthless." "You will never amount to anything." Comments such as these make a child feel inadequate. They harm the child's self-respect and are considered abusive. Emotional abuse should not be confused with constructive criticism. Responsible adults also look at their other behaviors to determine if they are forms of emotional abuse. For example, suppose a parent, stepparent, or guardian pushes a child to excel in beauty pageants, athletics, or other activities without allowing the child to have a healthful, normal childhood. Does pushing a child in these ways cause emotional harm? Are these actions examples of child abuse? These actions are examples of harmful emotional abuse.

Sexual abuse is a topic that is very difficult for most people. The thought of a parent, stepparent, or guardian having sexual contact with a child is upsetting. However, both males and females are abused by adult family members. Sexual abuse often is a family secret. Family members may not talk about the abuse and may hide the abuse from people outside the family. There are different forms of sexual abuse. **Incest** is having sexual intercourse with a family member. Many people believe incest and sexual abuse are synonymous. But, acts other than incest can be considered sexual abuse. Showing young people pornographic pictures or taking pornographic pictures of them is sexual abuse. Inappropriate touching of body parts is sexual abuse. These actions are inappropriate behaviors.

Neglect covers a wide range of actions. There are laws that further define neglect. For example, children under a certain age must have adult supervision. If parents, stepparents, or guardians work, children must be in the care of a responsible adult—children cannot be left at home alone. If children are not supervised, parents, stepparents, or guardians are guilty of neglect. Most likely you have read articles or seen television reports of other actions that show neglect. Some children have not been given food or clothing. Some children require medical care and their parents, stepparents, or guardians do not obtain it for them. These actions can be considered neglect.

Why would parents, stepparents, or guardians abuse their children? Don't these adult family members "love" their children? There is something important you should know about "love." If you look in a dictionary, you will learn that "love" is both a feeling and an action.

1. **A parent may have loving feelings AND loving actions.**

2. **A parent may have little or no loving feelings AND loving actions.**

3. **A parent may have loving feelings AND unloving actions.**

4. **A parent may have unloving feelings AND unloving actions.**

Parents, stepparents, or guardians can fall into any of these four categories. Responsible parents, stepparents, or guardians have loving feelings and loving actions.

You will want to be a responsible parent if you choose to be a parent some day. Did you know that there are some indications now of your future parenting behavior? Consider your behavior right now. Are you able to control your anger? Are you able to express your feelings without trying to control others? Were you raised in a home without violence and abuse? Do you recognize how important it is for you to graduate from high school, get the skills you need for employment (and/or college or vocational school), and get a job before marrying and having children?

Suppose you have been raised in a home with violence and abuse. Teens who have been abused are at risk for abusing others. The **cycle of abuse** is the repeating of abuse from one generation to the next. Teens who have been abused learned to interact with others in much the same way as their family members interact. They want to control others and they use wrong actions to do so. They practice the wrong actions they have learned. This is one reason why people who have been abused often need help before they are ready to have children. They need to sort through the confusion, secrecy, and wrong actions that occurred while they were growing up. Then the cycle of abuse can be stopped.

Every child deserves parents, stepparents, or guardians who have loving feelings AND loving actions.

Lesson 24 will include more information on the risks associated with teen parenthood.

Lesson 19
Review

Vocabulary Words

Write a separate sentence using each of the vocabulary words listed on page 152.

Objectives

1. What are the three "Rs" to consider before becoming a parent? **Objective 1**

2. What does it mean to be a responsible parent? **Objective 2**

3. What are four ways to discipline children? **Objective 2**

4. What are five actions parents take to effectively teach their children self-discipline and self-control? **Objective 2**

5. What is child abuse and how can a person break the cycle of abuse? **Objective 3**

Responsible Decision-Making

A classmate discusses with you her relationship with her boyfriend. Her boyfriend is two years older and is beginning to pull away from the relationship. She confides in you that she is thinking about "trapping" him into marriage by getting pregnant. Write a response to this situation.

1. Describe the situation that requires your classmate to make a decision.
2. List possible decisions your classmate might make.
3. Name two responsible adults with whom your classmate might discuss your decisions.
4. Evaluate the possible consequences of your classmate's decisions. Determine if each decision will lead to actions that:
   - promote health,
   - protect safety,
   - follow laws,
   - show respect for your friend and others,
   - follow the guidelines of your friend's parents and of other responsible adults,
   - demonstrate good character.
5. Decide which decision is most responsible and appropriate for your classmate.
6. Tell two results your classmate can expect if (s)he makes this decision.

Effective Communication

Prepare a 30-second public service announcement for radio to educate the public about the difference between physical abuse and discipline.

Self-Directed Learning

Browse through a magazine written for parents. Find an article of interest to you. Read the article and write a short summary. Include at least two facts or ideas you have learned.

Critical Thinking

Suppose a teen has broken curfew and twice has been late getting home. His/her parent is angry. Explain how the parent might use the following forms of discipline to deal with the teen's behavior: preventive discipline, behavior modification, logical consequences discipline, physical punishment. Which form of discipline would be most effective and why?

Responsible Citizenship

Laws protect children from being abused. Responsible citizens report child abuse to authorities. Find out what laws govern child abuse in your community. Also find out to what agencies you can report child abuse.

You Can Adjust to Family Changes

Life Skill **I will make healthful adjustments to family changes.**

Family relationships are the connections a person has with family members, including extended family members. **Extended family members** are the members of a family in addition to parents, brothers, and sisters. An extended family may include grandparents, aunts, uncles, cousins, stepparents, stepbrothers, and stepsisters. This lesson discusses changes that may occur within family relationships. You will learn ways teens can adjust if parents divorce, a teen lives in a single-custody family, a parent remarries, a parent loses a job, or a parent goes to jail.

The Lesson Outline

If Parents Divorce

If a Teen Lives in a Single-Custody Family

If a Parent Remarries

If a Parent Loses a Job

If a Parent Goes to Jail

Objectives

1. List and explain the six stages in the divorce process. **pages 161–162**

2. List and explain five suggestions for teens who live in single-custody families. **page 164**

3. Discuss the sources of conflict in a blended family. **page 165**

4. List and explain three suggestions for teens who have a parent who loses a job. **page 166**

5. List and explain four suggestions for teens who have a parent in jail. **page 167**

Vocabulary Words

family relationships

extended family members

marital conflict resolution

marital separation

divorce

annulment

dissolution

single custody

custodial parent

joint custody

visitation rights

grandparents' rights

single-custody family

remarriage

blended family

stepfamily

downsize the workforce

foster care

If Parents Divorce

In order for marriages to succeed and be satisfying, married partners need to pay attention to the status of their relationship. When a marriage is taken for granted, the quality of the marriage declines and intimacy is lost. The most common stressors in marriage are changes in financial status, changes in living arrangements, changes in work situations, illness of a family member, abuse, infidelity, poor communication, and alcohol and other drug dependency.

If Parents or Stepparents Have Conflict

Marital conflict resolution is a process in which married partners identify their problems, agree upon solutions, and reestablish intimacy. The attitude of each partner is important in marital conflict resolution. In a healthful and caring marriage, each partner is willing to work on problems. Marital conflict resolution is impossible if one or both partners are not committed to restoring the quality of the marriage.

Sometimes marriage partners need help with marital conflict resolution. They may need assistance identifying their problems or finding solutions. In some cases, one partner is aware there is a problem and has resolved to do something about the situation, but the other partner does not recognize there is a problem. This is often the case in a marriage in which one partner abuses drugs. The partner who abuses drugs denies a problem exists. Outside intervention may be needed to help resolve the problem.

A married couple may recognize a problem but not be able to solve it. A marriage counselor, such as a member of the clergy, psychologist, psychiatrist, or social worker, may help present possible solutions. If the solution involves new ways of behaving, the counselor may help assist one or both partners to change behavior. Again, the importance of attitude and commitment is obvious. A counselor cannot help marriage partners change ways of behaving if they do not want to do so.

What to Know About the Divorce Process

Married couples are not always able to solve problems and reestablish intimacy. About two-thirds of all first marriages end in marital separation and/or divorce. **Marital separation** is the living apart of marriage partners. **Divorce** is a legal way to end a marriage in which a judge or court decides the terms with respect to property, custody, and support. Most married couples who divorce experience a six-stage process. Marital separation may occur at any time during the six stages, but it often occurs in an earlier stage.

In the first stage of divorce, the marriage deteriorates and partners show less affection and begin to detach from one another. One or both partners do not meet the needs of the other. The first stage may last up to several years. In the second stage of divorce, one or both partners seek legal counsel. This begins the process of discussing the grounds for the divorce and issues regarding property, custody of children, and financial support. During this stage of divorce, the different options for ending the marriage are examined. An **annulment** is a legal way to end a marriage in which it is decided that what was a legally binding marriage actually is not. A **dissolution** is a legal way to end a marriage in which the marriage partners decide the terms with respect to property, custody, and support.

In the third stage of divorce, issues regarding property and support payments are finalized.

The property in a marriage usually refers to the home and household furnishings the couple owns, jewelry, cars, life insurance, money in savings accounts, stocks, and other investments. One partner may agree to pay spousal support to the other. Usually, the partner paying spousal support is the partner who has the greater ability to earn money. Spousal support often is based on the potential earning power of one partner versus the other, the length of the marriage, and the other assets in the marriage.

In the fourth stage of divorce, issues of custody, visitation rights, and child support are negotiated. **Single custody** is an arrangement in which one parent keeps legal custody of a child or children. The **custodial parent** is the parent with whom a child or children live and the parent who has the legal right to make decisions about the health and well-being of a child or children. Sometimes the parents or the court decide upon joint custody of a child or children. **Joint custody** is an arrangement in which both partners keep legal custody of a child or children. A child or children may live with one parent or may alternate living arrangements, spending time with one parent and then the other. In joint custody, both parents maintain the legal right to make decisions about the health and well-being of a child or children. This arrangement requires that meaningful communication between the parents be maintained after the marriage has ended.

Visitation rights are guidelines set for the visitation of children by the parent who does not have custody. In some cases, visitation rights are very specific and include the exact number of days and a specific amount of time during which the parent can spend time with a child or children. Some guidelines may be set with regard to a parent moving to a new location and the effects of the move on visitation. Recently, the court has begun to look at other aspects of visitation such as grandparents' rights. **Grandparents' rights** are the visitation rights with grandchildren courts have awarded grandparents when their son's or daughter's marriage ends.

In the fifth stage of divorce, each of the partners establishes a new identity with family, friends, and co-workers. This stage often is difficult. In fact, some people going through divorce delay telling others about the divorce because they fear it will affect their relationships with them. These former relationships may have been based on being part of a couple. Some family members and friends may take sides and feel angry or disappointed with one or both partners.

In the sixth stage of divorce, each of the partners makes emotional adjustments to the new lifestyle that results from being divorced. This stage of divorce affects both marriage partners and their children.

Suggestions for Teens Whose Parents Divorce

1. Practice stress management skills. Remember, you have experienced a major life stressor.

2. Avoid using alcohol and other drugs to numb your painful feelings. You need to work through your anger, disappointment, and sadness without using drugs.

3. Recognize that becoming sexually active WILL NOT fill the empty feelings you experience as a result of your family's breakup. In most cases, this behavior will make you feel even more empty and alone.

4. Choose healthful ways to express your anger over your family's breakup. Participating in delinquent behavior will make life even more difficult for you.

5. Be aware of your feelings of rejection and betrayal and ask for help. Do not allow your feelings to keep you from forming healthful friendships and dating relationships. Responsible adults can help you learn to connect with others.

What Kinds of Adjustments to Expect

Divorce is intended to fulfill at least two purposes for the married partners involved. First, divorce is intended to end a marriage that at least one spouse believed was intolerable. Second, separation and divorce are intended to be the beginning of building a new life. This second task is of particular importance to both the formerly married partners and their child or children.

Adjustments made by formerly married partners. Often, one marriage partner has a more difficult time adjusting to the divorce than the other. Usually, one partner feels that (s)he is much better off for getting divorced, while the other partner feels (s)he is not better off. Usually, the partner who initiated the divorce feels as though (s)he is better off.

The immediate response of partners varies. Some people become very involved in work, others begin to date excessively to be reassured of their attractiveness, others withdraw, and others are too depressed to function. Females who divorce usually require three years to regain balance in their lives. Males who divorce usually require two to two-and-one-half years. Females usually must make more economic adjustments than males. Many females experience a drop in their standard of living. They must adjust to living on much less money. Both females and males who divorce are more at risk for health problems because of added stress.

Adjustments made by children after parents separate and divorce. Separation and divorce are very different experiences for children and adults. At least one of the married partners wanted the divorce and felt it was for the best. Children do not have this kind of control over their situation. They usually feel that they have had no control over a decision that influences something fundamental to their development— an intact family structure.

The initial reactions of all children to separation and divorce are usually similar. They feel very vulnerable and fearful. Young children exhibit these fears by having difficulty sleeping or having nightmares. Teens exhibit these fears through a loss of concentration and a need either to cling to others or to withdraw from others.

Divorced parents may spend less time with their children. Most divorced fathers do not have custody of their children. They have infrequent or no contact with their children. Any lack of parenting takes its toll on the children. Many have a decline in their grades. Many are at risk for becoming depressed, becoming sexually active, abusing alcohol and other drugs, and having delinquent behavior.

Some children may have to adjust to parental dating. This can stress them out. If parental dating begins before or soon after the divorce, children may feel angry. They may believe the new person caused the breakup. Children often fantasize about their parents getting back together. They may continue to hope for a reconciliation for many years.

When parents date, children may resent the time and attention given to someone new. They may be jealous of the people the parent dates. They may set out to disrupt the relationship and to regain the parent's attention.

Children of divorce have two traits in common— fear of rejection and fear of betrayal. These traits affect all their relationships. For example, teen females whose parents divorce often fear abandonment. As a result, they may try to have many boyfriends at the same time so there will always be a backup. They may seek an older boyfriend to be the father figure they do not have. They are more likely to get into harmful relationships and not end them. Teen males whose parents divorce often feel awkward with females. These teens often hold back their feelings in dating and have difficulty trusting others. In some cases, they throw themselves into sports and/or work, rather than into developing and maintaining relationships.

If a Teen Lives in a Single-Custody Family

A **single-custody family** is a family in which a child or children live with one parent who has custody. This term, rather than "single-parent" family, is used because a child or children may have two living parents. However, only one of the parents has custody or responsibility for them. When both parents have custody and responsibility, a child or children live in a joint-custody family.

There often are differences between living in a single-custody family and living in a joint-custody family. In most cases, children raised in a single-custody family live with their mothers. They are more likely to be economically disadvantaged. This means they will lack many of the resources that other families have available. These resources range from good medical care to clothing. These families might lack resources such as food and shelter. This makes living in a single-custody family more stressful than living in a two-parent family.

In a two-parent, or joint-custody family, there is a role model for both male and female children. After divorce, many teens who live in single-custody families have little or no contact with their fathers. Unless there is another male figure, such as a grandfather in their lives, these teens do not experience the benefits of having a male role model.

The single-custody parent has the sole responsibility for supervising his/her children. If (s)he works outside the home, there is less time for supervising children and for being involved in their academic performance. This accounts for the finding that teens whose parents divorce spend less time with parents and are at risk for getting poorer grades.

Suggestions for Teens Who Live in a Single-Custody Family

1. Recognize the financial pressures your parent has. Discuss ways to control expenses.

2. Schedule time to be with your parent. Your parent will have many demands for his/her time. If you arrange a set time to be together, you will have time to which you can look forward.

3. Look for a mentor to serve as a role model. Try to find a mentor who is the same sex as the parent with whom you have little or no contact. Having a mentor means having an adult who can care about you. Organizations, such as Big Brothers and Big Sisters, will give you contact with an adult who can provide support and advice.

4. Pay attention to your academic performance. You do not have two parents to be interested in your schoolwork. You will need to take more responsibility for yourself. You might want to think about a tutor or additional after-school help.

5. Discuss your fears and concerns about your parent's dating. Your parent can reassure you of your importance and that his/her dates do not replace you. Your parent can discuss other concerns you have.

If a Parent Remarries

A **remarriage** is a marriage in which a previously married person marries again. A **blended family** or **stepfamily** is a family consisting of the marriage partners, children that one or both of them had previously, and the children that they have by their marriage to one another. Blended families often include a stepfather whose new wife has custody of her children. At the same time, he may have visitation rights for children of his former marriage. In some blended families, the father has custody of his children, but this is not a common arrangement. Some blended families include joint custody arrangements.

The two greatest sources of conflict in a blended family are determining which set of rules the children will follow and adjusting to a new budget. Often, children have been raised with specific rules that may not be the same as those they are now expected to follow. Suppose one set of children in a blended family was raised with very clear guidelines in which consequences were identified for inappropriate behavior. However, the other children in the family had little discipline and were allowed to behave as they pleased. Blending these two sets of children into one framework for discipline will likely cause conflict.

Another issue is the rules for children who live with the other parent and come to visit the blended family. All parents and stepparents involved need to communicate about the ways to blend these children into the family during visitation, rules the children must follow, and how to discipline the children.

Decisions about the budget in a blended family can be challenging. Parents and stepparents have many decisions to make about how to spend money. When money is spent on one child for a birthday or other special circumstances, it may not be available for the needs of other children. The two sets of children may have been used to having different guidelines for spending money.

Other issues that are important in blended families arise from the new relationships that are formed. The success of the blended family often depends on how step-siblings interact. Clear guidelines for interaction must be set by parents. For example, teens from different families who are living together may find each other attractive. Parents must establish that acting on the attraction is not acceptable. Guidelines for resolving conflict also must be set for the family.

Many teens who live in blended families resent their stepparent. They may think that their stepparent does not like them, or that their stepparent does not treat them well. However, with effective communication and mutual respect they can establish a healthful relationship with their stepparent.

Suggestions for Teens Whose Parents Remarry

1. Respect the new guidelines for your behavior. Although you may not like the new rules, you must obey them.

2. Help your family follow a budget. Recognize that your parents have the challenging task of providing for a larger family.

3. Interact in healthful ways with your stepbrothers and stepsisters. Discuss guidelines for behavior when interacting with new siblings.

4. Interact in healthful ways with your stepparent. Use effective communication skills and mutual respect to establish a healthful relationship with stepparents.

If a Parent Loses a Job

A teen's parent might lose his/her job. There are a number of reasons this can happen. One reason is that the company or factory at which the parent worked may have downsized. To **downsize the workforce** is to reduce the number of employees in a company. Downsizing often affects people who have performed well at their jobs. Downsizing may not have been tied to job performance but rather to economics.

Another reason a parent may lose a job has to do with job performance. A parent may not have had the appropriate skills for the job. Or, the parent might have had problems, such as alcoholism, that resulted in a poor work record. These are only a few of the reasons why a parent might lose a job. There are many others.

The loss of a job can be devastating to a parent and very stressful for the family. The parent who loses the job may become depressed and disappointed. (S)he may lose self-confidence and feel embarrassed. (S)he may worry that family members and friends will lose respect for him/her. (S)he may be anxious and worried about how the family will survive. There may be an adjustment period before (s)he feels energized and ready to find another job. (S)he may need training or other help before getting another job.

Teens who have a parent who has lost a job also may be anxious and worried. They may wonder: "What should I say to my parent?" "What should I say to other people?" "What changes will this bring about in where and how we live?" "How will the loss of income affect me?"

Suggestions for Teens Who Have a Parent Who Loses a Job

1. Give your parent emotional support. Remember, you are on the same team. Encourage your parent.

2. Discuss what to say to people outside the family. Your parent(s) can offer suggestions. You can discuss which family discussions are private and what information can be shared with others.

3. Discuss what changes will occur in the family budget. Recognize that money might be tight. Do not spend money on things you do not need. Perhaps you can contribute money from a part-time job.

If a Parent Goes to Jail

When a parent is sentenced to jail, his/her family experiences a great deal of stress. One of the most immediate stressors may be a shortage of money, if the parent was the main source of income for the family. Legal fees can be very expensive, and arrangements must be made to pay these fees. The family may be eligible for money from the government for rent and food stamps. However, the family may be left with no source of support.

The loss of income may result in other changes. The family may have to move to another place or move in with relatives. Suppose the parent who goes to jail is a single parent. Teens who live with this parent may end up living with other relatives or be placed in foster care. **Foster care** is an arrangement in which another unrelated adult assumes temporary responsibility for a child.

Teens who have a parent who is sentenced to jail may have to deal with the response from society. If the crime was widely publicized, people may make cruel remarks. They may be angry because of the behavior of the teen's parent's. This may require a teen to be resilient. It can be very embarrassing to listen to comments about the wrong behavior of a parent. Other people may assume that the teen is like the parent who committed a crime and that the teen also will participate in criminal behavior.

Teens who have a parent who is sentenced to jail must recognize that they are not responsible for what has happened. Their guilty parents chose wrong actions for which there are consequences. These teens did not choose this behavior. They do not have to behave in similar ways. They can choose to follow the law.

Suggestions for Teens Who Have a Parent in Jail

1. Discuss your feelings with a trusted adult. Teens who have a parent in jail often feel ashamed, angry, confused, betrayed, and anxious. Share your feelings with another parent, a teacher, or a counselor.

2. Ask about changes that might result. Ask your other parent, a teacher, a counselor, a social worker, or a legal advisor any questions you may have. Questions you might ask include:
   - Will there be any changes in my living arrangements?
   - Will my family's financial situation change?
   - Will my family responsibilities change (such as looking after younger siblings)?
   - What kind of contact am I allowed to have with my parent?
   - When will my parent be eligible for parole or release from jail?

3. Do not accept blame for the parent's illegal actions. Some teens blame themselves for their parent's imprisonment. They might wonder if they could have prevented the parent's criminal behavior if they had noticed wrong behavior sooner or done something differently. This is faulty thinking. In some cases, the parent may be imprisoned based on an action a teen took, such as calling the police. If this is your case, recognize that your action may have protected innocent people. Remember, you did not commit a crime. Your parent committed a crime and must pay the consequences.

4. Pledge that you will not engage in illegal behavior. Teens who have a parent in jail are more at risk for committing a crime themselves. It is important to understand that you do not have to behave in similar ways. You can make responsible decisions that follow the law.

Activity

Toss Out the TRASH

Life Skill: I will make healthful adjustments to family changes.

Materials: paper, pencil, trash bag

Directions: Teens have different feelings when they must adjust to family changes. Some of these feelings are listed below and make up the acronym TRASH. The acronym TRASH is used as a reminder that these emotions should be dealt with and not allowed to collect and become serious problems. For good health, these feelings must be examined and shared. Complete the following activity with classmates.

T: Threatened
R: Regretful
A: Angry
S: Sad
H: Helpless

 Select one of the letters from the acronym **TRASH.** For best results, have classmates select different letters so each emotion will be selected.

 Select one of the family changes about which you have just learned. You might select: separation and divorce, living in a single-custody family, having a parent who remarries, having a parent who loses a job, or having a parent who goes to jail.

 Write the feeling and the family change you selected on one side of a sheet of paper.

 On the other side of the paper, explain why a teen might have this feeling during the family change you selected.

 Share what you have written with your classmates.

 Wad the sheet of paper and throw it into the trash bag.

 Write a one-page paper explaining why it is important for teens to share their feelings with a parent or trusted adult when there are family changes.

Lesson 20

Review

Vocabulary Words

Write a separate sentence using each of the vocabulary words listed on page 160.

Objectives

1. What are the six stages in the divorce process? **Objective 1**

2. What are five suggestions for teens who live in single-custody families? **Objective 2**

3. What are the sources of conflict in a blended family? **Objective 3**

4. What are three suggestions for teens who have a parent who loses a job? **Objective 4**

5. What are four suggestions for teens who have a parent in jail? **Objective 5**

Responsible Decision-Making

Suppose you have a friend whose parents are going through a difficult divorce. The parents have several disagreements over dividing the property, financial support, and custody of the children. Your friend seems very depressed. You suspect that your friend is using alcohol and other drugs to cope with his/her emotions. Write a response to this situation.

1. Describe the situation that requires you to make a decision.

2. List possible decisions you might make.

3. Name two responsible adults with whom you might discuss your decisions.

4. Evaluate the possible consequences of your decisions. Determine if each decision will lead to actions that:
   • promote health,
   • protect safety,
   • follow laws,
   • show respect for yourself and others,
   • follow the guidelines of your parents and of other responsible adults,
   • demonstrate good character.

5. Decide which decision is most responsible and appropriate.

6. Tell two results you expect if you make this decision.

 Effective Communication

Pretend you are a teen who has experienced one of the family changes identified in the lesson. Write a letter to an advice columnist asking for suggestions about coping with this change. Then pretend you are the advice columnist and write a response to the teen.

 Self-Directed Learning

Check the library or Internet to locate information on new aspects of custody and visitation the courts have considered recently. Make a copy of the information you find and share it with your classmates.

 Critical Thinking

Your friend's parent has gone to prison for committing a serious crime. The details of the case are all over the newspapers and TV. At school, your other classmates start making fun of your friend and calling him/her names. How might your friend deal with the situation? What other suggestions might you give your friend to cope with the situation?

 Responsible Citizenship

Do you know someone who has experienced one of the family changes discussed in this lesson? If so, give this person suggestions about how (s)he might cope with the situation.

Responsible Decision–Making

You go to a party with someone who is 18. When you decided to be in this person's company, you expected friendship and nothing else. At the party, this person "hits" on you. The person begins to make sexual advances. The person says (s)he is older and can teach you a lot about sex. You are very uncomfortable with this person's behavior. What would you do?

1. Describe the situation that requires you to make a decision.
2. List possible decisions you might make.
3. Name two responsible adults with whom you might discuss your decisions.
4. Evaluate the possible consequences of your decisions. Determine if each decision will lead to actions that:
   • promote health,
   • protect safety,
   • follow laws,
   • show respect for yourself and others,
   • follow the guidelines of your parents and of other responsible adults,
   • demonstrate good character.
5. Decide which decision is most responsible and appropriate.
6. Tell two results you expect if you make this decision.

Health Behavior Inventory of Life Skills

Number from 1 to 10 on a sheet of paper. Read each life skill carefully. Write YES or NO next to the same number on your paper. Each YES response indicates a life skill you practice to promote your health status. Each NO response indicates a life skill you do not practice. Plan to begin practicing these life skills.

1. I will develop healthful family relationships.
2. I will work to improve difficult family relationships.
3. I will use conflict resolution skills.
4. I will develop healthful friendships.
5. I will develop dating skills.
6. I will practice abstinence.
7. I will recognize harmful relationships.
8. I will develop skills to prepare for marriage.
9. I will develop skills to prepare for parenthood.
10. I will make healthful adjustments to family changes.

Multicultural Health

Obtain permission from your parent or guardian to E-mail a teen who lives in another country. Ask this teen about the dating practices of teens in his/her country. At what age do teens begin to date? What social activities are available to enjoy while dating? Write a short summary of the information you obtain from your pen pal. Share your summary with classmates.

Family Involvement

As a family, make The Top Ten List of Healthful Activities Our Family Enjoys Together. Rank order your list so that the activity your family enjoys most is #1 on the list.

Health Behavior Contract

Copy and complete the following health behavior contract. Evaluate your progress.
Share the results with your family.

Health Behavior Contract

1. Name_____ Date_____

2. **Life Skill:** I will develop healthful friendships.

3. **Effects on Health Status:** A friendship is a special relationship with someone I like.
Having close friendships allows me to have others with whom I can share my interests. I
can share my successes as well as my disappointments. Having close friendships contributes to my health and well-being.

4. **Plan and Method to Record Progress:** I will take time to develop a new friendship. First, I will make a background check. I will answer the following questions in the
space provided.

- What do I know about this person?
- Does this person have good character?
- Do my parents or guardian know this person?
- Will my parents or guardian approve of my spending time with this person?

I will make plans to get together with this person if this person has good character and my
parents or guardian approve. I will contact this person and suggest two different social
activities we can enjoy together. I recognize that this person may suggest that we do something different.

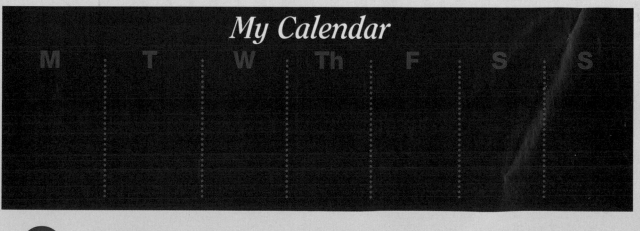

My Calendar

M   T   W   Th   F   S   S

5. **Evaluation:** I will describe my feelings about our interactions and about my desire to
get together again_____
_____

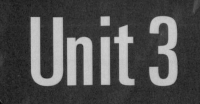

Growth and Development

You Can Have a Healthy Body

Life Skill **I will keep my body systems healthy.**

Your body is made of cells, tissues, and organs that form body systems. A **cell** is the smallest living part of the body. A **tissue** is a group of similar cells that work together. An **organ** is a body part consisting of several kinds of tissue that do a particular job. A **body system** is a group of organs that work together to perform a main body function. This lesson will help you review information about body systems.

Objectives

1. Identify seven ways to keep the nervous system healthy. **pages 178–179**

2. Identify six ways to keep the cardiovascular system healthy. **pages 180–181**

3. Identify five ways to keep the immune system healthy. **page 182**

4. Identify seven ways to keep the respiratory system healthy. **page 183**

5. Identify seven ways to keep the skeletal system healthy. **page 184**

6. Identify seven ways to keep the muscular system healthy. **page 185**

7. Identify three ways to keep the endocrine system healthy. **pages 186–187**

8. Identify five ways to keep the digestive system healthy. **pages 188–189**

9. Identify two ways to keep the urinary system healthy. **page 190**

10. Identify eight ways to keep the integumentary system healthy. **pages 191–192**

Vocabulary Words

See the Body Systems Crossword Puzzle Activity on page 177 for the vocabulary words in this lesson.

The Lesson Outline

What to Know About the Nervous System

What to Know About the Cardiovascular System

What to Know About the Immune System

What to Know About the Respiratory System

What to Know About the Skeletal System

What to Know About the Muscular System

What to Know About the Endocrine System

What to Know About the Digestive System

What to Know About the Urinary System

What to Know About the Integumentary System

Activity

Body Systems Crossword Puzzle

Life Skill: I will keep my body systems healthy.

Materials: paper, ruler, pencil or pen

Directions: The vocabulary words for this lesson are listed below. Design a crossword puzzle using at least 15 of these words. Exchange your crossword puzzle with a classmate.

cell	atrium	ligament	esophagus
tissue	ventricle	joint	peristalsis
organ	vena cava	muscular system	stomach
body system	aorta	voluntary muscle	small intestine
nervous system	heart rate	involuntary muscle	villi
central nervous system	pulse	smooth muscle	enzyme
peripheral nervous system	blood pressure	skeletal muscle	liver
brain	immune system	cardiac muscle	gallbladder
cerebrum	lymph	tendon	large intestine
cerebellum	lymph node	endocrine system	rectum
brain stem	spleen	gland	anus
spinal cord	immunity	hormone	urinary system
neuron	antibody	pituitary gland	kidney
cell body	thymus gland	thyroid gland	urine
axon	T cell	thyroxin	ureter
dendrites	B cell	metabolism	urinary bladder
sensory neurons	respiratory system	parathyroid glands	urethra
motor neurons	mucus	pancreas	integumentary system
reflex action	mucous membrane	insulin	melanin
cardiovascular system	pharynx	diabetes	epidermis
plasma	epiglottis	diabetes mellitus	dermis
red blood cell	trachea	adrenal glands	sweat gland
hemoglobin	cilia	adrenaline	sebaceous gland
white blood cell	bronchi	ovaries	sebum
pathogen	lungs	ova	subcutaneous layer
platelet	bronchioles	estrogen	wart
artery	alveoli	testes	ringworm
vein	skeletal system	testosterone	keratin
capillary	bone	digestive system	hair
coronary artery	periosteum	digestion	hair follicle
pulmonary artery	bone marrow	salivary glands	
heart	cartilage	saliva	

What to Know About the
Nervous System

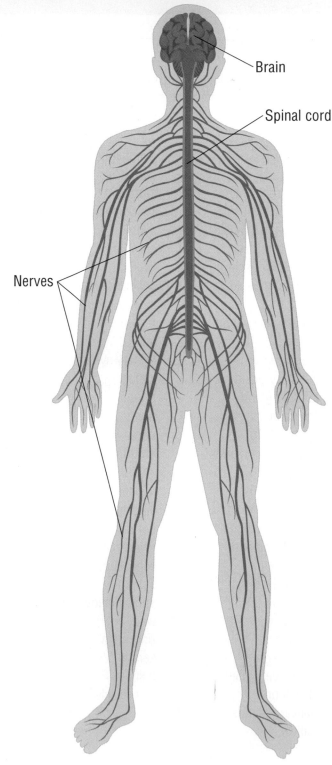

Brain

Spinal cord

Nerves

The **nervous system** carries messages to and from the brain and spinal cord and all other parts of the body. The nervous system is composed of two divisions: the central nervous system and the peripheral nervous system.

The **central nervous system** consists of the brain and spinal cord. The **peripheral nervous system** consists of nerves that branch out from the central nervous system to the muscles, skin, internal organs, and glands. Your sense organs continually send messages such as odors, sights, or tastes to your brain through the peripheral nervous system. These messages go to your central nervous system. Your central nervous system in turn relays responses to these messages to your muscles and glands as your body responds to changes in your environment.

Brain

The **brain** is a mass of nerve tissue that acts as the control center of the body. The human brain weighs about three pounds (1.35 kilograms) and can store more information than all the libraries in the world put together. Your brain creates ideas and controls thinking, reasoning, movement, and emotions. The brain has three major parts: the cerebrum, the cerebellum, and the brain stem.

The **cerebrum** is the largest part of the brain and controls the ability to memorize, think, and learn. The cerebrum also determines a person's intelligence and personality. It consists of two halves, called hemispheres, divided by a deep groove. The right hemisphere controls the left side of the body and the left hemisphere controls the right side of the body. The **cerebellum** is the part of the brain that controls and coordinates muscle activity. It also helps you maintain your balance. Your ability to catch a ball is a function of your cerebellum. The **brain stem** is the part of the brain that controls the functions of the internal organs.

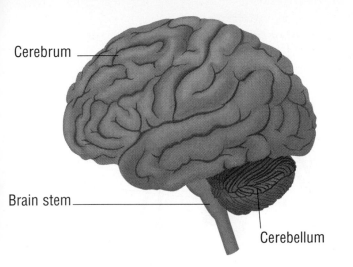

Cerebrum

Brain stem

Cerebellum

Spinal Cord

The **spinal cord** is a thick column of nerve cells that extends from the brain through the spinal column. Your spinal cord carries messages to and from your brain and body. It keeps your brain informed of changes in your body and in your environment, often creating changes in your movement and organ function. Your spinal cord is protected by your backbone.

Nerve Cells

The nervous system is composed of cells called neurons. A **neuron** is a nerve cell that is the structural and functional unit of the nervous system. Some neurons in the spinal cord may be several feet long. A neuron consists of a cell body, an axon, and dendrites. A **cell body** is the main body of the neuron. An **axon** is an elongated fiber that carries impulses away from the cell body to the dendrites of another neuron. **Dendrites** are branching fibers that receive impulses and carry them to the cell body.

Sensory and motor neurons work together to help you respond to your environment. **Sensory neurons** carry impulses from the sense organs to the spinal cord and brain. **Motor neurons** carry responding impulses to muscles and glands from the brain and spinal cord. Motor neurons tell muscles and glands what to do.

Reflex Action

Have you ever touched something hot and pulled away from it? If so, you have experienced a reflex action. A **reflex action** is an involuntary action in which a message is sent to the spinal cord, is interpreted, and is responded to immediately. Sensory neurons carry a message to your spinal cord and brain. The brain interprets the message. Motor neurons carry the message back to your muscles. You respond quickly and move your hand. Reflex actions do not involve conscious thought and take only a fraction of a second. Reflex actions help keep you safe.

Keep Your Nervous System Healthy

1. Wear a protective helmet for sports.
2. Avoid diving into shallow water or water of unknown depth.
3. Use a safety restraint system when riding in a motor vehicle.
4. Follow safety rules when taking part in physical activities.
5. Follow directions for taking any medications that affect the nervous system.
6. Avoid drinking alcohol and using other drugs that impair the nervous system.
7. Follow directions for using household products containing chemicals that may affect the nervous system.

What to Know About the
Cardiovascular System

The **cardiovascular system** transports nutrients, gases, hormones, and cellular waste products throughout the body. The cardiovascular system consists of the blood, blood vessels, and heart.

Blood

Your blood carries nutrients, oxygen, carbon dioxide, and cellular waste products to and from cells. The average-sized adult has about ten pints (4.7 liters) of blood. Blood is composed of plasma and blood cells. **Plasma** is the liquid component of blood that carries blood cells and dissolved materials. It is about 95 percent water. Plasma contains two major types of blood cells: red blood cells and white blood cells. A **red blood cell** is a blood cell that transports oxygen to body cells and removes carbon dioxide from body cells. Red blood cells contain large quantities of hemoglobin. **Hemoglobin** is an iron-rich protein that helps transport oxygen and carbon dioxide in the blood. New red blood cells are constantly produced in bone marrow, which is the spongy interior of some bones. A **white blood cell** is a blood cell that attacks, surrounds, and destroys pathogens that enter the body and prevents them from causing infection. A **pathogen** is a germ that causes disease. The number of white blood cells in your blood increases when you have an infection. White blood cells will be discussed more in the section on the immune system. Plasma also consists of particles called platelets. A **platelet** is a particle that helps the blood clot. Blood clots stop the bleeding when blood vessels are injured.

Platelets

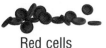

Red cells

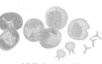

White cells

Heart

Vein

Artery

Blood Vessels

There are three major types of blood vessels: arteries, veins, and capillaries. An **artery** is a blood vessel that carries blood away from the heart. Arteries have thick muscular walls that move the blood between heartbeats. A **vein** is a blood vessel that returns blood to the heart. Veins have thinner walls than arteries. A **capillary** is a tiny blood vessel that connects arteries and veins. Capillaries have thin walls that allow the transfer of nutrients, oxygen, carbon dioxide, and cellular waste to and from blood and body cells.

A **coronary artery** is a blood vessel that carries blood to the heart muscles. Coronary arteries supply the heart with food and oxygen. A **pulmonary artery** is a blood vessel that carries blood from the heart to the lungs to pick up oxygen and release carbon dioxide.

Heart

The **heart** is a four-chambered muscle that pumps blood throughout the body. The chambers are called atria and ventricles. An **atrium** is one of the upper two chambers of the heart. A **ventricle** is one of the lower two chambers of the heart. The heart is divided into the right atrium and ventricle and the left atrium and ventricle. Blood returning from the body flows constantly into the right atrium and into the right ventricle.

A **vena cava** is one of two large veins that returns blood rich in carbon dioxide to the right atrium. Carbon dioxide is a waste product of body cells. This blood flows from the right atrium into the right ventricle. From the right ventricle, the blood is pumped through the pulmonary arteries to the lungs, where carbon dioxide is released and oxygen is absorbed as the blood circulates in capillaries around the air sacs in the lungs. This oxygen-rich blood returns in pulmonary veins to the left atrium and flows into the left ventricle. Contractions of the heart muscle pump the blood through the aorta to the body. The **aorta** is the main artery in the body. The aorta branches into smaller arteries through which blood flows to all parts of the body.

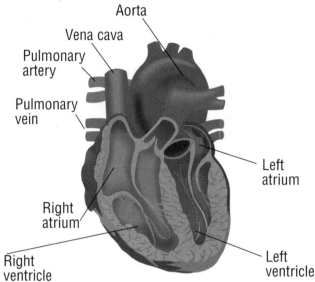

Heart diagram labels: Aorta, Vena cava, Pulmonary artery, Pulmonary vein, Right atrium, Right ventricle, Left atrium, Left ventricle

Heart rate is the number of times the heart contracts each minute. **Pulse** is the surge of blood that results from the contractions of the heart. **Blood pressure** is the force of blood against the artery walls.

Keep Your Cardiovascular System Healthy

1. Reduce the amount of fat in your diet.
2. Reduce the amount of salt in your diet.
3. Exercise regularly to strengthen your heart muscles.
4. Avoid using tobacco products because they increase blood pressure.
5. Maintain a healthful weight.
6. Practice stress management skills.

What to Know About the Immune System

The **immune system** removes harmful organisms from the blood and combats pathogens. The immune system is composed of lymph, lymph nodes, lymph vessels, tonsils, thymus, and spleen. The immune system protects your body from pathogens. A pathogen is a germ that causes disease. When white blood cells attack pathogens, the pathogens are filtered into the lymph. **Lymph** is a clear liquid that surrounds body cells and circulates in lymph vessels. Lymph carries harmful pathogens and other small particles to lymph nodes. A **lymph node** is a structure that filters and destroys pathogens. Pathogens also are removed by the spleen. The **spleen** is an organ on the left side of the abdomen that filters foreign matter from the blood and lymph.

The immune system plays an important role in immunity. **Immunity** is the body's resistance to disease-causing agents. An **antibody** is a special protein that helps fight infection. The **thymus gland** is a gland that causes white blood cells to become T cells. A **T cell** is a white blood cell that destroys pathogens. A **B cell** is a white blood cell that produces antibodies. Antibodies cover the surface of pathogens and make it difficult for them to attack the body.

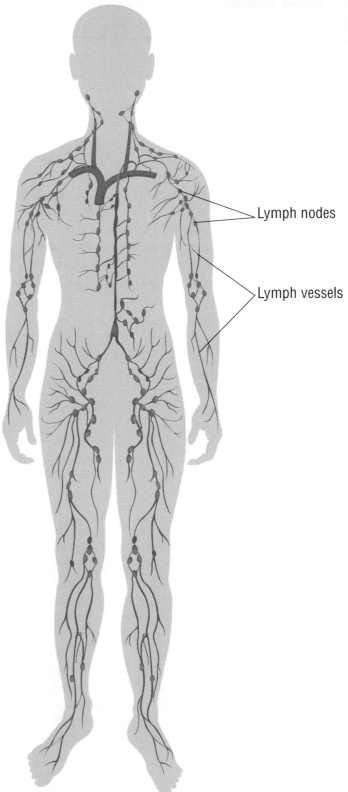

Lymph nodes

Lymph vessels

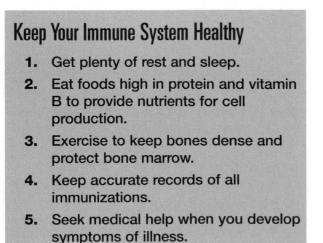

Keep Your Immune System Healthy

1. Get plenty of rest and sleep.
2. Eat foods high in protein and vitamin B to provide nutrients for cell production.
3. Exercise to keep bones dense and protect bone marrow.
4. Keep accurate records of all immunizations.
5. Seek medical help when you develop symptoms of illness.

What to Know About the
Respiratory System

The **respiratory system** provides body cells with oxygen and removes carbon dioxide that cells produce as waste. Air enters your respiratory system through your nose or mouth when you inhale. Mucus in the nasal passages and sinuses warms and moistens the air and traps dust particles and pathogens. **Mucus** is a thick secretion that moistens, lubricates, and protects mucous membranes. A **mucous membrane** is a type of tissue that lines body cavities and secretes mucus.

Air moves from your nose or mouth through your pharynx to your trachea. The **pharynx** is the throat. The **epiglottis** is a flap that covers the entrance to the trachea when a person swallows foods or beverages. When you inhale, the epiglottis opens and air flows into the trachea. The **trachea** (TRAY·kee·uh) is a tube through which air moves to the lungs. The trachea is sometimes called the windpipe. The trachea is lined with cilia. **Cilia** (SIH·lee·uh) are hair-like structures that remove dust and other particles from the air.

Next the air enters the bronchi. The **bronchi** are two tubes through which air moves to the lungs. The **lungs** are the main organs of the respiratory system. As the bronchi enter each lung, they branch into smaller tubes called bronchioles. The **bronchioles** are small tubes divided into the alveoli. The **alveoli** (al·vee·OH·ly) are microscopic air sacs. The walls of the alveoli are so thin that gases can easily pass through them. Two exchanges take place in the alveoli. Oxygen passes through the walls of the alveoli into your capillaries. At the same time, carbon dioxide passes from your capillaries through the walls of the alveoli into the alveoli. When you exhale, carbon dioxide passes out of your body. Blood rich in oxygen flows from your lungs to your heart, where it is pumped to your body cells.

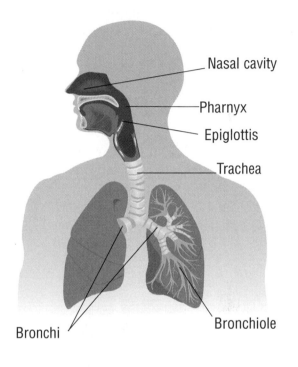

- Nasal cavity
- Pharnyx
- Epiglottis
- Trachea
- Bronchi
- Bronchiole

Keep Your Respiratory System Healthy

1. Do not smoke.
2. Avoid breathing secondhand smoke.
3. Do not inhale harmful drugs.
4. Avoid breathing polluted air.
5. Exercise regularly.
6. Avoid inhaling harmful chemicals.
7. Seek medical help for respiratory infections.

What to Know About the
Skeletal System

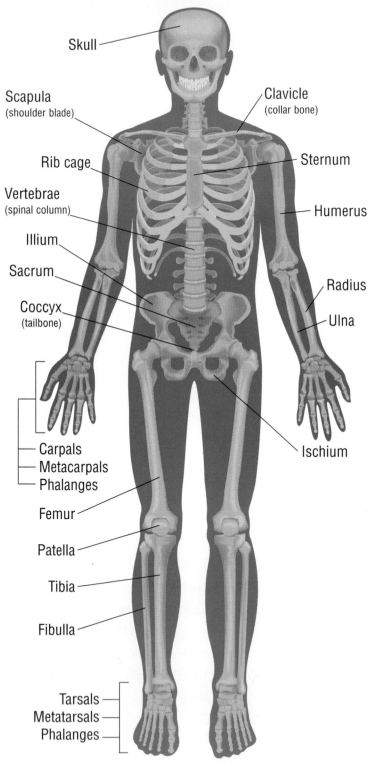

Skull

Scapula
(shoulder blade)

Clavicle
(collar bone)

Rib cage

Sternum

Vertebrae
(spinal column)

Humerus

Illium

Sacrum

Coccyx
(tailbone)

Radius

Ulna

Carpals
Metacarpals
Phalanges

Ischium

Femur

Patella

Tibia

Fibulla

Tarsals
Metatarsals
Phalanges

The **skeletal system** serves as a support framework, protects vital organs, works with muscles to produce movement, and produces blood cells. There are 206 bones in the skeletal system of an adult. **Bone** is the structural material of the skeletal system. **Periosteum** (per·ee·AHS·tee·um) is a thin sheet of outer tissue that covers bone. It contains nerves and blood vessels. The nerves cause you to feel pain when you suffer a blow to the bone. **Bone marrow** is the soft tissue in the hollow center area of most bones where red blood cells are produced.

Cartilage is a soft, connective tissue on the ends of some bones. It acts as a cushion where bones meet. For example, the disks between vertebrae are cartilage and serve as shock absorbers. Cartilage forms a cushion in the knee and hip joints. A **ligament** is a tough fiber that connects together bones. Sprained ankles and knees are caused by stretched or torn ligaments. A **joint** is the point where two bones meet. There are several types of joints in your body.

Keep Your Skeletal System Healthy

1. Select foods and beverages rich in calcium, phosphorus, and vitamin D.

2. Wear protective equipment when participating in sports.

3. Exercise regularly to strengthen joints and ligaments.

4. Sit, stand, and walk with correct posture.

5. Warm up before participating in physical activity.

6. Participate in screening for scoliosis, an irregular curvature of the spine.

7. Wear properly fitting, well-cushioned shoes.

What to Know About the
Muscular System

The **muscular system** consists of muscles that provide motion and maintain posture. There are more than 600 muscles in your body. Muscles are divided into two major groups. A **voluntary muscle** is a muscle a person can control. Muscles in your arms and legs that help you move are voluntary muscles. An **involuntary muscle** is a muscle that functions without a person's control. Muscles in your stomach and other internal organs are involuntary muscles.

There are three types of muscle tissue in your body. **Smooth muscle** is involuntary muscle tissue found in many internal organs. **Skeletal muscle** is muscle tissue that is attached to bone. Skeletal muscles help move your body. **Cardiac muscle** is muscle tissue found only in the heart. It is unique from other muscle tissue because of its structure. The contractions in cardiac muscles are generated by nerve stimulation.

A **tendon** is tough tissue fiber that attaches muscles to bones. Muscles work in pairs to move your body. One muscle in the pair contracts and shortens, while the other relaxes and lengthens.

Sternocleidmastoid (neck)

Trapezius (upper back and neck)

Deltoid (shoulder muscle)

Pectoralis (chest muscle)

Triceps brachii

Biceps brachii

Rectus abdominis (abdominal muscles)

Quadriceps (four muscles)

Gastrocnemius (calf muscle)

Keep Your Muscular System Healthy

1. Discontinue exercise if you have a muscle injury.
2. Warm up and stretch before vigorous exercise.
3. Exercise different muscle groups regularly.
4. Maintain your desirable weight.
5. Bend at the knees and keep your back straight when lifting heavy objects.
6. Select foods and beverages containing carbohydrates and proteins for energy and muscle development.
7. Sleep on a firm mattress.

What to Know About the
Endocrine System

The **endocrine system** consists of glands that control many of the body's activities by producing hormones. A **gland** is a group of cells or an organ that secretes hormones. A **hormone** is a chemical messenger that is released directly into the bloodstream. Hormones control many of your body's activities.

Pituitary Gland

The **pituitary** (pi·TOO·i·tehr·ree) **gland** is an endocrine gland that produces hormones that control growth and other glands. It is located just below the hypothalamus in the brain and is about the size of a pea. Hormones from the pituitary gland influence growth, metabolism, development of the reproductive organs, uterine contractions during childbirth, and many other body functions.

Thyroid Gland

The **thyroid gland** is an endocrine gland that produces thyroxin. **Thyroxin** is a hormone that controls metabolism and calcium balance in the body. **Metabolism** (muh·TAB·uh·liz·uhm) is the rate at which food is converted into energy in body cells. The thyroid gland is located near the upper portion of the trachea.

Parathyroid Gland

The **parathyroid glands** are endocrine glands that secrete hormones that control the amount of calcium and phosphorus in the body. There are four parathyroid glands. The parathyroid glands are located on the thyroid gland.

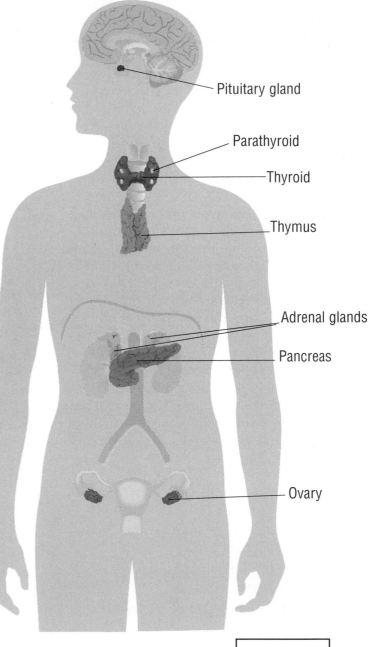

Pituitary gland

Parathyroid

Thyroid

Thymus

Adrenal glands

Pancreas

Ovary

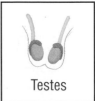

Testes

Lesson 67 will include more information about diabetes mellitus.

Pancreas

The **pancreas** is a gland that produces digestive enzymes and insulin. **Insulin** is a hormone that regulates the blood sugar level. If the pancreas fails to produce enough insulin, a person develops diabetes mellitus. **Diabetes**, or **diabetes mellitus** (dy·uh·BEE·teez me·LY·tuhs), is a disease in which the body produces little or no insulin.

Adrenal Glands

The **adrenal glands** are endocrine glands that secrete several hormones, including adrenaline. **Adrenaline** is a hormone that prepares the body to react during times of stress or in an emergency. The adrenal glands also secrete hormones that affect the body's metabolism. There are two adrenal glands in the body located on the kidneys.

Ovaries

The **ovaries** are female reproductive glands that produce ova and estrogen. **Ova** are egg cells, or female reproductive cells. There are two ovaries in the female body. **Estrogen** is a hormone produced by the ovaries that stimulates the development of female secondary sex characteristics and affects the menstrual cycle.

Testes

The **testes** are male reproductive glands that produce sperm cells and testosterone. There are two testes in the male body. **Testosterone** (te·STAH·stuh·rohn) is a hormone that produces the male secondary sex characteristics.

Pituitary Gland

The pituitary gland often is called the master gland because it releases hormones that affect the working of the other glands. The hormones:

- regulate the development of bones and muscles;
- affect the reproductive organs;
- affect the functioning of the kidney, the adrenal gland, and the thyroid glands;
- stimulate the uterus to contract during childbirth.

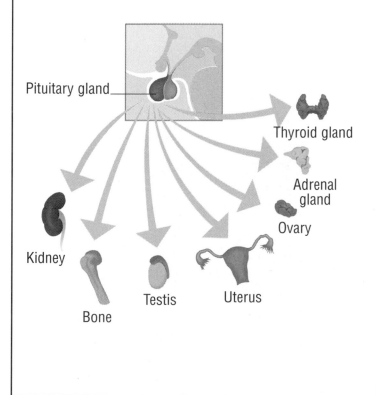

Pituitary gland

Thyroid gland

Adrenal gland

Ovary

Kidney

Testis

Uterus

Bone

Keep Your Endocrine System Healthy

1. Have regular medical checkups.
2. Perform testicular self-examinations each month (males).
3. Keep track of the length and dates of your menstrual cycles (females).

What to Know About the
Digestive System

The **digestive system** breaks down food into nutrients that can be used by the body. The digestive system also allows nutrients to be absorbed by body cells and eliminates waste from the body. **Digestion** is the process by which food is changed so that it can be absorbed by the body's cells.

Mouth

When food is chewed in the mouth, the teeth break it into smaller pieces. The **salivary glands** are glands in the mouth that release saliva that contains a chemical to begin the digestion of carbohydrates. **Saliva** is a fluid that helps soften food so that it can be swallowed more easily.

Esophagus

When you swallow, food moves into the esophagus. The **esophagus** is a tube connecting the mouth to the stomach. Food passes to your stomach by the process of peristalsis. **Peristalsis** (per·uh·STOHL·suhz) is a series of involuntary muscle contractions. Peristalsis can move food to your stomach even if you are standing on your head.

Stomach

The **stomach** is an organ that releases acids and juices that mix with the food and produce a thick paste called chyme (KIME). Your stomach produces a layer of mucus to protect its lining from the strong acids that it releases. After about four hours of churning the food, muscles in the stomach force the food into the small intestine.

Small Intestine

The **small intestine** is a coiled tube in which the greatest amount of digestion and absorption take place. The small intestine is about 21 feet (6.3 meters) long and is lined with villi. **Villi** are small folds in the lining of the small intestine. The villi increase the surface area and allow more food to be absorbed. Several enzymes are produced in the lining of the small intestine. An **enzyme** is a protein that regulates chemical reactions.

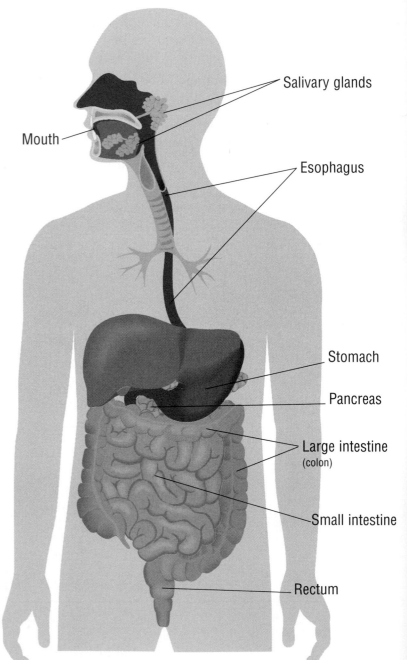

Salivary glands

Mouth

Esophagus

Stomach

Pancreas

Large intestine
(colon)

Small intestine

Rectum

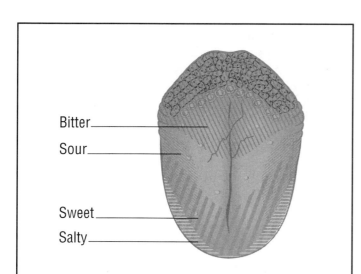

Bitter

Sour

Sweet

Salty

Approximately 10,000 microscopic taste buds located on the tongue pick up four basic flavor sensations. Each sensation is detected on a certain part of the tongue, although there is some overlap. Sweet is tasted at the tip, salty on the front sides, sour on the middle sides, and bitter at the back.

Liver

The **liver** is a gland that releases bile to help break down fats, maintain blood sugar level, and filter poisonous wastes. Bile flows to the small intestine to help in the digestion of fats. The **gallbladder** is an organ that stores bile. The liver produces bile, which is transported to the small intestine. Bile aids in digestion. The pancreas produces several enzymes that aid digestion in the small intestine.

Pancreas

The pancreas is a gland that produces digestive enzymes and insulin. A portion of your pancreas produces enzymes for the digestive system, while another portion produces hormones for the endocrine system. Enzymes from your pancreas break down proteins, starches, and fats in your small intestine.

Large Intestine

After food passes through the small intestine, it enters the large intestine, also called the colon. The **large intestine** is a tube extending from the small intestine in which undigested food is prepared for elimination from the body. When the large intestine is full, it contracts, and solid wastes leave the body through the rectum and anus. The **rectum** is a short tube at the end of the large intestine that stores wastes temporarily. The **anus** is the opening to the outside of the body at the end of the rectum.

Keep Your Digestive System Healthy

1. Eat plenty of foods containing fiber.
2. Eat slowly.
3. Practice stress management skills to avoid indigestion.
4. Drink at least six to eight glasses of water each day.
5. Seek proper medical care if vomiting occurs after eating.

What to Know About the
Urinary System

The **urinary system** removes liquid wastes from the body and maintains the body's water balance. The organs of the urinary system are the kidneys, ureters, bladder, and urethra.

Kidneys

A **kidney** is an organ that filters the blood and excretes waste products and excess water in the form of urine. **Urine** is a pale yellow liquid composed of water, salts, and other waste products. The body has two kidneys. They lie on either side of the spinal column just above the waist.

Ureters

A **ureter** (YU·ruh·ter) is a narrow tube that connects the kidneys to the urinary bladder. The ureters carry urine from the kidneys to the urinary bladder.

Urinary Bladder

The **urinary bladder** is a muscular sac that stores urine. As the urinary bladder fills with urine, it expands. When it reaches its capacity, the urinary bladder releases urine into the urethra.

Urethra

The **urethra** (yu·REE·thruh) is a narrow tube extending from the urinary bladder to the outside of the body through which urine passes out of the body.

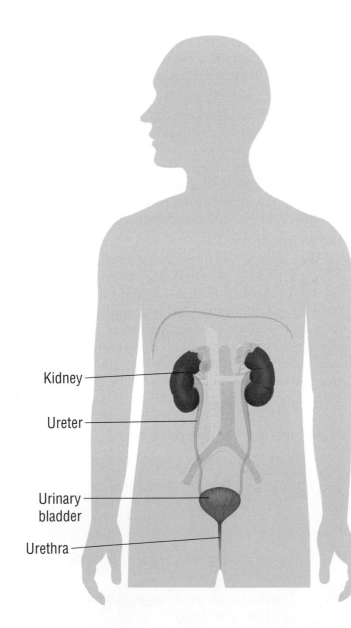

Kidney

Ureter

Urinary bladder

Urethra

Keep Your Urinary System Healthy

1. Drink at least six to eight glasses of water each day.

2. Maintain a healthful blood pressure, because high blood pressure damages the kidneys.

What to Know About the
Integumentary System

The **integumentary** (in·TEH·gyuh·ment·tuh·ree) **system** covers and protects the body and consists of skin, glands associated with the skin, hair, and nails.

Your skin is the largest organ in your body. It has nerve cells that help you detect pain, pressure, touch, heat, and cold. The skin protects some body parts against injury, serves as a protective layer that keeps microorganisms from entering your body, and helps you maintain a healthful body temperature. Your skin helps with the removal of wastes from the body and helps you sense the environment. It also helps protect you from ultraviolet radiation because of the presence of melanin. **Melanin** is a pigment that gives the skin its color and protects the body from the ultraviolet rays of the sun.

The skin is made up of two layers. The **epidermis** is the outer layer of skin cells. These cells are constantly shed and replaced. The epidermis does not contain blood vessels or nerve endings. New skin cells are produced in the deepest layer of the epidermis. The **dermis** is a thick layer of cells below the epidermis that contains sweat glands, hair follicles, sebaceous (oil) glands, blood vessels, and nerves. A **sweat gland** is a gland that aids the body in getting rid of wastes, such as salt. Sweat glands also help cool your body by releasing sweat through your pores to evaporate on the surface of your skin. A **sebaceous gland** is a small oil-producing gland that helps protect the skin. **Sebum** is the oil produced by sebaceous glands. Your skin has several types of nerve cells that help you detect pain, pressure, touch, heat, and cold. Below the dermis is the subcutaneous layer. The **subcutaneous layer** is a layer of fatty tissue located below the dermis. A large portion of the body's fat is stored in this layer.

Because your skin is the largest organ in your body, it also is the most vulnerable organ in your body. There are several types of conditions that affect the skin. Common skin conditions include birth marks and scars. A birth mark is an area of discolored skin that is present at birth. Birth marks include different types of freckles and moles and may be removed by a physician. A scar is a mark left on damaged tissue after the tissue has healed. If a person is cut or has a severe burn, (s)he may develop a scar. Some people are more likely than others to develop scars. These people may get large, thick scars from small cuts or burns.

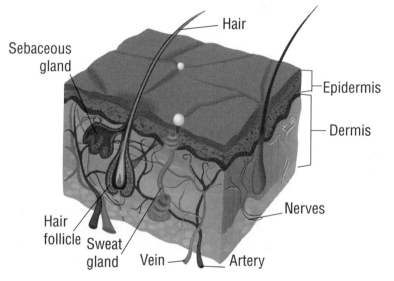

Warts and ringworm are other common skin conditions. A **wart** is a contagious growth that forms on the top layer of the skin. Warts are caused by a viral infection. They usually grow in groups and can be spread by contact. Warts can be treated with over-the-counter drugs. However, if warts spread, they should be treated by a physician. **Ringworm** is a skin condition that causes small, red, ring-shaped marks on the skin. Ringworm is caused by a fungal infection and can be spread by physical contact. Physicians usually treat ringworm with ointments or creams. However, severe cases of ringworm may require treatment with antifungal tablets.

Lesson 21

Review

Nails and hair also are part of the integumentary system. Nails are made up of dead cells and keratin. **Keratin** is a tough protein that makes up nails and hair. **Hair** is a thread-like structure consisting of dead cells filled with keratin. Hair protects your skin from harmful sun rays and helps you maintain your body temperature. Hair varies in color, texture, and amount for each person. From 100,000 to 200,000 hairs may be on your head. Each hair grows from a follicle. A **hair follicle** is a pit on the surface of the skin that contains nutrients a hair needs to grow. The roots of your hair are made up of living cells. As new hair cells are produced, old hair cells are pushed up through the scalp.

Keep Your Integumentary System Healthy

1. Wear sunscreen with an SPF of at least 15 when you are exposed to the sun.
2. Examine skin monthly for any changes in moles, warts, or freckles.
3. Shower or bathe each day.
4. Follow directions when using make-up.
5. Eat foods containing vitamin A.
6. Seek proper medical care for skin rashes.
7. Wash hair often.
8. Treat dandruff.

Vocabulary Words

Write a separate sentence using 25 of the vocabulary words listed on page 177.

Objectives

1. What are seven ways to keep the nervous system healthy? **Objective 1**
2. What are six ways to keep the cardio-vascular system healthy? **Objective 2**
3. What are five ways to keep the immune system healthy? **Objective 3**
4. What are seven ways to keep the respiratory system healthy? **Objective 4**
5. What are seven ways to keep the skeletal system healthy? **Objective 5**
6. What are seven ways to keep the muscular system healthy? **Objective 6**
7. What are three ways to keep the endocrine system healthy? **Objective 7**
8. What are five ways to keep the digestive system healthy? **Objective 8**
9. What are two ways to keep the urinary system healthy? **Objective 9**
10. What are eight ways to keep the integumentary system healthy? **Objective 10**

Responsible Decision-Making

You stop to talk to a classmate after school. When (s)he opens his/her locker, you notice several tubes of glue. You ask if (s)he is working on a school art project. Your classmate explains that (s)he takes a big whiff of the glue between classes to get high. (S)he takes the cap off the glue, takes three big whiffs, and hands it to you. Write a response to this situation.

1. **Describe the situation that requires you to make a decision.**
2. **List possible decisions you might make.**
3. **Name two responsible adults with whom you might discuss your decisions.**
4. **Evaluate the possible consequences of your decisions. Determine if each decision will lead to actions that:**
   - promote health,
   - protect safety,
   - follow laws,
   - show respect for yourself and others,
   - follow the guidelines of your parents and of other responsible adults,
   - demonstrate good character.
5. **Decide which decision is most responsible and appropriate.**
6. **Tell two results you expect if you make this decision.**

Effective Communication

Prepare a 30-second public service announcement reminding people in your community to wear safety belts when riding in a motor vehicle. Record your announcement and send the tape to a local radio station.

Self-Directed Learning

Try to find information about kidney diseases and kidney transplants. Use a computer to access the web site for the Kidney Foundation or write a letter to the Kidney Foundation. Share with your classmates the information you receive from the foundation.

Critical Thinking

Your school has a rule that a student must attend school the day on which (s)he participates in a school-related athletic event. You are a member of an athletic team, the band, or the cheerleading squad. The day of a "big game" you wake up with swollen lymph nodes and a fever. Write a short essay explaining why you should stay home from school and miss the game when you have these symptoms.

Responsible Citizenship

A neighbor asks you to supervise his six-year-old son while he does errands. He has given his son permission to ride his bicycle. Shortly after the boy's father leaves, the boy takes off his bicycle safety helmet. As a committed health advocate, what would you say to the boy? What would you say to the boy's father when he returns from doing his errands?

You Can Learn About Female Reproductive Health

Life Skill **I will recognize habits that protect female reproductive health.**

During adolescence, a female's body matures. She develops secondary sex characteristics and has her first menstrual period. Her body becomes capable of reproduction even though she is not prepared to be a parent. This lesson discusses the physical and emotional changes in females during puberty. You will learn about the structure and function of the organs in the female reproductive system. You also will learn about the menstrual cycle and how a female can protect her reproductive health.

The Lesson Outline

What to Know About Puberty in Females

What to Know About the Female Reproductive System

What to Know About the Menstrual Cycle

What to Know About Female Reproductive Health

How Females Can Protect Reproductive Health

Objectives

1. Discuss the physical and emotional changes females experience during puberty. **page 195**

2. Name and give the function of the organs in the female reproductive system. **page 196**

3. Outline the physiological changes that occur in a menstrual cycle. **page 197**

4. Discuss information pertaining to female reproductive health, including products to absorb the menstrual flow; menstrual cramps; toxic shock syndrome; a missed menstrual period; the pelvic examination; and breast self-examination. **pages 198–199**

5. Identify seven ways females can protect reproductive health. **page 199**

Vocabulary Words

puberty
estrogen
secondary sex characteristics
body image
female reproductive system
mons veneris
labia majora
labia minora
clitoris
hymen
ovaries
ovulation
Fallopian tube
uterus
cervix
vagina
menstrual cycle
menstruation
corpus luteum
progesterone
toxic shock syndrome (TSS)
premenstrual syndrome (PMS)
amenorrhea
pelvic examination
Pap smear
breast self-examination (BSE)

What to Know About
Puberty in Females

Puberty is the stage of growth and development when both the male and female body become capable of producing offspring. When a female is around eight years old, the pituitary gland increases its production of a hormone called FSH. FSH travels through the bloodstream to the ovaries and causes them to secrete estrogen. **Estrogen** is a hormone produced by the ovaries that stimulates the development of female secondary sex characteristics and affects the menstrual cycle. **Secondary sex characteristics** are physical and emotional changes that occur during puberty. During puberty, a female must learn to accept these physical changes and manage her emotions in responsible ways.

How to Manage Emotions

During puberty, a female may notice that she has sudden emotional changes and sexual feelings. Estrogen and other hormones cause these changes. Hormone levels fluctuate and as a result a female may experience sudden changes in her emotions. Everyday occurrences, such as school assignments or family responsibilities, may produce intense feelings. A female may be puzzled at some of her reactions. But she should know that most changes in mood are normal. Of course, she must take responsibility for behaving in responsible ways even though her emotional feelings may change rapidly.

The increase in estrogen also produces sexual feelings. Sexual feelings result from a strong physical and emotional attraction to another person. Females must set limits, stick to these limits, and practice abstinence. In Lesson 16, how to set limits and how to resist pressure to be sexually active was discussed in detail.

How to Accept Physical Changes

The physical changes that occur during puberty are listed below. These changes become noticeable between the ages of eight and 15. The maturing process that happens in puberty is affected by a female's heredity, diet, health habits, and health status. For example, a female with an inadequate diet may mature more slowly. A female who overtrains for a sport may have a delayed menstrual cycle.

During puberty, a female must become comfortable with her maturing body. **Body image** is the perception a person has of his/her body's appearance. A female is more likely to have a positive body image when she is well-educated about her anatomy and physiology. Knowing that females mature at different rates can be comforting. A female should avoid comparing her body to that of other females the same age. She should ask her parents, guardian, or physician when she has questions about her growth and development.

Female Secondary Sex Characteristics

- Increase in height
- Widening of the hips
- Softer and smoother skin
- Increase in breast size
- Growth of pubic hair and underarm hair
- Enlargement of external genitals
- Formation of mature ova
- Beginning of menstruation

What to Know About the Female Reproductive System

The **female reproductive system** consists of organs in the female body that are involved in producing offspring. The external female reproductive organs are called the vulva. The vulva consist of the mons veneris, the labia majora, the labia minora, the clitoris, and the hymen. The **mons veneris** is the fatty tissue that covers the front of the pubic bone and serves as a protective cushion for the internal reproductive organs. During puberty, hair begins to cover both the mons veneris and the labia majora. The **labia majora** are the heavy folds of skin that surround the opening of the vagina.

The **labia minora** are two smaller folds of skin located within the labia majora. The clitoris and the openings of the urethra and the vagina are located within the labia minora. The **clitoris** is a small, highly sensitive structure located above the opening of the urethra. The clitoris is richly supplied with blood vessels and nerve endings.

The **hymen** is a thin membrane that stretches across the opening of the vagina. The hymen has small openings in it. Some females do not have a hymen. Other females often break or tear the hymen when they ride bicycles or horses or exercise strenuously.

The internal female reproductive organs are the ovaries, Fallopian tubes, uterus, and vagina. The **ovaries** are female reproductive glands that produce ova and estrogen. A female is born with between 200,000 and 400,000 immature ova in her ovaries. About 375 of these ova will mature and be released in a female's lifetime. During puberty, the ova begin to develop. Each developing ova is enclosed in a small, hollow ball called a follicle. Each month during the menstrual cycle, an ovum matures and is released from its follicle. **Ovulation** is the release of a mature ovum from one of the two ovaries.

When an ovum is released from an ovary it enters one of the Fallopian tubes. A **Fallopian tube** is a four-inch-(ten-centimeter) long tube that connects an ovary to the uterus. A female has two Fallopian tubes—one connected to each ovary. During the menstrual cycle, a mature ovum moves through a Fallopian tube to the uterus. If fertilization occurs, it usually occurs in a Fallopian tube. An ovum that is not fertilized either disintegrates in the uterus or leaves the body in the menstrual flow. The **uterus** is a muscular organ that receives and supports the fertilized egg during pregnancy and contracts during childbirth to help with delivery. The **cervix** is the lowest part of the uterus that connects to the vagina. The **vagina** is a muscular tube that connects the uterus to the outside of the body. The vagina serves as the female organ for sexual intercourse, as the birth canal, and as the passageway for the menstrual flow.

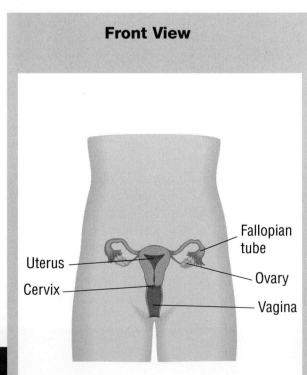

Front View

Uterus

Cervix

Fallopian tube

Ovary

Vagina

What to Know About the
Menstrual Cycle

The **menstrual cycle** is a monthly series of changes that involves ovulation, changes in the uterine lining, and menstruation. **Menstruation** is the period in the menstrual cycle in which the unfertilized egg and the lining of the uterus leave the body in a menstrual flow. Females often describe menstruation as their "period." The menstrual cycle occurs over 28 days. This means a female will have her period every 28 days. However, many teens have irregular cycles. The length of their menstrual cycle varies. The menstrual flow usually is about five days. However, the number of days also may vary. In the box to the right, the series of changes that occur during a 28-day menstrual cycle is outlined. The next section of this lesson discusses female reproductive health and how to protect it.

The Menstrual Cycle

Days 1–5

Menstruation or the menstrual flow leaves the body. The menstrual flow consists of about two ounces (56 grams) of blood. Some females may notice small particles. These are small pieces of uterine lining. At the same time, a new ova is maturing in the ovary.

Days 6–12

The uterine lining begins to thicken. The uterus prepares ahead for ovulation and the possibility that an ovum will be fertilized.

Days 13–14

Ovulation occurs. A follicle in an ovary bursts, and an ovum is released into one of the Fallopian tubes.

Days 15–20

The corpus luteum secretes hormones to support a pregnancy. The corpus luteum is formed when the remains of the burst follicle close. The **corpus luteum** is a temporary gland that secretes progesterone. **Progesterone** is a hormone that changes the lining of the uterus. As the uterine lining changes, it prepares to support a fertilized ovum. If an ovum is fertilized, the corpus luteum continues to secrete progesterone throughout pregnancy.

Days 21–28

The corpus luteum disintegrates if an ovum is not fertilized. No more progesterone is secreted. The cells in the lining of the uterus die without progesterone. The unfertilized ovum disintegrates. The menstrual cycle begins again.

Side View

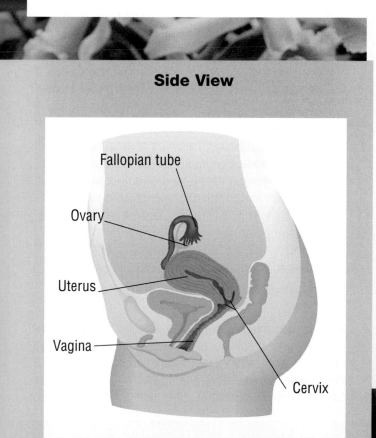

Fallopian tube

Ovary

Uterus

Vagina

Cervix

What to Know About
Female Reproductive Health

Q A

Answers to the questions that follow provide information on female reproductive health.

Q: What products can be used to absorb the menstrual flow?

A: Pads, panty shields or liners, and tampons are products that can be used to absorb the menstrual flow. A pad is a thick piece of cotton that absorbs the menstrual flow as it leaves the vagina. A pad should be changed every four to six hours. A panty shield or liner is a thin strip of cotton that is worn inside underpants to collect the menstrual flow. It is usually worn on days when flow is light and may be worn with a tampon for extra protection. A tampon is a small tube of cotton placed inside the vagina to absorb the menstrual flow. The tampon collects the menstrual flow before any of the flow leaves the vagina. A female who wears a tampon can swim during her period without fear that the menstrual flow will get on her bathing suit or into the water. Tampons should be changed at least every four to six hours.

Q: How can menstrual cramps be reduced?

A: Some females have painful menstrual cramps in the lower abdomen caused by contractions of the uterus. A warm bath and moderate exercise may relieve the cramps. Reducing the amount of caffeine and sodium in the diet also may reduce menstrual cramps. A female can speak with her parents, guardian, or physician about using medications, such as ibuprofen, that reduce menstrual cramps.

Q: What is toxic shock syndrome (TSS)?

A: Toxic shock syndrome (TSS) is a severe illness resulting from infection with toxin-producing strains of *Staphylococcus*. Early flu-like symptoms of TSS include a high fever of more than 102°F (39°C), vomiting, diarrhea, dizziness, fainting, and a rash like a sunburn. These symptoms may progress to a sudden drop in blood pressure. Complications of TSS include kidney and heart failure and difficulty in breathing. About 95 percent of TSS cases occur in females having

their menstrual period. Bacteria in the vagina secrete a toxin that gets into the bloodstream. Females should be careful when using tampons and change them at least four or five times a day. Regular tampons changed often are better than superabsorbent tampons worn for longer periods of time. A pad should be worn at night. Tampon use should be discontinued if fever or other signs appear. Prompt medical care is needed if symptoms occur.

Q: What is premenstrual syndrome (PMS)?

A: Premenstrual syndrome (PMS) is a combination of physical and emotional symptoms that affect a female a week to ten days prior to menstruation. These symptoms may include weight gain, bloating, swollen breasts, headaches, backache, constipation, mood swings, cravings, anxiety, and depression. A female can help reduce weight gain, bloating, and swelling by avoiding caffeine and salt. This reduces the chances that she will retain fluids. She also can exercise regularly to produce beta-endorphins that improve mood and reduce anxiety and depression. A physician can prescribe medications to lessen the symptoms of PMS.

Q: What causes a missed menstrual cycle?

A: Amenorrhea (ah·me·nuh·REE·uh) is the absence of menstruation. The menstrual cycles of some females do not begin at puberty. This type of amenorrhea may be caused by underdeveloped female reproductive organs, poor general health, and/or emotional stress. Some females miss additional menstrual cycles after their first menstrual cycle. This type of amenorrhea is often caused by pregnancy or by a reduction in red blood cell levels resulting from stress, overtraining, eating disorders, drastic weight loss, and anemia.

Q: What does a pelvic examination include?

A: A **pelvic examination** is an examination of the internal female reproductive organs. A Pap smear usually is done when this examination is performed. A **Pap smear** is a screening test in which cells are scraped from the cervix and examined to detect cervical cancer.

How Females Can Protect Reproductive Health

1. **Keep a calendar in which you record information about your menstrual cycle.** Keep track of the number of days in each cycle. Keep track of the number of days that you have a menstrual flow. Know the date of your last menstrual period (LMP). Make a note of any questions you have about cramps, mood swings, or heavy menstrual flow. Share this information with your parents or guardian and your physician.

2. **Practice good menstrual hygiene habits.** Change your pad, panty shield, or tampon every four to six hours. Wear a pad or panty shield at night to reduce the risk of TSS. Change underwear often and wash your genitals daily to avoid vaginal odor.

3. **Choose habits to prevent or lessen menstrual cramps.** Exercise regularly and reduce the amount of caffeine and salt in your diet.

4. **Perform monthly breast self-examinations.** Begin the habit of monthly breast self-examination (BSE). Perform BSE each month after your menstrual flow stops.

5. **Have regular medical checkups.** Bring the calendar in which you have recorded information about your menstrual cycles to your checkup. Go over the recorded information with your physician. Your parents or guardian and your physician will determine the appropriate age for you to begin to have a pelvic examination and Pap smear.

6. **Seek medical attention when you show signs of infection.** Vaginal discharge, lumps, and rashes are symptoms of infection. You may be infected with a sexually transmitted disease.

7. **Practice abstinence from sex.** Abstinence from sex is choosing not to be sexually active. Practicing abstinence prevents teen pregnancy and infection with sexually transmitted diseases.

Lesson 63 will include more information on STDs.

Breast Self-Examination

All females should perform a breast self-examination. A **breast self-examination (BSE)** is a screening procedure for breast cancer in which a female checks her breasts for lumps and changes. A physician or a nurse performs BSE when a female has checkups. Below are four basic steps to follow for a breast self-examination. A female should check her technique with a physician or nurse to be certain she performs BSE properly.

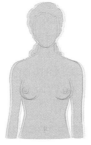

Stand in front of a mirror with arms at your sides. Examine breasts carefully for anything unusual—puckering, dimpling, changes in skin texture.

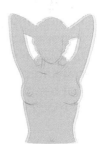

Clasp your hands behind your head. Press your hands forward. Look carefully for changes in size, shape, and contour of each breast.

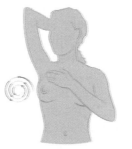

Raise your left arm. Use the fingers of the other hand to examine the left breast. Start at the outermost top edge of the breast. Go in circles toward the nipple. Fingers flat, press gently in small circles. Move the circles slowly around the breast. Include the area between the breast and the armpit and the armpit itself. Raise your right arm, and examine the right breast.

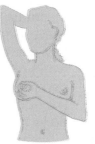

Gently squeeze each nipple between your thumb and index finger. Look for discharge.

Activity

Dear Physician

Life Skill: I will recognize habits that protect female reproductive health.

Materials: paper and pencil; computer (optional)

Directions: Suppose you are a physician who writes a column for a woman's magazine. You need to respond to the letters below from readers. Design a one-page advice column in which to place the letters and your responses. If possible, use a computer.

Dear Physician:

Every month, before her menstrual period begins, my sister complains of sharp pains in her lower abdomen. She stays at home and survives by drinking soda pop and pigging out on chocolates. But this does not seem to stop her pain. What should she do?

Concerned Brother

Dear Physician:

My family is going south for Spring break. I've trying to lose weight to get into my bathing suit. I skip breakfast and lunch and exercise for two hours every day. I feel tired and have missed my last two menstrual periods. I am not sexually active. Why haven't I had my period?

Starving and Exercising

Dear Physician:

My brother and sister-in-law live with us. The week before my sister-in-law gets her menstrual period, she usually suffers from PMS. She is really cranky. She complains that she feels sick and has headaches that won't go away. She ends up staying in bed for days and taking medication that her doctor prescribed. What else can she do to reduce the effects of PMS?

PMSed

Dear Physician:

My girlfriend has a calendar on which she records information about her menstrual cycles. Why does her physician want her to do this? What information does she record on her calendar?

Curious

Dear Physician:

I caught the tail end of a news report from the Centers for Disease Control and Prevention that discussed TSS. What is TSS and how can it be prevented?

Super News Watcher

Lesson 22

Review

Vocabulary Words

Write a separate sentence using each of the vocabulary words listed on page 194.

Objectives

1. What are eight female secondary sex characteristics? **Objective 1**

2. What are the organs in the female reproductive system and their functions? **Objective 2**

3. What are the physiological changes that occur in a menstrual cycle? **Objective 3**

4. What should females know about products to absorb the menstrual flow, menstrual cramps, toxic shock syndrome, a missed menstrual period, the pelvic examination, and breast self-examination? **Objective 4**

5. What are seven ways females can protect reproductive health? **Objective 5**

Responsible Decision-Making

You are at the mall with a friend. Your friend uses one of the restrooms. (S)he is gone a long time. You enter the restroom and find your friend writing slang terms about the female reproductive system on one of the stalls. Your friend hands you a marker and tells you a crude, slang word for a female reproductive organ. Write a response to this situation.

1. Describe the situation that requires you to make a decision.
2. List possible decisions you might make.
3. Name two responsible adults with whom you might discuss your decisions.
4. Evaluate the possible consequences of your decisions. Determine if each decision will lead to actions that:
   - promote health,
   - protect safety,
   - follow laws,
   - show respect for yourself and others,
   - follow the guidelines of your parents and of other responsible adults,
   - demonstrate good character.
5. Decide which decision is most responsible and appropriate.
6. Tell two results you expect if you make this decision.

 ## Effective Communication

Collect several old teen magazines. Cut out pictures of teen females and males. Make a collage by glueing the pictures to posterboard. Use the poster to illustrate teens at different stages in their growth spurt. Share the poster with your classmates.

 ## Self-Directed Learning

Locate an article in a medical journal that focuses on an aspect of female reproductive health. Read the article and write a one-or two-paragraph summary.

 ## Critical Thinking

Suppose you know a female gymnast. To prepare for the districts, she begins training long hours. She also begins a starvation diet. In confidence, she shares that she has missed several menstrual periods. She is not sexually active or pregnant. Why might she have missed several menstrual periods?

 ## Responsible Citizenship

Pretend that you work for the Cancer Society. Write or make a tape of a public service announcement that reminds females to perform monthly breast self-examinations.

You Can Learn About Male Reproductive Health

Life Skill **I will recognize habits that protect male reproductive health.**

During adolescence, a male's body matures. He develops secondary sex characteristics. His body becomes capable of reproduction even though he is not prepared to be a parent. This lesson discusses the physical and emotional changes in males during puberty. You will learn about the structure and function of the organs in the male reproductive system. This lesson also explains how a male can protect his reproductive health.

The Lesson Outline

What to Know About Puberty in Males

What to Know About the Male Reproductive System

What to Know About Male Reproductive Health

How Males Can Protect Reproductive Health

Objectives

1. Discuss the physical and emotional changes males experience during puberty. **page 203**

2. Name and give the function of the organs in the male reproductive system. **page 204**

3. Discuss information pertaining to male reproductive health, including circumcision, inguinal hernia, mumps, digital rectal examination, and testicular self-examination. **page 205**

4. Discuss seven ways to protect male reproductive health. **page 206**

Vocabulary Words

puberty

testosterone

male reproductive system

penis

scrotum

testes

sperm

seminiferous tubules

spermatogenesis

epididymis

vas deferens

seminal vesicles

ejaculatory duct

prostate gland

Cowper's glands

erection

ejaculation

semen

circumcision

smegma

inguinal hernia

sterility

digital rectal examination

testicular self-examination

What to Know About
Puberty in Males

Puberty is the stage of growth and development when both the male and female body become capable of producing offspring. During puberty the male's pituitary gland increases its production of a hormone called LH. LH travels through the bloodstream to the testes and causes them to secrete testosterone. **Testosterone** is a hormone that produces male secondary sex characteristics. The secondary sex characteristics are physical and emotional changes that occur during puberty. During puberty, a male must learn to accept these changes.

How to Manage Emotions

During puberty, a male may notice that he has sudden emotional changes and sexual feelings. Testosterone is responsible for causing these changes. Testosterone levels fluctuate, and a male experiences sudden changes in his emotions.

A male may become angry or say things he does not mean to say. He may feel insecure or edgy for no reason. A male may be puzzled when he has such intense feelings. But, he should know that changes in emotions are normal during puberty. Teen males are accountable for the way they respond to emotional changes. Lesson 8 explains how to express emotions in healthful ways.

The increase in testosterone also produces sexual feelings. Sexual feelings result from a strong physical and emotional attraction to another person. Males must set limits, stick to these limits, and practice abstinence. Lesson 16 explains how to set limits and how to resist pressure to be sexually active.

How to Accept Physical Changes

The physical changes that occur during puberty are listed below. These changes become noticeable between the ages of 12 and 15. The maturing process that happens in puberty is affected by heredity, diet, health habits, and health status. For example, a male who lifts weights may develop a more muscular body than a male who does not. A male who is short for his age may have biological relatives who are short.

During puberty, a male must become comfortable with his maturing body. Body image is the perception a person has of his/her body's appearance. A male is more likely to have a positive body image when he is knowledgable about male anatomy and physiology. For example, the growth spurt in males occurs later than it does in females. Also, males mature at very different rates. A male who is short in stature suddenly may have a growth spurt of several inches. A male should ask his parents, guardian, or physician questions he has about growth and development. He should avoid comparing his body to those of other males. For example, a teen male should not compare his body to a professional athlete's body. Professional athletes are older and have completed training programs that have affected their bodies.

Male Secondary Sex Characteristics

• ►

- Increase in height
- Longer and heavier bones
- Broader shoulders
- Thicker and tougher skin
- Deepened voice
- Growth of facial hair, pubic hair, and body hair
- Enlargement of penis, scrotum, and testes
- Formation of sperm

What to Know About the
Male Reproductive System

The **male reproductive system** consists of organs in the male body that are involved in producing offspring. The external organs of the male reproductive system are the penis and the scrotum. The **penis** is the male sex organ used for reproduction and urination. The **scrotum** is a sac-like pouch that holds the testes and helps regulate their temperature. The **testes** are male reproductive glands that produce sperm cells and testosterone. The scrotum hangs from the body so that the testes have a lower temperature than the rest of the body. This allows the testes to produce sperm. **Sperm** are male reproductive cells.

The internal male reproductive organs include the testes, seminiferous tubules, epididymis, vas deferens, seminal vesicles, ejaculatory duct, prostate gland, Cowpers' glands, and urethra. The testes are divided into several sections that are filled with seminiferous tubules. The **seminiferous** (se·muh·NI·fuh·ruhs) **tubules** are a network of coiled tubules in which sperm are produced. **Spermatogenesis** (spur·muh·toh·JEN·uh·sis) is the process by which sperm are produced.

After sperm are produced in the seminiferous tubules, they move to the epididymis. The **epididymis** (e·puh·DI·duh·mus) is a comma-shaped structure along the upper rear surface of the testes where sperm mature. Some sperm are stored in the epidiymis, but most move to the vas deferens after they mature.

The **vas deferens** are two long, thin tubes that act as a passageway for sperm and a place for sperm storage. They extend from the epididymis in the scrotum up into the abdomen. The walls of the vas deferens are lined with cilia. The contractions of the vas deferens along with the action of the cilia help transport sperm. In the abdomen, the vas deferens circle the bladder and connect with the ducts of the seminal vesicles to form the ejaculatory duct. The **seminal vesicles** are two small glands that secrete a fluid rich in sugar that nourishes and helps sperm move. The **ejaculatory duct** is a short, straight tube that passes into the prostate gland and opens into the urethra. The urethra serves as a passageway for sperm and urine to leave the body.

The **prostate gland** is a gland that produces a fluid that helps keep sperm alive. The prostate gland is located beneath the bladder and surrounds the urethra. Without the fluid from the prostate gland, fertilization would be almost impossible because many sperm would die. The Cowper's glands are located beneath the prostate gland. The **Cowper's glands** are two small glands that secrete a clear, lubricating fluid into the urethra.

An **erection** is a process that occurs when the penis swells with blood and elongates. An erection may be acccompanied by ejaculation. **Ejaculation** is the passage of semen from the penis and is a result of a series of muscular contractions. **Semen** is the fluid that contains sperm and fluids from the seminal vesicles, prostate gland, and Cowper's glands. After ejaculation, the penis returns to a nonerect state.

Front View

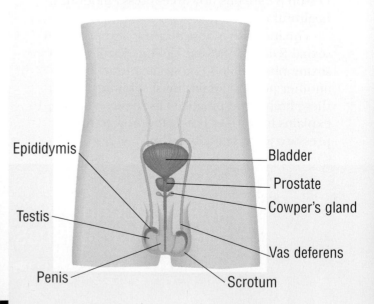

Epididymis
Bladder
Prostate
Cowper's gland
Testis
Vas deferens
Penis
Scrotum

What to Know About
Male Reproductive Health

Answers to the questions that follow provide information on male reproductive health.

Q: What is circumcision?

A: The end of the penis is covered by a piece of skin called the foreskin. **Circumcision** is the surgical removal of the foreskin from the penis. This procedure usually is performed on the second day after birth. Circumcision may reduce the risk of urinary infections and cancer of the penis. Males who are not circumcised should pull the foreskin back and cleanse the penis regularly to prevent smegma from collecting. **Smegma** (SMEG·muh) is a substance that forms under the foreskin consisting of dead skin and other secretions.

Q: What causes an inguinal hernia?

A: In a developing fetus, the testes pass from the abdomen into the scrotum through the inguinal canal during the seventh month of pregnancy. Then the inguinal canal closes to keep the intestines from also passing into the scrotum. In some males, the inguinal canal does not completely close off. The intestines pass into the inguinal canal and the male develops an inguinal hernia. An **inguinal hernia** is a hernia in which some of the intestine pushes through the inguinal canal into the scrotum. Lifting heavy objects sometimes stresses this area and is the cause of the hernia. An inguinal hernia may be painful and can be repaired surgically.

Q: How can having mumps after puberty cause sterility?

A: Mumps is a viral infection that affects the salivary glands. Mumps usually occurs in childhood. There is a vaccine to prevent mumps. But, some people do not get mumps in childhood, and they do not get the mumps vaccine. If a male has mumps after puberty, the virus can affect the testes. The virus causes swelling in the testes. The seminiferous tubules may be crushed and become incapable of producing sperm. This causes sterility. **Sterility** is the inability to produce offspring.

Q: Why should males have a digital rectal examination?

A: Prostate cancer is the second most common cancer in males. A major symptom of prostate cancer is an enlarged prostate. Physicians use digital rectal examinations to examine males for symptoms of prostate cancer. A **digital rectal examination** is an examination in which the physician inserts a finger into the rectum and examines the internal reproductive organs and the rectum for irregularities. The American Cancer Society recommends that males over the age of 40 have a digital rectal examination annually.

Q: What is testicular self-examination?

A: Testicular cancer is one of the most common cancers among males between the ages of 15 and 34. The best way to detect testicular cancer is by doing regular testicular self-examinations. A **testicular self-examination** is a screening procedure for testicular cancer in which a male checks his testes for lumps or tenderness. If detected early, testicular cancer has a high rate of curability. Teen males should begin the habit of performing testicular self-examination.

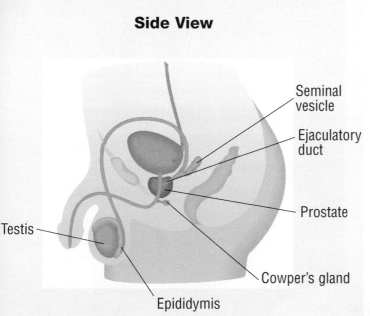

Side View

Seminal vesicle

Ejaculatory duct

Prostate

Cowper's gland

Testis

Epididymis

How Males Can Protect Reproductive Health

1. **Bathe or shower daily.** Keep your external reproductive organs clean to prevent infection and odor.

2. **Bend at the knees and keep your back straight when lifting heavy objects.** Using the correct technique when lifting heavy objects can help prevent the risk of an inguinal hernia.

3. **Wear protective clothing and equipment when participating in sports and physical activities.** Some sports have athletic supporters that provide extra support for the penis and testes. You should wear protective equipment, such as a cup, to prevent injury to these organs.

4. **Perform testicular self-examinations.** Testicular cancer is one of the most common cancers in younger males. Teen males should examine their testes for lumps and tenderness.

5. **Have regular medical checkups.** Your physician will examine you and discuss the ways your body is changing. Your physician also will answer any questions you have.

6. **Seek medical attention when you show signs of infection.** A discharge from the penis, tenderness in the scrotum, lumps, and rashes are symptoms of infection with sexually transmitted diseases (STDs).

7. **Practice abstinence from sex.** Abstinence from sex is choosing not to be sexually active. Practicing abstinence prevents teen pregnancy and infection with sexually transmitted diseases, including HIV.

Lesson 63 will include more information about STDs.

Lesson 23

Review

Vocabulary Words

Write a separate sentence using each of the vocabulary words listed on page 202.

Objectives

1. What are eight male secondary sex characteristics? **Objective 1**

2. What causes emotional changes during puberty? **Objective 1**

3. What are the organs in the male reproductive system and their functions? **Objective 2**

4. What should males know about circumcision, inguinal hernia, mumps, digital rectal examination, and testicular self-examination? **Objective 3**

5. What are seven ways males can protect reproductive health? **Objective 4**

Responsible Decision-Making

A classmate tells you he is very attracted to one of your friends. He brags about how he is going to put the moves on her. He says he intends to "go all the way" with her this weekend. You are not comfortable with his attitude or behavior. Write a response to this situation.

1. Describe the situation that requires you to make a decision.
2. List possible decisions you might make.
3. Name two responsible adults with whom you might discuss your decisions.
4. Evaluate the possible consequences of your decisions. Determine if each decision will lead to actions that:
   - promote health,
   - protect safety,
   - follow laws,
   - show respect for yourself and others,
   - follow the guidelines of your parents and of other responsible adults,
   - demonstrate good character.
5. Decide which decision is most responsible and appropriate.
6. Tell two results you expect if you make this decision.

Effective Communication

Illustrate the correct technique to use when lifting heavy objects. (The correct technique helps prevent inguinal hernia.)

Self-Directed Learning

Contact a physician or nurse or call the local health department. Find out at what age the mumps vaccine is recommended and where a person can go in your community to get vaccinated.

Critical Thinking

Suppose you have a brother who is physically active. He says wearing an athletic supporter is uncomfortable and unnecessary. Why is it recommended that males wear an athletic supporter for strenuous physical activity?

Responsible Citizenship

Pretend you work for the Cancer Society. Write or make a tape of a public service announcement that reminds males to perform frequent testicular self-examinations.

You Can Learn About Pregnancy and Childbirth

Life Skill **I will learn about pregnancy and childbirth.**

This unit contains information on growth and development. The most rapid growth and development occurs shortly after a single cell is formed from the union of the sperm and egg. The single cell divides into trillions of cells to become a baby. You are not ready to marry and have a baby right now. But you do need to know some facts. The habits you choose right now may affect your ability to be a parent in the future. The habits you choose also may affect the health of your offspring. This lesson will include many facts about pregnancy and childbirth. You will learn about conception and heredity. You will learn how pregnancy is determined and why prenatal care is needed. You will learn about the three stages of childbirth. This lesson also discusses complications that can occur during pregnancy and childbirth.

The Lesson Outline

What to Know About Conception

What to Know About Pregnancy

What to Know About Childbirth

Objectives

1. Explain how a baby is conceived and how the baby's sex and inherited traits are determined. **page 209**
2. Explain how pregnancy is determined and why prenatal care is important. **pages 210–211**
3. Discuss the three stages of labor. **pages 212–213**

Vocabulary Words

conception

fertilization

heredity

chromosome

gene

sex-linked characteristics

genetic counseling

amniocentesis

amniotic sac

ultrasound

embryo

fetus

placenta

umbilical cord

prenatal care

premature birth

low birth weight

fetal alcohol syndrome (FAS)

miscarriage

labor

crowning

afterbirth

Apgar score

postpartum period

What to Know About
Conception

Conception or fertilization is the union of an ovum and a sperm. One ovum matures and is released from an ovary each month. Ovulation usually occurs on about the fourteenth day before the expected beginning of the next menstrual period. Once an ovum is released, it enters a Fallopian tube. As the ovum moves through the Fallopian tube, it can be fertilized if sperm are present. Conception usually occurs in the upper third of a Fallopian tube.

At conception, heredity is determined. Heredity is the passing of characteristics from biological parents to their children. All body cells, except sperm and ova, contain 23 pairs of chromosomes. A chromosome is a threadlike structure that carries genes. A gene is a unit of hereditary material. In a female, the 23 pairs of chromosomes are identical. In a male, one pair of chromosomes is not made up of identical chromosomes. In both males and females, one pair is called the sex chromosomes. In females, the pair of sex chromosomes is identical and is called XX. Every ovum produced by a female contains an X chromosome. In males, the pair of sex chromosomes is not identical and is called XY. Sperm produced by a male contain either an X chromosome or a Y chromosome. The presence of a Y chromosome is essential for the development of male characteristics.

The sex of a baby is determined by the sex chromosome it receives from the father. When a sperm fertilizes an ovum, a full complement of 46 chromosomes (23 from the father and 23 from the mother) is present in the resulting cell. If a sperm with an X chromosome fertilizes an ovum, the resulting cell will have an XX pair of sex chromosomes. A fertilized ovum with an XX set of chromosomes develops into a female. If a sperm with a Y chromosome fertilizes an ovum, the resulting cell will have an XY pair of sex chromosomes. A fertilized ovum with an XY set of chromosomes develops into a male.

All chromosomes carry genes that contain hereditary material. Sex-linked characteristics are hereditary characteristics transmitted on the sex chromosomes. The X chromosome carries genes for traits such as color vision and blood clotting. The Y chromosome does not carry matching genes for those or other traits. Therefore, when the X and Y chromosomes are present together, the genes on the X chromosome control the traits.

A couple may receive genetic counseling to prepare for parenthood. In some cases, a physician may recommend that a pregnant female have a test for possible genetic defects. Genetic counseling is a process in which a trained professional interprets medical information concerning genetics to prospective parents. Amniocentesis (am·nee·oh·sen·TEE·suhs) is a diagnostic procedure in which a needle is inserted through the uterus to extract fluid from the amniotic sac. The amniotic sac is a pouch of fluid that surrounds a fetus. Cells extracted from the amniotic fluid are analyzed to determine if any genetic defects are present. Ultrasound is another diagnostic procedure used to monitor the fetus. Ultrasound is a procedure in which high-frequency sound waves are used to provide an image of the developing baby. The image of the developing baby is evaluated by the physician. Knowing ahead about the presence of a birth defect is helpful in planning how to care for the baby after birth.

What to Know About
Pregnancy

After conception, a fertilized egg continues to divide and move through the Fallopian tube. The cell divisions are a cluster of cells by the time they reach the uterus. These cells attach to the endometrium, the lining of the uterus. **Embryo** is the name given a developing baby through the second month of growth after conception. **Fetus** is the name given a developing baby from the ninth week until birth. The outer cells of the embryo and the cells of the endometrium form the placenta. The **placenta** is an organ that anchors the embryo to the uterus. Other cells form the umbilical cord. The **umbilical cord** is a ropelike structure that connects the embryo to the placenta. Blood from the mother-to-be carries nutrients and oxygen to the embryo through the cord. Waste products from the embryo move to the mother-to-be's bloodstream through the cord to be excreted.

How Pregnancy Is Determined

The first sign that indicates pregnancy is the absence of a menstrual period. However, a missed period does not always indicate pregnancy. A female may skip her menstrual period because of stress, diet, physical activity, or illness. If conception has occurred, she usually has other symptoms of pregnancy. She may have tenderness in her breasts, fatigue, a change in appetite, and morning sickness. Morning sickness is nausea and vomiting during pregnancy. Some pregnant females have spotting or light irregular menstrual flow.

A female who misses a period and also has other symptoms of pregnancy should have a pregnancy test. A physician or nurse practitioner can administer this test and send it to a lab for confirmation. Some pregnancy tests also are sold in drugstores. However, a pregnancy should be confirmed by a physician or nurse.

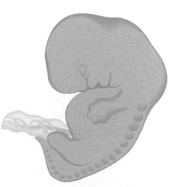

5–6 weeks
Actual size=1/2 inch (1.3 centimeters)

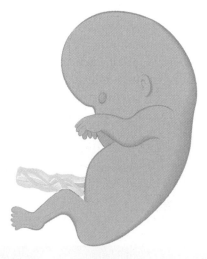

8–9 weeks
Actual size=2 inches (5 centimeters)

Why Prenatal Care Is Needed

Prenatal care is the care that is given to the mother-to-be and baby before birth. Prenatal care includes routine medical examinations, proper nutrition, reasonable exercise, extra rest and relaxation, childbirth and child care education, avoidance of drugs and other risk behaviors, and the practice of common sense.

A pregnant female needs a well-balanced diet. Premature birth or low birth weight may result when a developing baby does not receive adequate nutrients. **Premature birth** is the birth of a baby before it is fully developed; less than 38 weeks from time of conception. A **low birth weight** is a weight at birth that is less than 5.5 pounds (2.5 kilograms). Premature birth and low birth weight are associated with mental retardation and infant death.

A pregnant female needs to check with her physician before taking any prescription or over-the-counter drugs. Drugs present in her bloodstream can pass into the developing baby's bloodstream. They can harm the developing baby. For example, tranquilizers taken early in pregnancy can cause birth defects. Some drugs prescribed for acne also can cause birth defects. Hormones, such as those in birth control pills, can cause birth defects. Aspirin may interfere with blood clotting in both the pregnant female and her developing baby.

A female should not drink alcohol during pregnancy. **Fetal alcohol syndrome (FAS)** is the presence of severe birth defects in babies born to mothers who drink alcohol during pregnancy. FAS includes damage to the brain and to the nervous system, facial abnormalities, small head size, below normal I.Q., poor coordination, heart defects, and behavior problems.

A pregnant female should not smoke or inhale the smoke from tobacco products. Females who smoke have smaller babies in poorer general health than babies of nonsmoking females. Smoking and breathing smoke increase the risk of complications, miscarriage, and stillbirth during pregnancy. A **miscarriage** is the natural ending of a pregnancy before a baby is developed enough to survive on its own. Babies born to mothers who smoke also may be at risk for heart disease in adulthood.

A pregnant female should not use other harmful drugs, such as marijuana, crack, cocaine, or heroin. Babies born to mothers who use these drugs can be born prematurely and have low birth weight. These babies may be born addicted to drugs. Some research indicates that caffeine may be linked to birth defects. Caffeine is found in coffee, chocolate, cola drinks, tea, and some prescription and over-the-counter drugs. A mother-to-be should follow her physician's advice about caffeine.

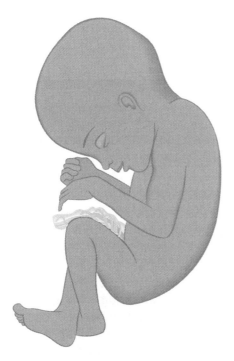

16–18 wks
Actual size=5 1/2 inches (13.8 centimeters)

Lesson 25

You Can Recognize the Risks of Teen Pregnancy and Parenthood

Life Skill **I will practice abstinence to avoid the risks of teen pregnancy and parenthood.**

How would your life change if you became pregnant or got someone pregnant? What would it be like to be a parent right now? Unfortunately, some teens do not think ahead about the consequences of pregnancy and parenthood. More than three out of ten teen females become pregnant before age 20. Of those who become pregnant before age 15, 60 percent will become pregnant more than once. Teen mothers and fathers are less likely to graduate from either high school or college. They have difficulty earning enough money to support their families because they have no skills. Babies who are born to teen parents are more likely to have birth defects and to be raised in poverty. This lesson will examine the faulty thinking that can result in teen pregnancy. You will learn the risks of teen pregnancy for the mother, the father, and the baby.

Vocabulary Words

faulty thinking

generational cycle of teen pregnancy

unnecessary risk

low birth weight

anemia

toxemia of pregnancy

The Lesson Outline

Why Teens Become Pregnant

Why Teen Pregnancy and Parenthood Are Risky

Objectives

1. List and discuss six examples of faulty thinking that can result in teen pregnancy. **pages 217–218**

2. Outline the risks associated with being a baby born to teen parents, being a pregnant teen, being a teen mother, and being a teen father. **pages 219–220**

Why Teens Become Pregnant

Do you usually consider the consequences of your behavior? Do you gather facts before you act? **Faulty thinking** is a thought process in which a person ignores or denies facts or believes false information. Faulty thinking is dangerous. It can lead to actions that cause you and others harm. It is a factor in teen pregnancy and parenthood. The following examples of faulty thinking explain why three out of ten teen females become pregnant.

FAULTY THINKING: I can have a baby now; my mother had a baby when she was a teen and she managed OK.

The **generational cycle of teen pregnancy** occurs when a teen whose mother was a teen parent becomes pregnant. This cycle has heartbreaking consequences. According to the Alan Guttmacher Institute, only 70 percent of teen females who have babies finish high school. The likelihood that any of these teen females will get a higher education is very slim. As a result, the downward cycle of low income and poverty begins for a teen mother and her baby. She is less likely to marry or stay married to the baby's father than is a female who has her first baby in her twenties. By the time her baby is five years old, a teen mother is less likely to own a home or have savings in the bank. Now, suppose the teen mother has a daughter and raises her with limited financial resources AND then the daughter also becomes pregnant as a teen. The cycle of low income and poverty is perpetuated and continues from one generation to the next.

If you are female, and your mother was a teen parent, do not repeat this pattern. Your mother loves you and is glad she has you. However, if you wait to have a daughter or son to love, you are more likely to have the resources to raise your child. Wait to finish school, get a job, get married, and then have a baby.

FAULTY THINKING: I'll be the center of attention if I have a baby.

Perhaps you have read about an unmarried actress who has a baby. Her pregnancy received a lot of publicity. Keep in mind that she also may have a full-time nanny, cook, and housekeeper to care for her needs and the needs of her baby. She is not frazzled and struggling to make ends meet. After all, she is rich and famous—which is a major reason she is the center of attention as an unmarried mother. Perhaps you know a teenager who has a baby. Maybe everyone makes a fuss over the baby when the mother is around. This makes the teen mother the center of attention—but only for a brief moment. Consider what a teen mother's life is like most of the time. She must spend time preparing formula, changing diapers, and comforting a crying baby who will not sleep. She has little, if any, social life.

The brief moments of attention you might receive if you have a baby right now are just that—brief. After the novelty wears off, you have a baby who is depending upon you to meet his/her every need. As a teen, you have many needs of your own. You have needs to stay in school, enjoy social activities, and to learn skills for a career. You can't meet those needs and also meet the needs of a baby.

FAULTY THINKING: He won't leave me if I have his baby.

If you have a fantasy that for mom and dad a baby means "living happily ever after," guess again. More than 25 percent of teen mothers have never lived with their baby's father. By the time a child of a teen mother reaches grade school, more than half of teen mothers no longer live with their child's father. Although laws are being passed to require teen fathers to support their babies financially, to this point in time only 20 percent of never-married mothers receive child support.

Guess again if you think pregnancy cements a teen relationship. On the contrary, pregnancy stresses a teen relationship. The teen couple usually does not stay together. The baby is raised without living with a father. As fatherless children grow older, they are more likely than children raised with a father to take drugs, drop out of school, get involved in crime, and become teen parents.

FAULTY THINKING: I (she) won't get pregnant if we have sex.

Remember, three out of ten females become pregnant before the age of 20. And, how many of these females planned on getting pregnant? Very, very few. Every day there are teens who become pregnant who believed "it won't happen to me." The fact is that a female can become pregnant the first time she has sex. She can become pregnant if she has sex only once. She can become pregnant even if she is "being careful." She can become pregnant even if he says he is "being careful."

Don't take chances and do not allow someone else to persuade you to take chances. "Being careful" is not an option. Practice abstinence. When you practice abstinence, a female will not get pregnant. A male will not get a female pregnant.

FAULTY THINKING: I can drink alcohol and still stay in control of my decisions about sex.

Alcohol is a depressant drug that numbs the part of the brain that controls reasoning and judgment. The inner voice that says, "I want to practice abstinence" is dulled when you drink alcohol. Drinking alcohol is very risky AND is illegal for someone your age. Drinking alcohol is especially risky when you choose abstinence and your partner is trying to pressure you to be sexually active.

Most teens who are sexually active were drinking alcohol the first time they had sex. They didn't plan to have sex. Do not drink alcohol or try to get someone to drink alcohol in order to persuade the person to have sex. If someone wants you to drink alcohol so that your decision-making ability will be affected, recognize how little respect that person has for you.

FAULTY THINKING: It's up to her to set the limits; after all, "boys will be boys."

For conception to occur, a sperm must fertilize an egg. In other words, "it takes two to have a baby." Although the female carries the unborn child, the male also is responsible for the pregnancy. AND, the male is responsible for the baby when it is born. If you are a male, think ahead about the need a baby has for a father. The close bonding of a baby with a father helps the baby develop self-confidence. In addition to emotional support, a father helps provide financial support for his family. Can you really justify "boys will be boys"? Do you really believe that a female is the only person responsible when pregnancy occurs? Are you aware that laws have been passed that require you to financially support a baby who is yours?

A teen male should be proud of the way he lives his life. He must value respectful relationships, the institution of marriage, and fatherhood. He must treat every female with respect. He should not see "how far he can go." He must take responsibility, set limits, and practice abstinence. A teen male must recognize the significance of fatherhood. A teen male is not ready to provide the emotional and financial support a mother and baby need.

Why Teen Pregnancy and Parenthood Are Risky

An **unnecessary risk** is a chance that is not worth taking after the possible outcomes are considered. The possible outcomes of teen pregnancy and parenthood are included in the discussion that follows. These outcomes are reasons why you should practice the life skill, I will practice abstinence to avoid the risks of teen pregnancy and parenthood.

Risks Associated with Being a Baby Born to Teen Parents.

A discussion of teen pregnancy and parenthood often begins with the risks to the teen mother and father. But, let's begin with the correct focus. A loving, caring, and responsible person considers the effects of his/her behavior on others. Teens are at-risk for producing unhealthy babies.

A teen female's body is still developing and maturing. For proper growth, her body needs adequate and balanced nutrition. Many teen females do not have healthful habits. Since a developing baby relies on the mother-to-be for its nutrition, whatever the mother-to-be eats, smokes, or drinks gets into the baby's bloodstream. Even if a teen female changes her habits as soon as she knows she is pregnant, the developing baby already has relied on her until her pregnancy was confirmed. This means the baby may have been inadequately nourished for six to eight weeks or more. Most pregnant teens delay getting prenatal care and many do not receive any prenatal care. As a result, teen mothers are at-risk for having a baby with a low birth weight. A **low birth weight** is a weight at birth that is less that 5.5 pounds (2.5 kilograms). Low birth weight babies are more likely to have physical and mental problems than do babies of normal birth weights.

The health habits of a teen father-to-be also affect a developing baby. The habits of the father-to-be affect the the quality of the hereditary material contained in his sperm. Some substances that can damage a male's sperm are related to poor lifestyle choices such as smoking, drinking alcohol, and taking other drugs. Lead, pesticides, benzene, and anaesthetic gases also can damage sperm. Males who plan to be fathers should avoid these substances for at least three months prior to conception. Since most teen pregnancies are not planned, a teen female should understand that the habits of a father-to-be may seriously affect the quality of his sperm.

Babies born to teen parents are at-risk for having parents with inadequate parenting skills. Parenting takes knowledge and skill. Any parent has a 24-hour job. However, a teen has responsibilities that include school, his/her social development, and other learning experiences. Having a baby in addition to those responsibilities can be overwhelming to a teen. In addition, as an infant becomes a toddler, a firm value system is required in order to discipline the toddler. This is hard work and many teen parents become frustrated with the process. This explains why the incidence of child abuse is very high in teen parents. A child deserves to be raised by parents equipped to handle frustration and who will not be abusive.

Risks Associated with Being a Pregnant Teen and Teen Mother

Pregnancy places many demands on a female's body. The demands on a female who is a teen are even greater because her body is still growing. A pregnant teen is at-risk for developing anemia and toxemia of pregnancy. **Anemia** is a condition in which the oxygen-carrying pigment in the blood is below normal. If the pregnant teen is anemic, the developing baby will be seriously affected because the baby depends on the mother's blood for oxygen and nutrients. **Toxemia of pregnancy** is a disorder of pregnancy characterized by high blood pressure, tissue swelling, and protein in the urine. If severe, toxemia of pregnancy can progress to seizures and coma.

Pregnant teens and teen mothers are at-risk in other ways. Pregnancy and parenthood disrupts education and career plans. Dating opportunities are limited for an unmarried teen raising a child. She does not have as much time or money as her peers. Males, other than the baby's father, may not want to get involved with someone who has a baby.

Risks Associated with Being a Teen Father

Teen fathers have the responsibility of providing for the care of their babies. Some states have passed laws that require teen fathers to pay child support until their child is 18. Many teen fathers drop out of school to earn money to provide child support. They are less likely to graduate from high school or college than their peers who did not become fathers when they were teens. Teen fathers usually do not marry the mother of their children. If they do marry the mother of their child, they often divorce within five years. As a result, teens who become fathers spend little time with their children. Only one in three fathers who live apart from their children visit their children at least once a week. Children do not thrive when there is a lack of contact with their father. Fathers also can feel the emptiness of not being close to their children.

Activity

Write Your Own Success Story

Life Skill: I will practice abstinence to avoid the risks of teen pregnancy and parenthood.

Materials: paper, pen or pencil

Directions: The decisions you make help create the success you will achieve. Complete the following activity to learn how being a teen parent might interfere with your goals and dreams.

 1. **Outline your success story.** Assume that you are 30 years old and consider yourself a success. Make an outline that includes this information:

- Your marital status
- Number of children you have
- Education and training you have completed
- Jobs you have had, including homemaker
- Your income, including that of a spouse
- Your hobbies and leisure activities
- Awards or recognitions you have received

 2. **Cross out items listed in your success story that would not be a reality if you became a teen parent.**

 3. **Write a paragraph summarizing why it is risky to be a teen parent.**

Lesson 25

Review

Vocabulary Words

Write a separate sentence using each of the vocabulary words listed on page 216.

Objectives

1. What are six examples of faulty thinking that can result in teen pregnancy? **Objective 1**

2. Why is it important to stop the generational cycle of teen pregnancy? **Objective 1**

3. What are the risks associated with being a baby born to teen parents? **Objective 2**

4. What are the risks associated with being a pregnant teen and teen mother? **Objective 2**

5. What are the risks associated with being a teen father? **Objective 2**

Responsible Decision-Making

Suppose a person you date pressures you to have sex. (S)he says (s)he will "be careful". Write a response to this situation.

1. Describe the situation that requires you to make a decision.
2. List possible decisions you might make.
3. Name two responsible adults with whom you might discuss your decisions.
4. Evaluate the possible consequences of your decisions. Determine if each decision will lead to actions that:
   - promote health,
   - protect safety,
   - follow laws,
   - show respect for yourself and others,
   - follow the guidelines of your parents and of other responsible adults,
   - demonstrate good character.
5. Decide which decision is most responsible and appropriate.
6. Tell two results you expect if you make this decision.

 ## Effective Communication

Divide a sheet of paper in half. On one half, list the six examples of faulty thinking that can result in teen pregnancy. On the second half, change each example to reflect correct thinking.

 ## Self-Directed Learning

Laws have been passed to require fathers to pay child support for their children who are under 18 years of age. Research the child support laws of the community where you live.

 ## Critical Thinking

A male classmate has a macho attitude. He brags he can have any girl he wants. He says he doesn't care if a girl gets pregnant. He says it is the girl's responsibility to avoid pregnancy. Write a paragraph explaining why his thinking is wrong.

 ## Responsible Citizenship

Be a health advocate for responsible parenthood. Tape-record a baby's wish list. The wish list should include five qualifications a baby desires his/her parents to have. For example, one qualification might be "I want my parents to be married and to love one another."

You Can Provide Responsible Care for Infants and Children

Life Skill I will provide responsible care for infants and children.

Have your parents or guardian ever asked you to look after a younger brother or sister? Has a neighbor ever asked you to look after his/her children? A **childsitter** is a person who provides care for infants and children with the permission of a parent or guardian. This lesson describes how to prepare to be a childsitter. You will learn how to care for infants and toddlers from birth to three years old. You will learn how to care for young children three to eight years old. The activity in this lesson helps you create a job description if you want to be a childsitter.

Vocabulary Words
childsitter

time out

The Lesson Outline

How to Prepare to Be a Childsitter

How to Care for Infants and Toddlers (Birth to Three Years)

How to Care for Young Children (Three to Eight Years)

Objectives

1. List 25 things a childsitter must do to be prepared to childsit. **page 223**

2. List seven skills a responsible childsitter for infants and toddlers must have. **page 225**

3. List five skills a responsible childsitter for young children three to eight years old must have. **page 225**

How to Prepare to Be a Childsitter

The Childsitter's Check Sheet ✓

A responsible childsitter is prepared. It is your responsibility to obtain the information you nead before you childsit. Use The Childsitter's Check Sheet to make sure you are prepared. Copy the check sheet on a separate piece of paper. **DO NOT WRITE IN THIS BOOK.** ✓

1.	I have taken a First Aid course, and I am familiar with universal precautions.	
2.	I have taken a childsitting course offered by the American Red Cross or by another organization.	
3.	I have a parent's or guardian's approval to childsit.	
4.	I have checked to make sure I am available to childsit.	
5.	I have discussed with the parents or guardian the hours I will childsit and the payment.	
6.	I have arranged for transportation to and from the job.	
7.	I have met the child or children and learned their name(s) and age(s).	
8.	I have familiarized myself with the house and where everything is.	
9.	I have discussed pets and rules for them.	
10.	I have discussed what privileges I will have in regard to such things as the telephone, food, and visitors.	
11.	I know the address and telephone number of the home where I will be childsitting.	
12.	I know what time to arrive.	
13.	I know what time the parents or guardian will be home.	
14.	I know the address and telephone number of the parents or guardian.	

15.	I know whom to contact if the parents or guardian cannot be reached.	
16.	I know emergency telephone numbers, including police, fire, and poison control.	
17.	I know if 9-1-1 service is available.	
18.	I know the name and telephone number of the child's physician.	
19.	I know the child's mealtime(s).	
20.	I know the child's naptime(s) and bedtime.	
21.	I know what health problems the child has.	
22.	I know what medications the child needs.	
23.	I know what allergies the child has.	
24.	I know what the child is and is not allowed to do.	
25.	I know what the child's favorite activities and toys are.	

Tips

A responsible childsitter is:

- Observant and alert
- Calm during emergencies
- Able to follow instructions
- Trained in first aid
- Able to recognize safety hazards
- Able to communicate with adults
- Able to communicate with young children
- Able to supervise young children
- Patient
- Friendly

How to Care for Infants and Toddlers
(Birth to Three Years)

Infants, or babies, share some common characteristics. So do toddlers. Learn the common characteristics so you will know what to expect from infants and toddlers in your care.

I know what to do when a baby cries. I determine why the baby is crying. I ask myself if the baby is too warm, too cold, or hungry, teething, or ill. Is the diaper wet or soiled? Does the baby want company or attention? Then I take the appropriate action.

I know what to do if I think an infant or toddler is sick. I call the parents or guardian. I tell them the signs and symptoms I have observed. I follow the parents' or guardian's instructions.

I know how to diaper a baby. I follow universal precautions and wear rubber gloves. I have everything ready I will need—diaper, baby wipes or a washcloth, ointment, water, cotton balls, (for cloth diapers) safety pins. I take off the soiled or wet diaper and clean the baby's bottom with a baby wipe or damp washcloth. I place the baby on the new diaper and bring the bottom of the diaper up between the baby's legs. First, I bring one side across the front. Then, I bring the other side across the front and fasten the diaper. I dispose of the soiled diaper appropriately.

Newborns to one-year-olds:
• Need to feel secure
• Like to be with people
• Cry when they are hungry or uncomfortable
• Like to touch and hold things
• Like to look at hands and faces
• Like to put things in their mouths

One-year-olds to three-year-olds:
• Need to feel secure
• Want to be independent
• Want to eat, drink, and get dressed without help
• Like to play, build things, and watch what others are doing
• Like to do the same thing over and over again
• May have temper tantrums if they don't get what they want

A responsible childsitter never leaves an infant or toddler alone. A responsible childsitter never shakes or hits an infant or toddler. You need to consult a parent or guardian if an infant or child persists in a behavior you find difficult or inappropriate.

You need certain skills to provide responsible care for an infant or toddler. Consult The Childsitter's List of Skills for Infant and Toddler Care to make sure you have the skills you need.

The Childsitter's List of Skills for the Care of Infants and Toddlers

I know how to bathe a baby. If the baby still has an umbilical cord, I give the baby only a sponge bath. Otherwise, I bathe the baby in a plastic baby tub or a sink. I warm the room, have ready water, a soft washcloth, and baby soap. I fill the baby tub or a sink with several inches of warm water. I place the baby on a flat surface and undress him/her. I place the baby in the water, supporting the baby's head and keeping the baby's face out of the water. I wash the entire body and rinse the baby with clean, warm water from a cup. When I am finished, I wrap the baby in a towel to dry. I make sure the baby's head is covered.

I know how to give a baby a bottle. I ask the parents or guardian for instructions. I follow the instructions about preparing the bottle. I pick up the baby and hold him/her in my arms to feed. I make sure the bottle nipple is always full of milk.

I know how to burp a baby. I put a towel or diaper on my shoulder and pick up the baby. I hold the baby upright with his/her head resting on my shoulder. I support the baby's head and back. I pat the baby's back gently with my other hand. Or, I lay the baby stomach down on my lap. I place one hand on the baby's bottom and use the other hand to gently pat the his/her back. Or, I sit the baby on my lap. I support the baby's chest with one hand. I gently pat the baby's back with my other hand.

How to Care for Young Children
(Three to Eight Years)

Three-to-five-year-old children share common characteristics, as do five-to-eight-year-olds.

Three-to-five-year-olds:
- Enjoy playing with friends and communicating with others
- Like to learn numbers and play simple games
- Like to be independent and do things for themselves
- Like to learn new words and names for things
- Can be very active
- Can be very aggressive

Five-to-eight-year-olds:
- Need to socialize with others besides family members
- Want to be a part of conversations with family members
- Usually have more self-confidence than do three-to-five-year-olds
- Like to ask questions about almost everything
- Are influenced by what adults say and do

A responsible childsitter never leaves a young child alone. A responsible childsitter never shakes or hits a young child. You need to consult a parent or guardian if a young child persists in a behavior you find difficult or inappropriate.

You need certain skills to provide responsible care for young children who are three to eight years old. Consult The Childsitter's List of Skills for the Care of Young Children to make sure you have the skills you need.

The Childsitter's List of Skills for the Care of Young Children

I know what to do when a child is afraid. I talk quietly with the child and show the child that I am not afraid. I find out exactly why the child is afraid. If an object frightens the child, I move it out of the child's sight. I give the child a favorite toy or stuffed animal to hold.

I know how to pick up and hold a baby. I slide my arm under the baby's body. I cradle the baby against my body. Or, I support the baby against my shoulder. I support the baby's head with one hand. I also support the shoulders. I am very careful when touching the two soft spots on the top of the baby's head.

I know what to do if a child has a tantrum. I ask the parents or guardian ahead of time how to respond to a tantrum. I find out why the child is angry. Quietly and calmly I tell the child that a tantrum is not appropriate or acceptable. I tell the child that I will not pay attention to his/her wants until the tantrum stops. If it does not stop in a short amount of time, I tell the child that (s)he will have time out. **Time out** is a calming-down period of time. I tell the child that (s)he may play again after becoming calm.

I know how to help a young child learn. I smile at the child. I talk to and play games with the child. I use safe toys and games that interest the child.

I know what to do when a child refuses to go to bed. I find out if the child does not want to be left alone or is afraid of the dark. I read the child a story to help the child relax. Or I sit and quietly talk to the child for a short period of time. I assure the child that I will be close by and will check him/her again very soon.

I know what to do if I think a young child is sick. I call the parents or guardian. I describe the signs and symptoms I have observed. I follow the parents' or guardian's instructions about what steps to take.

Activity

Creating a Job Description for a Responsible Childsitter

Life Skill: I will provide responsible care for infants and children.

Materials: paper, pen or pencil, computer (optional)

Directions: Parents and guardians want responsible care for their children. They want a childsitter who is mature, responsible, and has healthful habits. They want a childsitter who is neat and organized, in good health, with good judgment and common sense. Follow each of the steps below to create a job description for a responsible childsitter.

 Follow your teacher's instructions to select a classmate to be your partner.

 Make a list of possible characteristics of a responsible childsitter. Think about the tasks you might have to perform to care responsibly for an infant, toddler, or young child. Work with your partner to brainstorm a list of characteristics, or qualities, a responsible childsitter should have. Choose five characteristics from the list to use in your job description.

Write a job description for a responsible childsitter. Your description should be one or two paragraphs. It should include the following:

- number and ages of the infants and children who need care
- number of hours the childsitter is needed
- day(s) of week the childsitter is needed
- length of time the childsitter is needed for (week, month, year)
- descriptions of the five qualities the childsitter should have

 Prepare a handout or printout of the job description to share with the class. Following your teacher's instructions, share your job description with your classmates. Explain why you think each of the five characteristics is important.

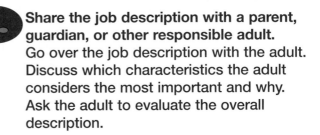 Share the job description with a parent, guardian, or other responsible adult. Go over the job description with the adult. Discuss which characteristics the adult considers the most important and why. Ask the adult to evaluate the overall description.

Lesson 26
Review

Vocabulary Words

Write a separate sentence using each of the vocabulary words listed on page 222.

Objectives

1. What must you do to be prepared to childsit? **Objective 1**

2. What are seven skills you need to be a responsible childsitter for infants and toddlers? **Objective 2**

3. What are the characteristics of newborn to one-year-olds? **Objective 2**

4. What are five skills you need to be a responsible childsitter for young children three to eight years old? **Objective 3**

5. What are the characteristics of young children three to eight years old? **Objective 3**

Responsible Decision-Making

You agree to childsit for a neighbor's baby. You are giving the baby a bath when the telephone rings. The phone is just in the next room. The water in the baby's plastic tub is not very deep. Write a response to this situation.

1. Describe the situation that requires you to make a decision.
2. List possible decisions you might make.
3. Name two responsible adults with whom you might discuss your decisions.
4. Evaluate the possible consequences of your decisions. Determine if each decision will lead to actions that:
   • promote health,
   • protect safety,
   • follow laws,
   • show respect for yourself and others,
   • follow the guidelines of your parents and of other responsible adults,
   • demonstrate good character.
5. Decide which decision is most responsible and appropriate.
6. Tell two results you expect if you make this decision.

 ## Effective Communication

Your younger sister has accepted her first job as a childsitter. Write her a note that explains the five most important things she should know to be a responsible childsitter.

 ## Self-Directed Learning

Call the local hospital, local chapter of the American Red Cross, health center, or community center. Find out if the organization offers a course in childsitting. Arrange to attend the classes. Share with your parents or guardian the skills you have learned to help you be a responsible childsitter.

 ## Critical Thinking

Evaluate your skills as a childsitter. Which skills do you possess that help make you a responsible childsitter? Which skills do you need to acquire?

 ## Responsible Citizenship

Contact a neighborhood youth center or community center. Offer to prepare a pamphlet on ways to be a responsible childsitter.

Lesson 27

You Can Work to Become a Responsible Adult

Life Skill **I will achieve the developmental tasks of adolescence.**

Adolescence is the period of growth between childhood and adulthood. During adolescence, you must master tasks that help you become independent. To be **independent** is to be able to rely on oneself.

Your parents or guardian guide you through childhood and adolescence. They want you to become an independent and responsible adult. At times, you may wish they did not interfere in your life. But, deep down inside you are grateful for their guidance and support. This lesson focuses on eight developmental tasks of adolescence. You will learn how you can master these tasks. This lesson also explains how to set goals and make plans to reach them. You will examine eight keys that can help you unlock the door to a successful future.

The Lesson Outline

How to Achieve Developmental Tasks

How to Set Goals and Make Plans to Reach Them

How to Plan for a Successful Future

Objectives

1. List and discuss ways to achieve the eight developmental tasks of adolescence. **pages 229–230**

2. Explain how to set goals and make plans to reach them. **page 231**

3. Discuss eight keys to unlock the door to a successful future. **page 232**

Vocabulary Words

adolescence

independent

developmental tasks of adolescence

sex role

body image

intimacy

self-disclosure

social conscience

goal

short-term goal

long-term goal

action plan

work ethic

How to Achieve Developmental Tasks

The **developmental tasks of adolescence** are achievements that need to be mastered to become a responsible, independent adult. Robert Havighurst, a sociologist, identified eight developmental tasks that you need to master:

Task 1: Develop healthful friendships with members of both sexes.

Healthful friendships involve mutual respect, flexibility, trust, honesty, and the opportunity to share feelings. Through healthful friendships, you learn how to communicate effectively, cooperate, and resolve conflict. These skills will help you in the workplace and if you marry. Friends provide support and companionship throughout life.

To achieve Task 1:

1. Initiate a new friendship with a responsible person.
2. Evaluate the friendships you already have to make sure they are healthful.
3. Make an effort to be a good friend to others.

Task 2: Become comfortable with your maleness and femaleness.

A **sex role** is a way a person acts and the feelings and attitudes (s)he has about being male or female. Your sex role was influenced by the way adults in your life have related to one another. As a result, you have beliefs about the ways males and females should behave toward one another. Adolescence is a good time to test your attitudes and beliefs. The social activities you enjoy provide an opportunity to observe and react to how you interact with others.

To achieve Task 2:

1. Participate in a variety of social activities.
2. Consider what you expect males to be like.
3. Consider what you expect females to be like.
4. Discuss unrealistic, uncertain, or uncomfortable expectations about sex roles with a responsible adult, such as a parent or guardian.

Task 3: Become comfortable with your body.

Adolescence is a period of transition that involves physical, social, emotional, and intellectual changes. You experience secondary sex characteristics, and your body becomes adult-like. You are capable of producing offspring, although you are not ready to marry and have children. During adolescence, you must become comfortable with the ways in which your body changes. You must develop a positive body image. **Body image** is the perception a person has of his/her body's appearance. Being proud that your body is male or female is an important part of developing healthy sexuality.

To achieve Task 3:

1. Discuss any concerns you have about your body with a responsible adult.
2. Maintain a healthful appearance.
3. Practice habits that will keep your body in top condition.
4. Perform regular breast self-examinations or testicular self-examinations.

Task 4: Become emotionally independent from adults.

Your parents or guardians have provided emotional security throughout your childhood. They have shielded you and helped you sort out things. As an adult, you can still stay close to them. However, the balance of responsibility now starts to shift to you. You may still ask for feedback but must become responsible for yourself and independent from your parents or guardian.

To achieve Task 4:

1. Use The Responsible Decision-Making Model when you make a decision.
2. Keep a journal. Note decisions that did not turn out as you expected. Analyze what you might have done differently.
3. Stay close to your parents or guardian by sharing your decisions and emotions with them.

Task 5: Learn skills you will need later if you marry and become a parent. As an adolescent, you are learning about intimacy. **Intimacy** is a deep and meaningful kind of sharing between two people. **Self-disclosure** is the act of making thoughts and feelings known to another person. During adolescence, you practice self-disclosure. Self-disclosure may bring you closer to someone. Sometimes the other person disappoints you. These kinds of experiences help you learn to trust your instincts about people. You learn with whom you can share feelings. Later on, this helps you select a marriage partner with whom you can be intimate. During adolescence, you also can practice relating to infants and young children. You can learn skills that will help you if you become a parent.

To achieve Task 5:

1. Analyze whether you make wise choices about with whom you share your thoughts and feelings.

2. Review your relationships that have not been healthful and supportive.

3. Discontinue all relationships that have been destructive.

4. Practice relating to infants and children.

Task 6: Prepare for a career. During adolescence, you gain skills and knowledge about yourself to help you prepare for a career. Consider what you want to do next. Do you need to continue your education to be able to get the kind of job and income you want? Will you attend college or a vocational school? Is there some other training in which you are interested? Make careful selections when planning your high school courses. Talk to adults engaged in the type of career that interests you. You may want to be a volunteer or get a part-time job to gain experience.

To achieve Task 6:

1. Work with your high school guidance counselor to select the right courses to prepare for the career in which you are interested.

2. Study hard.

3. Get your high school diploma.

4. Speak with adults who have careers of interest.

5. Participate in volunteer opportunities.

6. Get a part-time job.

Task 7: Have a clear set of values to guide your behavior. Your parents or guardian have taught you a set of values to guide your behavior. During adolescence, these values must move from your head to your heart. As a child, you learned what values were important. You knew what behaviors were expected of you. To know about values is to have values in your head. But, as you mature, values must be in your heart as well. You must believe in these values and want them to guide your behavior. To want to practice values because you believe in them is to have values in your heart.

To achieve Task 7:

1. Examine how the values you have learned from your parents or guardian have guided your behavior.

2. Identify what you want to stand for.

3. Examine whether your behavior is consistent with the values you say are important to you.

Task 8: Understand and achieve socially responsible behavior. To be a responsible adult, you must have a social conscience. A **social conscience** is a desire to contribute to society and to live a socially responsible life. To do this, you must move beyond thinking about yourself to thinking about the lives of others. What can you do to enrich the quality of life within your home, school, family, community, nation, and world?

To achieve Task 8:

1. Participate in volunteer activities that benefit others, such as collecting food for the needy.

2. Join clubs at school that volunteer in the community.

3. Look for ways to help out a home.

How to Set Goals and Make Plans to Reach Them

Is there something you want to achieve now or in the future? Wishing and hoping will not help you accomplish what you have named. You need to set goals. A **goal** is a desired achievement toward which a person works. A **short-term goal** is something a person plans to achieve in the near future. A **long-term goal** is something a person plans to achieve after a period of time. Setting and achieving personal goals need not be an overwhelming task. There are seven steps you can take to successfully reach a goal. Those steps are outlined below.

1. **State your goal.** Write your goal in a short sentence. Be as specific as possible. Share your goal with your parents or guardian. Is the goal clear? Is it realistic? Is it achievable?

2. **Make an action plan.** An **action plan** is a detailed description of the steps a person will take to reach a goal. You may need to identify short-term goals to help you make progress toward a long-term goal.

3. **Identify obstacles to your plan.** Brainstorm obstacles that might interfere with your plan. Ask yourself what might keep you from being able to do what you plan to do.

4. **Set up a timeline.** When will you begin your plan? When do you hope to achieve your goal? Have you taken into consideration all your obligations and responsibilities? Is this a realistic timeline?

5. **Keep a chart or diary in which you record progress toward your goal.** Seeing progress will encourage you to stick to your goal.

6. **Build a support system.** Consider people who will help you reach your goal. Ask them for ideas and help.

7. **Revise your goal, plan, or timeline if necessary.** Sometimes you realize that your plans are not working out as you expected and changes must be made. If you need to make changes in your plan, do so. Do not give up on your goal. When you make changes in your plan, do not lower your standards.

Successful Future

There are eight keys that can help you unlock the door to a successful future.

Key 1: Assess your strengths.

Try to find where your strengths lie. You can take tests prepared by professionals to assess your strengths. Talk to your parents or guardian, school counselor, and other responsible adults.

Key 2: Assess your interests.

There are interest inventories to help you determine what you like to do. This lesson includes a sample interest inventory. Your school counselor will answer any questions you have.

Key 3: Identify and use resources.

You must make things happen for yourself. Go out and find people who can advise you about and help you reach your goals. Use resources in your community, such as the library or youth center, to help you reach your goals.

Key 4: Set goals and make plans to reach them.

This lesson has discussed how to set goals and make plans to reach them. Always consider ways to improve yourself. Set new short-term and long-term goals.

Key 5: Develop a work ethic.

A **work ethic** is an attitude of discipline, motivation, and commitment toward tasks. When you have a work ethic, you increase your self-respect. Others know they can count on you. You are committed and motivated.

Key 6: Keep your priorities in order.

The ability to prioritize will help you be successful. You may need to give up some things in order to reach your goal. Carefully pick and choose what your priorities are. Which things must you do and which can you give up?

Key 7: Manage your time wisely.

Time management is critical in school, on the job, and in your personal life. Create a realistic schedule that you can follow. Determine how much time you need to spend on school and work to be successful. Consider how much time you need for your family responsibilities. Then you will know how much time you have for your social life.

Key 8: Develop a positive attitude.

Remember, what you believe you can achieve. Be an "I can" person.

Lesson 27

Review

Vocabulary Words

Write a separate sentence using each of the vocabulary words listed on page 228.

Objectives

1. What are the eight developmental tasks of adolescence? **Objective 1**

2. What are three steps you can take to become emotionally independent from adults? **Objective 1**

3. What are six steps you can take to prepare for a career? **Objective 1**

4. What are seven steps to take to successfully reach your goals? **Objective 2**

5. What are eight keys to unlock the door to a successful future? **Objective 3**

Responsible Decision-Making

You need to raise your grade in math to remain eligible to play basketball. A friend who is a math ace offers to give you his/her answers to the homework assignment. Write a response to this situation.

1. Describe the situation that requires you to make a decision.
2. List possible decisions you might make.
3. Name two responsible adults with whom you might discuss your decisions.
4. Evaluate the possible consequences of your decisions. Determine if each decision will lead to actions that:
   • promote health,
   • protect safety,
   • follow laws,
   • show respect for yourself and others,
   • follow the guidelines of your parents and of other responsible adults,
   • demonstrate good character.
5. Decide which decision is most responsible and appropriate.
6. Tell two results you expect if you make this decision.

 ### Effective Communication

Create a poster or design a graphic on your computer to depict the eight keys to unlock the door to a successful future.

 ### Self-Directed Learning

Select a biography of a successful person. Read the biography and write a report identifying this person's key to success.

 ### Critical Thinking

One of your goals should be to receive your high school diploma. What are three short-term goals that will help you reach your goal to graduate?

 ### Responsible Citizenship

Identify three successful people in your community. Select one to interview. Ask this person what (s)he believes people your age can do to make the community a better place.

You Can Develop Your Learning Style

Life Skill **I will develop my learning style.**

During adolescence, you experience many physical, mental, and social changes. You also experience rapid intellectual growth as your brain stores and interprets vast amounts of new information. You may gain and process information in a different way than your classmates do. A **learning style** is the way a person gains and processes information. This lesson will describe different learning styles. You will be given tips that will help you gain and process information. This lesson also will discuss learning disabilities. You will learn about four different learning disabilities. As a result, you will understand that your classmates may have different learning styles. You will be sensitive to those who learn in different ways.

The Lesson Outline

What to Know About Learning Styles

What to Know About Learning Disabilities

Objectives

1. Discuss the four learning styles and tips for each. **page 235**
2. Discuss four common learning disabilities and the learning support available for people with them. **page 236**

Vocabulary Words

learning style

visual learner

auditory learner

kinesthetic learner

global learner

learning disability

dyslexia

Attention Deficit Disorder (ADD)

Attention Deficit Hyperactive Disorder (ADHD)

hyperactive

tracking disorder

tutor

What to Know About
Learning Styles

Educators have identified four kinds of learners. These kinds of learners are described in the discussion that follows. You may recognize yourself as one of these kinds of learners. Pay attention to the list of tips that maximize learning for your learning style. Then you will be able to make a plan to learn that emphasizes your strengths.

Visual Learners. A **visual learner** is a person who learns best by seeing or creating images and pictures. A visual learner:

- pictures the words (s)he reads or hears,
- stores what (s)he sees, reads, or hears in images or pictures rather than in words; for example, a visual learner is more likely to remember the face rather than name of a person (s)he has met for the first time,
- performs better on written tests than on oral tests.

Tips for Visual Learners

1. Take notes and review them often.
2. Color code or highlight notes to be reviewed.
3. Make a mental picture of key words.
4. Remember lists by using a mnemonic, or memory assisting, device or code.

Auditory learners. An **auditory learner** is a person who learns best by listening or by discussing a topic. An auditory learner:

- remembers what (s)he hears,
- can repeat word for word what someone else says,
- can remember every word of a song,
- would rather listen than take notes,
- performs better on oral tests than on written tests.

Tips for Auditory Learners

1. Tape record information you need to recall.
2. Play the tape several times when studying.
3. Read or say information aloud to yourself.
4. Study by having someone give you an oral test.
5. Make a song of words or facts you need to remember.

Kinesthetic Learners. A **kinesthetic learner** is a person who learns best by acting out something, touching an object, or repeating a motion. People who are blind often become kinesthetic learners. For example, they may recall a location by using their cane to feel a sidewalk or curb. A kinesthetic learner:

- remembers objects (s)he has touched,
- remembers facts from being in role play,
- performs better on tests requiring demonstration rather than on oral or written tests,
- can act out a story or concept.

Tips for Kinesthetic Learners

1. Associate information with a feeling or smell.
2. Role play situations in which you recall facts.
3. Demonstrate concepts you have learned.
4. Make a story to help you remember facts.

Global Learners. A **global learner** is a person who learns best by combining visual, auditory, and kinesthetic ways of learning.

Tips for Global Learners

1. Assess which learning style works best for specific situations.
2. Experiment with the tips given for the other types of learners.

What to Know About
Learning Disabilities

A **learning disability** is a disorder in which a person has difficulty acquiring and processing information. You or someone you know may have one of the following learning disabilities.

Dyslexia. **Dyslexia** is a learning disability in which a person has difficulty spelling, reading, and writing. People who have dyslexia may reverse letters and numbers. They may read from right to left.

Attention Deficit Disorder. **Attention Deficit Disorder (ADD)** is a learning disability in which a person is restless and easily distracted. People who have ADD cannot keep their attention focused on what they are doing. They have difficulty completing tasks. They may daydream.

Attention Deficit Hyperactive Disorder. **Attention Deficit Hyperactive Disorder (ADHD)** is a learning disability in which a person is easily distracted and also is hyperactive. To be **hyperactive** is to not be able to sit or stand still. People who have ADHD cannot keep their attention focused on what they are doing. They are restless and fidgety. They may be impulsive.

Tracking Disorder. **Tracking disorder** is a learning disability in which a person has difficulty following a series of words or images. People who have tracking disorder have difficulty staying on the same line as they read. Or, they may have difficulty catching a baseball thrown from the outfield to home plate.

People who have difficulty acquiring and processing information can take diagnostic tests to find out if they have a learning disability. If they have a learning disability, a plan to increase learning can be made. A variety of professionals will work with the person and his/her parents or guardian. These professionals may include a counselor, school psychologist, teacher, and tutor.

Schools may offer special education classes for students with learning disabilities. The curriculum and teaching techniques are adapted to the needs of students who require help in order to learn to their full capacity. There may be fewer students in the class to allow the teacher more time with each student. Many students with learning disabilities remain in the same classroom with other students. Their teachers provide special help when needed. For example, a student who has dyslexia may take an oral test rather than a written one. Some students with learning disabilities may get extra help outside the classroom. For example, a student may work with a speech pathologist or a reading specialist after school. Many students have a tutor. A **tutor** is a person who works with individual students to help them with schoolwork.

You will be more sensitive to people with learning disabilities if you understand the following five facts. If you have a learning disability, these facts may help you understand yourself more fully.

People with learning disabilities:
1. are capable of learning,
2. can learn strategies that help them acquire and process information,
3. may need special education classes and/or a tutor,
4. need support and encouragement from classmates and family members,
5. can be very successful.

Lesson 28

Review

Vocabulary Words

Write a separate sentence using each of the vocabulary words listed on page 234.

Objectives

1. What are tips to maximize the strengths of a visual learner? **Objective 1**

2. What are tips to maximize the strengths of an auditory learner? **Objective 1**

3. What are tips to maximize the strengths of a kinesthetic learner? **Objective 1**

4. What are tips to maximize the strengths of a global learner? **Objective 1**

5. What are four common learning disabilities and the learning support available for people with them? **Objective 2**

Responsible Decision-Making

Suppose you have a test tomorrow. Your friend calls you and suggests studying together. Your friend suggests that you can quiz each other out loud. However, you know you study best when you outline the material you need to learn. Write a response to this situation.

1. Describe the situation that requires you to make a decision.
2. List possible decisions you might make.
3. Name two responsible adults with whom you might discuss your decisions.
4. Evaluate the possible consequences of your decisions. Determine if each decision will lead to actions that:
   - promote health,
   - protect safety,
   - follow laws,
   - show respect for yourself and others,
   - follow the guidelines of your parents and of other responsible adults,
   - demonstrate good character.
5. Decide which decision is most responsible and appropriate.
6. Tell two results you expect if you make this decision.

 Effective Communication

Obtain permission from your parent, guardian, or teacher to interview a professional who works with students who have learning disabilities. Prepare by making a list of at least five questions to ask. Share the questions and answers with classmates.

 Self-Directed Learning

Check the library or Internet to locate the name of a successful person who has a learning disability. Write a short report about this person's learning disability. Explain why you believe this person became successful.

 Critical Thinking

What is your learning style? What changes can you make in the way you study to maximize learning?

 Responsible Citizenship

Obtain permission from your parents or guardian and from your teacher. Help a younger student or a student who is blind prepare for a test.

You Can Age in a Healthful Way

Life Skill **I will develop habits that promote healthful aging.**

To **age** is to grow older. There are several ways to measure a person's age. **Chronological age** is the number of years a person has lived. **Biological age** is a measure of how well a person's body systems are functioning. **Social age** is a measure of a person's involvement in leisure activities. Nothing can be done to change a person's chronological age. However, your health habits can affect your biological and social age. This lesson will include facts about aging. You will learn about the physical, mental, and social changes that occur in middle and late adulthood. You also will learn factors to consider if you are a caregiver for an older member of the family. This lesson also identifies ten habits that promote healthful aging. You can develop these habits and stay in top condition.

The Lesson Outline

What to Know About Aging

What to Know About Being a Caregiver

How to Promote Healthful Aging

Objectives

1. Describe the physical, mental, and social changes that occur in middle and late adulthood. **pages 239–240**

2. Discuss factors and resources to consider if you are a caregiver. **page 241**

3. Identify ten habits that promote healthful aging. **page 242**

Vocabulary Words

age

chronological age

biological age

social age

gerontology

gerontologist

Parkinson's disease

chronic disease

chronic bronchitis

emphysema

arthritis

osteoporosis

diabetes

diabetes mellitus

male climacteric

menopause

estrogen replacement therapy (ERT

dementia

Alzheimer's disease

clinical depression

caregiver

hospice

What to Know About
Aging

Gerontology is the study of aging. A **gerontologist** is a person who specializes in the study of aging. Some gerontologists believe that aging begins the day you are born. Others believe that aging begins when you stop growing. Physical, mental, and social changes occur during middle and late adulthood.

Physical Changes in Middle and Late Adulthood

As a person ages, body systems also age. Some changes are due to a person's heredity. Other changes may be due to one of the other factors that influence health status. Changes occur in each body system.

The Nervous System. As people age, reaction time slows. Eyesight changes. Muscles that make adjustments for seeing clearly may not be as strong. Body senses change because of a loss of nerve cells. Touch, taste, smell, and hearing may be affected. Some short term memory may be lost, but intelligence is not affected. The loss and degeneration of nerve cells also may cause Parkinson's disease. **Parkinson's disease** is a brain disorder that causes muscle tremors, stiffness, and weakness. To lessen changes to the nervous system, older people should exercise their minds and bodies regularly.

The Cardiovascular System. As people age, their hearts may become less efficient. Blood may not circulate as well. Blood vessels may lose their elasticity and become clogged, causing increased blood pressure. Resting heart rate may increase and oxygen consumption decrease. To lessen changes to the cardiovascular system, older people should maintain a desirable weight, exercise regularly, and eat a low-fat diet.

The Immune System. As people age, their immune system becomes less efficient in protecting the body. Older people have less resistance to communicable diseases and are more likely to develop chronic diseases. A **chronic disease** is an illness that develops and lasts over a long period of time. To lessen changes to the immune system, older people should have regular physical examinations, eat a healthful diet, and get regular flu shots if advised by a physician.

The Respiratory System. As people age, their lungs become less elastic. They may not be able to hold the same volume of air as in earlier years and may get short of breath. They have an increased risk of chronic bronchitis, emphysema, and flu. **Chronic bronchitis** is a recurring inflammation of the bronchial tubes. **Emphysema** is a condition in which the alveoli lose most of their ability to function. To lessen changes to the respiratory system, older people should avoid secondhand smoke, use caution in severe weather, exercise regularly, and not smoke.

The Skeletal System. As people age, their bones become less dense and, when broken, take longer to heal. There may be less fluid between the bones in the spinal column so an older person may become shorter with age. As people age, they may develop arthritis. **Arthritis** is a painful inflammation of the joints. Some older people, especially females, develop osteoporosis. **Osteoporosis** (ahs·tee·oh·puh·ROH·sis) is a condition in which the bones become thin and brittle. To lessen changes in the skeletal system, older people should maintain a desirable weight, exercise regularly, and eat foods with calcium.

The Muscular System. As people age, muscle mass and strength decrease. Body composition changes. The percentage of body fat increases. To lessen changes to the muscular system, older people should exercise regularly and lift objects correctly.

The Endocrine System. As people age, there may be changes in the secretions of hormones. Some people who are overweight or who have an hereditary tendency may develop diabetes mellitus. **Diabetes** or **diabetes mellitus** is a disease in which the body produces little or no insulin. To lessen changes to the endocrine system, older people should maintain a desirable weight and have regular blood tests.

The Digestive System. As people age, their metabolism slows and their weight may increase. Fewer nutrients are absorbed from foods. The liver may be less effective as it breaks down toxic substances. Some older people have difficulty digesting fatty foods. Gum disease and the loss of teeth may make it difficult to eat. Some older people may lose their appetites, eat less, and become malnourished. To lessen changes to the digestive system, older people should maintain a desirable weight, eat a balanced diet, limit alcohol consumption, and eat smaller meals more often.

The Urinary System. As people age, their bladder may decrease in size so that they have to urinate more frequently. Their kidneys also may produce less urine. To lessen changes to the urinary system, older people should drink at least eight glasses of water each day.

The Integumentary System. As people age, their skin becomes drier and may wrinkle. Age spots may appear on the skin. Extended exposure to sunlight earlier in life may affect how skin ages. Hair thins and grays. Some males become bald, and some females develop bald spots. To lessen changes to the integumentary system, older people should regularly check their skin and hair for signs of aging, wear sunblock and a hat to reduce exposure to ultraviolet radiation, and use lotions to keep skin from being dry.

The Reproductive System. As people age, their bodies produce fewer sex hormones. **Male climacteric** is a decrease in testosterone in males accompanied by symptoms such as hot flashes, depression, insomnia, and fatigue. **Menopause** is a decrease in estrogen in females and the cessation of the menstrual cycle. During menopause, some females experience hot flashes, depression, insomnia, headaches, fatigue, and short-term memory loss. A female's risk of developing heart disease increases as her ovaries secrete less estrogen. Some females choose estrogen replacement therapy. **Estrogen replacement therapy (ERT)** is synthetic estrogen given as a drug to reduce the symptoms of menopause and to help prevent osteoporosis.

Mental Changes in Middle and Late Adulthood

As people age, they may lose some short-term memory. Some older people develop dementia. **Dementia** is a general decline in all areas of mental functioning. Dementia is usually due to brain disease or mental impairment. Alzheimer's disease is a type of dementia. **Alzheimer's disease** is a progressive disease in which the nerve cells in the brain degenerate and the brain shrinks in size. Symptoms vary, but there are usually three stages. In the first stage, people are forgetful, lose interest, and feel anxious and depressed. In the second stage, people are disconnected and restless and have increased memory loss, especially for recent events. In the third stage, people become very disoriented, confused, and completely dependent on others. Older people should work to stay mentally sharp by using their mental skills, drink at least eight glasses of water each day, limit intake of alcohol, and not abuse drugs. They should be cautious and try to avoid accidents that may affect their mental functions.

Social Changes in Middle and Late Adulthood

People who are aging have the same needs as younger adults. They need friends with whom they can talk and engage in social activities. Most older people who stay active socially have better mental and physical health. Some older people suffer from depression. **Clinical depression** is long-lasting feelings of hopelessness, sadness, or helplessness. Exercise, therapy, and prescription medications are used to treat clinical depression.

What to Know About
Being a Caregiver

As people age, they may develop chronic diseases or other health conditions and require special care. Most older people turn to family members and friends for assistance and support. These family members and friends are caregivers. A **caregiver** is a person who provides care for a person who needs assistance. Most people are caregivers for an elderly family member at some time in their lives. You and your parents or guardian may be providing care for a grandparent or other relative right now. Your family may help with everyday tasks, such as bathing, dressing, cooking, and paying bills. Your family may provide transportation for an elderly relative who cannot drive.

Resources for Caregivers

Senior centers. Senior centers are facilities where older people can be involved in classes and social activities. Most senior centers provide meals.

Transportation assistance. Some community agencies and senior centers provide buses or vans to transport older people to a physician, grocery store, or senior center.

Friendly visitors or companions. Friendly visitors or companions are volunteers who regularly visit older people who are alone. They check on their needs and provide companionship.

Telephone reassurance programs. Telephone reassurance programs are staffed by volunteers who regularly call older people who are alone. They check on the older person's needs and provide companionship by telephone.

Home delivered meal programs. Organizations such as Meals-on-Wheels deliver food to older people who are shut-ins.

There are six factors to consider when you are a caregiver for a family member:

- the type of care the family member needs,
- the type of care the family member will accept,
- the cost of the type of care needed,
- the insurance coverage and financial resources of the family member,
- the type of care you can provide,
- the type of care provided by resources in the community.

Gatekeeper and home observation programs. Service people who work for the postal service or public utilities company may be trained to notice changes that might affect the needs of the elderly and to report these changes for investigation and action.

Home health care organizations. Home health care organizations offer a variety of services including nursing care, medical treatment, and therapy in the home.

Personal emergency response devices. Personal emergency response devices are mechanical devices that help older people call for help even if they are not able to reach or dial the telephone.

Adult day care programs. Adult day care programs provide health care, social activities, meals, therapy, and transportation.

Respite care. Respite care is care provided by someone who is relieving a family member of caregiving responsibilities. Adult day care programs are examples of respite care.

Nursing homes or convalescent centers. Nursing homes or convalescent centers are facilities that provide 24-hour care. Medical care is provided at nursing homes.

Hospice care. **Hospice** is a facility for people who are dying and their families.

Lesson 30

You Can Express Feelings About Dying and Death

Life Skill **I will share with my family my feelings about dying and death.**

The reality is that everyone will die some day. Death is a normal part of the life cycle. Acknowledging and accepting this reality can give your life meaning and purpose. Fear of death is natural. However, you will be more accepting of death if you take the time to sort out the meaning and purpose of life and learn the facts about death. This lesson discusses facts you need to know about death. You will learn the legal definition of death. You also will learn about issues surrounding death that must be considered. This lesson also deals with grief. You will learn about the five stages of grief. You will learn how to express your grief when someone you care about dies. You also will learn how to comfort someone who is grieving.

The Lesson Outline

What to Know About Dying and Death

What to Know About Grief

Objectives

1. Discuss death and issues surrounding death: life support systems, living wills, and hospice. **page 245**

2. Discuss the five stages of grief, how to express grief, and how to comfort someone who is grieving. **pages 246–247**

Vocabulary Words

hospice

terminal illness

death

life support system

legal death

brain death

living will

coma

request for medical nonintervention

grief

five stages of grief

anticipatory grief

eulogy

Dying and Death

Many people discuss the way they want to die. Some people want to be near family members and close friends at the time of their death. These people can use hospice. **Hospice** is a facility for people who are dying and their families. Two criteria must be met before a person is eligible to use hospice. A person must have a terminal illness. A **terminal illness** is an illness that will result in death. A person also must be expected to die in less than six months. Hospices can provide support at a hospital, another facility, or in someone's home. When away from home, hospice provides a home-like atmosphere. When possible, hospice provides care in the person's home. Usually medications are given to keep the person as comfortable as possible. Family members and friends stay with the person who is dying. Hospice volunteers assist the family in caring for the person.

Death is the permanent cessation of all vital organs. At one time, a person was pronounced dead when his/her heart and lungs stopped functioning. But today, life support systems can prolong life by keeping the heart and lungs functioning. A **life support system** is mechanical or other means to support life. An example is the use of a respirator to force air into the lungs.

Life support systems brought about a need to define death in legal terms. **Legal death** is brain death or the irreversible stopping of circulatory and respiratory functions. **Brain death** is the irreversible cessation of all functions of the entire brain, including the brain stem.

People are living longer than they did in the past. This has made people think more about issues related to life support systems and legal death. People now have the right to make living wills. A **living will** is a document that tells what treatment a person wants in the event that (s)he no longer can make decisions. A living will differs from a regular will. A regular will tells how a person wants his/her possessions to be distributed. For example, a regular will may state exactly how much money to spend on care for children or other relatives.

A living will focuses on issues of medical treatment. A person may name someone to make decisions about medical treatment if (s)he cannot do so. For example, a person may be in a coma. A **coma** is a state of unconsciousness. A person in a coma cannot make his/her own decisions. In a living will, a person may make a request for medical nonintervention. A **request for medical nonintervention** is a person's refusal of specific life support systems when there is no reasonable expectation of recovering or regaining a meaningful life. A person can state which life support systems (s)he does not want. These may include antibiotics, machine or forced feedings or fluids, cardiac resuscitation, respiratory support, or surgery. The request also may state that treatment be limited to providing comfort, such as the administration of painkillers.

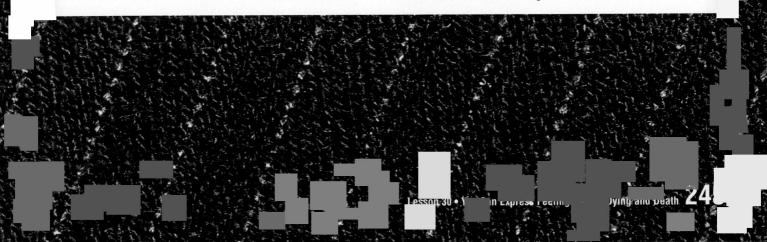

What to Know About
Grief

Grief is intense emotional suffering caused by a loss, disaster, or misfortune. When someone dies, people who have been close to this person grieve. People who are dying grieve the loss of their own life. There are five stages of grief. The **five stages of grief** are psychological stages of grieving that include denial, anger, bargaining, depression, and acceptance. The five stages of grief are outlined in the chart on the next page.

When someone close to you is dying both you and the person who is dying experience anticipatory grief. **Anticipatory grief** is grief experienced prior to a loss. The person who is dying grieves the loss of his/her life. You grieve the loss of the person you care about or love.

The time you have left to be together and share becomes very special. You can make wise use of the precious moments you have.

Suppose a person about whom you care is in a coma. The time you have left to be together and share is still very important. Frequent visits may be helpful to you and to the person who is dying. Many people who have come out of a coma remember words spoken to them. They also remember being comforted. You might hold this person's hand and speak to him/her. Expressing your feelings will help you and the person who is in a coma.

At other times, you may know someone who is grieving the loss of a close friend or loved one. You also can comfort this person.

When Someone Close to You Is Dying:

1. Spend time with the friend or family member who is dying.
2. Share your loving feelings and memories.
3. Share your feelings of loss and pain.
4. Encourage the person to talk about his/her death.
5. Listen carefully to the person's feelings and thoughts about the past, present, and future.
6. Reassure the person with affection; hold hands or hug.
7. Share your grief with family members and friends.
8. Continue your daily routine if possible.
9. Consider what you will do to keep alive the memory of the person.
10. Allow yourself time to grieve.

When Someone Who You Know Is Grieving a Loss:

1. Make yourself available. Remember, friends support one another during difficult times.
2. Do something thoughtful for the person. You might send a card or call the person. You might offer to help the person with meals or errands.
3. Attend memorial services, with permission of your parents or guardian.
4. Have empathy for the person's loss. Do not lessen the loss by making statements such as, "She would have wanted it this way." Instead say, "I am sorry you feel sad. I am here to support you."
5. Encourage the person to talk about his/her grief.
6. Recognize signs of grief that are not healthy. A person who remains severely depressed, or who relies on alcohol or other drugs may need help. **Tell a responsible adult if you notice any such behaviors.**

Five Stages of Grief

Ways People Who Are Dying Grieve

Stage 1: ## Denial
- People who are dying refuse to believe that they are dying.

Stage 2: ## Anger
- People who are dying are angry. They may direct their anger at family members, friends, their physician, or other medical professionals.

Stage 3: ## Bargaining
- People who are dying try to avoid death by making deals and promises.

Stage 4: ## Depression
- People who are dying become very sad when bargaining does not work. They know they will die and will not be around for future events.

Stage 5: ## Acceptance
- People who are dying begin to say good-bye and to share special feelings and thoughts.

Ways People Grieve When They Know a Family Member or Friend Is Dying

Stage 1: ## Denial
- Family members and friends of someone who is dying refuse to believe a person they care about or love is dying.

Stage 2: ## Anger
- Family members and friends of someone who is dying are angry and direct their anger at the person who is dying, other people who are close to them, or medical professionals.

Stage 3: ## Bargaining
- Family members and friends of someone who is dying make deals and promises hoping this will allow the person they care about to survive.

Stage 4: ## Depression
- Family members and friends of someone who is dying become very sad when bargaining does not work. They imagine what life will be like without that person.

Stage 5: ## Acceptance
- Family members and friends of someone who is dying begin to say good-bye and to share special feelings and thoughts.

The authors have developed their own interpretation of the five stages of grief based on the work of Elisabeth Kübler-Ross.

Activity

Writing a Eulogy

Life Skill: I will share with my family my feelings about dying and death.

Materials: paper, pen or pencil

Directions: There is a saying, "Death gives meaning to life." Accepting the fact that you will die someday can help you decide how you want to live. When people die, someone may give a eulogy. A **eulogy** is a formal speech about someone who has recently died. Suppose you died and someone were to give a eulogy about you. What would you want that person to say? Follow the directions below to write a eulogy about yourself.

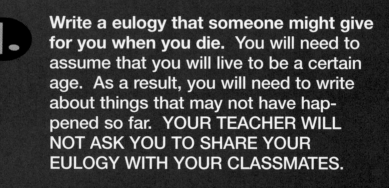 **1.** Write a eulogy that someone might give for you when you die. You will need to assume that you will live to be a certain age. As a result, you will need to write about things that may not have happened so far. YOUR TEACHER WILL NOT ASK YOU TO SHARE YOUR EULOGY WITH YOUR CLASSMATES.

 2. Include at least three to five reasons why your life benefitted both the people you loved and humankind in general.

 3. Review what you have written in your eulogy.

 4. List three actions you can take right now to be worthy of the respect you included in your eulogy.

 5. Share your eulogy and list of three actions with your parents or guardian.

Lesson 30

Review

Vocabulary Words

Write a separate sentence using each of the vocabulary words listed on page 244.

Objectives

1. Why was it necessary to define death in legal terms? **Objective 1**
2. Why might a person have a living will? **Objective 1**
3. What is the purpose of hospice? **Objective 1**
4. What are the five stages of grief? **Objective 2**
5. What are ten things you might do if someone you care about is dying or is grieving? **Objective 2**

Responsible Decision-Making

Your friend's grandmother is terminally ill. Your friend does not visit his/her grandmother at the hospital because it gives him/her "the creeps" to be around someone who is dying. Your friend's parents expect him/her to visit the hospital this evening. Your friend tells you that (s)he is going to make up a story and say (s)he has a big test tomorrow. Write a response to this situation.

1. Describe the situation that requires your friend to make a decision.
2. List possible decisions your friend might make.
3. Name two responsible adults with whom your friend might discuss his/her decisions.
4. Evaluate the possible consequences of your friend's decisions. Determine if each decision will lead to actions that:
   • promote health,
   • protect safety,
   • follow laws,
   • show respect for your friend and others,
   • follow the guidelines of your friend's parents and of other responsible adults,
   • demonstrate good character.
5. Decide which decision is most responsible and appropriate for your friend.
6. Tell two results your friend can expect if (s)he makes this decision.

Effective Communication

Suppose a parent of one of your friends dies unexpectedly in an automobile accident. Write a letter to your friend expressing sympathy and offering your help.

Self-Directed Learning

Different cultures have different ways of expressing grief and mourning the loss of a family member. Choose a culture different from your own. Talk to someone of that culture or research at the library or on the Internet how grief is expressed and mourning is carried out. Write a report about that culture's traditions about death. Share your report with your classmates.

Critical Thinking

The five stages of grief may be experienced whenever a person has a loss, disaster, or misfortune. Select a situation other than dying and death in which a person experiences a loss, disaster, or misfortune. Write an essay explaining what a person in this situation experiences based on the five stages of grief.

Responsible Citizenship

Look in your local telephone directory and locate hospices. You might look under "hospices" or "hospitals." Obtain permission from your parents or guardian to volunteer for a hospice.

Responsible Decision-Making

Your classmate tells you she wants to become pregnant. She says that her mother became pregnant when she was a teen so it is OK for her to get pregnant. Write a response to this situation.

1. Describe the situation that requires your friend to make a decision.
2. List possible decisions your friend might make.
3. Name two responsible adults with whom your friend might discuss his/her decisions.
4. Evaluate the possible consequences of your friend's decisions. Determine if each decision will lead to actions that:
   - promote health,
   - protect safety,
   - follow laws,
   - show respect for your friend and others,
   - follow the guidelines of your friend's parents and of other responsible adults,
   - demonstrate good character.
5. Decide which decision is most responsible and appropriate for your friend.
6. Tell two results you expect if your friend makes this decision.

Health Behavior Inventory of Life Skills

Number from 1 to 10 on a sheet of paper. Read each life skill carefully. Write YES or NO next to the same number on your paper. Each YES response indicates a life skill you practice to promote your health status. Each NO response indicates a life skill you do not practice. Plan to begin practicing these life skills.

1. I will keep my body systems healthy.
2. I will recognize habits that protect female reproductive health.
3. I will recognize habits that protect male reproductive health.
4. I will learn about pregnancy and childbirth.
5. I will practice abstinence to avoid the risks of teen pregnancy and parenthood.
6. I will provide responsible care for infants and children.
7. I will achieve the developmental tasks of adolescence.
8. I will develop my learning style.
9. I will develop habits that promote healthful aging.
10. I will share with my family my feelings about dying and death.

Multicultural Health

Create a world map using poster paper and markers or computer graphics. Research the life span of people in ten different countries. Illustrate this information on your world map. Which factors influence the life spans of the people living in the ten countries you selected?

Family Involvement

Discuss the Ten Habits That Promote Healthful Aging, page 242, with your parents or guardian. Which habits are practiced by your biological relatives? Which habits are not practiced by your biological relatives? How do each of the habits influence the health of your biological relatives?

Health Behavior Contract

Copy and complete the following health behavior contract. Evaluate your progress. Share the results with your family.

Health Behavior Contract

 1. Name_____Date_____

 2. **Life Skill:** I will develop habits that promote healthful aging.

3. **Effects on Health Status:** My chronological age is the number of years I have lived. My biological age is a measure of how well my body systems are working. Nothing can be done to change my chronological age. However, my habits affect my biological age. The habits I develop right now will affect my biological age in middle and late adulthood. If I develop healthful habits, I can keep my biological age lower than my chronological age.

4. **Plan and Method to Record Progress:** I will develop ten habits that promote healthful aging. I will write the number for each habit I practice in the space provided for each day of the week.

1. Eat a healthful, balanced breakfast each day.
2. Follow the Dietary Guidelines.
3. Exercise regularly.
4. Do not smoke or use other tobacco products.
5. Get plenty of rest and sleep.
6. Have regular physical examinations.
7. Balance work with play.
8. Choose activities to keep your mind alert.
9. Develop healthful relationships with family members and friends.
10. Practice stress management skills.

My Calendar

M	T	W	Th	F	S	S

 5. **Evaluation:** _____
_____
_____

Unit 4

Nutrition

You Can Select Foods That Contain Nutrients

Life Skill **I will select foods that contain nutrients.**

Are the foods and beverages you consume in a day healthful? **Nutrition** is the study of what people eat and of eating habits and how these affect health status. To obtain optimal health status, you must pay attention to getting the nutrients your body needs. A **nutrient** is a substance in food that helps with body processes, helps with growth and repair of cells, and provides energy. Energy is measured in calories. A **calorie** is a unit of energy produced by food and used by the body. This lesson discusses the six classes of nutrients: proteins, carbohydrates, fats, vitamins, minerals, and water. You will learn the functions and sources for each of these nutrients.

The Lesson Outline

What to Know About Proteins

What to Know About Carbohydrates

What to Know About Fats

What to Know About Vitamins

What to Know About Minerals

What to Know About Water

Objectives

Vocabulary Words

nutrition
nutrient
calorie
protein
complete protein
amino acids
essential amino acids
incomplete protein
carbohydrate
simple carbohydrates
complex carbohydrates
starch
fiber
fat
fat-soluble vitamin
saturated fat
cholesterol
unsaturated fat
visible fat
invisible fat
vitamin
water-soluble vitamin
mineral
water
dehydration
diuretic

What to Know About
Proteins

A **protein** is a nutrient that is needed:

- for growth;
- to build, repair, and maintain body tissues;
- to regulate body processes;
- to supply energy.

Proteins form part of every cell in your body. Proteins make up more than 50 percent of your total body weight. Your skin, nails, and hair are mostly proteins. Proteins help your body maintain strength and resist infection. Each gram of protein provides four calories. A daily diet deficient in proteins may stunt your growth, affect the development of certain tissue, and affect your mental development. Excess protein is burned as energy or stored as fat.

There are two kinds of proteins: complete proteins and incomplete proteins.

1. A **complete protein** is a protein that contains all of the essential amino acids. **Amino acids** are the building blocks that make up proteins. Examples of complete proteins are meat, fish, poultry, milk, yogurt, and eggs. The soybean is the only plant food that provides all nine of the essential amino acids. Your body needs 20 amino acids to function properly. Your body can produce only 11 of these amino acids. **Essential amino acids** are the nine amino acids the body cannot produce. These nine essential amino acids must come from the foods you eat.

2. An **incomplete protein** is a protein from plant sources that does not contain all of the essential amino acids. Incomplete proteins from plant sources fall into three general categories: grains (whole grains, pastas, and corn), legumes (dried beans, peas, and lentils), and nuts and seeds. Different plant sources of incomplete proteins can be combined to obtain all of the essential amino acids you need.

eggs

poultry

meat

fish

seeds

nuts

tofu

grains

yogurt

beans

milk

What to Know About
Carbohydrates

A **carbohydrate** (KAHR·boh·hy·drayt) is a nutrient that is the main source of energy for the body. Carbohydrates include sugars, starches, and fiber. Carbohydrates supply four calories of energy per gram of food. Your body can store only limited amounts of carbohydrates. Excess carbohydrates are stored as fat. Sources of carbohydrates include vegetables, beans, potatoes, pasta, breads, rice, bran, popcorn, and fruit.

apples

potatoes

carrots

cereals

whole-wheat breads

popcorn

brown rice

beans

oranges

There are two types of carbohydrates: simple carbohydrates and complex carbohydrates.

1. **Simple carbohydrates** are sugars that enter the bloodstream rapidly and provide quick energy. Sugars are found naturally in fruits, honey, and milk. Processed sugar, or table sugar, is added to food during processing. Processed sugar is found in cakes, candy, and other sweet desserts as well as in ketchup, spaghetti sauce, and soda pop. Simple carbohydrates provide calories but few vitamins and minerals.

2. **Complex carbohydrates** are starches and fiber. Most of the calories in your diet come from complex carbohydrates. Sources of complex carbohydrates include grains, such as bread and pasta, and vegetables, such as potatoes and beans. **Starch** is a food substance that is made and stored in most plants. Starches provide long-lasting energy.

   Fiber is the part of grains and plant foods that cannot be digested. Fiber also is known as roughage. Fiber helps move food through the digestive system. Fiber helps prevent constipation and other intestinal problems. When you eat foods that contain fiber, you feel full. Eating foods with fiber reduces your blood cholesterol level and your risk of developing heart disease. Good sources of fiber include wheat, bran, cereals, fruit, and vegetables.

   When you eat complex carbohydrates, they are changed by saliva and other digestive juices to a simple sugar called glucose. Some glucose is used by cells to provide energy and heat. The remaining glucose is changed to glycogen. Glycogen is stored in the muscles. When you need energy, glycogen is converted to gluclose.

pears

What to Know About
Fats

A **fat** is a nutrient that provides energy and helps the body store and use vitamins. One gram of fat supplies nine calories of energy. Fats supply more than twice the number of calories supplied by proteins and carbohydrates. Fats store and transport fat-soluble vitamins. A **fat-soluble vitamin** is a vitamin that dissolves in fat and can be stored in the body. Fat-soluble vitamins include vitamins A, D, E, and K. Fats are stored as fat tissue that surrounds and cushions internal organs. Fats contribute to the taste and texture of many foods. The body needs fats to maintain body heat, store and use vitamins, maintain an energy reserve, and build brain cells and nerve tissues.

There are two main types of fats: saturated fats and unsaturated fats.

1. **Saturated fat** is a type of fat from dairy products, solid vegetable fat, and meat and poultry. Saturated fats usually are in solid form when at room temperature. Saturated fats contribute to the level of cholesterol that is in a person's blood. **Cholesterol** (Kuh·LES·tuh·rohl) is a fat-like substance made by the body and found in certain foods. Cholesterol in food is called dietary cholesterol. Dietary cholesterol is found in foods of animal origin, such as meats and dairy products. A person's blood cholesterol level is a combination of dietary cholesterol and cholesterol produced by the body. Blood cholesterol level can be lowered by eating fewer saturated fats. Maintaining a healthful cholesterol level lowers the risk of heart disease and some cancers.

2. **Unsaturated fat** is a type of fat obtained from plant products and fish. Unsaturated fats are usually liquid at room temperature. There are two types of unsaturated fats: polyunsaturated fats and monounsaturated (mahn·oh·uhn·SACH·uh·rayt·id) fats. Polyunsaturated fats include sunflower, corn, and soybean oils. Monounsaturated fats include olive and canola oils.

Visible fat is fat that can be seen when looking at food. For example, you can see fatty areas on some meats and grease on potato chips. **Invisible fat** is fat that cannot be seen when looking at food. For example, a piece of cake contains eggs and shortening.

nuts butter margarine salad dressing oils meat egg yolks sour cream pastries milk ice cream cheese

What to Know About
Vitamins

A **vitamin** is a nutrient that helps the body use carbohydrates, proteins, and fats. There are two types of vitamins: fat-soluble vitamins and water-soluble vitamins.

A fat-soluble vitamin is a vitamin that dissolves in fat and can be stored in the body. There are four fat-soluble vitamins: A, D, E, and K.

A **water-soluble vitamin** is a vitamin that dissolves in water and cannot be stored by the body in significant amounts. Examples of water-soluble vitamins are B complex and C. You need foods and beverages each day that are sources of water-soluble vitamins.

The chart that follows identifies vitamins and their functions and lists their sources.

VITAMIN	FUNCTIONS	SOURCES
Vitamin A	Keeps eyes, skin, hair, teeth, and gums healthy	Milk, cheese, egg yolk, green and yellow vegetables, liver, fruits
Vitamin D	Necessary for formation of bones and teeth	Dairy products, fish-liver oils, tuna, egg yolk
Vitamin K	Necessary for normal blood clotting	Leafy, green vegetables; liver; cheese; pork
Vitamin B₁ (Thiamin)	Necessary for function of nerves	Whole-grain cereals and breads, poultry, eggs, wheat germ, pasta
Vitamin B₁₂	Necessary for formation of red blood cells	Beef, poultry, fish, eggs, cheese, milk
Vitamin C	Helps heart, cells, and muscles function	Citrus fruits, green vegetables, potatoes, tomatoes, cantaloupe
Vitamin B₃ (Riboflavin)	Helps body use energy	Yeast, wheat germ, fish, eggs, milk, cheese
Vitamin B₆	Helps body use fats and take in protein	Liver, whole grains, vegetables
Vitamin E	Helps form and maintain cells	Green vegetables, whole-grain cereals and breads, nuts
Folacin	Necessary for formation of hemoglobin in red blood cells; necessary for production of genetic material	Green vegetables, liver, whole-grain cereals and breads, legumes
Vitamin B₂	Necessary for function of nerve cells; necessary for a healthy appetite; helps cells produce energy	Milk; eggs; whole-grain products; leafy, green vegetables; dried beans; enriched breads; cereals; pasta
Biotin	Necessary for normal metabolism of carbohydrates and other B vitamins	Organ meats, egg yolks, green vegetables, dried beans, bananas, peanuts, some fruits
Pantothenic acid	Necessary for production of RNA, DNA, and normal red blood cells	Liver, kidney, milk, yeast, wheat germ, whole-grain cereals and breads, green vegetables

What to Know About
Minerals

A **mineral** is a nutrient that regulates many chemical reactions in the body. There are two types of minerals: macro minerals and trace minerals. Macro minerals are required in amounts greater than 100 milligrams. Examples of macro minerals are calcium and sodium. Trace minerals are needed in very small amounts. Examples of trace minerals are iron and zinc. Trace minerals are as important to the body as macro minerals.

The following chart identifies minerals and their functions and sources.

MINERALS	FUNCTIONS	SOURCES
MACRO MINERALS		
Calcium	Builds up bones and teeth	Milk; cheese; legumes; soybean products; clams; oysters; leafy, green vegetables
Magnesium	Necessary for chemical reactions during metabolism	Milk; dairy products; leafy, green vegetables
Phosphorus	Builds bones, teeth, and cells	Milk, whole-grain cereals, meats, poultry, legumes, cheese
Potassium	Keeps fluids balanced within cells	Whole-grain cereals and breads, green vegetables, legumes, fruit
Sodium	Necessary for water balance in cells and tissues and for nerve cell conduction	Table salt, high-salt meats, cheese, crackers
Sulfur	Builds hair, nails, and skin	Meats, milk, eggs, legumes, nuts, cheese, brown sugar
TRACE MINERALS		
Copper	Necessary for production of hemoglobin in red blood cells	Red meat, liver, seafood, whole grains, poultry, nuts, legumes
Iodine	Necessary for production of the thyroid gland hormone	Iodized salt, milk, cheese, fish, whole-grain cereals and breads
Iron	Aids red blood cells	Liver, red meats, fish, eggs, legumes, whole-grain cereals
Manganese	Aids in synthesis of cholesterol and normal function of nerve tissue	Whole-grain products; leafy, green vegetables; fruits; legumes; nuts
Zinc	Necessary for digestive enzymes and healing of wounds	Seafood, red meats, milk, poultry, eggs, whole-grain breads and cereals

You Can Follow the Food Guide Pyramid

Life Skill I will eat the recommended number of servings from the Food Guide Pyramid.

You need to eat a variety of foods to obtain the nutrients your body needs for optimal health. A careful selection of foods is required. The United States Department of Agriculture and the United States Department of Health and Human Services created the Food Guide Pyramid to help you select foods. This lesson explains the Food Guide Pyramid. You will learn about each food group in the pyramid. You will learn how many servings from each food group you need each day. This lesson also discusses vegetarian diets. You will learn about different kinds of vegetarian diets. You will learn how a person who follows a vegetarian diet can get the nutrients needed for optimal health.

The Lesson Outline

How to Use the Food Guide Pyramid

What to Know About Each Food Group

What to Know About Vegetarian Diets

Objectives

1. Identify the recommended number of daily servings for each food group in the Food Guide Pyramid. **page 265**

2. List examples of foods from each of the food groups in the Food Guide Pyramid. **pages 266–267**

3. Explain how to follow a vegetarian diet. **page 268**

Vocabulary Words

food group
Food Guide Pyramid
vegetarian diet
vegan diet
lacto-vegetarian diet
lacto-ovo-vegetarian diet
semi-vegetarian diet

How to Use the Food Guide Pyramid

A **food group** is a category of foods that contain similar nutrients. The **Food Guide Pyramid** is a guide that tells how many servings from each food group are recommended each day. The number of servings recommended for you depends on your age, sex, size, and activity level.

Examine the Food Guide Pyramid. A balanced diet includes servings of foods from different food groups. The greatest number of servings of food you eat each day should come from the bottom of the pyramid. The fewest number of servings you eat each day should come from the top of the pyramid.

It is important to eat a variety of foods from each food group because foods within the same group have different combinations of nutrients. For example, some vegetables are good sources of vitamin C, while others are good sources of vitamin A.

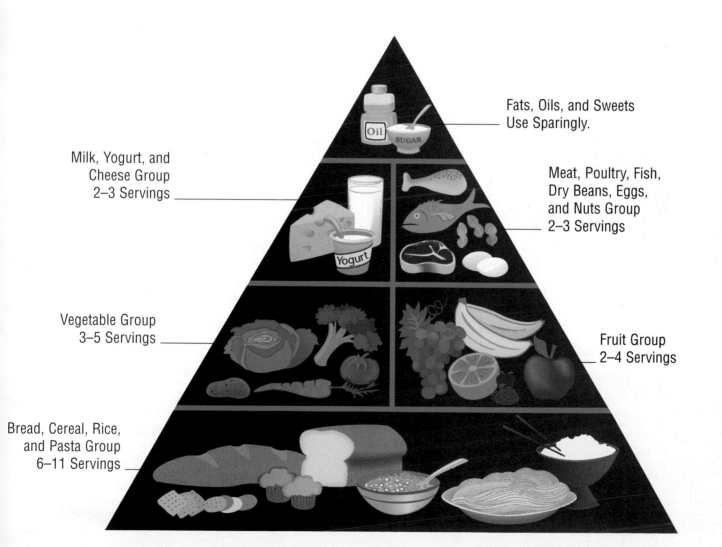

Fats, Oils, and Sweets
Use Sparingly.

Milk, Yogurt, and
Cheese Group
2–3 Servings

Meat, Poultry, Fish,
Dry Beans, Eggs,
and Nuts Group
2–3 Servings

Vegetable Group
3–5 Servings

Fruit Group
2–4 Servings

Bread, Cereal, Rice,
and Pasta Group
6–11 Servings

What to Know About Each
Food Group

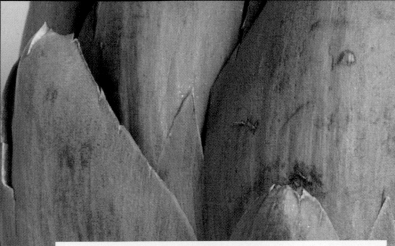

Vegetable Group

You need three to five servings each day from the vegetable group. Foods from this food group are low in fat and calories. They are good sources of vitamins A and C and minerals. Starchy vegetables, such as potatoes, are good sources of complex carbohydrates and fiber.

One serving =

- 1 cup raw, leafy vegetables

  or

- 1/2 cup cooked or raw vegetables

  or

- 3/4 cup vegetable juice

Bread, Cereal, Rice, and Pasta Group

You need six to 11 servings each day from the bread, cereal, rice, and pasta group. Foods from this food group are good sources of vitamins, minerals, and complex carbohydrates. They provide fiber, iron, and vitamin B.

One serving =

- 1 slice of bread

  or

- 1 ounce (28 grams) of ready-to-eat cereal

  or

- 1/2 cup cooked cereal, rice, or pasta

Fruit Group

You need two to four servings each day from the fruit group. Foods from this food group are low in fat. They are good sources of vitamins A and C, potassium, and carbohydrates. Fruits with skins you can eat also supply fiber.

One serving =

- 1 medium apple, banana, or orange

  or

- 1/2 cup chopped, cooked, or canned fruit

  or

- 3/4 cup 100 percent fruit juice

Milk, Yogurt, and Cheese Group

You need two to three servings each day from the milk, yogurt, and cheese group. Foods from this food group are good sources of calcium and protein. These foods may contain high levels of fat, but choosing low-fat and fat-free versions of these foods can help limit fat intake.

One serving =

- **1 cup milk**

  or

- **1 1/2 ounces (42 grams) of natural cheese**

  or

- **2 ounces (56 grams) of processed cheese**

  or

- **1 cup of yogurt**

Meat, Poultry, Fish, Dry Beans, Eggs, and Nuts Group

You need two to three servings each day from the meat, poultry, fish, dry beans, eggs, and nuts group. Foods from this food group are good sources of protein, B vitamins, iron, and zinc. These foods also may contain high levels of fat. Choosing lean meats and poultry without the skin and limiting the egg yolks, nuts, and seeds you consume can help limit fat intake.

One serving =

- **2 to 3 ounces (56 to 84 grams) of cooked lean meat, poultry, or fish**

  or

- **1/2 cup of dry beans**

  or

- **1 egg**

  or

- **2 tablespoons of peanut butter**

Fats, Oils, and Sweets

You should limit the amount of fats, oils, and sweets you eat. These foods provide few vitamins and minerals and are high in sugars and fats. Foods that belong to this food group are candy, butter, margarine, salad dressing, soda pop, table sugar, cream, cookies, pies, and doughnuts.

A food is high in sugars if one of the ingredients listed below is at the top of an ingredients list on a food label. The food also may be high in sugars if several of the ingredients are listed on the food label itself.

- ● **Corn sweetener**
- ● **Corn syrup**
- ● **Fructose**
- ● **Fruit juice concentrate**
- ● **Glucose**
- ● **High-fructose corn syrup**
- ● **Honey**
- ● **Lactose**
- ● **Molasses**

How to Use the Dietary Guidelines

To have a healthful diet, you must select the correct number of servings from the Food Guide Pyramid each day. When you make your selections, use the Dietary Guidelines. For example, you must select two to three servings each day from the Milk, Yogurt, and Cheese Group. Pay close attention to Dietary Guideline 3—*Choose a diet low in fat, saturated fat, and cholesterol.* Suppose one of the foods you want to select is ice cream.

After considering this guideline, you may substitute low-fat yogurt or low-fat ice cream for whole-milk ice cream. You also must select six to 11 servings from the Bread, Cereal, Rice, and Pasta Group. When you make your selections, pay attention to Dietary Guideline 5—*Choose a diet moderate in sugars.* After considering this guideline, you may substitute sugarless oatmeal for a sugared cereal.

Activity

Dietary Guidelines Self-Check

Life Skill: I will follow the Dietary Guidelines.

Materials: paper, red pen or marker, blue pen or marker

Directions: A careful evaluation of your food selections is important. Complete the directions for the following activity to learn if you are getting the servings you need from each food group and are following the Dietary Guidelines.

1. **Draw an outline on a sheet of paper of the Food Guide Pyramid.**

2. **Keep track of what you eat and drink for one day.** Write the name and number of servings of each food and beverage in the appropriate space on the Food Guide Pyramid. If a food or beverage falls into more than one group, separate the ingredients into the different spaces. For example, a turkey sandwich contains turkey (Meat, Poultry, Fish, Dry Beans, Eggs, and Nuts Group) and bread (Bread, Cereal, Rice and Pasta Group).

 Record the number of servings you have eaten from each food group. Write and circle the number in the appropriate space on the Food Guide Pyramid.

 Indicate the Dietary Guidelines you followed. Use a blue pen or marker to draw arrows from the foods and beverages you wrote in each food group to indicate the Dietary Guideline you followed. For example, suppose you wrote "egg-substitute omelet." Draw a line from "egg-substitute omelet" to Dietary Guideline 3.

 Indicate the Dietary Guidelines you did not follow. Use a red pen or marker to draw arrows from the foods and beverages you wrote in each food group that did not follow Dietary Guidelines. For example, suppose you wrote "cake" on the Food Guide Pyramid. Draw a line to Dietary Guideline 5.

 Write a one-page summary discussing what you have learned.

Lesson 33

Review

Vocabulary Words

Write a separate sentence using each of the vocabulary words listed on page 270.

Objectives

1. What are the seven Dietary Guidelines? **Objective 1**

2. Why is it important to balance the food you eat with physical activity? **Objective 1**

3. Why is it important to choose a diet with plenty of grain products, vegetables, and fruits? **Objective 1**

4. Why is it important to choose a diet moderate in sugars? **Objective 1**

5. How are the Dietary Guidelines used when making food selections from the Food Guide Pyramid? **Objective 2**

Responsible Decision-Making

Your class has studied nutrients, the Food Guide Pyramid, and the Dietary Guidelines. You discuss what you have learned with a classmate. Your classmate says (s)he believes beer is a healthful choice because it is a source of carbohydrates. (S)he offers you a beer and suggests that you "drink your carbohydrates" instead of eating your sandwich for lunch. Write a response to this situation.

1. Describe the situation that requires you to make a decision.
2. List possible decisions you might make.
3. Name two responsible adults with whom you might discuss your decisions.
4. Evaluate the possible consequences of your decisions. Determine if each decision will lead to actions that:
   - promote health,
   - protect safety,
   - follow laws,
   - show respect for yourself and others,
   - follow the guidelines of your parents and of other responsible adults,
   - demonstrate good character.
5. Decide which decision is most responsible and appropriate.
6. Tell two results you expect if you make this decision.

Effective Communication

Prepare a list of five actions you can take to make it possible for you to follow the seven Dietary Guidelines more closely. Share the list with a responsible adult. Ask for advice and support in performing the actions.

Self-Directed Learning

At the local library, select a video, book on tape, or book about diet. View, listen to, or read the item you selected. Write a summary statement of the information you learned and tell how it relates to the Dietary Guidelines.

Critical Thinking

Suppose you follow the Food Guide Pyramid but ignore the Dietary Guidelines. Would your diet be healthful? Explain why or why not.

Responsible Citizenship

Review the Food Guide Pyramid and the Dietary Guidelines with a parent or guardian. Together, plan a meal that contains at least one serving from each food group in the Food Guide Pyramid and follows all seven Dietary Guidelines.

Lesson 34

You Can Plan a Healthful Diet That Reduces the Risk of Disease

Life Skill ▶ **I will plan a healthful diet that reduces the risk of disease.**

Your diet affects your health status right now as well as in the future. If you have a healthful diet, you obtain the nutrients you need for growth and development. You have energy for your daily activities—including physical activity. Having a healthful diet right now helps reduce your risk of developing certain diseases as an adult. This lesson explains how to plan a diet to reduce the risk of these diseases: cancer, cardiovascular diseases, diabetes, hypoglycemia, and osteoporosis. You also will learn what to do about food allergies and intolerances.

The Lesson Outline

What to Know About Diet and Cancer

What to Know About Diet and Cardiovascular Diseases

What to Know About Diet, Diabetes, and Hypoglycemia

What to Know About Diet and Osteoporosis

What to Know About Food Allergies and Intolerances

Objectives

1. Discuss dietary guidelines to reduce the risk of developing cancer. **page 275**

2. Discuss dietary guidelines to reduce the risk of developing cardiovascular diseases. **pages 276–277**

3. Discuss diet recommendations for people with diabetes or hypoglycemia. **page 279**

4. Discuss dietary guidelines to reduce the risk of developing osteoporosis. **page 279**

5. Discuss ways to avoid reactions to food allergies and intolerances, including lactose intolerance and celiac sprue, and reactions to MSG and yellow dye. **page 280**

Vocabulary Words

obesity

antioxidant

cruciferous vegetables

fiber

cardiovascular disease

cholesterol

plaque

atherosclerosis

embolism

olestra

diabetes

diabetes mellitus

insulin

hypoglycemia

osteoporosis

food allergy

food intolerance

lactase deficiency

celiac sprue

What to Know About
Diet and Cancer

The National Academy of Sciences, the National Cancer Institute, and the American Cancer Society are organizations that have examined the role of diet in preventing cancer. You can reduce the risk of developing cancer by practicing the following dietary guidelines.

1. **Avoid obesity. Obesity** is a body weight that is 20 percent or more than desirable body weight. Being obese increases the risk of developing cancers of the uterus, breast, gallbladder, prostate gland, and colon.

2. **Eat a variety of foods.** When you eat a variety of foods, your body has a combination of nutrients. A combination of nutrients is helpful in reducing the risk of cancer. For example, different foods contain antioxidants. An **antioxidant** (an·ty·AHKS·uh·dent) is a substance that protects cells from being damaged by oxidation. Antioxidants prevent cell damage and repair damaged cells. Their actions help prevent healthy cells from becoming cancerous cells. Vitamins C, E, and A and the mineral selenium are antioxidants. When you eat a variety of foods, you are more likely to get the right combination of antioxidants.

3. **Eat several servings and a variety of fruits and vegetables each day.** Fruits and vegetables contain vitamins C, E, and A, antioxidants that help prevent cancer. Pay particular attention to choosing cruciferous vegetables. **Cruciferous** (kru·SIF·ehr·us) **vegetables** are vegetables that belong to the cabbage family, such as cauliflower, broccoli, and brussels sprouts. Fruits and vegetables reduce the risk of developing cancers of the colon, rectum, prostate, stomach, esophagus, and lung.

4. **Eat several servings of fiber-rich foods, such as whole-grain cereals, legumes, vegetables, and fruits**. **Fiber** is the part of grains and plant foods that cannot be digested. Eating fiber-rich foods helps you have a daily bowel movement. Having regular bowel movements reduces the risk of developing cancer of the colon and rectum.

5. **Limit fat intake, especially the intake of saturated fats.** A diet high in fatty foods may cause you to gain weight. When you eat too many fatty foods, you may not eat enough fruits and vegetables. Limiting the amount of fat you eat helps reduce the risk of developing cancers of the breast, prostate gland, and colon.

6. **Limit consumption of foods that are smoked, salted, or nitrite-cured.** By-products that result from the way these foods are prepared may increase the risk that healthy cells will become abnormal. Read labels and limit the number of foods you purchase that are smoked, salted, or nitrite-cured. When you eat out, ask if foods are smoked, salted, or nitrite-cured. Limiting your consumption of these foods helps reduce the risk of developing cancers of the esophagus and stomach.

7. **Do not drink alcohol as a teen.** Adults should avoid drinking alcohol. Or, they should only drink alcohol in moderation. Drinking too much alcohol may cause changes in body cells. Alcohol consumption robs the body of vitamins needed for optimal health. When you avoid drinking alcohol, you reduce the risk of developing cancers of the liver, throat, mouth, breast, and stomach.

Lesson 68 will include more information on cancer.

What to Know About
Diet and
Cardiovascular Diseases

A **cardiovascular disease** is a disease of the heart and blood vessels. Another term for cardiovascular disease is heart disease. Cardiovascular diseases are a leading cause of premature death and disability. You can reduce the risk of developing premature cardiovascular diseases by practicing the following dietary guidelines.

1. **Limit fat intake, especially the intake of saturated fats and foods high in cholesterol.** **Cholesterol** is a fat-like substance made by the body and found in certain foods. Eating foods that are high in saturated fats and contain cholesterol may cause plaque to form on artery walls. **Plaque** is hardened deposits. **Atherosclerosis** (ath·uh·roh·skluh·ROH·sis) is a disease in which fat deposits on artery walls. When a person has atherosclerosis, the diameter of the arteries become narrow because of the plaque buildup. Blood pressure must increase to get the same amount of oxygen and nutrients to cells. A person may develop high blood pressure. A piece of the plaque may break off, circulate in the bloodstream, and lodge in the bloodstream. An **embolism** is the blockage of an artery by a clump of material traveling in the bloodstream. If the blockage is in an artery in the brain, a person has a stroke. A blockage in the lung is called pulmonary embolism.

How to Limit Fat Intake

- Limit your intake of cooked lean meat, poultry, and fish to two three-ounce (84 grams) servings per day.

- Broil, bake, or steam food rather than fry it.

- Trim fat from meats before cooking.

- Trim fat from poultry before cooking.

- Limit your intake of egg yolks; consider using egg substitutes.

- Limit your intake of high-fat processed meats, such as hot dogs and bologna.

- Substitute turkey, such as turkey hot dogs and turkey chili, for red meat.

- Substitute nonfat or low-fat dairy products for whole-milk dairy products, such as low-fat yogurt for ice cream, skim milk for whole milk, reduced-fat mayonnaise for regular mayonnaise, low-fat or nonfat cheese for regular cheese.

- Substitute fruits and low-fat yogurt for high-fat desserts.

- Substitute fruits and vegetables for high-fat snacks, such as potato chips.

2. Increase your intake of foods and beverages containing antioxidants.
Antioxidants help prevent wear and tear in blood vessels.

How to Obtain Antioxidants in Your Diet

- Eat carrots, sweet potatoes, and squash to obtain vitamin A.

- Eat citrus fruits, such as oranges and pineapples, to obtain vitamin C.

- Eat green vegetables, nuts, and whole-grain cereals and breads to obtain vitamin E.

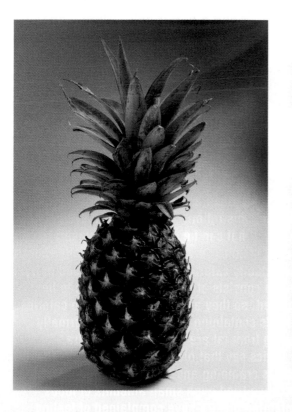

3. Limit your intake of sodium. Sodium is a mineral your body needs only in small amounts. The recommended daily allowance of sodium is three grams. Many teens consume ten times this amount. Too much sodium can affect people in different ways. It may cause some people to retain body fluid and, as a result, have increased blood pressure.

How to Limit Your Sodium (Salt) Intake

- Eat fresh rather than canned foods. Salt is usually added to canned foods as a preservative.

- Read food labels for sodium content. Sodium appears in food as sodium bicarbonate, monosodium glutamate, sodium nitrite, sodium propionate, and sodium citate.

- Select prepared foods that are labeled low-salt or salt-free, such as canned corn that is low-salt and unsalted potato chips.

- Avoid eating foods on which you can see the salt, such as pretzels and nuts coated with pieces of salt.

- Taste food before adding salt.

- Do not add salt to food.

- Season foods with herbs and spices rather than with salt.

- Limit your intake of salty foods, such as bacon, barbecue sauce, chips, crackers, hot dogs, processed meats, ketchup, canned meat, mustard, pepperoni, pizza, pickles, canned soup, and soy sauce.

- Limit your intake of salt-cured foods.

What to Know About
Food Allergies and Intolerances

You may have felt ill after eating a food and wondered if you were allergic to it. A **food allergy** is an abnormal response to food that is triggered by the immune system. Food allergies can cause severe illness. In some cases, food allergies may be deadly.

A person who suspects (s)he has a food allergy should see a physician. The physician first may consider other possibilities that lead to the symptoms. If a food allergy is diagnosed, the physician may recommend that the person completely avoid the food causing the allergy. Or, (s)he may recommend some other treatment, such as some medication.

The most common foods that cause allergic reactions in adults are shellfish, peanuts, fish, and eggs. In children, foods such as eggs, milk, and peanuts commonly cause allergic reactions.

Symptoms of food allergies include:

- Vomiting
- Diarrhea
- Abdominal cramps
- Hives
- Swelling
- Sneezing
- Asthma
- Difficulty breathing
- Itching
- Nausea

Food Intolerances

What many people think are food allergies are actually food intolerances. A **food intolerance** is an abnormal response to food that is not caused by the immune system. It merely means that a food is not tolerated well.

Lactase deficiency. Lactase deficiency (LAK·tays dee·FEE·shuhn·see) is a condition in which lactase, an enzyme that breaks down the milk sugar present in the cells of the small intestine, is missing. This condition results in the inability to digest lactose, which is found in most dairy products. This is called lactose intolerance. As the undigested lactose moves through the lower gastrointestinal tract, it releases products that are gaseous and cause discomfort. The symptoms of lactase deficiency include abdominal pain, bloating, and diarrhea.

Lactase deficiency is the most common form of food intolerance. Many people become lactose intolerant as adolescents or adults. They feel ill or uncomfortable after eating or drinking dairy products. Some people feel a little uncomfortable after eating a lot of dairy foods. Others have severe problems after eating even a small amount of foods containing lactose. Drinking skim or low-fat milk will not help. It is not the fat, but the lactose, that causes the symptoms. Some people with lactose intolerance find relief of symptoms through over-the-counter lactose remedies. Others choose to drink and eat lactose-free products, such as soybean milk or milk substitute. Lactose also is found in foods that are not considered dairy foods. For example, some cold cuts and baked products contain lactose.

Celiac sprue. Celiac sprue (SEE·lee·ak SPROO) is a condition in which a person is intolerant to gluten. Gluten is a part of wheat, rye, and certain other grains. The symptoms of celiac sprue include tiredness, breathlessness, weight loss, diarrhea, vomiting, and abdominal pain. People with celiac sprue must stick to a restricted diet and avoid eating any form of gluten.

Abnormal reaction to substances added to food. Food additives can cause allergic reactions. Monosodium glutamate (MSG) is a common cause of food intolerance. A flavor enhancer added to many foods, it can cause headaches, feelings of warmth, and chest pain in some people. MSG is often added to Chinese and other Asian foods.

Coloring agents, such as yellow dye number 5, also have been associated with food intolerance. Coloring agents may cause a rash or digestive problems. Sulfites added to foods also may cause food intolerance. Sulfites can be found in wines, potatoes, and packaged foods. Sulfites are especially harmful to people with asthma, who might react by going into shock.

Lesson 34

Review

Vocabulary Words

Write a separate sentence using each of the vocabulary words listed on page 274.

Objectives

1. What are seven dietary guidelines to follow to reduce the risk of developing cancer? **Objective 1**

2. What are three dietary guidelines to follow to reduce the risk of developing cardiovascular diseases? **Objective 2**

3. What are four dietary recommendations for people with diabetes or hypoglycemia? **Objective 3**

4. What foods can teens eat to reduce the risk of developing osteoporosis when they are adults? **Objective 4**

5. What are ways to avoid reactions to food allergies and food intolerances including lactose intolerance and celiac sprue, and reactions to MSG and yellow dye? **Objective 5**

Responsible Decision-Making

Suppose you have lactase deficiency. You accept a dinner invitation at a friend's house and forget to mention that you have a lactose intolerance. The main dish is lasagna heavy with cheese. Pudding made with skim milk is the dessert. Write a response to this situation.

1. **Describe the situation that requires you to make a decision.**
2. **List possible decisions you might make.**
3. **Name two responsible adults with whom you might discuss your decisions.**
4. **Evaluate the possible consequences of your decisions. Determine if each decision will lead to actions that:**
   - **promote health,**
   - **protect safety,**
   - **follow laws,**
   - **show respect for yourself and others,**
   - **follow the guidelines of your parents and of other responsible adults,**
   - **demonstrate good character.**
5. **Decide which decision is most responsible and appropriate.**
6. **Tell two results you expect if you make this decision.**

 Effective Communication

Design a pamphlet that includes at least ten ways to limit fat intake and reduce blood cholestrol.

 Self-Directed Learning

Check the library or the Internet to find two articles in medical journals about antioxidants. Write a short summary of the facts in the articles. Include correct bibliographical references.

 Critical Thinking

Pizza is one of your favorite foods. What are some ways pizza might be prepared so you can follow dietary guidelines to reduce the risk of developing heart disease and cancer?

Responsible Citizenship

Your family invites one of your friends to go on vacation. Your friend has diabetes. How might you consider your friend's dietary needs as you plan ahead for the vacation? List actions you might take.

How to Be Food Label Savvy

Along with Nutrition Facts, other information can be found on a food label. This information may be included on the Nutrition Facts panel. Or, it may be found elsewhere on the packaging. Included in this information is a listing of ingredients, food additives, and other important facts.

The food label is NOT required on: fresh fruits and vegetables; food served in restaurants; food sold by vendors; bakery, deli, and candy products; spices; coffee and tea; fresh meats; foods in very small packages.

Ingredients Listing

> **INGREDIENTS:** DICED TOMATOES, TOMATO PUREE, HIGH FRUCTOSE CORN SYRUP, SALT, EXTRA VIRGIN OLIVE OIL, DEHYDRATED ONIONS, DEHYDRATED GARLIC, BASIL, LEMON PEEL, CALCIUM CHLORIDE, DEHYDRATED RED BELL PEPPERS, CITRIC ACID, OREGANO, MODIFIED CORNSTARCH, NATURAL FLAVOR.

Almost all foods must have an ingredients listing. Ingredients are the parts that make up the particular food. The **ingredients listing** is the list of ingredients in a food. Ingredients are listed by weight, beginning with the ingredient that is present in the greatest amount. This listing is not a part of the Nutrition Facts label but is found somewhere else on the label.

Check the Dates!

Information involving dates may be included on the food label.

Sell By: The last date by which the product should be sold (although it can be stored past this date)

Best If Used By: The date by which the product should be used to ensure quality

Expiration Date: The date after which the product should not used

Food Additives

Food labels must list additives. **Food additives** are substances intentionally added to food. Food additives may add nutrients, flavor, color, or texture. They may prevent spoilage or help foods age quickly. They also improve taste and appearance.

Foods may be enriched or fortified to add to the nutrient value. An **enriched food** is a food in which nutrients lost during processing are added back into the food. A **fortified food** is a food in which nutrients not usually found in the food are added. For example, some orange juice products are fortified with calcium.

Know the Terms for Health Claims on Food Labels

The Term	What It Really Means
Healthy =	Low in total fat, low in saturated fat, and no more than 60 milligrams cholesterol per serving
Fat Free =	Less than .5 grams of fat per serving
Low Fat =	3 grams of fat (or less) per serving
Lean =	Less than 10 grams of fat, 4.5 grams of saturated fat, and no more than 95 milligrams of cholesterol per serving
Light =	1/2 fewer calories or no more than 1/2 the fat or sodium of the regular version
Lite =	The same as Light (but spelled incorrectly)
Cholesterol Free =	Less than 2 milligrams of cholesterol and 2 grams of fat or less of saturated fat per serving
___Free =	No amount or only a negligible amount of fat, saturated fat, cholesterol, sodium, sugar, and/or calories per serving
___Less =	At least 25 percent less of a nutrient or calories than the regular version
High =	Supplies 20 percent or more of the Percent Daily Value of a particular nutrient per serving
Fresh =	Raw, unprocessed, containing no preservatives, and has never been frozen or heated

Lesson 35

Review

Vocabulary Words

Write a separate sentence using each of the vocabulary words listed on page 282.

Objectives

1. What are the five elements required on all food labels? **Objective 1**

2. What information other than the five required elements are found on food labels? **Objective 2**

3. Why are food additives added to foods? **Objective 2**

4. What are definitions for the 11 terms for health claims used on food labels? **Objective 2**

5. What are three types of dated information that may be included on food labels? **Objective 2**

Responsible Decision-Making

Your father asks you to purchase a half-gallon of milk for the family. Today's date is March 1. The milk container is stamped with an expiration date of February 27. You check out other milk containers and they also have this expiration date. Write a response to this situation.

1. Describe the situation that requires you to make a decision.
2. List possible decisions you might make.
3. Name two responsible adults with whom you might discuss your decisions.
4. Evaluate the possible consequences of your decisions. Determine if each decision will lead to actions that:
   - promote health,
   - protect safety,
   - follow laws,
   - show respect for yourself and others,
   - follow the guidelines of your parents and of other responsible adults,
   - demonstrate good character.
5. Decide which decision is most responsible and appropriate.
6. Tell two results you expect if you make this decision.

 ## Effective Communication

Obtain the recipe for making one of your favorite foods. Pretend you are a food manufacturer who is preparing this food to sell. Create a food label for this food.

 ## Self-Directed Learning

On a sheet of paper, list the terms from the Know the Terms for Health Claims on Food Labels chart on page 284. Go to the grocery store to look at food labels. Next to each term listed on your sheet of paper, write the name and brand of a food whose label contains that term.

 ## Critical Thinking

To follow dietary guidelines, you want to eat cereal that is fiber-rich and does not contain sugar. What part of the food label on cereal will tell you about the ingredients in the cereal?

 ## Responsible Citizenship

Make a poster by hand or on the computer that shows your food label savvy. Go to a local grocery store or supermarket. Introduce yourself to the manager. Explain that you have been studying nutrition in school. Request permission to post your poster in a store window or other prominent place in the store so that customers can learn how to read a food label.

Lesson 36

You Can Develop Healthful Eating Habits

Life Skill **I will develop healthful eating habits.**

Consider your eating habits. Do you eat breakfast every morning? Do you eat healthful foods for lunch and dinner? Do you have a healthful snack between meals? Does your exercise or sport routine require that you change your eating habits? This lesson includes information to help you develop healthful eating habits. You will examine what motivates you to eat in different situations. You will learn how to plan a healthful breakfast, lunch, dinner, and snacks. The lesson also includes information on nutrition and sports. You will learn how different eating practices and foods and beverages affect performance in sports.

The Lesson Outline

What Motivates You to Eat

How to Plan a Healthful Breakfast and Lunch

How to Plan a Healthful Dinner and Snacks

What to Know About Nutrition and Sports

Objectives

1. Explain the difference between hunger and appetite. **page 287**
2. List guidelines to follow when planning a healthful breakfast and lunch. **page 288**
3. List guidelines to follow when planning a healthful dinner and snacks. **page 289**
4. Discuss how the following affect performance in sports: vitamin supplements, salt tablets, sports drinks, energy bars, carbohydrate loading, and protein loading. **page 291**

Vocabulary Words

hunger

appetite

metabolism

snack

megadosing

electrolyte

carbohydrate loading

protein loading

What Motivates You to Eat

Hunger is the physiological need for food. Sometimes you eat because you are hungry. At other times, you eat even though you are not hungry. Your appetite influences your decision to eat. **Appetite** is a desire to eat that comes from factors other than hunger. Do you decide to eat because you are hungry or because of your appetite?

Consider the following situations in which you decide to eat something.

1. You have not eaten since last night. You eat breakfast.

2. You are stressed about a test tomorrow. You pig out on chips.

3. You played in a soccer game and burned many calories. You eat a sports nutrition bar.

4. You feel rejected when you are not invited to a party. You treat yourself to a large order of fries.

5. You are growing rapidly. You eat an extra serving of vegetables for dinner.

6. You feel insecure at a party. You nibble on snack mix.

7. You have a lunch break at school. You eat the lunch you packed this morning.

8. You feel depressed. You scarf down a carton of ice cream.

9. You cannot eat for several hours before taking a physical exam. You eat shortly after the exam.

10. You just ate dinner. Your friends order a pizza to share. You eat several slices of the pizza.

Each of the odd numbers is a situation in which hunger motivates you to eat. Each of the even numbers is a situation in which appetite motivates you to eat.

You need to eat when you are hungry. You also need to eat to obtain the nutrients necessary for good health. But you do not need to eat to satisfy appetite.

- **You do not need to eat to manage stress.**
- **You do not need to eat when the sight or smell of food tempts you.**
- **You do not need to eat when you feel rejected, depressed, anxious, bored, or lonely.**
- **You do not need to eat to have something to do at a party where you feel uncomfortable.**
- **You do not need to eat because people around you are eating.**

To develop healthful eating habits, you must understand why you eat. You must plan breakfast, lunch, dinner, and snacks to satisfy hunger. You must recognize when you are eating for reasons other than hunger. Then you must evaluate whether eating for this reason promotes health or harms health. Suppose you eat a few slices of pizza with friends after you just ate dinner. You have eaten extra calories but probably have caused no harm. But, suppose you ate the pizza because you wanted to be like your friends. This is not a healthful reason to eat pizza.

Suppose you feel rejected, depressed, anxious, bored, or lonely. There are better ways to handle these feelings than by eating. When you rely on eating to cope, you develop harmful eating habits. Some teens develop eating disorders when they focus on eating or starving as a way of coping.

Lesson 40 will include more information on eating disorders.

How to Plan a Healthful
Breakfast and Lunch

The word breakfast means "break the fast." Your body has been fasting (going without food for several hours) and is running out of energy. Eating a healthful breakfast gives you the energy you need to begin your day. Eating a healthful breakfast also "jump starts" your metabolism. **Metabolism** is the rate at which food is converted into energy in body cells. Your metabolism has slowed from the day before. As your body begins to use the nutrients in foods, your metabolism speeds up. Eating a healthful breakfast helps you feel alert. A healthful breakfast provides some of the servings you need from the Food Guide Pyramid. Follow the Dietary Guidelines when choosing foods and beverages for breakfast.

If you eat a healthful breakfast, you have begun your day in a healthful way. But, remember, lunch also is a must. A well-balanced lunch provides energy for your afternoon activities. You remain alert and able to do schoolwork. If you have activities after lunch, you will be ready to participate in them. If you skip lunch, you may experience a mid-afternoon slump. Plan lunch carefully. A healthful lunch provides some of the servings you need from the Food Guide Pyramid. Follow the Dietary Guidelines when choosing foods and beverages for lunch.

Please—No Excuses

Possible Excuse	Get the Facts Straight!
I have no time to eat breakfast.	• Prepare breakfast the night before.
	• Choose foods that are easy to prepare, such as skim milk, juice, and low-fat peanut butter on whole-grain bread.
I will lose weight if I skip breakfast.	• Eating breakfast "jump starts" metabolism and burns calories.
	• Skipping breakfast usually causes a person to eat more calories during the rest of the day.
	• A breakfast containing protein, such an omelet made from egg substitute, helps maintain energy level throughout the morning and is low in calories.
I don't like breakfast foods.	• Eat other healthful foods for breakfast, such as tuna fish, veggie pizza, or beans and rice.

BREAKFAST AND LUNCH DOs AND DON'Ts

DO

Eat foods high in proteins.

Eat fruits or drink fruit juice.

Eat vegetables or drink vegetable juice.

Eat foods, such as cereal or bread, that are sources of grains and fiber.

DON'T

Skip foods that are a source of protein.

Survive on a doughnut or sweet roll.

Eat fatty foods, greasy foods, or fried foods.

Pig out on salt-cured foods, such as ham or bacon.

How to Plan a Healthful
Dinner and Snacks

Breakfast will help you start your day. Dinner will help "fuel" you to complete it. A healthful dinner helps you complete your daily nutrition requirements. Plan your snacks as well. It is as important for snacks to be nutritious as it is for your breakfast, lunch, and dinner.

Eating a Healthful Dinner

Plan your dinner. Evaluate the foods you have eaten during the day. Then, for dinner, select foods that provide the nutrients you did not eat at breakfast, lunch, and between meals. Because you may be less physically active in the evening, dinner should not make up more than one-third of your daily calorie intake.

Having Healthful Snacks

A **snack** is a food that is eaten between meals. When you eat snacks, you should do so to stop hunger and to get the needed servings from the Food Guide Pyramid. Do not snack because you are bored, lonely, anxious, or depressed. Do not snack just to take a break from hard work such as homework. Snacking for these reasons leads to harmful eating habits. Always follow the Dietary Guidelines when choosing snacks.

Making the Most of the Munchies

1. Select snacks that provide the servings you need from the Food Guide Pyramid. For example, if you have not eaten three to five servings of vegetables during the day, you might choose to snack on raw carrots.
2. Limit snacks that have a high level of sugar.
3. Limit snacks that have a high level of fats and saturated fats.
4. Limit snacks that have a high salt content.
5. Carry healthful snacks with you so you won't be tempted to go to the vending machine.

Snack Attack:
Healthful Snack Choices

fat-free yogurt	rice cakes
fruit	low-fat peanut butter
plain popcorn	cottage cheese
low-salt pretzels	bagels
veggies	bean dip
low-fat granola	shrimp
low-sugar cereals	juice
crackers	low-fat cheese

DINNER DOs AND DON'Ts

DO
Round out daily requirements.

Eat a variety of foods.

Eat early in the evening rather than close to bedtime.

DON'T
Eat dinner too close to bedtime.

Drink caffeine if you have difficulty falling asleep.

Eat spicy foods, if you have difficulty sleeping.

Activity

Creating a Top Ten List of Your Favorite Foods

Life Skill: I will develop healthful eating habits.

Materials: paper, pen or pencil

Directions: Complete the following activity to learn more about your eating habits.

 Examine the list of the ten foods children and teens selected as their favorites.

 Make a list of your favorite foods. Include more than ten foods.

 Evaluate each food on the list. Is the food:
   a) low in fat?
   b) low in sodium content?
   c) low in sugar?
   d) rich in vitamins?
   e) rich in minerals?
   f) rich in fiber?

 Select ten healthful foods from your list of favorite foods.

 Create a Top Ten List of Favorite Foods. List the ten healthful foods you selected.

The Ten Favorite Foods of Children and Teens

1. Pizza
2. Chicken nuggets
3. Hot dogs
4. Cheeseburgers
5. Macaroni and cheese
6. Hamburgers
7. Spaghetti and meatballs
8. Fried chicken
9. Tacos
10. Grilled cheese sandwiches

The Peoplepedia, Henry Holt and Company, New York, 1996.

Nutrition and Sports

Suppose you are physically active, enjoy sports, or are a member of an athletic team. You may have questions about the best diet for you. You may want to know if certain foods or eating habits will improve your performance. Be certain to get answers to your questions from professionals who are well-qualified to answer them. Your physician or a dietitian can provide answers. Carefully evaluate ads that say specific foods and beverages enhance performance. Remember, these ads are designed to sell you foods and beverages. Read food labels to learn nutrition information.

Vitamin supplements. A supplement is something that is added to the diet to enhance performance. For example, a teen might take extra vitamins to improve performance. **Megadosing** is taking vitamins in excessive amounts. To date, there is no evidence that megadosing will improve your performance in sports. Taking specific vitamins in excess can be harmful to your health.

Salt tablets. A teen also might try to enhance performance by taking salt tablets. The teen may notice that his/her skin is salty during physical activity and believe the salt must be replaced. The teen may believe that salt is needed to keep the body from losing too much water. Most teens get ten times the salt that is needed. However, many teens do not replace the water they lose through physical activity. Forget the salt tablets and drink plenty of water.

Sports drinks. Perhaps you have seen ads on TV for sports drinks. Ads may claim that sports drinks help replace electrolytes lost during physical activity. An **electrolyte** is a nutrient that becomes electrically charged when in a solution such as a body fluid. Sodium and potassium are electrolytes. They need to be in just the right balance for you to have a normal heartbeat. Use sports drinks to replace fluid, but do not try to figure out your electrolyte balance. A physician or dietitian can advise you on your electrolyte balance. And, remember that many sports drinks are high in sugar and calories. The best (and least expensive) choice is to eat foods with potassium, follow the Dietary Guidelines for salt intake, and drink plenty of water.

Energy bars. There are a variety of energy bars that look like candy bars. They are supposed to contain ingredients that enhance performance. Always read the food label before purchasing an energy bar. Many energy bars contain similar ingredients to candy bars—sugars. They are high in calories. Some energy bars are made from fruits, nuts, and grain. These energy bars are mostly carbohydrate and provide quick energy. The nuts are a source of protein, but usually the amount is too small to provide long-lasting energy. Some energy bars contain more grams of protein. These energy bars provide longer-lasting energy than the energy bars made of sugar.

Carbohydrate loading. **Carbohydrate loading** is an eating strategy in which a few days of a very low carbohydrate intake is followed by a few days of a very high carbohydrate intake. This strategy is supposed to load the muscle with glycogen prior to strenuous physical activity. It is referred to as "carbo loading." Experts have mixed opinions about the advantages of carbohydrate loading.

Protein loading. **Protein loading** is an eating strategy in which extra protein is eaten to increase muscle size. Eating extra protein does not increase muscle size; exercise increases muscle size. A physician or dietitian can tell you how much protein to eat. If you eat too much protein, it is converted to fat, not muscle.

Before the Big Game

It is generally recommended that a pre-game meal should be eaten two-to-three hours before competition. However, eating directly before a competition can decrease an athlete's performance. Foods to avoid in a pre-game meal include:

● **spicy foods, which might cause gastrointestinal problems;**

● **fried foods, which might cause gastrointestinal problems;**

● **sugary foods, which might cause gastrointestinal problems;**

● **caffeine, which may increase nervousness and stimulate the flow of urine.**

Making Weight

There is pressure for participants in some sports to maintain a certain weight. Athletes in sports such as wrestling or boxing may need to "make weight." Other sports in which participants may be overly concerned about weight include gymnastics, swimming, dancing, cheerleading, and running. Excessive concern about weight can lead to harmful eating disorders.

Lesson 40 will include more information on eating disorders.

Lesson 36

Review

Vocabulary Words

Write a separate sentence using each of the vocabulary words listed on page 286.

Objectives

1. What is the difference between hunger and appetite? **Objective 1**

2. What are some guidelines to follow when planning a healthful breakfast and lunch? **Objective 2**

3. What are some guidelines to follow when planning a healthful dinner and snacks? **Objective 3**

4. How do the following affect performance in sports: vitamin supplements, salt tablets, sports drinks, and energy bars? **Objective 4**

5. What are carbohydrate loading and protein loading? **Objective 4**

Responsible Decision-Making

Suppose you have a friend who is on an athletic team that requires him/her to maintain a certain weight. Your friend tries many techniques to cut weight, including exercising non-stop, trying various diets, and regularly using the sauna and the steam room. One day you walk into the bathroom after lunch and you find your friend forcing himself/herself to vomit. Write a response to this situation.

1. Describe the situation that requires you to make a decision.
2. List possible decisions you might make.
3. Name two responsible adults with whom you might discuss your decisions.
4. Evaluate the possible consequences of your decisions. Determine if each decision will lead to actions that:
   - promote health,
   - protect safety,
   - follow laws,
   - show respect for yourself and others,
   - follow the guidelines of your parents and of other responsible adults,
   - demonstrate good character.
5. Decide which decision is most responsible and appropriate.
6. Tell two results you expect if you make this decision.

 ## Effective Communication

Interview an athletic trainer or a dietitian who focuses on sports nutrition. Prepare ahead by identifying five questions you want to have answered by the person you plan to interview.

 ## Self-Directed Learning

Locate an article on a specific aspect of sports nutrition such as carbohydrate loading, megadosing, or pre-game meals. Write a one-page summary of the article. Include the complete bibliographical reference for the article. Share the summary with your classmates.

 ## Critical Thinking

Suppose a teen eats high-calorie foods, such as chocolates, peanuts, and potato chips when (s)he is stressed. Why is this pattern of eating harmful?

 ## Responsible Citizenship

Compile a list of breakfast, lunch, and dinner DOs and DON'Ts. Hang the list in a visible place in your home—on the refrigerator, on a cupboard door, or on a bulletin board in the kitchen.

Lesson 37

You Can Follow the Dietary Guidelines When You Go Out to Eat

Life Skill **I will follow the Dietary Guidelines when I go out to eat.**

You eat at places other than your home. You eat in cafeterias, in restaurants, and in friends' and relatives' homes. This lesson tells you how to have style and grace when you are eating in these places. This lesson also suggests ways to follow the Dietary Guidelines when you go out to eat. You will learn how to order from a restaurant menu and how to order fast foods. You also will learn how to make healthful selections when you eat in ethnic restaurants.

Vocabulary Words
fast food
ethnic restaurant

The Lesson Outline

How to Have Table Manners

How to Order from a Restaurant Menu

How to Order Fast Foods

What to Know About Ethnic Foods

Objectives

1. Identify and describe ten table manners to practice. **page 295**

2. Discuss five guidelines to follow when ordering from a restaurant menu. **pages 296–297**

3. Discuss three guidelines to follow when ordering fast foods. **pages 298–299**

4. List three examples of healthful foods that can be ordered at ethnic restaurants: Mexican, French, Japanese, Chinese, Italian, and Indian. **page 300**

How to Have
Table Manners

Table manners are polite ways to eat. When you have table manners, you know how to make a special request when eating at a restaurant. You know how to refuse a dish without offending a host or hostess. Table manners help you to be confident when you are eating with others. The Teen's Guide to Table Manners includes ten suggestions for polite ways to eat.

The Teen's Guide to Table Manners

- **Say, "No, thank you" politely when you are offered a food you do not wish to eat.** Making a big issue and announcing that you don't eat a certain food is not appropriate.

- **Discuss special diet restrictions with your host or hostess when (s)he first invites you out to eat.** While the meat dish is being served is not the appropriate time to announce that you are a vegetarian.

- **If a food is not prepared the way you asked, politely send it back.** Loudly announcing that your order is not to your liking is inappropriate.

- **Don't speak with your mouth full.** Chances are people will not be able to understand what you are saying. Even worse, pieces of your food may fall out and offend other people.

- **If you knock over your glass, just pick it up.** Don't make a big deal out of it or be embarrassed. Apologize if it spills on someone else.

- **If you want to make a special request at a restaurant, ask the server politely.** Complaining to the server that you can't find anything decent on the menu is not appropriate.

- **Taste a food before deciding you don't like it.** Try a small amount if you are served a food you do not recognize. Or, you may refuse it politely. Do not make offensive comments, such as "This looks disgusting."

- **Keep your elbows off the table.** Keeping your elbows on the table increases the chances that you will spill your food or drink.

- **Wait until everyone has been served before you begin eating, unless someone else tells you to go ahead and eat.** Starting to eat before everyone else is served is inappropriate. However, it is OK to begin if people not yet served tell you not to wait for them.

- **Do not reach across someone's plate.** Ask to have something, such as the butter, passed to you by the person who is closest.

How to Order from a Restaurant Menu

Suppose you are at a favorite restaurant. The waiter or waitress gives you a few minutes to glance at the menu before taking your order. There are five guidelines to follow when ordering from a restaurant menu.

1. Order foods and beverages that help you get the appropriate number of servings from each food group in the Food Guide Pyramid.

2. Follow the Dietary Guidelines and choose foods that are low in fat, saturated fat, cholesterol, sugar, and salt; include fruits, vegetables, and grains.

3. Check the menu to see if there are foods that are designated as "heart healthy" or "light."

4. Ask questions when you are uncertain about the ingredients in foods. This helps you avoid foods to which you may have a food allergy or food intolerance.

5. Request that your food be prepared in a healthful way. For example, ask if a food can be prepared without butter or salt or broiled instead of fried. When ordering hamburger or ground sirloin, ask that it be cooked well-done.

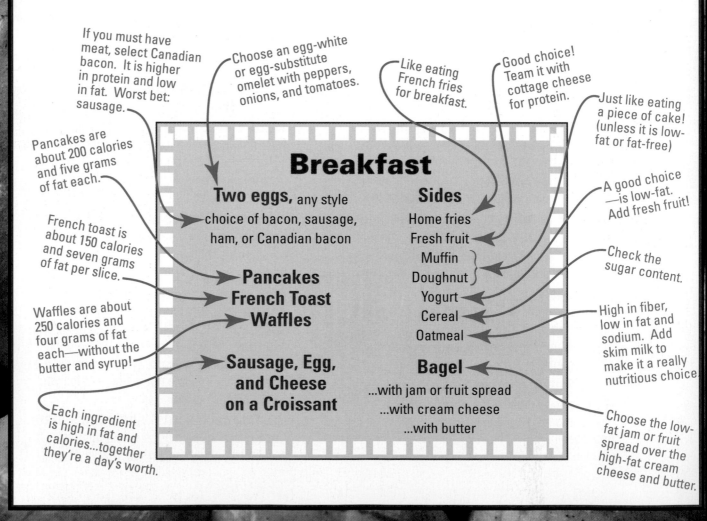

If you must have meat, select Canadian bacon. It is higher in protein and low in fat. Worst bet: sausage.

Choose an egg-white or egg-substitute omelet with peppers, onions, and tomatoes.

Like eating French fries for breakfast.

Good choice! Team it with cottage cheese for protein.

Just like eating a piece of cake! (unless it is low-fat or fat-free)

Pancakes are about 200 calories and five grams of fat each.

French toast is about 150 calories and seven grams of fat per slice.

Waffles are about 250 calories and four grams of fat each—without the butter and syrup!

Each ingredient is high in fat and calories...together they're a day's worth.

A good choice —is low-fat. Add fresh fruit!

Check the sugar content.

High in fiber, low in fat and sodium. Add skim milk to make it a really nutritious choice.

Choose the low-fat jam or fruit spread over the high-fat cream cheese and butter.

Breakfast

Two eggs, any style
choice of bacon, sausage, ham, or Canadian bacon

Pancakes
French Toast
Waffles

Sausage, Egg, and Cheese on a Croissant

Sides
Home fries
Fresh fruit
Muffin
Doughnut
Yogurt
Cereal
Oatmeal

Bagel
...with jam or fruit spread
...with cream cheese
...with butter

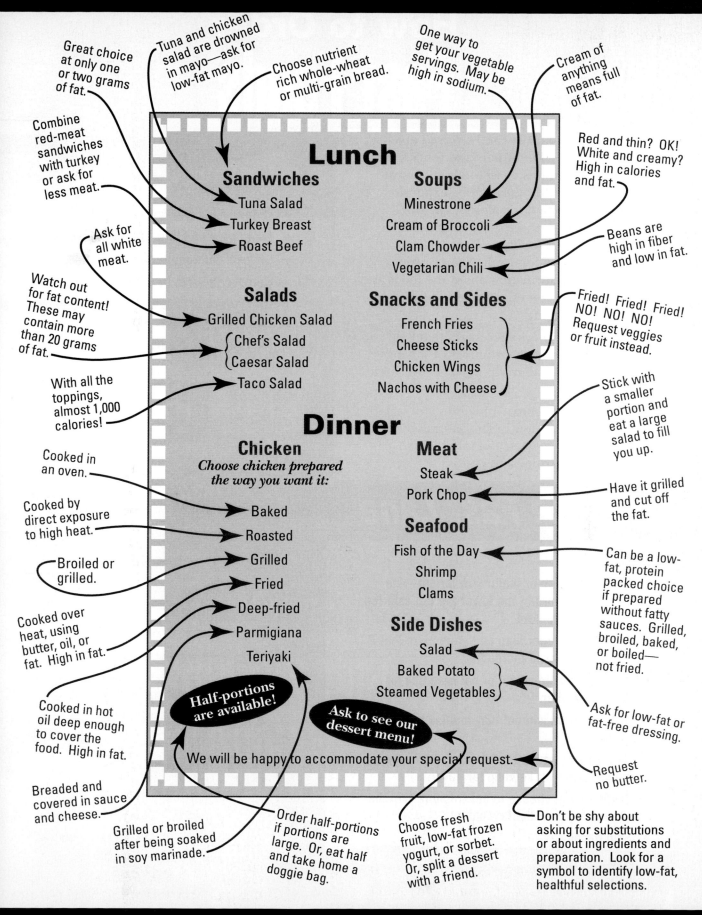

Great choice at only one or two grams of fat.

Tuna and chicken salad are drowned in mayo—ask for low-fat mayo.

Choose nutrient rich whole-wheat or multi-grain bread.

One way to get your vegetable servings. May be high in sodium.

Cream of anything means full of fat.

Combine red-meat sandwiches with turkey or ask for less meat.

Red and thin? OK! White and creamy? High in calories and fat.

Ask for all white meat.

Beans are high in fiber and low in fat.

Watch out for fat content! These may contain more than 20 grams of fat.

Fried! Fried! Fried! NO! NO! NO! Request veggies or fruit instead.

With all the toppings, almost 1,000 calories!

Stick with a smaller portion and eat a large salad to fill you up.

Cooked in an oven.

Have it grilled and cut off the fat.

Cooked by direct exposure to high heat.

Broiled or grilled.

Can be a low-fat, protein packed choice if prepared without fatty sauces. Grilled, broiled, baked, or boiled— not fried.

Cooked over heat, using butter, oil, or fat. High in fat.

Ask for low-fat or fat-free dressing.

Cooked in hot oil deep enough to cover the food. High in fat.

Request no butter.

Breaded and covered in sauce and cheese.

Grilled or broiled after being soaked in soy marinade.

Order half-portions if portions are large. Or, eat half and take home a doggie bag.

Choose fresh fruit, low-fat frozen yogurt, or sorbet. Or, split a dessert with a friend.

Don't be shy about asking for substitutions or about ingredients and preparation. Look for a symbol to identify low-fat, healthful selections.

Lunch

Sandwiches
Tuna Salad
Turkey Breast
Roast Beef

Soups
Minestrone
Cream of Broccoli
Clam Chowder
Vegetarian Chili

Salads
Grilled Chicken Salad
Chef's Salad
Caesar Salad
Taco Salad

Snacks and Sides
French Fries
Cheese Sticks
Chicken Wings
Nachos with Cheese

Dinner

Chicken
Choose chicken prepared the way you want it:
Baked
Roasted
Grilled
Fried
Deep-fried
Parmigiana
Teriyaki

Meat
Steak
Pork Chop

Seafood
Fish of the Day
Shrimp
Clams

Side Dishes
Salad
Baked Potato
Steamed Vegetables

Half-portions are available!

Ask to see our dessert menu!

We will be happy to accommodate your special request.

How to Order
Fast Foods

Fast food is food that can be served quickly. Fast food includes TV dinners and foods served at fast-food restaurants. Fast foods are convenient and quick. But, they can be expensive. They also can be high in calories, fat, and sodium. There are three guidelines to follow when ordering fast foods.

1. Ask if the fast-food restaurant provides nutrition information about the foods and beverages it serves. Read the information before ordering.

2. Choose foods and beverages that help you get the appropriate number of servings from each food group in the Food Guide Pyramid.

3. Follow the Dietary Guidelines and order foods that are low in fats, saturated fats, cholesterol, sugars, and salt; include vegetables, fruits, and grains.

Chicken Choices

- Order grilled chicken.
- Avoid fried and breaded chicken.
- Choose white meat over dark meat.
- Remove the skin or order skin-free.
- Order chicken sandwiches without mayonnaise and special sauces.
- Choose a whole-wheat or oat bran bun for additional fiber.
- Skip the fried and fattening chicken wings.

Chicken Trivia: Extra crispy usually means extra fattening.

In the Fast Lane

Burger Bests

- Order the small or junior size burger—the smaller the burger, the lower the fat, calories, and sodium content.
- Order your burger lean and emphasize that it should be cooked thoroughly.
- Choose a whole-wheat or oat bran bun for additional fiber.
- Order burgers without mayonnaise and special sauces.
- Use a small amount of mustard, barbecue sauce, salsa, or ketchup for flavor.
- Order low-fat cheese to get calcium; skip the cheese to lower the fat content.
- Skip bacon.

Burger Bit: The average single burger at a fast-food restaurant ranges from 10 to 26 grams of fat. A double bacon cheeseburger or deluxe burger can be as high as 70 grams of fat.

Pizza Picks

- Try pizza without cheese.
- Avoid pepperoni, sausage, and bacon.
- Order vegetables such as broccoli, peppers, mushrooms, or spinach.
- Add pineapple for an extra serving of fruit.
- Skip extra cheese; it adds extra fat.

Pizza Pop Quiz: Did you know that two slices of a stuffed-crust pizza may contain more than two times the amount of calories of a thin-crust pizza?

Salad Smarts

- Load up on fresh vegetables.
- Choose fat-free or low-fat salad dressings.
- Add fresh fruit.
- Order low-fat or fat-free cheese.
- Choose dark green lettuce instead of iceberg lettuce.
- Add beans as a protein source.
- Add grilled chicken as a protein source.

Salad Spot: Just because it says salad, it doesn't mean low-fat. Tuna, chicken, potato, and pasta salads may contain lots of mayonnaise. A Caesar salad contains eggs, oils, and cheese. A chef's salad contains cheese and ham.

Breakfast Bets

- Order a fiber-rich, low-sugar cereal with skim or low-fat milk.
- Choose a low-fat bran muffin instead of a doughnut.
- Have a bagel or English muffin instead of a croissant or biscuit.
- Choose Canadian bacon rather than bacon or sausage.
- Drink fruit juice or eat fresh fruit.
- Order an omelet made of egg whites or egg substitute.

Breakfast Bit: A muffin may have as many calories and grams of fat as a piece of cake. Order your muffin low-fat or fat-free.

In the Fast Lane

Side Dish Selections

- Eat a salad with low-fat or fat-free dressing.
- Choose a plain baked potato instead of French fries.
- Skip the sour cream, bleu cheese, and bacon bits on baked potatoes.
- Have a side of steamed vegetables without butter, such as corn.
- Choose vegetable soup on the side.
- Limit fried sides, such as onion rings.
- Don't add extra salt.

Side Dish Suggestion: Choose several side dishes, such as a side salad and baked potato for a filling but low-calorie meal.

Dessert and Drink Decisions

- Limit soda pops.
- Choose fat-free or low-fat yogurt shakes and sundaes.
- Drink fruit juice.
- Top yogurt sundaes with fresh fruit.
- Limit pies, cakes, and other fatty desserts.

Dessert and Drink DOs: If it is sweet, it probably is sugary. Watch out for the sugar content in fast-food desserts and beverages.

What to Know About
Ethnic Foods

An **ethnic restaurant** is a restaurant that serves food that is customary for people of a specific culture. When you eat at an ethnic restaurant, choose foods and beverages that help you get the appropriate number of servings from each food group in the Food Guide Pyramid. Follow the Dietary Guidelines and choose foods that are low in fat, saturated fat, cholesterol, sugars, and salt. The Guide to Ethnic Food Choices identifies foods offered at Mexican, French, Japanese, Chinese, Italian, and Indian restaurants. Foods in the first column meet the Dietary Guidelines. Foods in the second column are high in fat, saturated fat, cholesterol, sugar, or salt.

Guide to Ethnic Food Choices

Mexican

Sí*	No**
Whole beans	Refried beans
Rice	Heavy cheese
Salsa	Sour cream
Grilled chicken and fish	Deep-fried dishes
Corn and flour tortillas	Fried tortilla chips and shells

Fajitas and burritos without cheese are usually lower in fat and calories than enchiladas and empanadas.

French

Oui*	Non**
Steamed seafood	Pâté
Chicken with light sauces	Au gratin dishes
"Nouvelle" (new, light) dishes	Heavy sauces and gravy
Fresh fruit	Croissants and pastries
Sorbet	Souffle

Ratatouille helps provide servings of vegetables. Duck a l'orange and Quiche Lorraine can contain 60 percent fat.

Japanese

Hai*	Iya**
Steamed rice	Peanut and soy sauce
Broiled fish	Deep-fried tempura
Tofu	Pickled foods
Miso (bean paste) soup	Stir-fried dishes
Ramen noodles	

Soy sauce and pickled foods are high in sodium content.

Chinese

Duì/bushì*	Bù duì/bushì**
Stir-fry vegetables	Extra soy sauce
Brown rice	Egg rolls
Skinless chicken dishes	Spare ribs
Wonton soup	Salty soups
Steamed or boiled fish dishes	Fried noodles and rice
Tofu dishes	Egg dishes

One eggroll has about ten grams of fat.

Italian

Si*	No**
Pasta with vegetables	Italian sausages
Pasta with marinara sauce	Deep-fried dishes
Broiled fish dishes	Cheese-stuffed dishes
Salads and antipasto without oily dressing	Salads with oily dressing
Italian ices	Cream sauces
	Spumoni

Fettucini Alfredo and fried mozzarella sticks contain about 45 grams of fat per serving.
Meatless spaghetti with tomato sauce contains only one gram of fat—add extra vegetables.

Indian

Jee Haan*	Je Naheen**
Tandoori chicken	Deep-fried meats
Chickpeas Ghee (butter)	Curry sauce
Chutney	

Creamy curries may have a higher fat content than tomato-based curries.

*Yes   **No

Lesson 37

Review

Vocabulary Words

Write a separate sentence using each of the vocabulary words listed on page 294.

Objectives

1. What are ten table manners to practice? **Objective 1**

2. What are five guidelines to follow when ordering form a restaurant menu? **Objective 2**

3. What are three guidelines to follow when ordering fast foods? **Objective 3**

4. What are three tips for ordering hamburgers? Chicken? Pizza? Salad? Side dishes? **Objective 3**

5. What are three healthful foods to order at these ethnic restaurants: Mexican, French, Japanese, Italian, and Indian? **Objective 4**

Responsible Decision-Making

You accept a dinner invitation from your best friend. The appetizer is a vegetable soup that you find tasty. The main dish is a casserole with your least favorite vegetable in it. The sight, smell, and taste of this vegetable does not appeal to you. Write a response to this situation.

1. Describe the situation that requires you to make a decision.
2. List possible decisions you might make.
3. Name two responsible adults with whom you might discuss your decisions.
4. Evaluate the possible consequences of your decisions. Determine if each decision will lead to actions that:
   • promote health,
   • protect safety,
   • follow laws,
   • show respect for yourself and others,
   • follow the guidelines of your parents and of other responsible adults,
   • demonstrate good character.
5. Decide which decision is most responsible and appropriate.
6. Tell two results you expect if you make this decision.

Effective Communication

Make a menu for your favorite type of ethnic food. Use computer graphics or another artistic form to create your menu. If you have never eaten ethnic food, make a menu of ethnic foods you would like to try.

Self-Directed Learning

Obtain a pamphlet or listing of nutritional information from a fast-food restaurant. Make a list of items that contain a healthful amount of fat and sodium. Share the information with your classmates.

Critical Thinking

Suppose you are having lunch at a restaurant that offers a salad bar. Begin with lettuce. Then add ten items to create a salad that follows the Dietary Guidelines and has at least one serving from each of the food groups. What are the ten items?

Responsible Citizenship

Good table manners show respect for yourself and for others. Add two suggestions for table manners that are not in the guide. Make a copy of The Teen's Guide to Table Manners and share it with your friends and family members.

Lesson 38

You Can Protect Yourself from Food-Borne Illnesses

Life Skill **I will protect myself from food-borne illnesses.**

Have you ever felt ill after you have eaten? Perhaps you thought, "It must have been something I ate." You may have contracted a food-borne illness. A **food-borne illness** is an illness caused by consuming foods or beverages that have been contaminated with pathogens. A food-borne illness is referred to as food poisoning. This lesson explains how to protect yourself from food-borne illnesses. You will learn about four serious food-borne illnesses and how they are spread. This lesson also discusses ways people spread germs to one another when they share foods and beverages. You will learn to protect yourself from food-borne illnesses when you are in social situations.

Vocabulary Words

food-borne illness

salmonellosis

botulism

E. coli

gastroenteritis

The Lesson Outline

How to Protect Yourself from Food-Borne Illnesses

How to Share Food without Spreading Germs

Objectives

1. Outline ways to protect yourself from food-borne illnesses. **page 303**
2. Explain five ways germs can be spread when people share food. **page 304**

How to Protect Yourself from
Food-Borne Illnesses

A food-borne illness may develop from one-half hour to several hours after eating food contaminated with germs. Common symptoms of food-borne illness are cramps, nausea, diarrhea, vomiting, and fever. If symptoms are severe, or the person is young, elderly, or pregnant, prompt medical care is needed. Treatment includes drinking fluids and bed rest.

There are four serious food-borne illnesses:

1. **Salmonellosis** (sal·muh·NEH·loh·suhz) is a food-borne illness in which the bacterium *Salmonella* contaminates undercooked chicken, eggs, and meats.

2. **Botulism** (BAH·chuh·li·zuhm) is a food-borne illness in which the bacterium *Clostridium botulinum* contaminates improperly canned foods.

3. **E. coli** is a food-borne illness in which a specific strain of the bacterium *Escherica coli* contaminates undercooked meat, especially hamburger.

4. **Gastroenteritis** (gas·tro·en·tuh·RI·tuhz) is a food-borne illness in which the bacterium *Campylobacter jejuni* contaminates animal products, especially chicken.

The Guide to Food Safety outlines ways to prevent food-borne illnesses.

Look Over Leftovers

Are your leftovers OK to eat? How long will they last? If foods or beverages look or smell unusual, throw them out. Check the following list for storage times for specific foods.

- **Milk:** Four to five days after the sell-by date
- **Orange juice:** Up to a week after opening
- **Refrigerated raw chicken:** Three days
- **Hard cheese:** One to two months after opening
- **Cold cuts and hot dogs:** Three to five days
- **Eggs:** Three to five weeks
- **Restaurant doggie bags:** Three days

The Guide to Food Safety

At the Store
- Check expiration dates, and do not buy outdated foods.
- Choose canned foods and packages that are free of dents, cracks, rust, holes, bulges, and tears.
- Check that products marked "keep refrigerated" are stored in a refrigerated case and that frozen foods are frozen solid.
- Open egg cartons to check that eggs are whole, clean, and chilled.

In the Refrigerator
- Keep your refrigerator temperature between 35°F (2°C) and 45°F (8°C).
- Keep your freezer thermometer at or below 0°F (-20°C).
- Pay attention to the "use by" date and "keep refrigerated" instructions on any food.
- Don't store food in metal cans.

In the Kitchen
- Wash your hands with hot, soapy water for at least 20 seconds before preparing food.
- Wash hands, cooking utensils, and surfaces after contact with raw eggs, raw chicken, and raw meats. Keep raw meat, chicken, and fish juices from contact with other foods.
- Do not use the same sponge or towel on other surfaces or items such as cooking utensils after cleaning surfaces on which there was raw food.
- Cover cuts or sores with bandages or plastic gloves before preparing food.
- Thaw frozen foods in the microwave or in the refrigerator—never at room temperature.
- Wash fruits and vegetables with running water.
- Cook eggs until they are firm, not runny.
- Do not taste foods that are not cooked thoroughly.

On the Table
- Place cooked food in a clean dish for serving.
- Do not use the same unwashed plate for both preparing and serving foods.
- Rinse utensils before using.
- Do not let cooked food sit at room temperature for more than two hours.
- Keep hot foods hot and cold foods cold.

How to Share Food without Spreading Germs

There are many situations when you eat with other people. That means many opportunities to contaminate foods and beverages with germs. Beware of the following food safety offenders.

1. The "double dipper" puts a piece of food into a dip and takes a bite. Then, (s)he puts the same piece of food back in the dip and finishes it. Double dipping contaminates food with germs. Other people who eat the same dip ingest these germs. Don't double dip: put a scoop of dip on your own plate to use for dipping.

2. The "pop swapper" drinks from another person's can, glass, or bottle. Germs get on the can, glass, or bottle. Another person drinks from the same can, glass, or bottle. This person ingests germs. Don't pop swap: pour a beverage into a separate glass when you share a beverage.

3. The "careless cook" tastes foods as (s)he prepares them. Germs get into the foods as they are prepared. Don't be a careless cook: use a clean utensil each time you taste foods you are preparing.

4. The "container contaminator" takes a sip or bite from a container of food and puts it back for others. This person contaminates foods and beverages with his/her germs. Don't be a container contaminator: use a glass or clean utensil to take a sip or bite of food.

5. The "bite burglar" takes a bite of another person's food and gives it back or takes bites off another person's plate. This person contaminates other people's food with his/her germs. Don't be a bite burglar: cut off a piece of food or use a clean utensil and put a portion on your own plate before eating.

Activity

Recognizing a Most Wanted Food-Safety Criminal

Life Skill: I will protect myself from food-borne illnesses.

Materials: paper and pencil; props (optional)

Directions: Complete the following activity to gain skill in recognizing ways food-borne illnesses are spread.

1. Following your teacher's instructions, form groups of three or four. Brainstorm a list of five food-safety criminals and describe their offenses. For example, a food-safety criminal might be a "Bite Burglar" who takes a bite from another person's hamburger. Do not use any of the names used in this lesson.

2. Select one food-safety criminal and plan a skit to depict this criminal's offense. Your skit should show the food-safety criminal in action. You might use props.

3. Perform your skit at the time specified by your teacher.

4. Ask classmates to identify the specific offense of the food-safety criminal in your skit. After classmates have identified the specific offense, tell them the name you have given the food-safety criminal.

Lesson 38
Review

Vocabulary Words

Write a sentence using the vocabulary word listed on page 302.

Objectives

1. What are four serious food-borne illnesses? **Objective 1**

2. What are some ways to protect yourself from food-borne illnesses? **Objective 1**

3. What is the appropriate storage time for milk? Juice? Eggs? Tuna? Refrigerated raw chicken? **Objective 1**

4. What are five ways people can contaminate foods or beverages that other people will eat or drink? **Objective 2**

5. How might germs be spread when two people share a can of soda pop? **Objective 2**

Responsible Decision-Making

Suppose you come home from school for lunch one day. You look in the refrigerator and find a leftover deli sandwich. The sandwich looks fine, but you are not sure how long it has been in the refrigerator. When you smell the sandwich, it smells a little strange. But, it may be your imagination. There is nothing else in the house you want to to eat. Write a response to this situation.

1. Describe the situation that requires you to make a decision.
2. List possible decisions you might make.
3. Name two responsible adults with whom you might discuss your decisions.
4. Evaluate the possible consequences of your decisions. Determine if each decision will lead to actions that:
   • promote health,
   • protect safety,
   • follow laws,
   • show respect for yourself and others,
   • follow the guidelines of your parents and of other responsible adults,
   • demonstrate good character.
5. Decide which decision is most responsible and appropriate.
6. Tell two results you expect if you make this decision.

Effective Communication

Design a warning label for a can of soda pop. The warning label should advise that germs are spread when two people drink from the same can.

Self-Directed Learning

Check the library or the Internet to locate a news story about food-borne illness. Make a copy of the information, including correct bibliographical references, and share it with your classmates.

Critical Thinking

You are at a party where low-fat chips and salsa are served. You observe someone double dipping. Should you put a scoop of dip on your plate and eat the chips and salsa? Explain why or why not.

Responsible Citizenship

Investigate the rules and laws that govern food safety. Include information on regulations that govern the storage and transportation of food and restaurant cleanliness. Make a list of these regulations. Share the list with your family members and classmates.

Activity

How to Calculate Your Daily Caloric Needs

Life Skill: I will maintain my desirable weight and body composition.

Materials: paper, pen or pencil

Directions: Your daily caloric needs depend on your basal metabolic rate, your activity level, and the number of calories you need to digest food. Complete the following activity to get an estimate of your daily caloric needs. Use a separate sheet of paper. DO NOT WRITE IN THIS BOOK.

 Calculate the number of calories your body uses at rest (your BMR). A physician or dietitian can perform an accurate, actual BMR. The following calculations provide an estimate.

Females: Multiply your body weight in
pounds X 10 = calories for BMR

Males: Multiply your body weight in
pounds X 11 = calories for BMR

 Calculate the number of calories you use for physical activity. If you are...

Inactive: Multiply .3 X the calories for BMR = calories for physical activity

Moderately active: Multiply .5 X the calories for BMR = calories for physical activity

Very active: Multiply .75 X the calories for BMR = calories for physical activity

 Calculate the number of calories your body needs to digest food. (calories for BMR + calories for physical activity) X (.1) = calories to digest food

 Calculate the number of calories you need each day.
Add: calories for BMR (step 1) +
calories for physical activity (step 2) +
calories to digest food (step 3) =
Total calories you need per day

Example:
A teen male weighs 150 pounds and is moderately active.
150 lbs. X 11 = 1650.0 calories for BMR
.5 X 1650 = 825.0 calories
for physical activity
(1650 + 825) X .1 = 247.5 calories
to digest food
1650 + 825 + 247.5 = 2722.5
2722.5 total calories needed per day

How to
Gain Weight

Underweight is a body weight that is 10 percent or more below desirable body weight. People who are underweight may be malnourished. **Malnutrition** is a condition in which the body does not get the nutrients required for optimal health. In most cases, people who are malnourished have inadequate vitamin and mineral intake. Teens who are malnourished may not have the nutrients needed for proper growth. They may lack energy. There are other reasons why teens may be underweight. They may have a disease or an eating disorder. Teens who are underweight should have a physical examination to determine the cause. They should work with a physician and/or dietitian to develop a healthful plan for weight gain.

Steps to Healthful Weight Gain

1. **Have a physical examination.**

2. **Have a physician or dietitian determine the number of pounds you need to gain.**

3. **Have a physician or dietitian help you design a plan for weight gain.** Remember, one pound of body fat is equal to 3,500 calories. Suppose you want to gain five pounds. You may want to gain one pound a week for five weeks. You will need to increase your caloric intake by 3,500 calories a week to gain a pound each week. This means you need to take in 500 more calories each day (3,500 calories divided by seven days = 500 calories).

4. **Increase the number of servings from each food group in the Food Guide Pyramid. Eat extra servings from the:**
   - Bread, Cereal, Rice, and Pasta Group.
   - Vegetable Group.
   - Fruit Group.
   - Milk, Yogurt, and Cheese Group.
   - Meat, Poultry, Fish, Dry Beans, Eggs, and Nuts Group.

5. **Follow the Dietary Guidelines and do not develop harmful eating habits.** Even though you want to gain weight, you must follow Dietary Guidelines. Choose low-fat and lean foods from the Meat, Poultry, Fish, Dry Beans, Eggs, and Nuts Group. Select broiled, baked, steamed or poached foods rather than fried foods. Use egg substitutes. Choose low-fat or fat-free foods from the Milk, Yogurt, and Cheese Group. You do not want to develop harmful eating habits that are difficult to break. For example, you do not want to pig out on French fries with lots of salt.

6. **Eat snacks between meals.**

7. **Exercise to increase muscle mass.**

8. **Drink plenty of fluids.**

9. **Ask for the support of family members and friends.**

10. **Keep a journal of food and beverage intake and weight gain.** Review the information in your journal with a physician or dietitian.

How to
Lose Weight

Overweight is a body weight that is 10 percent or more than desirable body weight. **Obesity** is a body weight that is 20 percent or more than desirable body weight. People who are overweight or obese need to have a physical examination. Usually their condition is caused by overeating and lack of physical activity. However, there may be other causes.

A physician can check for other causes, such as an underactive thyroid gland.

People who are overweight and obese are at risk for developing cardiovascular diseases, diabetes, and certain cancers. They also have more accidents and more injuries. They are less likely to be satisfied with their relationships.

Steps to Healthful Weight Loss

1. **Have a physical examination.**

2. **Have a physician or dietitian determine the number of pounds you need to lose.**

3. **Have a physician or dietitian help you design a plan for weight loss.** Remember, one pound of body fat is equal to 3,500 calories. Suppose you want to lose ten pounds. You may want to lose two pounds a week for five weeks. This means you need to use 1,000 more calories than you take in. The physician or dietitian can advise you how best to make this change. Most likely, they will recommend that you decrease caloric intake AND increase physical activity. For example, you might reduce your caloric intake by 500 calories and engage in physical activity to burn 500 calories.

4. **Select the appropriate number of servings from the Food Guide Pyramid.** Do not leave out any food group. Each food group contains nutrients that are needed for optimal health. Instead, select low-calorie foods and beverages from each food group. Read food labels to determine serving sizes and calories.

5. **Follow the Dietary Guidelines.** Be especially careful to choose low-fat and fat-free foods that also are low-calorie. Trim fat from foods. Select broiled, baked, poached, and steamed foods rather than fried foods. Limit sugars and salt.

6. **Keep available ready-to-eat, low-calorie snacks.** Keep snacks such as celery sticks and carrots in the refrigerator. Carry snacks such as an apple or celery sticks with you to eat between classes. Satisfy your appetite with these snacks rather than being tempted to eat high-calorie foods.

7. **Participate in regular physical activity.** Physical activity increases BMR. Try to engage in physical activity early in the morning and again later in the day. Physical activity tones muscle. When you engage in vigorous physical activity, your body secretes beta-endorphins. These hormones improve mood. They keep you from feeling down when you are dieting.

8. **Drink plenty of fluids.** Your body needs plenty of water to burn fat. You may develop gall stones if you do not drink enough water.

9. **Ask for the support of family members and friends.** Discuss the changes in lifestyle that your diet will require. For example, your friends may eat pizza on Fridays. You will not be eating pizza. They may volunteer to make some changes that will make it easier for you to stick to your diet. Ask for encouragement.

10. **Keep a journal of food and beverage intake and weight loss.** Your physician or dietitian will recommend a way of keeping a record of your food and beverage intake and weight loss. Review this information with the physician or dietitian.

What to Know About Weight Loss Strategies

The Steps to Healthful Weight Loss are suggestions for gradual weight loss and should be followed after checking with a physician and/or dietitian. Following the steps allows a person to develop healthful eating habits. After reaching desirable weight, a person gradually adds more calories to his/her diet to maintain weight.

Some people try other strategies for losing weight. You should know the following facts about other weight loss strategies.

Fad diets

A **fad diet** is a quick weight loss strategy that is popular for a short time. The grapefruit diet and the cabbage soup diet are examples of fad diets. Some people try one fad diet after another. They try such varied diets that they never develop healthful eating habits. They lose weight and gain it back when they resume their former eating habits. Some fad diets are dangerous. Remember, a person needs a balanced diet for optimal health. The only way to obtain a balanced diet is to get the correct number of servings from each food group in the Food Guide Pyramid.

Liquid diets

A **liquid diet** is a diet in which beverages are substituted for some or all meals. Some liquid diets are obtained only at a diet center, hospital, or physician's office and must be followed under medical supervision. Before beginning a medically supervised liquid diet, a person has a physical examination and extensive blood tests. An electrocardiogram is required to check the condition of the heart.

While on the liquid diet, a person has medical supervision with blood tests at set intervals. (S)he must drink plenty of fluids and will urinate frequently. (S)he may take an over-the-counter product to help with bowel movements. The person may attend classes to learn more about eating habits. When the weight loss goal is reached, a maintenance plan must be followed. The maintenance plan is designed to help the person practice healthful eating habits.

Some liquid diets are sold in supermarkets and drugstores and do not require medical supervision. Using these liquid diets can be dangerous. These diets usually contain few calories. People who use them may have side effects. They do not learn healthful eating habits and often gain back weight.

Reason 3:

Some teens are perfectionists.

"I need to be perfect." **Perfectionism** is a compelling need to be accurate. Teens who are perfectionists are overly critical of themselves. Perfectionism is the result of feeling inadequate and insecure. Some teens become perfectionists because adults had unrealistic expectations of them during their childhood. When teens who are perfectionists begin a diet, they may go overboard. The result is an eating disorder.

Reason 4:

Some teens feel their lives are out of control.

"I need to be in control." Some teens feel compelled to control every situation. These teens may have had traumatic childhoods. Perhaps they were raised in families with alcoholism or abuse and were not able to rely on responsible adults to protect them. They might never know when a parent, guardian, or adult family member might be drinking or be physically or sexually abusive. As a result, these teens have difficulty trusting the unknown and feel more secure when they control situations. They diet or exercise to extremes as a way to show control.

Reason 5:

Some teens are not able to express their emotions.

"I do not know how to express my emotions." They have difficulty when they feel frustrated, lonely, depressed, or anxious. They substitute other behaviors for the healthful expression of these emotions. For example, suppose a teen feels lonely and rejected. This teen may have a sundae to comfort himself/herself. Suppose a teen is frustrated when doing algebra. This teen may reach for a bag of chips and pig out. These teens turn to food for comfort. They rely on excessive eating as a way to satisfy their emotional needs. Other teens starve when they have emotional needs.

Warning:

These behaviors may indicate that you are at risk for developing an eating disorder.

Read each of the following statements. If one or more describe you, talk to your parents, guardian, or other responsible adult.

1. I constantly compare myself to others.
2. I am unhappy with my physical appearance.
3. I wear baggy clothes to hide my body changes, such as my breasts. (females)
4. I think it is disgusting to have menstrual periods. (females)
5. I am never satisfied with anything I do.
6. My parent or guardian is never satisfied with anything I do.
7. I felt unsafe during my childhood (from alcoholism, physical abuse, or sexual abuse in the family).
8. I only feel secure when I can control a situation.
9. I do not know what to do when I feel lonely, frustrated, rejected, or depressed.
10. I reach for food, starve, exercise, or rid myself of food when I am uncomfortable.

What to Know About
Anorexia Nervosa

Anorexia nervosa is an eating disorder in which a person starves himself/herself and weighs 15 percent or more below desirable weight. The person also may exercise to extremes, vomit, and use laxatives and diuretics. Anorexia nervosa is usually referred to as anorexia. Teens with anorexia are obsessed with being thin. They do not recognize when they are dangerously thin. When they look at their bodies in the mirror, they see themselves as fat even when they are very thin. Many teens with anorexia are obsessed with exercise. Most are perfectionists. They often are good students and are obedient and respectful. They often have a parent or guardian who set very high expectations for them. As a result, they feel inadequate and controlled. To gain back control, they starve themselves. The one thing they can control is whether or not they eat. When their parents or guardian pressure them, they become even more committed to starving. Teens with anorexia deny their behavior.

How Anorexia Nervosa Harms Health

There are many physical problems associated with anorexia. Teens with anorexia may have:

- a weight loss of 15 percent or more below desirable weight;
- dehydration and constipation;
- abdominal pain and nausea;
- hair loss;
- hormonal changes;
- damage to heart, kidneys, and other body organs;
- decrease in heart rate and blood pressure;
- impaired immune system function;
- absence of menstruation in females;
- malnutrition.

Without treatment, 10 percent of teens with anorexia will die. Other teens with anorexia will have permanent damage to body organs.

Teens with anorexia may:

- have negative self-confidence,
- lack self-respect,
- have frequent bouts with depression,
- withdraw from others,
- be at risk for making suicide attempts.

Treatment for Anorexia Nervosa

Treatment for anorexia involves a team of professionals—physicians, nurses, dietitians, and mental health professionals. A treatment plan is developed that deals with physical and emotional health problems. A hospital stay may be necessary to treat for dehydration and malnutrition. Intravenous feedings may be required to supply nutrients. Tests are required to assess and treat damage to body organs. Mental health professionals work with the teen who is anorexic and with his/her family. The teen must recognize and deal with the motional problems that caused the eating disorder. Often, the family is involved in therapy. The teen may need to achieve independence from a controlling parent or guardian.

What to Know About
Bulimia

Bulimia is an eating disorder in which a person binges and purges. The bingeing involves eating large amounts of food in a short period of time. This is followed by purging, or ridding the body of foods that were eaten. Teens with bulimia may vomit or use laxatives or diuretics to purge.

Bulima is far more common than anorexia nervosa. Most cases of bulimia occur in teen females who want to lose weight. They are obsessed with their body shape and size. They try to follow a diet but are unsuccessful. So they turn to starvation to lose weight. Then they feel compelled to eat and go on a binge. After the binge, they feel guilty and worry about weight gain. Then they feel compelled to purge. A binge-purge cycle dominates their lives.

Teens who have a negative body image are at risk for bulimia. Other teens at risk include those teens who were raised in families in which there was alcoholism or abuse. These teens are insecure and depressed. They hide their insecurity and depression from others. Denying their feelings increases the likelihood that they will binge and purge.

Behaviors of Teens With Bulimia

Unlike teens with anorexia, teens with bulimia usually know they have a problem. They feel guilty and ashamed but are unable to change their behavior. At first, they find purging disgusting. Then they get used to it. Usually they do not want anyone to know they binge and purge. They hide their behavior. They may not eat at their friends' homes. If they eat out, they choose restaurants where they can vomit without anyone knowing. Some teens do not hide their bulemic behavior. They become friends with other teens who have bulimia. They binge and purge together. They share laxatives and diuretics.

Teens with bulimia may:

- binge in private, eating regular amounts when with others;

- have one secret place in which to binge, such as closet;

- steal food or hide it in a secret place;

- think about food constantly and plan each binge carefully;

- buy or steal special treats or elaborate dishes for a binge;

- gulp or stuff food quickly while bingeing so as not to be discovered;

- steal money to purchase food or steal food from the stores;

- exercise and diet excessively between binges.

How Bulimia Harms Health

There are many physical problems associated with bulimia. Teens with bulimia may have:

- dissolved tooth enamel;
- tooth decay;
- sore gums;
- enlarged salivary glands;
- swollen cheeks;
- water loss;
- depletion of potassium;
- increase in blood pressure;
- damage to the colon, heart, and kidneys;
- impaired bowel function.

Teens with bulimia may:

- have a negative body image,
- lack self-respect,
- be insecure and depressed,
- deny their feelings.

Treatment for Bulimia

It is difficult to diagnose bulimia in teens. Teens with bulimia often have desirable weight and are successful at hiding their behavior. Treatment for bulimia involves a team of professionals—physicians, nurses, dentists, dietitians, and mental health professionals. A treatment plan is developed that deals with physical and emotional health problems. Tests are required to assess and treat damage to body organs. A dentist may repair teeth and treat gums. Tests for basal metabolic rate may be used. Some teens with bulimia have a metabolic condition. They do not feel full after eating. This condition is corrected.

Teens with bulimia need help with their emotional health. They need to recognize the reasons why they developed bulimia. Teens who have been raised in families with alcoholism, physical abuse, or sexual abuse must sort out their feelings. They must develop new ways of coping. Teens with a negative body image and who lack self-respect must gain self-confidence.

Anorexia vs. Bulimia: What's the Difference?

Teens with anorexia and bulimia have some characteristics in common. There are some differences too.

Teens with anorexia...	Teens with bulimia...
• Are often females age 14 to 18	• Are often females age 15 to 24
• Are very thin	• May have normal weight
• Deny their behavior	• Are aware of their behavior and feel guilty but cannot change
• Deny they are hungry	• Recognize they are hungry and and want to eat
• Withdraw from others	• May be outgoing and social
• Do not have menstrual periods	• May have irregular menstrual periods
• Resist treatment	• Are more likely to get help when they are confronted with their behavior

What to Know About Binge Eating Disorder and Obesity

Binge eating disorder is an eating disorder in which a person cannot control eating and eats excessive amounts. The diagnosis is made when a person binges two or more times per week for six months. When food is in front of teens with binge eating disorder, they cannot resist the urge to eat. They eat too much, too often. They are obsessed with eating.

Binge eating disorder is more common in females. Teens with this disorder have difficulty expressing emotions and coping. They turn to food as a substitute for coping. After a time, they are addicted to food. They may stuff themselves in private while pretending to diet when they are with others. But, they are not successful at hiding their disorder. Most teens with binge eating disorder are overweight. Family and friends know they have a weight problem but may not realize that the cause is an eating disorder.

Teens with binge eating disorder may not understand that they need medical and psychological help. They may think they will lose weight if they can find the right diet. But, their attempts at weight loss are never successful. Until they are treated for binge eating disorder, they will continue to be overweight. Binge eating disorder is the most common cause of obesity. **Obesity** is a body weight that is 20 percent or more than desirable body weight.

How Binge Eating Disorder and Obesity Harm Health

There are many physical problems associated with binge eating disorder and obesity. Teens who are overweight or obese may have:

- skeletal difficulties due to need for bones to support extra weight,
- increase in heart rate and blood pressure,
- increased risk of developing cardiovascular diseases, high blood pressure, diabetes, and certain types of cancer.

More than 80 percent of teens who are obese are obese as adults.

Teens with binge eating disorder may:

- lack self-respect,
- have negative self-esteem,
- have a negative body image,
- have frequent bouts of depression,
- not feel accepted by peers,
- withdraw from social activities,
- substitute eating for relationships.

Treatment for Binge Eating Disorder and Obesity

Treatment for binge eating disorder and obesity involves a team of health care professionals. A treatment plan is developed that deals with physical and emotional problems. A complete physical examination is required. Blood tests and an electrocardiogram are needed. Existing health conditions are treated.

A weight loss plan is designed. The person on the diet has medical supervision with blood tests at set intervals. Obese people are placed on liquid diets. They see a physician each week, have regular blood tests, and may have an electrocardiogram at set intervals. The FDA has approved anorectic drugs for patients who are obese. An **anorectic drug** is a drug that decreases appetite. It is a prescription drug. Patients receiving these drugs must meet certain restrictions and be supervised by a physician.

After weight loss, patients must learn new eating habits. Patients are put on a maintainence plan. They are supervised on the maintainence plan to prevent relapse. To change eating habits, patients need to examine the reasons why they developed binge eating disorder. If not, they will relapse and begin to overeat again. Therapy, nutrition classes, and support groups are helpful.

Lesson 40

Review

Vocabulary Words

Write a separate sentence using each of the vocabulary words listed on page 314.

Objectives

1. What are five reasons why some teens are at risk for developing eating disorders? **Objective 1**

2. What are the facts about anorexia nervosa: the causes, symptoms, associated health problems, and treatment? **Objective 2**

3. What are the facts about bulimia: the causes, symptoms, associated health problems, and treatment? **Objective 3**

4. How do teens with anorexia differ from teens with bulimia? **Objectives 2 and 3**

5. What are the facts about binge eating disorder and obesity: the causes, symptoms, associated health problems, and treatment? **Objective 4**

Responsible Decision-Making

Perhaps you need to make weight for a wrestling match. Or, perhaps you need to lose weight to fit into your favorite outfit. You have a friend who is being treated for obesity. (S)he takes a prescription drug, follows a specific diet, and is supervised by a physician. You tell your friend you cannot lose weight. Your friend offers you a handful of his/her prescription pills. Write a response to this situation.

1. Describe the situation that requires you to make a decision.
2. List possible decisions you might make.
3. Name two responsible adults with whom you might discuss your decisions.
4. Evaluate the possible consequences of your decisions. Determine if each decision will lead to actions that:
   • promote health,
   • protect safety,
   • follow laws,
   • show respect for yourself and others,
   • follow the guidelines of your parents and of other responsible adults,
   • demonstrate good character.
5. Decide which decision is most responsible and appropriate.
6. Tell two results you expect if you make this decision.

 Effective Communication

Make a Top Ten List of Ways to Prevent Eating Disorders. Ask the school librarian for permission to post the list in the health section of the library.

 Self-Directed Learning

Locate a medical journal or other periodical that contains an article on obesity. Read the article. Write three facts you have learned on an index card.

 Critical Thinking

You are at a party with other teens. You feel self-conscious and left out of the conversation. A table of snacks is set up. You are tempted to place several snacks on a plate even though you have just eaten. Why might you want to do this? What might you do instead?

 Responsible Citizenship

Write a letter to the editor of a teen magazine. Explain why some teens place too much emphasis on their appearance.

Responsible Decision-Making

You go to the local pizza place with a group of friends on Saturday evening. After you finish eating your pizzas, one of your friends suggests that you "dine and dash." (S)he thinks it would be funny if the whole group left the restaurant without paying the bill. Some of your friends think this is a great idea. Others are not so sure. Write a response to this situation.

1. Describe the situation that requires you to make a decision.
2. List possible decisions you might make.
3. Name two responsible adults with whom you might discuss your decisions.
4. Evaluate the possible consequences of your decisions. Determine if each decision will lead to actions that:
   - promote health,
   - protect safety,
   - follow laws,
   - show respect for yourself and others,
   - follow the guidelines of your parents and of other responsible adults,
   - demonstrate good character.
5. Decide which decision is most responsible and appropriate.
6. Tell two results you expect if you make this decision.

Health Behavior Inventory of Life Skills

Number from 1 to 10 on a sheet of paper. Read each life skill carefully. Write YES or NO next to the same number on your paper. Each YES response indicates a life skill you practice to promote your health status. Each NO response indicates a life skill you do not practice. Plan to begin practicing these life skills.

1. I will select foods that contain nutrients.
2. I will eat the recommended number of servings from the Food Guide Pyramid.
3. I will follow the Dietary Guidelines.
4. I will plan a healthful diet that reduces the risk of disease.
5. I will evaluate food labels.
6. I will develop healthful eating habits.
7. I will follow the Dietary Guidelines when I go out to eat.
8. I will protect myself from food-borne illnesses.
9. I will maintain a desirable weight and body composition.
10. I will develop skills to prevent eating disorders.

Multicultural Health

Different cultures often have different table manners. For example, in some cultures people use chopsticks, while in others they use forks. Interview someone in your community of a culture different from your own to research the table manners of his/her culture. Write a short essay describing the eating habits of this culture. Be prepared to share your essay with your classmates.

Family Involvement

Your eating habits are influenced by your family's eating habits. Evaluate your family's eating habits using the information you have learned in this unit. Does your family have healthful eating habits? What types of foods does your family usually eat? What can your family do to improve its eating habits? Share your evaluation with family members.

Health Behavior Contract

Copy and complete the following health behavior contract. Evaluate your progress. Share the results with your family.

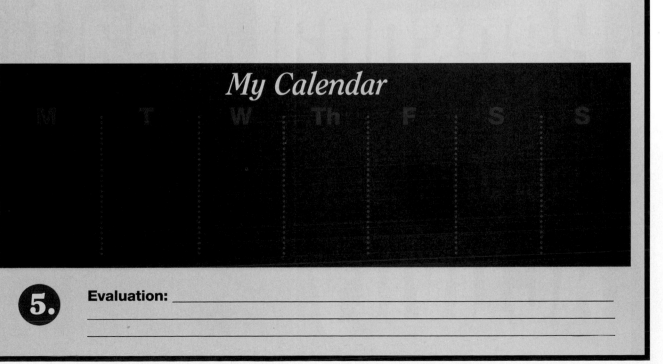

Health Behavior Contract

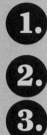

1. Name_____Date_____

2. **Life Skill:** I will develop healthful eating habits.

3. **Effects on Health Status:** Eating habits are patterns in my behavior regarding when and what I eat. My eating habits can be either healthful or harmful. When I practice healthful eating habits, I will be less likely to develop certain diseases. I will be less likely to eat as a way to cope with stressful situations. I will also be less likely to develop eating disorders.

4. **Plan and Method to Record Progress:** I will practice healthful eating habits when I make food selections for breakfast, lunch, dinner, and snacks.

My Calendar

M	T	W	Th	F	S	S

5. **Evaluation:** _____
_____
_____

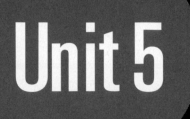

Unit 5

Personal Health and Physical Activity

You Can Have Regular Examinations

Life Skill **I will have regular examinations.**

Health care is the professional medical and dental help that promotes a person's health. The kind of health care available to you and the way you use it affects your health status. For example, to maintain and improve health status, you need regular examinations. During these examinations, your physician or other health care professional will discuss proper health care. This lesson explains what you need to know about physical examinations. You will learn what is included in a physical examination. You will learn what symptoms require you to see a physician. This lesson also will cover eye care and ear care. You will learn about conditions affecting the eyes and ears and how these conditions are treated. You also will learn ways to protect your vision and hearing.

The Lesson Outline

What to Know About Physical Examinations

What to Know About Eye Care

What to Know About Ear Care

Objectives

1. Discuss physical examinations: how often to have them, what they include, and symptoms that require them. **page 329**
2. Discuss health care for the eyes: eye examinations, visual acuity, correcting visual acuity, eye conditions and diseases, and eye protection. **pages 330–332**
3. Discuss health care for the ears: ear examinations, hearing loss, and assistive hearing devices. **pages 333–334**

Vocabulary Words

health care
physical examination
health history
symptom
diagnosis
ophthalmologist
optometrist
visual acuity
refractive error
retina
myopia
hyperopia
astigmatism
cornea
presbyopia
bifocals
conjunctivitis
glaucoma
optic nerve
cataract
audiologist
audiometer
Eustachian tube
conductive hearing loss
sensorineural hearing loss
acoustic nerve
assistive hearing device
hearing aid

What to Know About
Physical Examinations

Teens need a physical examination at least every two years. A **physical examination** is a series of tests that measure health status. Physical examinations may be performed by a physician with assistance from other health care professionals.

During a physical examination, a health history is taken. A **health history** is a record of a person's health habits, past health conditions and medical care, allergies and drug sensitivities, and health facts about family members. You and your parents or guardian may be asked many questions. Bring health-related information with you to the examination so you can give accurate answers to the questions. This information becomes a part of your permanent health record. A health record is a file that includes a health history and the results of the physical examination. Your health record is updated each time you visit your physician.

In a typical physical examination, the physician checks your height, weight, body temperature, pulse rate, respiratory rate, blood pressure, general appearance, skin, eyes, ears, nose, mouth, neck, lungs, heart, breasts, lymph nodes, back, reproductive organs, rectum, legs, feet, bones, joints, and reflexes. A physical examination may include an electrocardiogram and a number of different laboratory tests such as urinalysis and blood tests. An electrocardiogram (ECG) (ee·lek·troh·KAHR·dee·uh·gram) is a record of the electrical impulses of the heart that is used to diagnose disorders of the heart. A urinalysis (yohr·uh·NAHL·uh·sis) is a battery of tests on a person's urine. It can help check normal kidney function and detect urinary tract infections. A blood test is an analysis of blood for blood components, chemicals, pathogens, and antibodies.

Your physician will discuss the results of your physical examination with you and your parents or guardian. If the physician diagnoses any health problems or conditions, a treatment plan will be discussed. Be certain to ask questions if you do not understand something. Your physician also may advise you to change some of your health habits. Never put off adopting lifestyle changes that can improve your health status.

You may need to contact your physician between regularly scheduled physical examinations because you have symptoms that require prompt medical attention. A **symptom** is a change in a body function from the normal pattern. Your physician will make a diagnosis after reviewing your symptoms. A **diagnosis** is the determination of a person's problem after taking a health history, studying symptoms, or getting test results. Your physician may recommend a treatment plan or refer you to a specialist for further diagnosis or treatment. You, your parents or guardian, physician, and other professionals must work together to make a plan for your health care.

Symptoms Alert. . .

Contact your physician if you have any of these symptoms:

- Shortness of breath
- Loss of appetite for no obvious reason
- Blood in the urine or in a bowel movement
- Blood in the mucus or saliva
- A constant cough
- Fever of 100°F (37.7°C) or higher for more than one day
- Swelling, stiffness, or aching in the joints
- Severe pain in any body part
- Frequent or painful urination
- Sudden weight gain or loss
- Dizziness
- Any warning sign of cancer
- Any warning sign of heart attack or stroke

What to Know About
Eye Care

Your sense of sight adds to the quality of your life. If you have your sight, you use it to acquire more than 80 percent of your knowledge.

What to Know About Eye Examinations

Eye examinations are performed by ophthalmologists and optometrists. An **ophthalmologist** (ahp·thuh·MAHL·uh·jist) is a physician who specializes in medical and surgical care and treatment of the eyes. Ophthalmologists can diagnose and treat all types of eye conditions, test vision, perform surgery, and prescribe corrective lenses. An **optometrist** is an eye care professional who is specially trained in a school of optometry. Optometrists can test vision and prescribe corrective lenses.

During an eye examination, an eye care professional reviews your health history and examines your eyes for vision problems. (S)he checks your eyes for refractive errors, color blindness, lazy eye, crossed-eyes, eye coordination, depth perception, eye disease, and general eye health. This helps determine if correction is necessary.

What to Know About Visual Acuity

Visual acuity is sharpness of vision. Refractive errors may interfere with visual acuity. A **refractive error** is a variation in the shape of the eyeball that affects the way images are focused on the retina and blurs vision. The **retina** is the inner lining of the eyeball.

Refractive errors include myopia, hyperopia, astigmatism, and presbyopia. **Myopia**, nearsightedness, is a refractive error in which distant objects appear blurred and close objects are seen clearly. Eyes of nearsighted people are longer than average. The images they see are focused in front of the retina. As the body grows during adolescence, nearsightedness often worsens. **Hyperopia**, farsightedness, is a refractive error in which close objects appear

blurred and distant objects are seen clearly. Eyes of farsighted people are shorter than average. The images they see are focused behind the retina. **Astigmatism** is a refractive error in which irregular shape of the cornea causes blurred vision. The **cornea** is the transparent front part of the outer shell of the eyeball. Astigmatism affects both distant and close vision. You can have astigmatism and either myopia or hyperopia. **Presbyopia** (prez·bee·OH·pee·uh) is a refractive error caused by weakening of eye muscles and hardening of the cornea.

Ways to Correct Visual Acuity

Refractive errors may be corrected with eyeglasses or contact lenses. They help the eye focus images on the retina so that visual acuity is restored. People with presbyopia may wear bifocals. **Bifocals** are lenses that correct for both close and distant vision.

Eyeglasses usually are made of plastic or nonbreakable glass. A protective coating may be added to prevent glare and protect the eyes against ultraviolet radiation. Contact lenses can be hard or soft and are worn directly on the cornea. It is important to clean and store the lenses correctly to help prevent eye infection.

Myopia also can be corrected with surgery. Radial keratotomy (kur·uh·TOT·uh·mee) is a type of surgery that improves myopia by changing the curve of the cornea. The surgeon makes several incisions in the cornea that flatten it out and allow images to focus directly on the retina. Photorefractive keratectomy (kur·uh·TEHK·tuh·mee) is laser surgery that reshapes the cornea to improve myopia. Some risks may be involved in both types of surgery.

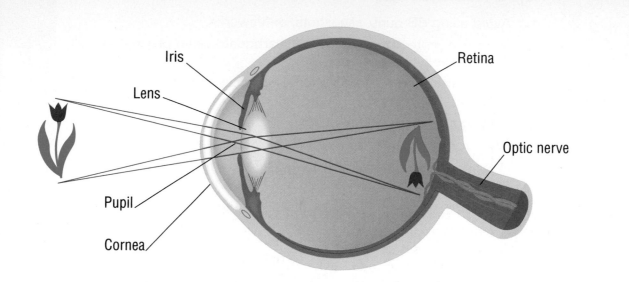

Iris
Lens
Pupil
Cornea
Retina
Optic nerve

What to Know About Eye Conditions and Diseases

Eyes can be affected by conditions and diseases. **Conjunctivitis** is an inflammation of the eye membranes that causes redness, discomfort, and discharge. Another name for conjunctivitis is pinkeye. The eyelids of a person who has conjunctivitis may stick together. Causes include bacterial infection, allergies, contact lenses, certain drugs, and secondhand smoke. Pinkeye caused by bacteria is highly contagious. Pinkeye usually is not serious unless the infection spreads to the deeper tissues in the eye. This may result in a permanent loss of vision.

Two eye conditions may affect visual acuity in middle and late adulthood. **Glaucoma** is a condition in which the pressure of the fluid in the eye is high and may damage the optic nerve. The **optic nerve** is the nerve fibers that transmit messages from the retina to the brain. Regular eye examinations are important for early detection. The increased pressure of glaucoma can be prevented with early treatment. A **cataract** is a clouding of the lens of the eye that obstructs vision. Seeing through an eye with a cataract in it is like trying to see through a steamy window. Images are hazy and out of focus. Cataract surgery involves removing the cloudy lens and implanting an artificial lens. Risks may be involved in both types of surgery.

How to Protect Your Eyes

Most eye injuries involve people under the age of 25. Ninety percent of eye injuries could be prevented if people protected their eyes.

Sports such as racquetball and hockey often cause eye injuries due to the high speed of the objects used in the sport. For example, a hockey puck travels at 90–100 miles (153–170 kilometers) per hour. Eye injuries in sports may be prevented by wearing eye protectors made of polycarbonate. Normal prescription eyeglasses, made of hardened glass or plastic, are not designed to withstand the force of a collision with the objects used in sports. Contact lenses can make sports-related eye injuries worse by scraping and cutting the surface of the eye.

Many eye injuries that can lead to permanent eye damage and loss of vision are caused by BB guns, slingshots, and fireworks. Chemicals, such as chlorine, also can damage your eyes. Chlorine and other substances in water irritate the eyes. Wearing goggles can protect your eyes from these substances when swimming. Safety goggles should be worn if you work around dangerous chemicals such as bleach, insecticides, or cleaning products that can splash into your eyes and cause injury. Long exposure to ultraviolet (UV) radiation in sunlight also causes severe eye damage. Wearing a wide-brimmed hat and sunglasses with 99–100 percent UV protection reduces risk of eye damage from UV radiation.

Ways to Protect Your Eyes

1. Avoid using BB guns, slingshots, or fireworks.

2. Wear eye protectors made of polycarbonate when playing sports that involve high-speed objects.

3. Do not wear normal prescription eyeglasses or contact lenses in place of eye protectors.

4. Wear goggles when swimming.

5. Wear safety goggles when working around dangerous chemicals.

6. Wear a wide-brimmed hat and sunglasses with 99–100 percent UV protection to protect against UV radiation.

Activity

Selecting the Proper Shades

Life Skill: I will have regular examinations.

Materials: paper, pen or pencil

Directions: Sunglasses are more than just a fashion statement. They are important for protecting your eyes from the sun. Complete this activity to make sure you are sunglass savvy.

 Go to a local drugstore that sells sunglasses. Look at the label information that accompanies the two pairs of sunglasses you like most. Write down the information on a sheet of paper.

 Match the label information to the label information and facts in the chart below.

Write and design an advertisement for the sunglasses you choose.

Label Information	Fact	Label Information	Fact
Blocks at least 99 percent of all UV light	Long exposure to UV light can cause eye damage.	Mirror-coated	Have a metallic finish on the lenses. Protect from glare. Usually offer little UV protection.
Blocks 90 percent of infrared light	Sunlight has low levels of infrared light. Infrared rays are not believed to be to the eyes.	Photochromatic	Darken in bright light. Become clear in weaker light. Do not always offer UV protection.
Blue-blocking	It is not known whether blue light is harmful to the eyes. Give a yellow or orange tint. Help vision in snow and haze.	Single-gradient lenses	Shaded at the top and but not at the bottom. Useful for driving.
Polarized	Cut reflected glare. Good for water sports and driving. May not have adequate UV protection.	Double-gradient lenses	Shaded at the top and the bottom but not in the middle. Useful for skiing, tennis, and sailing. Do not always block UV light.

What to Know About
Ear Care

Your sense of hearing adds to the quality of your life. You should have regular ear examinations and tests for hearing loss.

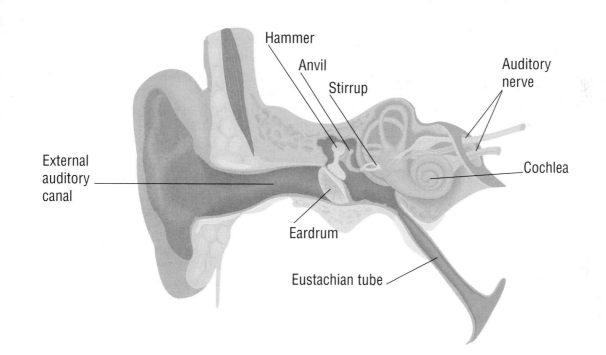

Hammer

Anvil

Stirrup

Auditory nerve

External auditory canal

Cochlea

Eardrum

Eustachian tube

What to Know About Ear Examinations

Ear examinations are performed by audiologists or by otolaryngologists. An **audiologist** (awh·dee·AH·luh·jist) is a specialist who diagnoses and treats hearing and speech-related problems. An otolaryngologist (ENT) (oh·toh·lahr·en·GAH·luh·jist) is a physician who diagnoses and treats disorders of the ears, nose, and throat. An ENT can diagnose ear conditions, test hearing, recommend hearing devices, and perform surgery.

A common way to test for hearing loss is to use an audiometer. An **audiometer** is a machine used to measure the range of sounds a person hears. The results provide data on the type and extent of hearing loss and show if the loss is due to problems in the middle or inner ear or to nerve damage. A tympanogram is a measure of the vibrations of the ear drum and air pressure in the Eustachian tube. The **Eustachian tube** is the tube that connects the middle ear and the back of the nose. It allows fluid to drain from the middle ear and regulates air pressure on both sides of the eardrum. If the middle ear fills with fluid, the eardrum will not vibrate as it should. Air pressure increases in the Eustachian tube and may affect hearing.

Symptoms Alert. . .

Contact your physician if you have any of these symptoms:

- Pain in your ears
- Drainage from your ears
- Difficulty hearing people talking to you
- Difficulty hearing on the telephone
- Need to turn up the volume on the TV to a point that others complain it is too loud
- Difficulty determining from what direction sounds are coming
- Difficulty understanding what is being said in a noisy room
- Difficulty hearing in social situations

What to Know About Hearing Loss

One in every ten people have hearing loss. Over half of all 18-year-olds have some hearing loss. Hearing loss ranges from mild to profound deafness. Causes of hearing loss include: premature birth, respiratory distress at birth, a birth defect, exposure to drugs or infection before birth, viral infections, middle ear infections, high fevers, and injuries.

Exposure to noise pollution also can lead to hearing loss. Noise pollution is a loud or constant noise that causes hearing loss, stress, fatigue, irritability, and tension. The intensity of noise pollution is measured in decibels. A decibel (dB) is a unit used to measure the loudness of sounds. Sounds of more than 70 decibels can cause discomfort and hearing loss.

Hearing loss is either conductive or sensorineural. **Conductive hearing loss** is hearing loss that occurs when sound is not transported efficiently from the outer to the inner ear. Conductive hearing loss is caused by excessive wax buildup, ear injury, birth defects, and middle ear infection. **Sensorineural** (sens·ree·NOOR·uhl) **hearing loss** is hearing loss that occurs when there is damage to the inner ear or acoustic nerve. The **acoustic nerve** is the nerve that connects the inner ear to the brain. Generally sensorineural hearing loss is permanent. Some people with sensorineural hearing loss receive cochlear implants. A cochlear (KAH·klee·uhr) implant is an electronic device that is implanted in the ear to restore partial hearing to the totally deaf.

What to Know About Assistive Hearing Devices

People who have hearing loss may use assistive hearing devices. An **assistive hearing device** is a device that helps a person with hearing loss communicate and hear. The most common assistive hearing device is the hearing aid. A **hearing aid** is an electronic device worn in or near the ear that improves hearing.

Even with a hearing aid, certain situations may pose problems for people with hearing loss. For example, using the telephone may be difficult. A person with hearing loss may need a telephone amplifier that increases the volume on the telephone.

Background noise also can cause problems for people with hearing loss—especially when listening to the TV, radio, or stereo. Increasing the volume to overcome the background noise may make the sound too loud for others. Headphones and other headsets can be connected directly to a TV, radio, or stereo. Television caption devices allow a person to read the audio portion of a TV program. Many people with hearing loss use signaling devices to deal with special circumstances. Flashing lights are used to alert a person that the phone is ringing, someone is at the door, or the smoke detector has been activated.

Ways to Protect Against Hearing Loss

1. Do not insert any objects, including cotton-tipped swabs, into your ears. These objects may puncture the eardrum.

2. Clean the outer ear with a soft, clean washcloth to avoid wax buildup.

3. Use the corner of a dry, clean towel to gently dry your ears after bathing or swimming.

4. Contact your physician if your ears become infected or you have signs of hearing loss.

5. Keep the volume of radios, compact disc players, stereos, and TVs at safe levels.

6. Avoid listening to music through headphones at unsafe levels.

7. Wear protective earplugs when operating loud machinery, using power tools, or attending rock concerts.

Lesson 41
Review

Vocabulary Words

Write a separate sentence using each of the vocabulary words listed on page 328.

Objectives

1. What do physical examinations include and for what 13 symptoms do you need prompt medical attention? **Objective 1**

2. What are the common refractive errors and how can they be corrected? **Objective 2**

3. What are six ways to protect the eyes? **Objective 2**

4. What are nine causes of hearing loss? **Objective 3**

5. What are eight symptoms that may indicate hearing loss and seven ways to protect ears against it? **Objective 3**

Responsible Decision-Making

You are invited to a classmate's house for a holiday. After you arrive, you discover his/her parents are not at home. The teens gathered at the house are lighting fireworks. You know that many eye injuries are caused by fireworks. Someone hands you a "bottle rocket" and a pack of matches and says, "Come on, join the party!" Write a response to this situation.

1. Describe the situation that requires you to make a decision.
2. List possible decisions you might make.
3. Name two responsible adults with whom you might discuss your decisions.
4. Evaluate the possible consequences of your decisions. Determine if each decision will lead to actions that:
   • promote health,
   • protect safety,
   • follow laws,
   • show respect for yourself and others,
   • follow the guidelines of your parents and of other responsible adults,
   • demonstrate good character.
5. Decide which decision is most responsible and appropriate.
6. Tell two results you expect if you make this decision.

 ### Effective Communication

Design a poster that illustrates ways to protect the eyes when playing sports. Ask one of the coaches at your school if you can display your poster in the gym and the locker room so all the athletes can see it.

 ### Self-Directed Learning

Sounds of more than 70 decibels can cause discomfort and hearing loss. Check the library or the Internet to find out how many decibels are produced by: a whisper, normal conversation, loud city traffic, a live rock concert, a jet engine at close range, a rocket launch site. Make a graph to illustrate your findings.

 ### Critical Thinking

One of your grandparents lives with you. Over the past few years, his/her hearing has worsened. (S)he plays the TV so loudly that it hurts your ears. What actions might you take to make both you and your grandparent more comfortable?

 ### Responsible Citizenship

Obtain permission from your parents or guardian to contact a local organization that works with people who are blind. Find out for what tasks the organization uses volunteers. Volunteer to perform one of the tasks, such as read to someone who is blind.

You Can Follow a Dental Health Plan

Life Skill **I will follow a dental health plan.**

A priority is something to be given attention. Your dental health plan should be a priority to you. After all, your permanent teeth must last you a lifetime. This lesson discusses your dental examination, including teeth cleaning, X-rays, whitening of teeth, dental sealants, and dental veneers. You will learn how to prevent and treat tooth decay and periodontal disease and how to correct maloclussion. This lesson also outlines ways to care for your teeth and gums. You will learn why you need to brush and floss teeth daily, obtain a source of fluoride, eat a healthful diet, and wear a mouthguard when participating in sports.

The Lesson Outline

What to Know About Dental Examinations

How to Keep the Teeth and Gums Healthy

Objectives

1. Discuss the dental examination, including teeth cleaning, X-rays, whitening of teeth, dental sealants, and dental veneers. **page 337**
2. Explain how to prevent and treat tooth decay and periodontal disease. **page 338**
3. Discuss the use of braces and a retainer to correct maloclussion. **page 338**
4. List and explain five actions to take to care for the teeth and gums. **pages 339–340**

Vocabulary Words

dental hygienist

dental plaque

calculus

dental sealant

dental veneer

cavity

dentin

filling

pulp

root canal

periodontal disease

gingivitis

malocclusion

orthodontist

braces

retainer

dental floss

fluoride

systemic fluoride

dietary fluoride supplement

topical fluoride

community water fluoridation

custom-made mouthguards

What to Know About
Dental Examinations

For good dental health, you need a dental examination every six months. Even if you are not aware of any dental problems, you should have a checkup. A dentist can find and correct problems before they become painful or obvious to you. When a dental problem has had time to develop, the treatment often is painful and costly.

Teeth Cleaning

A thorough cleaning by a dental hygienist is a part of a dental checkup. A **dental hygienist** is a trained dental health professional who works under the direction of a dentist to provide dental care. Dental plaque and calculus that have built up on your teeth will be removed. **Dental plaque** is an invisible, sticky film of bacteria on teeth, especially near the gum line. **Calculus** is hardened plaque. Plaque builds and continues to harden. Calculus is difficult to remove by yourself. Removal must be done by a trained dental health professional. A fluoride treatment may be given to help strengthen your teeth and help prevent cavities. The dental hygienist also will give you instructions for brushing and flossing your teeth.

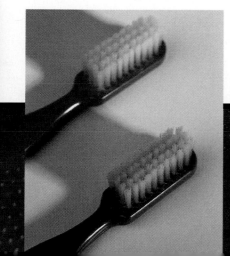

X-Rays

X-rays of your teeth may be taken to detect tooth decay or other dental problems. X-rays show the insides of the teeth, gums, and supporting bones. X-rays can detect problems that a dentist cannot see by examination alone. Dentists are very careful to minimize your exposure to radiation when taking X-rays. They will use lead aprons and shields to protect you.

Whitening

Human teeth naturally are somewhat yellow. As you age, your teeth will become more yellow. Using tobacco and drinking coffee are two habits that affect the color of teeth. The natural yellowing does not place you at higher risk of dental problems. There are treatments to whiten teeth. The only reason to get such treatment is cosmetic. Whitening kits are available over-the-counter, but there are possible side effects.

Dental Sealants

A **dental sealant** is a thin, plastic coating painted on the chewing surfaces of the back teeth to prevent tooth decay. The chewing surfaces of the back teeth are most susceptible to tooth decay. They are rough and uneven because they have small pits and grooves. Food and germs can get stuck in the pits and stay there a long time. Toothbrush bristles have a difficult time brushing away the food and germs.

Sealants are painted on as a liquid and quickly harden to form a shield over a tooth that keeps away from the teeth the food, bacteria, and acid leading to tooth decay. Many dentists recommend that children get sealants on their permanent molars before any decay occurs. The first molars come in between the ages of five and seven. The permanent molars come in between the ages of 11 and 14. Teenagers without decay or fillings also may get sealants.

Dental Veneers

A **dental veneer** is a thin shell of ceramic material used to cover teeth. Dental veneers are used to improve the appearance of the front teeth. They also are used to treat broken or chipped teeth, large gaps between teeth, permanently stained or discolored teeth, and crooked teeth.

Dental veneers are attached directly to the existing teeth. The dentist takes an impression of a person's tooth to make an exact copy. Bonding material is used to adhere the veneer to the tooth. Veneers can last for up to ten years, depending on how well a person takes care of them. They are resistant to stains and chipping. However, nail biting and chewing on hard objects such as ice and hard candies can damage them.

Tooth Decay

During a regular examination, a dentist will check for cavities and problems of the teeth and gums. A **cavity** is an area of tooth decay. The chief cause of dental decay is plaque. Dental plaque is an invisible, sticky film of bacteria on teeth, especially near the gum line. The bacteria found in plaque ingest sugars and starches. Then, the bacteria excrete an acid waste product that is corrosive to teeth. This acid causes tooth decay by dissolving the hard enamel and dentin of the teeth. **Dentin** is the hard tissue that forms the body of the tooth. A dentist may put a filling into a cavity. A **filling** is the material that a dentist uses to repair a cavity in a tooth.

Sometimes tooth decay progresses into the pulp of the tooth. The **pulp** is the living tissue within a tooth. If the pulp becomes irreversibly damaged or dies, a root canal must be performed. A **root canal** is a dental procedure performed to save a tooth in which the pulp has died or is severely diseased.

Periodontal Disease

When brushing and flossing are ignored, plaque and calculus buildup occurs. **Periodontal** (pehr·ee·oh·DAHN·tuhl) **disease** is a disease of the gums and other tissues supporting the teeth. Plaque formation and acid production by bacteria in the plaque can cause periodontal disease. This disease is the main cause of tooth loss in adults. The early stage of periodontal disease is called gingivitis. **Gingivitis** (jin·juh·VY·tuhs) is a condition in which the gums are red, swollen, and tender and bleed easily. The condition worsens if it is not treated. The gums pull away from the teeth. Pockets form between the teeth and gums. The pockets fill with more bacteria, pus, plaque, and calculus, which causes bad breath and infection. Particles of food also become trapped in the pockets and begin to decay. The supporting bones and ligaments that connect the root to the tooth can be destroyed. The teeth may loosen and fall out.

Malocclusion

During a dental examination you will be checked for malocclusion. **Malocclusion** (ma·luh·KLOO·zhuhn) is the abnormal fitting together of teeth when the jaws are closed. An **orthodontist** is a dental health professional who specializes in correcting malocclusion. Malocclusion can make it difficult for a person to bite and speak properly. It also affects a person's appearance. Malocclusion can make it difficult to clean teeth thoroughly, which can lead to gum disease.

Malocclusion usually is corrected by removing some teeth or by applying braces. **Braces** are devices that are placed on the teeth and wired together to help straighten teeth. Teeth with braces need to be cleaned very well in order to prevent cavities because food tends to collect under the braces. Braces usually are worn for 18 to 24 months. A dentist or orthodontist will give you an estimate of the time before beginning treatment.

After braces are removed, a retainer is usually worn. A **retainer** is a plastic device with wires that keep the teeth from moving back to their original places. If you have a retainer, do not forget to wear it and to keep it clean.

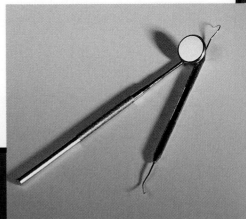

How to Keep the Teeth and Gums Healthy

For good dental health, you need to take care of your teeth and gums. If you don't take care of your teeth and gums, you may have dental problems, such as tooth decay and periodontal disease. You also may put yourself at risk for dental injuries. To keep teeth and gums healthy, you need to brush and floss teeth daily, obtain a source of fluoride, eat a healthful diet, and wear a mouthguard when you are participating in sports.

Toothbrushing

Daily toothbrushing helps remove plaque from the exposed surfaces of the teeth. It also freshens your breath. You should brush your teeth at least twice a day. If possible, brush after every meal. The toothbrush you select should be soft-bristled to prevent injury to the gums. The toothbrush also needs to be long enough to easily reach all of your teeth. Use a toothpaste that contains fluoride. Fluoride strengthens the teeth and helps prevent tooth decay. Take time to brush your teeth carefully. This means brushing the outer, inner, and chewing surfaces of your teeth and your tongue with gentle and short strokes.

Flossing

Flossing helps remove dental plaque and bits of food between teeth. Flossing can reach areas that brushing cannot. Flossing plays an important part in preventing gum disease. Wrap dental floss around two of your fingers. **Dental floss** is a string-like material used for flossing. Gently move the floss between your teeth to the gum line. Wrap the floss around each tooth and slide the floss up and down.

Fluoride

Fluoride can help prevent tooth decay. **Fluoride** is a mineral that strengthens the enamel of teeth. Teeth with strong enamel are resistant to tooth decay because they are able to withstand attacks from acid in the mouth. Fluoride also helps repair areas of teeth that have begun to be dissolved by acid. There are two sources of getting fluorides—by ingesting fluoride and through water treated with fluoride. **Systemic fluoride** is fluoride that is ingested into the body. A **dietary fluoride supplement** is product that is prescribed by a dentist or physician for prevention of tooth decay. Supplements come in the form of lozenges, drops, and tablets. They should be used only by children living in areas without water fluoridation. For best results, dietary fluoride supplements should begin when a child is six months old. Supplements should be taken until age 16. A **topical fluoride** is a fluoride product that is applied directly to the teeth. Fluoride toothpastes and mouth rinses are available for purchase without a prescription.

Community water fluoridation is the process of placing fluoride in community water supplies to a level that is optimal for dental health. The water supply of some communities does not need fluoridation because fluoride already appears naturally at an optimal level for dental health. The optimal level is .7 to 1.2 parts fluoride per million parts water. People without a fluoridated water supply can use dietary fluoride supplements.

Diet

Teeth-damaging acids form in your mouth every time you eat a sugary or starchy food. The acids continue to affect your teeth for at least 20 minutes before they are neutralized and can't do any more damage. The more times you eat sugary snacks during the day, the more often you feed bacteria the fuel they need to cause tooth decay. Certain kinds of sweets can do more damage than others. Gooey or chewy sweets spend more time sticking to the surface of your teeth. Because sticky snacks stay in your mouth longer than foods that you chew quickly and swallow, they give your teeth a longer sugar bath. Sugary foods such as candies, cakes, cookies, and soda pop are not the only culprits. Starchy snacks can also break down into sugars once they are in your mouth. You should think about when and how often you eat sugary and starchy snacks. Do you nibble on sugary snacks many times throughout the day? Or, do you usually eat these treats after a meal? You also should think about how long the sugary food stays in your mouth and whether it is chewy or sticky. There are many snacks that are less harmful to your teeth than chewy, sticky, and sugary foods. Low-fat choices like raw vegetables, fresh fruits, and whole-grain crackers or bread are smart choices. Eating foods that contain vitamin C keeps gums healthy. Eating healthful foods can help protect you from tooth decay and gum disease. So can brushing your teeth after snacks and meals.

Mouthguards

Your dentist will advise you to use mouthguards when playing sports to protect your teeth and face. Dentists see many oral and facial injuries that might have been prevented by the use of a mouthguard. You have choices when selecting a mouthguard. **Custom-made mouthguards** are mouthguards made from a cast model of the teeth. Usually they are more expensive than other types of mouthguards. However, they provide the best fit and protection. Custom-made mouthguards also prevent concussions caused by blows to the chin because they cushion the jaw. These mouthguards do not interfere with speech or breathing.

You can purchase ready-made commercial mouthguards in sporting goods stores. These are made of rubber or polyvinyl. They are the least expensive mouthguards. However, they also are the least effective in protecting the teeth and face. If you become unconscious, mouthguards that are not custom-fit may lodge in the throat and possibly cause an airway obstruction.

Another option is a mouthguard that you place in hot water, then in your mouth, and then bite down on to shape it. The mouthguard hardens. This kind of mouthguard tends to become brittle after being used for a while. People with braces find it difficult to wear mouthguards. They do not provide much protection to the tops of their teeth.

Mouthguards should be worn at all times during athletic competition. This includes practices as well as games. Mouthguards need to be kept clean. It is wise to rinse your mouthguard with water or mouthwash after each use. Never allow anyone else to use your mouthguard.

Sports That Require a Mouthguard

You should wear a mouthguard when participating in the following sports.

- **Acrobatics**
- **Badminton**
- **Baseball**
- **Basketball**
- **Bicycling**
- **Boxing**
- **Field hockey**
- **Football**
- **Gymnastics**
- **Handball**
- **Ice hockey**
- **Ice skating**
- **Lacrosse**
- **Martial arts**
- **Racquetball**
- **Rollerblading**
- **Roller hockey**
- **Roller skating**
- **Rugby**
- **Shotputting**
- **Skateboarding**
- **Skiing**
- **Skydiving**
- **Soccer**
- **Softball**
- **Squash**
- **Surfing**
- **Trampoline**
- **Volleyball**
- **Water polo**
- **Weightlifting**
- **Wrestling**

Lesson 42

Review

Vocabulary Words

Write a separate sentence using each of the vocabulary words listed on page 336.

Objectives

1. How does a dental hygienist clean teeth and why does (s)he take X-rays? **Objective 1**

2. What is the purpose of whitening teeth, applying dental sealants, or applying veneers? **Objective 1**

3. How can tooth decay and periodontal disease be prevented and treated? **Objective 2**

4. Why might teens wear braces and/or a retainer? **Objective 3**

5. What are five actions you can take to care for your teeth and gums? **Objective 4**

Responsible Decision-Making

You have been waiting all day for soccer practice to start. It is a beautiful, late September afternoon. Finally, your last class is over and you hurry to the practice field. You reach into your pack for your mouthguard. You thought that you put it in there before you left for school this morning. Now you discover that you left the mouthguard at home. Write a response to this situation.

1. Describe the situation that requires you to make a decision.
2. List possible decisions you might make.
3. Name two responsible adults with whom you might discuss your decisions.
4. Evaluate the possible consequences of your decisions. Determine if each decision will lead to actions that:
   • promote health,
   • protect safety,
   • follow laws,
   • show respect for yourself and others,
   • follow the guidelines of your parents and of other responsible adults,
   • demonstrate good character.
5. Decide which decision is most responsible and appropriate.
6. Tell two results you expect if you make this decision.

Effective Communication

Prepare a list of ten questions about oral health to ask a dental hygienist. Examples of questions might be: Does it matter what type of toothbrush I use? Can I damage my teeth if I don't brush the right way? Bring the ten questions with you to your next dental examination. Ask the dental hygienist for answers.

Self-Directed Learning

Conduct an observation survey by watching athletes at your school practice or play a game. Your goal is to determine what percent of teenagers playing sports are wearing mouthguards. Based on your survey, in which sports are teens most likely to wear mouthguards? Least likely? Share the results with the coaches.

Critical Thinking

Some people are resistant to the idea of community water fluoridation. Investigate the pros and cons of having a water supply fluoridated. List these on a sheet of paper. After looking at both sides of the issue, what is your stand? Do you support community water fluoridation? Why or why not?

Responsible Citizenship

Make up a puppet show for elementary children showing how tooth decay occurs. Include instructions on how to prevent tooth decay by brushing, flossing, and eating a healthful diet. Ask some other teens to help you perform the puppet show.

You Can Have a Clean and Healthful Appearance

Life Skill **I will be well-groomed.**

Grooming is keeping the body clean and having a neat appearance. Good grooming practices protect your health. When you keep your skin, hair, and nails clean, you help reduce the risk of infection from pathogens. Good grooming practices also improve the state of your social health. When you keep your body clean and have a neat appearance, other people find you more attractive. This lesson provides tips for good grooming. You will learn how to care for your hair, skin, and nails and what to do if you develop acne. This lesson outlines ways to dress for success. Remember, other people get a first quick impression of you based on how you look.

The Lesson Outline

How to Care for Your Hair

How to Care for Your Skin and Nails

How to Dress for Success

Objectives

1. Discuss how to keep hair clean, what to do about dandruff, products for hair care, and hair removal. **page 343**
2. Explain how you can prevent body odor, protect your skin, and care for your fingernails. **pages 344–345**
3. Discuss common foot problems, including athlete's foot, ingrown toenails, blisters, calluses, corns, bunions, and foot odor. **pages 344–345**
4. Discuss the types, causes, and treatment of acne. **page 345**
5. Discuss five guidelines that the well-dressed teen must consider. **page 346**

Vocabulary Words

grooming
shampoo
conditioner
dandruff
styling gel
hairspray
mousse
relaxer
curl activator
texturizing hair cream
razor
shaving cream
shaving gel
lice
sunburn
dermatologist
cuticle
hangnail
athlete's foot
ingrown toenail
blister
callus
corn
bunion
antiperspirant
deodorant
acne
designer label

How to Care for Your Hair

Your hair makes a statement about your personal style. Caring for your hair is an important part of grooming. Healthy hair is shiny and flexible. Unhealthy hair is dull, limp, or oily.

How to Wash and Style Hair

There are many products you can use to wash your hair. Choose one that meets the needs of your hair style and condition. **Shampoo** is a mild detergent for the hair. The more acid a shampoo has, the more it smoothes down the hair. Shampoos designed for oily hair have more detergent than shampoos for dry or normal hair. After using shampoo, some people use conditioner. **Conditioner** is a product that coats hair, helps detangle hair, and gives hair a smooth and shiny appearance. Some people use a shampoo to control dandruff. **Dandruff** is a condition in which dead skin is shed from the scalp producing white flakes.

To wash hair properly, wet it with warm water and work shampoo into a lather with your fingertips. If you have oily hair, do not rub your scalp vigorously. Rubbing can stimulate the oil glands in your scalp. Rinse well to remove suds and loosened scalp flakes. If you use a conditioner after the shampoo, rinse well to remove it. Squeeze extra water from the hair and pat dry with a towel. Comb wet hair gently. Brushing wet hair may cause it to break. If possible, let hair dry naturally or use a hair dryer on a warm or cool setting. Hair dryers set on hot can cause hair to become dry and brittle and have split ends. Curling irons and hot rollers also can damage the hair.

There are hair products to help hair keep its style. **Styling gel** is a jelly-like substance that gives hair body and keeps it in place. **Hairspray** is a spray that stiffens hair to keep it in place. **Mousse** is a foam that keeps hair in place. **Relaxer** is a product that helps take curl out of hair. **Curl activator** is a product that puts curl in a female's hair. **Texturizing hair cream** is a product that puts curl in a male's hair.

Ingredients in hair products may cause skin reactions and harm eyes. Incorrect use or overuse of hair products can damage hair.

How Fast Does Hair Grow?

The hair on the scalp grows an average of 1/2 inch (1.25 centimeters) per month. The rate of growth varies according to the hair length, the season, and a person's gender.

- Short hair grows faster than long hair.
- Hair cut infrequently grows more slowly.
- Hair grows faster during the day than at night.
- Hair grows faster in warm weather.
- Participating in physical activity may increase hair growth.

What to Know About Hair Removal

There are products available to remove hair:

- A **razor** is a device with a sharp blade used for shaving hair.
- **Shaving cream** is a foam placed on hair to make shaving easier.
- **Shaving gel** is a jelly-like substance placed on hair to make shaving easier.

Get permission from a parent or guardian before using any hair removal product. Some hair removal products can cause severe skin reactions in certain people. If they are not used correctly, the skin or hair follicles may be damaged.

What to Know About Head Lice

Lice are insects that pierce the skin and secrete a substance that causes itching and swelling. Head lice attach to hair on the head and other body parts. You can keep from being infected with head lice. Do not share brushes, combs, or hats with other people.

How to Care for Your Skin and Nails

Q: What can I do if I have smelly feet?

A: Foot odor is caused by bacteria that collect on the bottom of feet and between the toes. To prevent foot odor, wash your feet regularly with soap. Then scrub toenails with a nail brush. Dry feet well. Wear clean socks every day. Let shoes air out after you wear them.

Q: Why is it dangerous to sunbathe and go to tanning booths?

A: Limited exposure to sunlight is necessary for the body to produce vitamin D. Overexposure can have harmful effects on the skin. Short-term exposure can cause sunburn. **Sunburn** is a burn caused by overexposure to sunlight. Ultraviolet rays from the sun destroy cells in the outer layer of the skin and damage blood vessels. The affected skin becomes red and tender and may blister. Limit exposure to the sun to prevent sunburn, even if conditions are hazy.

- Long-term exposure to the sun's harmful rays increases the risk of developing skin cancer and premature wrinkles. Protect your skin by wearing protective clothing and applying sunscreen with a sun protective factor (SPF) of at least 15. Sunscreens work by absorbing or reflecting ultraviolet rays.

- Some people believe that tanning booths prevent future sunburn and are a safe alternative to sunbathing because they only emit a certain type of UV radiation. They are mistaken. Tanning booths are dangerous and a risk factor for developing premature wrinkles and skin cancer.

Q: Why do some grooming products make my skin red and itchy?

A: Some people have sensitive skin that reacts to grooming products. Products with strong scents often irritate skin and may cause allergic reactions. If you have a reaction, such as a rash, to a grooming product, stop using the product. If the rash does not clear up, contact a dermatologist or other physician. A **dermatologist** is a physician who specializes in the care of the skin.

Q: Why do I need to keep my fingernails well-groomed?

A: Your fingernails can collect dirt and bacteria. Trim them regularly to keep them clean. Trim nails straight across and not too close to the skin. Do not bite or pick at your nails or cuticles. A **cuticle** is the nonliving skin that surrounds the nails. If hands are dry, use moisturizing cream to avoid hangnails. A **hangnail** is a strip of skin torn from the side or base of a fingernail. Trim a hangnail with nail scissors and cover it until it heals. Picking at it can tear the skin and cause infection.

Q: What problems can affect my feet?

A: These problems can affect your feet.

- **Athlete's foot** is a fungus that grows on feet. Athlete's foot is treated by using special foot powders or creams.

- An **ingrown toenail** is a toenail that grows into the skin. An ingrown toenail may cause swelling and infection. Clip toenails straight across to reduce the risk of ingrown toenails.

- A **blister** is a raised area containing liquid that is caused by a burn or by an object rubbing against the skin. If a blister breaks and oozes fluid, clean the area, treat it with an antiseptic, and cover it with a sterile bandage.

- A **callus** is a thickened layer of skin caused by excess rubbing. Determine what causes the rubbing and make changes to stop it.

- A **corn** is a growth that results from excess rubbing of a shoe against the foot or from toes being squeezed together. Special pads can be used to reduce pain caused by corns.

- A **bunion** is a deformity in the joint of the big toe that causes swelling and pain. Wearing low-heeled shoes with a square toe or open toes helps prevent bunions.

Obtain medical help if a foot problem interferes with walking or lasts for a period of time.

Q: How can I prevent B.O.?

A: Body odor, or B.O., occurs when perspiration combines with dirt, oils, bacteria, and dead skin cells on the body. Sweat glands beneath the dermis allow perspiration to escape through the pores. Regular bathing and use of an antiperspirant or deodorant help prevent body odor. An **antiperspirant** is a product used to reduce the amount of perspiration. Most antiperspirants coat the skin and reduce the flow of sweat leaving the body. A **deodorant** is a product that reduces the amount of body odor, may reduce the amount of perspiration, and contains fragrance to cover up odor.

Q: What is acne?

A: Many teens develop acne. **Acne** is a skin disorder in which pores in the skin are clogged with oil. There are three main types of acne. Pimples: Pimples occur when a clogged pore becomes infected with bacteria. Whiteheads: Whiteheads occur when a clogged pore is not exposed to air. Blackheads: Blackheads occur when a pore becomes clogged with excess oil and dead skin cells.

Acne can appear on the face, neck, shoulders, upper arms, and chest. It usually appears first during puberty, when your oil glands produce and secrete more oil. Factors that make acne worse include: stress, certain medications, menstrual cycle, exposure to sun, oily or heavy cosmetics, popping or picking acne, perspiring, and putting pressure on the face for an extended period of time. Heredity plays a role in acne. The risk of developing acne is greater if your parents, brother, or sister had acne. Acne is not caused by foods or beverages such as chocolate, soda pop, or greasy foods. Acne is not caused by having a dirty face or body. Acne cannot be spread from one teen to another.

Q: How do you treat acne?

A: There is no cure for acne. However, there are many ways to treat acne.

1. Keep your skin clean. Wash it gently with a clean washcloth and rinse well.

2. Ask a physician to recommend a special soap or over-the-counter topical medication.

3. Do not squeeze, pick, scrub, or pop acne. These actions can cause infection and scars.

4. Keep hair away from your face. Hair touching skin causes excess oil.

5. Limit time in the sun to reduce perspiration.

6. Select cosmetics that are water-based.

Contact a dermatologist if you have severe acne, acne that does not clear up, or acne accompanied by signs of infection. Severe untreated acne may result in permanent scarring.

You Can Get Adequate Rest and Sleep

Life Skill **I will get adequate rest and sleep.**

The alarm clock rings. You jump out of bed, quickly shower and dress, rush through breakfast, and set off for school. Sound familiar? Most teens rush from one activity to the next. It seems like days are not long enough to get everything done. If you skimp on sleep, you will have extra hours to pack everything into your day. You might even want to brag about how little sleep you get. But, lack of rest and sleep will catch up with you. This lesson explains what you need to know about rest and sleep. You will learn about the body changes that occur during the sleep cycle and why you need to get adequate rest and sleep. This lesson will explain how rest and sleep affect your health status. You will learn ways to tell if you get enough rest and sleep. You also will learn seven tips for getting a good night's sleep.

Vocabulary Words

rest

sleep

rapid eye movement (REM) sleep

nonrapid eye movement (NREM) sleep

insomnia

tryptophan

The Lesson Outline

What to Know About the Sleep Cycle

How to Get Adequate Rest and Sleep

Objectives

1. Discuss the body changes that occur during the sleep cycle. **page 349**

2. Explain why you need adequate rest and sleep to protect your health status. **page 349**

3. Evaluate whether you are getting adequate sleep and rest. **page 350**

4. List seven tips for getting a good night's sleep. **page 350**

What to Know About the Sleep Cycle

Rest and sleep are essential to good health. They help the body rebuild and reenergize itself. **Rest** is a period of relaxation. You can be awake or asleep and be resting. **Sleep** is a state of deep relaxation in which there is little movement or consciousness. There are two kinds of sleep. **Rapid eye movement (REM) sleep** is the period of sleep characterized by rapid eye movements behind closed eyelids. Most dreaming occurs during REM sleep and is very vivid. **Nonrapid eye movement (NREM) sleep** is the period of sleep in which the eyes are relaxed. NREM sleep can range from very light to very deep sleep.

Sleep is an active state in which the brain continues to process information and the body continues to undergo changes. There are certain stages of sleep that you go through during each night of sleep. The first stage is a transition between being awake and asleep. Each stage progresses to deeper sleep and unresponsiveness. Heart rate slows by about ten to fifteen beats per minute. Blood pressure decreases. Fewer breaths are taken per minute. Muscles lose tension. Brain waves become much slower. It takes about one hour to get to the stage of deepest sleep.

When you are in the deepest stage of sleep, you begin REM sleep. Brain wave activity increases to the level of your brain when you are awake even though you arc sound asleep. Muscles of your face, arms, legs, and trunk remain relaxed. Your eyes dart back and forth in rapid motion. If you are awakened during REM sleep, you will recall a very vivid dream. Adults spend about one-fourth of a night's sleep in REM sleep. Infants spend half of their sleep in REM sleep. It takes about 90 minutes to go through the stages of sleep. After REM sleep, you start the sequence again. Throughout the night, you repeat the stages of sleep.

How to Get Adequate Rest and Sleep

You need to get adequate rest and sleep, or your ability to concentrate is affected. This influences your ability to perform well in school, in sports, and in other activities. Lack of sleep also increases your risk for certain illnesses. The immune system becomes weakened when people do not get enough sleep. People who lack sleep also become more accident-prone. Sleep is needed to restore your physical, emotional, and mental energy. Sleep is even critical to your growth. The growth hormone is released so that growth occurs during rest and sleep.

How to Evaluate Your Need for Rest and Sleep

The amount of rest and sleep needed varies from person to person according to a person's level of physical activity and usually decreases with age. As a teenager, you will often require extra sleep and rest because of your rapid physical growth. Most adults need about eight hours of sleep. Feeling rested and energetic during the day is a good sign that you have had enough sleep.

Signs That You Need More Rest and Sleep

You may need to get more rest and sleep if you answer yes to any of the following questions.

- Do you feel irritable during most of the time you are awake?
- Do you always have to have an alarm clock to wake up?
- Do you think about and crave more sleep during the day?
- Do you have to rely on caffeine to keep awake during the day?
- Do you find yourself dozing off during class?
- Do you doze off while watching television?
- Do you feel tired most of the day?
- Do you feel tired most of the time you are playing sports or participating in activities that you enjoy?

Ways to Relax and Rest

Take time for the things you enjoy doing. Participating in enjoyable activities such as hobbies, interests, and entertainment can energize you. These activities take your mind off your problems and worries. Participating in sports promotes relaxation by providing a physical outlet for stress and tension. If you are feeling uptight, try going for a walk, shooting some hoops, or kicking around a soccer ball.

Your Biological Sleep Clock

Your body is programmed to feel sleepy during the nighttime hours and to be active during the daylight hours. People who work at night and try to sleep during the day must constantly fight their biological sleep clock. The same is true for people who fly to other time zones. They get "jet lag" because they cannot maintain a regular sleep-wake schedule. They feel tired and sluggish and may have difficulty falling asleep.

Insomnia

At times, not being able to fall asleep is normal. Continual failure to be able to fall asleep may be insomnia. **Insomnia** is the prolonged inability to fall asleep, stay asleep, or get back to sleep once a person is awakened during the night. Insomnia becomes a pattern and can cause problems during the day, such as tiredness, a lack of energy, difficulty in concentrating, and irritability. Insomnia affects people of all ages.

Seven Tips for Getting a Good Night's Sleep

1. **Establish a sleep schedule.** Encourage getting a good night's sleep by establishing a regular time to go to bed at night and to get up in the morning.

2. **Engage in activities and nightly rituals that encourage sleep.** Read, take a warm bath, listen to relaxing music. Nightly rituals such as brushing teeth, setting the alarm clock, and organizing materials for the next day also encourage sleepiness. Reading also may help.

3. **Avoid napping too long.** Restrict naps during the day to 20 or 30 minutes. Avoid naps altogether if you have a lot of difficulty falling asleep at night.

4. **Create a comfortable place to sleep.** A medium-hard mattress supports a person's back and makes it easier to fall asleep and sleep restfully. A dark room, carpets and rugs that muffle sounds, and earplugs also can help.

5. **Avoid substances that can interrupt your sleep.** Limit liquid intake before bedtime to avoid having to get up and empty the bladder. Don't drink caffeinated beverages during the evening. Alcoholic beverages and some sleeping medications suppress REM sleep and cause restlessness. Nicotine in cigarettes is a stimulant.

6. **Watch what you eat before you go to bed.** Don't eat large amounts of food just before going to bed. Hunger pangs can keep you awake if you go to bed hungry.

7. **Get out of bed if you cannot sleep.** If you can't fall asleep after about half-an-hour, don't fight it anymore. Get out of bed and go into another room. Try reading, listening to relaxing music, doing a simple task, or having a glass of milk. Milk contains tryptophan. **Tryptophan** is an amino acid that helps promote relaxation.

Lesson 44

Review

Vocabulary Words

Write a separate sentence using each of the vocabulary words listed on page 348.

Objectives

1. What body changes occur during the sleep cycle? **Objective 1**

2. How do adequate rest and sleep protect your health status? **Objective 2**

3. What are eight questions you might answer to evaluate if you are getting adequate rest and sleep? **Objective 3**

4. What is your biological sleep clock? **Objective 3**

5. What are seven tips for getting a good night's sleep? **Objective 4**

Responsible Decision-Making

It has been a difficult week for you. You've been up late every night and feel drained. Next week promises to be just as busy. It is Friday and you have told your best friend that you are going to have to miss tonight's party. Your friend says you need more fun in your life. You agree but know that you also need to catch up on your sleep and that you have to work all day Saturday and Sunday. Write a response to this situation.

1. Describe the situation that requires you to make a decision.

2. List possible decisions you might make.

3. Name two responsible adults with whom you might discuss your decisions.

4. Evaluate the possible consequences of your decisions. Determine if each decision will lead to actions that:
   - promote health,
   - protect safety,
   - follow laws,
   - show respect for yourself and others,
   - follow the guidelines of your parents and of other responsible adults,
   - demonstrate good character.

5. Decide which decision is most responsible and appropriate.

6. Tell two results you expect if you make this decision.

Effective Communication

Write a poem or rap about how your dreams and sleep patterns have influenced your mental and physical health. Share with a classmate what you have written. Ask him/her to share with you.

Self-Directed Learning

Record the number of hours you sleep every night for two weeks. Draw a chart displaying the amount of sleep you got each night. Analyze your findings: Do you get a consistent amount of sleep every night? Or do you get more on weekends? Is there a relationship between how much sleep you get and how you perform in school?

Critical Thinking

Ask a pharmacist about advertisements in magazines and on television for over-the-counter medications to help you get a better night's sleep. How accurate are the claims? How effective are the medications? What risks do the medications pose? Explain why a person should or should not believe the advertisements.

Responsible Citizenship

The pressures and demands of parenthood often make it difficult for parents of young children to have time for relaxation or rest. Having a new baby can make it difficult for a young mother or father to get a good night's sleep. Volunteer to childsit for a young parent so (s)he can have some time to rest, relax, or sleep.

You Can Participate in Regular Physical Activity

Life Skill **I will participate in regular physical activity.**

Physical activity is any bodily movement produced by skeletal muscles that results in energy expenditure. This lesson contains information about physical activity from *Physical Activity and Health: A Report of the Surgeon General.* You will learn how regular physical activity improves health status. This lesson also explains how much physical activity is needed to improve health status. You will learn how to obtain a moderate amount of physical activity.

The Lesson Outline

How Regular Physical Activity Improves Health Status

How to Obtain a Moderate Amount of Physical Activity

Objectives

1. List and explain 11 benefits of regular physical activity. **pages 353–355**

2. Identify at least ten ways to obtain a moderate amount of physical activity. **page 356**

Vocabulary Words

physical activity

regular physical activity

life expectancy

premature death

cardiovascular disease

cardiac output

stroke volume

high density lipoproteins (HDLs)

low density lipoproteins (LDLs)

atherosclerosis

coronary thrombosis

coronary collateral circulation

non-insulin-dependent diabetes mellitus (NIDDM)

blood pressure

dynamic blood pressure

stroke

norepinephrine

beta-endorphins

body composition

osteoporosis

arthritis

moderate amount of physical activity

How Regular Physical Activity Improves Health Status

Regular physical activity is physical activity that is performed on most days of the week. According to *Physical Activity and Health: A Report of the Surgeon General:*

- People who are usually inactive can improve their health and well-being by becoming even moderately active on a regular basis.

- Physical activity need not be strenuous to achieve health benefits.

- Greater health benefits can be achieved by increasing the amount (duration, frequency, or intensity) of physical activity.

There are at least 11 benefits of regular physical activity.

Regular Physical Activity Reduces the Risk of Premature Death

Life expectancy is the number of years a person can expect to live. **Premature death** is death before a person reaches his/her predicted life expectancy. As a teen, you may not be thinking ahead to middle and late adulthood. However, you should know that participating in regular physical activity right now will affect the quality of your life in middle and late adulthood. No doubt there will be much you want to do and enjoy in your later years. Prepare now to live a long and healthful life.

Regular Physical Activity Reduces the Risk of Cardiovascular Diseases

Cardiovascular disease is a disease of the heart and blood vessels. During physical activity, cardiac output increases to provide muscle cells with oxygen. **Cardiac output** is the amount of blood pumped by the heart each minute. Cardiac output is equal to your heart rate multiplied by stroke volume. **Stroke volume** is the amount of blood the heart pumps with each beat. Regular physical activity makes the thread-like muscle fibers of the heart thicker and stronger. As a result, stroke volume increases. The heart does not have to beat as often to maintain the same cardiac output. Resting heart rate is lowered.

Regular physical activity influences blood lipid levels. **High density lipoproteins (HDLs)** are substances in the blood that carry cholesterol to the liver for breakdown and excretion. **Low density lipoproteins (LDLs)** are substances in the blood that carry cholesterol to body cells. Vigorous physical activity increases the number of HDLs, which reduces the risk of developing atherosclerosis. **Atherosclerosis** is a disease in which fat deposits on artery walls. The inside of the arteries become narrowed and blood flow is reduced.

Regular physical activity reduces the likelihood of developing coronary thrombosis. **Coronary thrombosis** is the narrowing of one of the coronary arteries by a blood clot. This causes a section of the heart muscle to die from lack of oxygen. Regular physical activity decreases the clumping together of platelets to form a blood clot. It also enhances the breakdown of blood clots.

Regular physical activity also improves coronary collateral circulation. **Coronary collateral circulation** is the development of additional arteries that can deliver oxygenated blood to the heart muscle. When you work out, your heart muscle needs oxygen. Small arteries branch off existing arteries to provide the additional blood flow. These additional routes for blood flow are helpful should you develop blockage in a coronary artery. You are less likely to die from a heart attack.

Regular Physical Activity Reduces the Risk of Developing Non-Insulin-Dependent Diabetes Mellitus (NIDDM)

Non-insulin-dependent diabetes mellitus (NIDDM) (dy·uh·BEE·teez me·luh·tuhs) is a type of diabetes in which the body produces insulin but it cannot be used by cells. More than 90 percent of people who have diabetes have NIDDM. People who are overweight are at risk for developing NIDDM. The risk is greatest in people with excess fat around the waist, abdomen, and upper body and within the abdominal cavity. People who are physically inactive have the greatest risk of developing NIDDM. They have higher blood glucose levels and insulin values than do people who are physically active.

Regular Physical Activity Reduces the Risk of Developing High Blood Pressure

Regular physical activity reduces the risk of developing atherosclerosis. When your arteries remain elastic, they can dilate when your body needs more oxygenated blood. Resting blood pressure stays in normal range. **Blood pressure** is the force of blood against the artery walls. When your arteries are elastic, your dynamic blood pressures remains low. **Dynamic blood pressure** is the measure of the changes in blood pressure during the day. Sudden changes in blood pressure can cause stroke. A **stroke** is a condition caused by a blocked or broken blood vessel in the brain.

Regular Physical Activity Reduces Blood Pressure in People Who Already Have High Blood Pressure

When people already have high blood pressure, they must pay attention to the risk factors over which they have control. They have control over their weight. Regular physical activity helps them to maintain desirable weight or to lose weight if needed. Regular physical activity helps prevent plaque from collecting in artery walls. When arteries are clear, they remain elastic. They are able to dilate when more oxygenated blood is needed. This helps prevent increases in blood pressure.

Regular Physical Activity Reduces the Risk of Developing Colon Cancer

Regular physical activity helps speed the movement of waste through the colon. As a result, a person is more likely to have daily bowel movements. Having daily bowel movements decreases the risk that a person will develop colon cancer.

Regular Physical Activity Reduces Feelings of Depression and Anxiety

Regular physical activity improves circulation to the brain. As a result a person feels more alert. Regular physical activity causes the body to produce higher levels of norepinephrine and beta-endorphins. **Norepinephrine** (NOR·ep·uh·nef·rin) is a substance that helps transmit brain messages along certain nerves. **Beta-endorphins** are substances produced in the brain that create a feeling of well-being. These two substances are helpful in reducing the risk of depression. They also provide some relief of symptoms in people who are suffering from depression.

Regular physical activity alters the body's response to stress. Regular physical activity counterbalances the bodily changes that occur in the first stage of stress by using up the adrenaline that is secreted. This helps the body return to its normal state and reduces the risk of stress-related diseases. Regular physical activity relieves anxiety by providing a physical outlet when a person is stressed.

Regular Physical Activity Helps Control Weight

Regular physical activity increases metabolic rate, burns calories, and shrinks fat cells. Regular physical activity also helps regulate the hypothalmus in the brain. As a result, appetite is decreased. Each of these factors is helpful in maintaining desirable weight. In fact, inactivity is a major factor contributing to overweight and obesity.

Regular physical activity also affects body composition. **Body composition** is the percentage of fat tissue and lean tissue in the body. Having too much fat tissue is a risk factor for cardiovascular diseases, diabetes, cancer, and arthritis. Regular physical activity also favorably affects fat distribution. It reduces the accumulation of fat in the abdominal area. This also reduces the risk of developing cardiovascular diseases.

Regular Physical Activity Helps Build and Maintain Healthy Bones, Muscles, and Joints

Weight-bearing physical activity is essential for normal skeletal development in children and teens. It continues to be essential for maintaing peak bone mass as young people age. A life-time habit of weight-bearing activities, such as running, walking, and rollerblading, prevents bones from becoming brittle. **Osteoporosis** is a condition in which the bones become thin and brittle. This condition can be prevented and managed with regular physical activity and diet. Females also may take estrogen replacement therapy after menopause.

Regular physical activity helps joints as well as bones. Stretching helps muscles lengthen. This allows the joints to move freely and easily through the full range of motion. Regular physical activity provides positive benefits for people who have arthritis. **Arthritis** is a painful inflammation of the joints. Moderate physical activity reduces the swelling around the joints. It increases the pain threshold and energy levels of people who have arthritis. As a result, people with arthritis are better able to cope with their condition.

Regular Physical Activity Helps Older Adults Become Stronger and Better Able to Move About without Falling

Regular physical activity may help prevent accidents by improving muscular strength, balance, and reaction time. Accidents, especially falls, are a primary cause of fractures and other injuries.

Regular Physical Activity Promotes Psychological Well-Being

People who participate in regular physical activity have higher levels of norepinephrine and beta-endorphins. These substances promote feelings of well-being. Regular physical activity promotes psychological well-being in other ways as well. Improved appearance from muscle tone and reduced body fat may boost self-confidence. The routine of regular physical activity increases self-discipline and promotes self-respect. Completing a workout gives a person a feeling of accomplishment.

Prevent and Improve Illnesses Through Regular Physical Activity

Millions of Americans suffer from illnesses that can be prevented or improved through regular physical activity.

- 13.5 million people have coronary heart disease.
- 1.5 million people suffer from a heart attack in a given year.
- 8 million people have adult-onset (non-insulin-dependent) diabetes.
- 95,000 people are newly diagnosed with colon cancer each year.
- 250,000 people suffer from hip fractures each year.
- 50 million people have high blood pressure.
- Over 60 million people (one-third of the U.S. population) are overweight.

Physical Activity and Health: A Report of the Surgeon General, U.S. Department of Health and Human Services, 1996.

How to Obtain a Moderate Amount of Physical Activity

A **moderate amount of physical activity** is roughly equivalent to physical activity that uses approximately 150 calories of energy per day, or 1000 calories per week. The amount of activity needed is a function of duration, intensity, and frequency. Short sessions of strenuous activity are not the only way to achieve physical activity. The same amount of activity can be obtained in longer sessions of moderately intense activities such as brisk walking. If you already participate in moderate physical activity, you can benefit even more by increasing the time or intensity of your activity.

The examples listed below show that a moderate amount of physical activity can be achieved in a variety of ways.

1. Washing and waxing a car for 45–60 minutes
2. Washing windows or floors for 45–60 minutes
3. Playing volleyball for 45 minutes
4. Playing touch football for 30–45 minutes
5. Wheeling self in wheelchair for 30–40 minutes
6. Walking 1 3/4 miles (2.8 kilometers) in 35 minutes
7. Shooting baskets for 30 minutes
8. Bicycling 5 miles (8 kilometers) in 30 minutes
9. Dancing fast (social) for 30 minutes
10. Pushing a stroller 1 1/2 miles (2.4 kilometers) in 30 minutes
11. Raking leaves for 30 minutes
12. Participating in water aerobics for 30 minutes
13. Swimming laps for 20 minutes
14. Playing wheelchair basketball for 20 minutes
15. Playing a game of basketball for 15–20 minutes
16. Bicycling 4 miles (6.4 kilometers) in 15 minutes
17. Jumping rope for 15 minutes
18. Running 1 1/2 miles (2.4 kilometers) in 15 minutes
19. Shoveling snow for 15 minutes
20. Stairwalking for 15 minutes

Physical Activity

Teens should engage in three or more sessions per week of physical activities that last 20 minutes or more at a time and that require moderate to vigorous levels of exertion.

The International Consensus Conference on Physical Activity Guidelines for Adolescents

Lesson 45

Review

Vocabulary Words

Write a separate sentence using each of the vocabulary words listed on page 352.

Objectives

1. What are 11 ways regular physical activity improves health status? **Objective 1**

2. How does regular physical activity reduce the risk of cardiovascular diseases? **Objective 1**

3. How does regular physical activity reduce the risk of high blood pressure and stroke? **Objective 1**

4. What are at least ten ways to obtain a moderate amount of physical activity? **Objective 2**

5. How can you benefit even more if you already participate in moderate physical activity? **Objective 2**

Responsible Decision-Making

You usually are busy with school, drama club, band, and a part-time job. You get a moderate amount of physical activity by walking to school every morning. Your friends ask you to ride to school with them. They say you will have more time to hang out before school starts. They do not understand why you walk to school when you could "hang out" with them. Write a response to this situation.

1. Describe the situation that requires you to make a decision.

2. List possible decisions you might make.

3. Name two responsible adults with whom you might discuss your decisions.

4. Evaluate the possible consequences of your decisions. Determine if each decision will lead to actions that:
   • promote health,
   • protect safety,
   • follow laws,
   • show respect for yourself and others,
   • follow the guidelines of your parents and of other responsible adults,
   • demonstrate good character.

5. Decide which decision is most responsible and appropriate.

6. Tell two results you expect if you make this decision.

 Effective Communication

Make a calendar for a family member that shows a different benefit of regular physical activity for every month of the year. Encourage the family member to whom you give the calendar to display the calendar in a place where (s)he will see it often.

 Self-Directed Learning

At the local library or video store, find a video about physical activity and health. Watch the video. List three new pieces of information you learned about physical activity and health.

 Critical Thinking

Suppose a person has several blood relatives who have non-insulin-dependent diabetes mellitus (NIDDM). Heredity is a risk factor that cannot be controlled. Although this person does not have NIDDM, what might (s)he do to reduce his/her risk of developing NIDDM?

 Responsible Citizenship

People who are elderly often need encouragement and support to participate in physical activity. Some elderly people may be fearful of going on a walk by themselves. Obtain permission from your parents or guardian, and ask a senior citizen to take a walk with you.

You Can Develop and Maintain Health-Related Fitness

Life Skill **I will develop and maintain health-related fitness.**

Physical fitness is the ability to perform physical activity and to meet the demands of daily living while being energetic and alert. There are several components of physical fitness. These components are grouped into health-related fitness and skill-related fitness. **Health-related fitness** is the ability of the heart, lungs, muscles, and joints to function at optimal capacity. This lesson discusses exercises that promote health-related fitness. You will learn about each of the five components of health-related fitness. The next lesson will discuss each of the components of skill-related fitness.

The Lesson Outline

What to Know About Exercises and Health-Related Fitness

What to Know About Cardiorespiratory Endurance

What to Know About Muscular Strength and Muscular Endurance

What to Know About Flexibility

What to Know About Healthful Body Composition

Objectives

1. List and discuss five kinds of exercises. **page 359**
2. Explain how to develop cardiorespiratory endurance using the FITT formula. **page 361**
3. Explain how to develop muscular strength and endurance using the FITT formula. **page 363**
4. Explain how to develop flexibility using the FITT formula. **page 364**
5. Explain how to develop a healthful body composition using the FITT formula. **page 365**

Vocabulary Words

physical fitness
health-related fitness
cardiorespiratory endurance
muscular strength
muscular endurance
flexibility
healthful body composition
exercise
aerobic exercise
anaerobic exercise
isometric exercise
isotonic exercise
isokinetic exercise
FITT formula
target heart rate
maximum heart rate
warm-up
cool-down
resistance exercise
repetitions maximum
repetitions
weight training
free weight
weight machine
static stretching
ballistic stretching
overfat

What to Know About Exercises and Health-Related Fitness

Five components of health-related fitness are:

1. **Cardiorespiratory endurance** is the ability of the circulatory and respiratory systems to supply oxygen during sustained physical activity.
2. **Muscular strength** is the maximum amount of force a muscle can produce in a single effort.
3. **Muscular endurance** is the ability of the muscle to continue to perform without fatigue.
4. **Flexibility** is the ability to bend and move the joints through the full range of motion.
5. **Healthful body composition** is a high ratio of lean tissue to fat tissue in the body.

Exercise is planned, structured, and repetitive bodily movement done to improve or maintain one or more components of physical fitness. There are five kinds of exercises: aerobic, anaerobic, isometric, isotonic, and isokinetic.

An **aerobic exercise** is one in which large amounts of oxygen are required continually for an extended period of time. Aerobic exercises are vigorous, continuous, and rhythmic. They improve cardiorespiratory endurance and help develop flexibility and muscular strength and improve body composition.

An **anaerobic exercise** is one in which the body's demand for oxygen is greater than what is available during exertion. Anaerobic exercises cause lactic acid to gather in the muscles. Lactic acid is a waste product that is produced when muscles work without the presence of oxygen. Running sprints and playing basketball are two examples of anaerobic exercises. Anaerobic exercises help improve muscular strength and endurance and flexibility.

An **isometric exercise** is one in which a muscle is tightened for about five to eight seconds and there is no body movement. Pressing the palms of the hands together at chest level for at least five seconds is an isometric exercise. Isometric exercises can be done almost anywhere and require little or no equipment. Holding your breath when you perform isometric exercises can cause your blood pressure to rise. Isometric exercises should not be performed by people with heart conditions.

An **isotonic exercise** is one in which a muscle or muscles move a moderate amount of weight eight to fifteen times. Weight lifting, push-ups, curl-ups, and jumping jacks are isotonic exercises. When performing isotonic exercises, increase resistance gradually. Isotonic exercises improve muscular strength and endurance and increase flexibility. Performing isotonic exercises at high intensity for a specified amount of time can improve cardiorespiratory endurance.

An **isokinetic exercise** is an exercise using special machines that provide weight resistance through the full range of motion. Isokinetic exercises promote muscular strength, muscular endurance, and flexibility.

The FITT Formula

The **FITT formula** is a formula in which each letter represents a factor for determining how to obtain fitness benefits from physical activity: F-Frequency, I-Intensity, T-Time, and T-Type.

F— Frequency is how often you will perform physical activities.

I— Intensity is how hard you will perform physical activities.

T— Time is how long you will perform physical activities.

T— Type is the kind of physical activities you will perform to develop a fitness component or obtain a specific benefit.

What to Know About
Cardiorespiratory Endurance

Q&A

Cardiorespiratory endurance is the ability of the circulatory and respiratory systems to supply oxygen during sustained physical activity.

Q: What are the benefits of cardiorespiratory endurance?

A: Cardiorespiratory endurance:

1. **Helps your heart and lungs function more efficiently.**

2. **Improves your metabolic rate.** Physical activities that promote cardiorespiratory endurance burn calories. They raise the resting metabolic rate for up to 12 hours.

3. **Promotes healthful aging.** Physical activities that promote cardiorespiratory endurance activate antioxidants. Antioxidants are substances that protect cells from being damaged by oxidation. Antioxidants also tie up free radicals. Free radicals are highly reactive compounds that can damage body cells. Free radicals are believed to be one cause of aging.

4. **Improves insulin sensitivity.** Physical activities that promote cardiorespiratory endurance improve insulin sensitivity. This helps with the metabolism of carbohydrates, fats, and proteins. The risk of developing diabetes is lowered.

5. **Reduces the harmful effects of the alarm stage of the GAS.** During the first stage of stress—the alarm stage—hormones are secreted. Epinephrine and cortisol are two hormones that are secreted and put the body in a state of emergency. Too much of these two hormones increases the risk of developing cardiovascular diseases. Too much of these two hormones can suppress the immune system. This increases the risk of developing certain kinds of cancers. Physical activities help prevent too much of these two hormones in the bloodstream.

6. **Improves the muscles' ability to use lactic acid.** Lactic acid is produced by muscles during vigorous exercise and is one of the factors that causes cramps. Physical activities that promote cardiorespiratory endurance provide a training effect. They lengthen the time people can exercise without feeling fatigue or cramping.

7. **Increases the number of high density lipoproteins and decreases the number of low density lipoproteins.** High density lipoproteins (HDLs) carry cholesterol to the liver for breakdown and excretion. Low density lipoproteins (LDLs) carry cholesterol to body cells. Physical activities that promote cardiorespiratory endurance increase HDLs and decrease LDLs. This reduces the risk of developing cardiovascular diseases.

8. **Improves the function of the immune system.** If you have cardiorespiratory endurance, you may have fewer colds and upper respiratory infections. (Caution: Strenuous physical activity may depress the function of the immune system.)

9. **Protects against some types of cancer.** Physical activities that promote cardiorespiratory endurance speed the movement of food through the gastrointestinal tract. You are more likely to have daily bowel movements. This decreases your risk of developing colon cancer.

10. **Improves psychological well-being.** Physical activities that promote cardiorespiratory endurance cause beta-endorphins to be secreted into the bloodstream. Beta-endorphins are substances produced in the brain that create a feeling of well-being.

Q: How do I develop a cardiorespiratory endurance program?

A: Follow the FITT formula.

F—Frequency: Participate in physical activity three to five days a week. Start with three days and work up to five days. Training less than three days a week does not produce fitness benefits. Training more than five days a week can lead to injury and can stress your immune system.

I—Intensity: Perform physical activity at your target heart rate. **Target heart rate** is a heart rate of 75 percent of maximum heart rate. **Maximum heart rate** is 220 beats per minute minus a person's age.

T—Time: The length of time you perform physical activity will depend upon the intensity. As a general rule, continue to perform physical activity until you have used 1.8 calories for each pound you weigh. For example, you might walk 45–60 minutes at four miles (6.4 kilometers) per hour. However, your workout will require less time if you pick up your pace and run. For example, you might run briskly for 20–25 minutes.

T—Type: Choose aerobic activities, such as: aerobic dancing, backpacking, badminton, basketball, bench-stepping, bicycling, cross-country skiing, field hockey, handball, hiking, hockey, in-line skating, jogging, karate, lacrosse, racquetball, jumping rope, rowing, rugby, running, soccer, stairwalking, swimming, walking.

Q: Do I need to warm up and cool down when I participate in physical activities/exercise to improve cardiorespiratory endurance?

A: A **warm-up** is a period of three to five minutes of easy physical activity to prepare the muscles to do more work. As you warm up, more blood flows to active muscles. Your muscles work better when their temperature is slightly above resting level. As you warm up, synovial fluid spreads throughout the joints. Synovial fluid is fluid that lubricates and provides nutrition to the cells on the surface of joints. These body changes enhance performance and decrease the chances of injury.

A **cool-down** is a period of five to ten minutes of reduced physical activity to help the body return to a nonexercising state. As you cool down, your heart rate, breathing, and circulation return to normal. You may include stretching exercises during cool-down.

Q: How do I maintain cardiorespiratory endurance?

A: You will notice steady improvement for about four to six weeks when you begin a training program. You have to gradually increase intensity and time during training sessions to become more fit. The more fit you become, the more difficult it will be to make gains. When you reach an acceptable level of cardiorespiratory fitness, begin a maintenance program. Continue training at the same intensity on at least three nonconsecutive days of the week.

Q: What is a test to measure cardiorespiratory endurance?

A: The one-mile walk test is a test to measure cardiorespiratory fitness based on the amount of time it takes a person to complete one mile (1.6 kilometers) of brisk walking and his/her heart rate at the end of the walk. Age, gender, and body weight also are considered. A fast time and a low heart rate are desirable. This test is included in the Activity at the end of this lesson.

What to Know About Muscular Strength and Muscular Endurance

Q & A

Muscular strength is the maximum amount of force a muscle can produce in a single effort. Muscular endurance is the ability of the muscle to continue to perform without fatigue.

Q: What are the benefits of muscular strength and endurance?

A: Muscular strength and endurance:

1. Help you perform everyday tasks, such as carrying schoolbooks, climbing stairs, and lifting objects
2. Help you maintain correct posture
3. Reduce the risk of low back pain
4. Reduce the risks of being injured
5. Help you enjoy physical activities without tiring
6. Improve body composition by increasing muscle mass and decreasing fat tissue
7. Improve self-image because your muscles are firm and your body is toned
8. Keep bones dense and strong
9. Make the surfaces of joints less susceptible to injury

Q: How do I develop a conditioning program for muscular strength and endurance?

A: Your conditioning program should include resistance exercises. A **resistance exercise** is an exercise in which a force acts against muscles. To obtain resistance, you can lift your own weight, lift free weights, or work with weights on a weight machine. A **repetitions maximum** is the maximum amount of resistance that can be moved a specified number of times. **Repetitions** are the number of times an exercise is performed in one set. A set is a group of repetitions followed by a rest period. You build muscular strength by doing exercises only a few times. You build muscular endurance with less resistance and more repetitions.

Weight training is a conditioning program in which free weights or weight machines provide resistance for muscles. Isometric, isotonic, and isokinetic exercises are used for weight training. You can do isometric exercises, such as tightening abdominal muscles, using an immovable object, such as a wall, to provide resistance. You can use your body to do isotonic or isokinetic exercises, such as push-ups or sit-ups, to strengthen muscles. You can use a free weight to do isotonic and isokinetic exercises. A **free weight** is a barbell or dumbbell. A collar is a device that secures weights to a barbell or dumbbell. Weight machines also can be used for isotonic and isokinetic exercises. A **weight machine** is an apparatus that provides resistance to a muscle or group of muscles. Obtain the advice of a coach or trainer when beginning to use free weights or a weight machine.

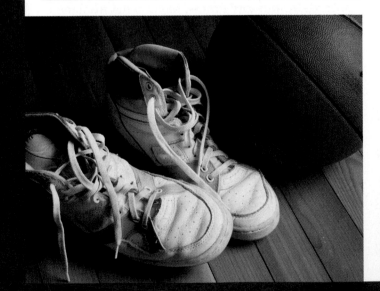

Follow the FITT formula.

F—Frequency: Train with weights two to four days a week. Schedule a day of rest between workouts.

I—Intensity: Keep a record of the amount of resistance and number of repetitions you do. Begin with a weight that you can move easily for 8–12 repetitions. Add more weight until you can do three sets of 10–12 repetitions. A heavy weight and a low number of repetitions (1–5) build muscular strength. A lighter weight and a high number of repetitions (20–25) build muscular endurance.

T—Time: Perform 8–12 repetitions of each exercise to build muscular strength and endurance. Perform at least one set of each exercise. Perform three sets for maximum fitness benefits.

T—Type: Choose exercises using your own body for resistance: abdominal crunch, bent arm hang, curl-up twist, dips, pull-ups, push-ups, side leg raises, sitting tuck, sit-ups, squats, stride jump. Choose exercises using free weights or weightmachines: bench press, bicep curl, decline press, flies, half squats, kickbacks, lateral pull-downs, lateral raises, leg curls, leg extensions, leg presses, seated overhead presses, seated rows, shrugs, squats, tricep extensions, tricep pull-downs.

Q: Do I need to warm up and cool down when I participate in a weight-conditioning program?

A: Before a weight-training session, warm-up by walking or easy jogging for three to five minutes. This prepares your muscles and joints for harder work. Warm up for different muscle groups before using free weights or weight machines. Do a set of 8–10 repetitions using a lot of lower weight resistance. For example, you may cut the weight resistance by half for your warm-up.

Cool down by walking or easy-jogging for five to ten minutes. Follow the cool-down with stretching exercises to prevent muscle soreness. (Also, consider stretching after completing the sets of repetitions you plan to do for each muscle group.)

Q: How do I maintain muscular strength and endurance?

A: You will improve rapidly during the first four to six weeks of training. After six weeks, you must evaluate your goals. Work with a trainer or coach to determine what you want to accomplish. Maintain muscular strength and endurance by continuing to train two to three days a week.

Q: What are tests to measure muscular strength and endurance?

A: Muscular strength is tested by measuring the maximum amount of weight a person can lift at one time. Muscular endurance is tested by counting the maximum amount of time a person can hold a muscular contraction or the maximum number of repetitions of a muscular contraction a person can do. Pull-ups also are used to measure muscular strengths and endurance. Pull-ups are included in the Activity at the end of this lesson.

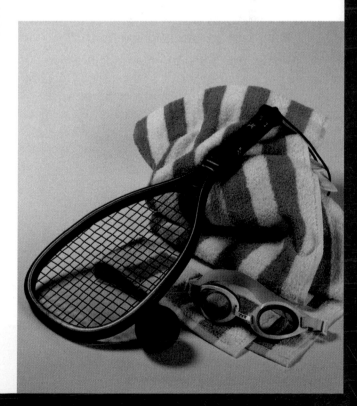

What to Know About
Flexibility

Q&A

Flexibility is the ability to bend and move the joints through the full range of motion.

Q: What are the benefits of flexibility?

A: Flexibility:

1. **Helps improve quality of life.** You can bend and move easily and without pain.
2. **Helps prevent and relieve symptoms associated with arthritis.**
3. **Helps prevent low-back pain.**
4. **Helps prevent injuries to muscles and joints.**
5. **Decreases the likelihood of having accidents, such as falls.**
6. **Improves performance in sports, such as golf and tennis, in which a range of motion is required.**

Q: Do I need to warm up and cool down when I do stretching exercises?

A: Warm up by walking or easy-jogging for three to five minutes. This increases blood flow to muscles to get them ready for more work. Begin gradually with slow stretches. Finish your workout with a cool-down period. Walking and easy jogging improve circulation. Easy stretches keep you from being sore.

Q: How do I develop flexibility?

A: Follow the FITT formula.

F—Frequency: Perform stretching exercises two to three times a week and as part of your cool-down for weight training.

I—Intensity: Hold each stretch for 15–30 seconds. Rest for 30–60 seconds between each stretch. Repeat each stretching exercise three to five times.

T—Time: Include exercises to stretch the muscles that work each of the major joints in the body. This will probably take you 15–30 minutes.

T—Type: Two techniques for stretching muscles that move joints are static stretching and ballistic stretching. **Static stretching** is stretching the muscle to a point where a pull is felt and holding the stretch for 15–30 seconds. Static stretching is safe and effective. **Ballistic stretching** is rapidly stretching the muscle with a bouncing movement. Fitness experts warn against ballistic stretching as it may cause injuries. Use free weights and weight machines to do stretching exercises for flexibility. Or, do stretching exercises on your own, such as: across-the-body, ankle flex, calf stretcher, lateral stretch, side launch, sit and reach, spine twist, step stretch, towel stretch, and upper back stretch.

Q: What test is used to measure flexibility?

A: There are a number of tests used to measure flexibility. The V-sit reach test assesses flexibility by measuring how far you can lean forward. The V-sit reach test is included in the Activity at the end of this lesson.

What to Know About
Healthful Body Composition

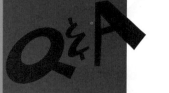

Healthful body composition is a high ratio of lean tissue to fat tissue in the body. **Overfat** is having a percentage of body fat that is not within a healthful range.

Q: What are the benefits of healthful body composition?

A: Healthful body composition:

1. Reduces the risk of obesity,
2. Reduces the risk of coronary heart disease,
3. Reduces the risk of developing diabetes,
4. Reduces the risk of developing high blood pressure,
5. Reduces the risk of having a stroke,
6. Improves appearance and self-image.

Percent Body Fat and Health Status

Percent Body Fat		Health Status
Males	Females	
5–10	8–15	Optimal Health
11–17	16–24	Healthful
18–25	25–32	Overfat
Over 25	Over 32	Obese

Q: Do I need to warm up and cool down when I participate in physical activities to develop and maintain healthful body composition?

A: You are performing the same physical activities used to develop cardiorespiratory endurance. Follow the same guidelines and warm up and cool down. Your warm-up should include three to five minutes of easy physical activity. Your cool-down should include five to ten minutes of reduced physical activity. You may include stretching exercises during cool-down.

Q: What are tests to measure my percentage of body fat?

A: One test uses calipers to measure the thickness of skinfolds. A more accurate test involves underwater weighing. To quickly determine if you have too much body fat, pinch a fold of skin on your upper arm. Estimate the thickness. You may have an excess of body fat if you pinch more than one inch (2.5 centimeters).

Q: How do I develop a program to develop and maintain a healthful body composition?

A: Eat a healthful diet and participate in physical activities to promote cardiorespiratory endurance. Follow the FITT formula.

F—Frequency: Participate in physical activity three to five days a week.

I—Intensity: Perform physical activity at your target heart rate.

T—Time: The length of time you perform physical activity will depend upon the intensity. As a general rule, continue to perform physical activity until you have used 1.8 calories for each pound you weigh.

T—Type: Choose aerobic activities, such as: aerobic dancing, backpacking, badminton, basketball, bench-stepping, bicycling, cross-country skiing, field hockey, handball, hiking, hockey, in-line skating, jogging, karate, lacrosse, racquetball, jumping rope, rowing, rugby, running, soccer, stairwalking, swimming, walking.

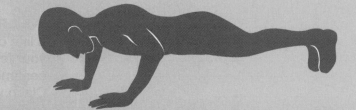

Males

Age	One-Mile Run (minutes/seconds)	Pull-Ups (number)	Curl-Ups (number)	V-Sit Reach (inches)
12	8:40	2	40	1.0
13	8:06	3	42	.5
14	7:44	5	45	1.0
15	7:30	6	45	2.0
16	7:10	7	45	3.0
17	7:04	8	44	3.0

Females

Age	One-Mile Run (minutes/seconds)	Pull-Ups (number)	Curl-Ups (number)	V-Sit Reach (inches)
12	11:05	1	35	3.5
13	10:23	1	37	3.5
14	10:06	1	37	4.5
15	9:58	1	36	5.0
16	10:31	1	35	5.5
17	10:22	1	34	4.5

Lesson 46

Review

Vocabulary Words

Write a separate sentence using each of the vocabulary words listed on page 358.

Objectives

1. What are five kinds of exercises?
   Objective 1

2. How can you develop cardiorespiratory endurance using the FITT formula?
   Objective 2

3. How can you develop muscular strength and endurance using the FITT formula?
   Objective 3

4. How can you develop flexibility using the FITT formula? **Objective 4**

5. How can you develop a healthful body composition using the FITT formula?
   Objective 5

Responsible Decision-Making

You have begun a weight-training program to improve muscular strength and reduce your percentage of body fat. Some teens from another school work out at the same place you do. They tell you they use steroids and suggest that you should use them too. Write a response to this situation.

1. Describe the situation that requires you to make a decision.
2. List possible decisions you might make.
3. Name two responsible adults with whom you might discuss your decisions.
4. Evaluate the possible consequences of your decisions. Determine if each decision will lead to actions that:
   - promote health,
   - protect safety,
   - follow laws,
   - show respect for yourself and others,
   - follow the guidelines of your parents and of other responsible adults,
   - demonstrate good character.
5. Decide which decision is most responsible and appropriate.
6. Tell two results you expect if you make this decision.

Effective Communication

Design a logo that might be used to represent the FITT formula.

Self-Directed Learning

Your target heart rate is a heart rate of 75 percent of your maximum heart rate. Your maximum heart rate is 220 beats minus your age. Compute your target heart rate.

Critical Thinking

You see an advertisement on television for a new piece of fitness equipment. The people demonstrating the equipment are very muscular and look fit. They say you can look like them in a few months if you use this piece of equipment. Write a short essay evaluating the ad. Do you think the information in the ad is reliable? Can the results described actually occur? Do you think the people in the ad are muscular and fit because they use the equipment?

Responsible Citizenship

Work with members of your family to make a list titled "Ten Physical Activities Our Family Can Enjoy Together to Become Fit."

You Can Develop Skill-Related Fitness

Life Skill **I will develop and maintain skill-related fitness.**

Physical fitness is the ability to perform physical activity and to meet the demands of daily living while being energetic and alert. Physical fitness is grouped into health-related fitness and skill-related fitness. Lesson 46 discussed health-related fitness. This lesson discusses the components of skill-related fitness. You will learn about fitness skills. This lesson also includes A Guide to Lifetime Sports and Physical Activities. This Guide will help you choose sports and physical activities to develop health-related fitness and skill-related fitness.

The Lesson Outline

What to Know About Skill-Related Fitness

What to Know About Lifetime Sports and Physical Activities

Objectives

1. List and discuss six fitness skills. **page 371**
2. Discuss the health-related and skill-related fitness benefits for these lifetime sports and physical activities: basketball, cross-country skiing, golf, in-line skating, martial arts, mountain biking, rock climbing and wall climbing, running and jogging, swimming, and walking. **pages 372–376**

Vocabulary Words

physical fitness

skill-related fitness

fitness skills

agility

balance

coordination

hand-eye coordination

reaction time

speed

power

lifetime sports and physical activities

What to Know About
Skill-Related Fitness

Skill-related fitness is the capacity to perform well in sports and physical activities. **Fitness skills** are skills that can be used in sports and physical activities. There are six fitness skills: agility, balance, coordination, reaction time, speed, and power. Heredity is an important influence on these fitness skills. However, most fitness skills can be developed and improved.

Agility is the ability to rapidly change the position of the body. Physical activities in which you change directions quickly require agility. For example, you need agility to change directions to hit a tennis ball. You need agility to make a jump shot when playing basketball.

Balance is the ability to keep from falling when a person is in a still position or moving. You need balance to keep from falling if you ski down a mountain slope or if you ride a bicycle. If you participate in gymnastics, you need balance to keep from falling off the balance beam. You need balance if you in-line skate.

Coordination is the ability to use the senses together with body parts during movement. For example, you may have heard the term hand-eye coordination. **Hand-eye coordination** is the use of the hands together with the eyes during movement. Suppose you are going to hit a tennis ball. You keep your eyes on the ball as you swing the racket with your hands. Suppose you play baseball and are the batter. You keep your eyes on the ball and swing the bat at the ball with your hands. Without hand-eye coordination, you would have difficulty playing sports such as tennis and baseball. There are other examples of coordination. Suppose you want to kick a soccer ball or a football. You would need foot-eye coordination. Your eyes must focus on the ball as you move your foot toward it to kick it.

Reaction time is the time it takes a person to move after (s)he hears, sees, feels, or touches a stimulus. The less time that elapses, the quicker your reaction time. Suppose a person is throwing a ball to you. The time it takes you to get into position to catch the ball is your reaction time. Suppose you are in the starting block for a race. A starting signal sounds for the race to begin. The time it takes you to begin to push off out of the starting block is your reaction time.

Speed is the ability to move quickly. Suppose you are playing basketball and have just grabbed a rebound under your opponent's basket. You use speed to dribble the length of the court to your team's basket. Or, suppose you are playing tennis and your opponent hits a drop shot close to the net. You need speed to get to the ball before it bounces twice. Many sports and physical activities require speed. You must run fast when you play soccer, football, lacrosse, and baseball.

Power is the ability to combine strength and speed. To throw a discus far requires power. If you are playing baseball, power is required to throw a fastball. If you make a high jump, you need power to lift your body high into the air.

What to Know About Lifetime Sports and Physical Activities

Lifetime sports and physical activities are sports and physical activities in which a person can participate throughout his/her life. There are many advantages to participating in lifetime sports and physical activities. Lifetime sports and physical activities often become long-lasting habits that ensure you will be physically active throughout your life. Participating in different lifetime sports and physical activities can help you improve different areas of physical fitness and different fitness skills. Social interaction with friends and family members is another important benefit of lifetime sports and physical activities. On the following pages is A Guide to Lifetime Sports and Physical Activities. Review this guide to learn more about the benefits of several lifetime sports and physical activities.

A Guide to Lifetime Sports and Physical Activities

Basketball

Basketball is a game that involves tossing an inflated ball through a raised basket. It usually is played between two teams of five players on a hard surface such as concrete, asphalt, or hardwood. Players must dribble, or bounce, the ball with their hands when they move with the ball. A player scores by successfully shooting the ball through the basket. Basketball is scored by keeping track of the number of successful shots each team makes. Variations of basketball called "pick-up" games can be played with fewer players. Playing basketball improves cardiorespiratory endurance and muscular endurance. Learning how to dribble, shoot, and pass the ball improves agility, balance, and coordination. When you play basketball, you burn between 500 and 600 calories per hour. Common basketball injuries include sprained ankles, sprained knees, and eye injuries. Avoid basketball injuries by wearing protective equipment such as a mouthguard, eye protection, and elbow and knee pads. Stretching and warming up before playing is another way to prevent injuries.

Cross-Country Skiing

Cross-country skiing is gliding over snow using specialized cross-country skis and poles. The skier uses the poles and the skis to push forward on the snow and to maintain balance. You can cross-country ski almost anywhere there is snow. Some golf courses and parks have cross-country ski trails during the winter. Cross-country skiing equipment includes skis, poles, boots, safety equipment, and the proper clothing. Your clothing depends on the climate and the difficulty of the terrain. In a cold and snowy climate, wear a hat, gloves, a waterproof and windproof jacket and pants, thermal underwear, insulated socks, and goggles or sunglasses.

Cross-country skiing helps maintain and improve fitness. The leg and arm movements involved in cross-country skiing improve muscular endurance and cardiorespiratory endurance. Depending on the difficulty of the terrain, cross-country skiing also improves balance, coordination, power, and reaction time. When you cross-country ski, you burn between 700 and 800 calories per hour. This activity reduces your percentage of body fat.

Safety is important when cross-country skiing. Be aware of natural dangers such as avalanches, freezing temperatures, and UV radiation from the sun. Know your physical abilities, skill level, and limitations. Know how to prevent and treat illnesses and injuries, such as hypothermia, frostbite, pulled muscles, and broken bones.

Golf

Golf involves using a club to hit a small, hard ball into a hole or cup. Golf is played on a course that has 9 or 18 holes. The distance to each hole may vary as well as the degree of difficulty. Golf is scored by keeping track of the number of strokes it takes to get the ball into each hole. A handicap system allows players with different levels of skill to play with one another. To play golf, you need golf clubs, golf balls, and tees. Most public golf courses rent golf clubs for a small fee. Many courses also require that you wear special shoes.

When you play golf you have two options: you can walk or ride in a golf cart. Walking the length of a golf course improves cardiorespiratory endurance. You burn close to 1,060 calories when you walk an 18-hole round of golf. Riding in a cart is less strenuous and burns much fewer calories. Hitting the ball also has fitness benefits. Learning how to hit the ball can improve balance, coordination, and power. The repeated swinging motion you use in a round of golf also improves your muscular endurance. To avoid injuries, always stretch before playing golf.

A Guide to Lifetime Sports and Physical Activities

In-Line Skating

In-line skating involves moving over asphalt, concrete, or other hard surfaces wearing in-line skates. In-line skating uses a motion similar to skiing and ice skating. You swing your arms back and forth as you push yourself forward on your skates. Bending your knees gives your legs a harder workout. Equipment for in-line skating includes skates, helmet, and knee and elbow pads. Several sports have developed out of in-line skating, such as in-line hockey and in-line speed skating.

In-line skating provides a vigorous cardiorespiratory workout in which you burn between 350 and 550 calories per hour. The wide range of movements improve muscular strength and muscular endurance and promote agility, balance, coordination, and power. Safety is an important factor of in-line skating. To in-line skate, you need to use the proper equipment and follow specific safety rules. The International In-Line Skating Association developed safety rules that can help protect you from potential injury. Also, remember to carry a water bottle to avoid dehydration and heat exhaustion.

Martial Arts

Martial arts are any of several methods of self-defense and combat developed in eastern Asia. Martial arts include karate, tae kwon do, judo, tai chi, and sumo. Training for martial arts includes physical, psychological, and emotional preparations. The physical preparations include stretching, running, practicing, and sparring. The psychological and emotional preparations vary. Martial arts usually do not require much equipment. For example, most dojos (centers for studying karate) require students to wear a white jacket and pants known as a karate-gi. The students also must wear a colored belt that designates their skill level. Students often wear padded gloves and mouthguards for protection.

Different martial arts promote different levels of physical fitness and fitness skills. Karate training combines vigorous cardiorespiratory workouts with skill training. The different movements involved in karate training improve agility, coordination, and reaction time. Most martial arts involve substantial physical contact resulting in frequent shoulder, elbow, and wrist injuries. Broken toes and fingers also are common. To avoid serious injuries, wear protective equipment and follow safety guidelines.

Rock Climbing and Wall Climbing

Rock climbing is scaling rocks or cliffs. Wall climbing is scaling indoor or outdoor walls that are made to resemble rocks and cliffs. To rock climb and wall climb, you need proper equipment, such as ropes, harnesses, protective equipment, and other specialized devices. Wear a safety helmet designed for these sports to prevent serious injuries.

When you climb a wall or rock, you use your arms to pull yourself up and to maintain your position. This improves muscular strength and muscular endurance. Agility, coordination, and reaction time are important in rock climbing and wall climbing because each move requires viewing the terrain, analyzing it, and using your abilities to climb it. When you rock climb and wall climb, you burn almost 600 calories per hour. Safety is always a concern when rock climbing and wall climbing. To avoid injuries and accidents, you should receive proper instruction and know the safety rules.

Mountain Biking

Mountain biking is riding an all-terrain bicycle, or mountain bike, on mountains or off-road trails. For mountain biking, you need a mountain bike and protective equipment. When you mountain bike you must wear a helmet. Buying mountain biking equipment can be an expensive investment. Rent and try out a bike before you commit to buying one.

The pedaling motion of mountain biking promotes muscular endurance, muscular strength, and cardiorespiratory endurance. Balance, coordination, and reaction time are important as you face steep trails and obstacles. To avoid injuries and accidents, you need to maintain control of your mountain bike, use proper equipment, and keep a watchful eye on other bikers.

Running and Jogging

Running is moving on foot at a moderate to fast pace. Jogging is running slowly at a pace of about 9 to 12 minutes per mile. When you begin running or jogging, do not overexert yourself. Start at a slow or conversational pace. As you improve, your speed and distance will improve. Shoes are the most important piece of equipment for runners and joggers. When you buy new running or jogging shoes, consider your body size, running style, skill level, and the comfort and shock absorption of the shoes.

Running and jogging improve health-related fitness. They improve cardiorespiratory endurance and also help reduce body fat and cholesterol levels. When you run at 12 miles (19.2 kilometers) per hour, you burn almost 1,500 calories per hour. When you jog at a moderate pace, you burn between 500 and 750 calories per hour. Running on hills or other inclines can triple the calories you burn depending on the incline. Watch out for injuries such as pulled muscles, tendonitis, and shin splints, that result from overuse of muscles. To avoid these and other types of injuries, you should always follow training principles. Carry a water bottle when you run or jog to avoid dehydration and heat exhaustion.

Lesson 48 will include more information about training principles.

How to Prevent, Recognize, and Treat Physical Activity-Related Injuries

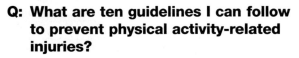

Q: What are ten guidelines I can follow to prevent physical activity-related injuries?

A: Follow these guidelines:

1. Have a medical examination before you begin vigorous physical activity or participate in a sport.

2. Participate in physical activities and sports with appropriate adult supervision.

3. Obtain appropriate instruction.

4. Develop and maintain proper conditioning. The diagram of the Fitness Training Zone illustrates the importance of proper progression.

5. Know and follow safety guidelines.

6. Review basic first aid procedures and CPR.

7. Practice precautions to prevent the spread of bloodborne pathogens.

8. Wear protective clothing and select equipment carefully.

   • Wear footwear appropriate for the activity.

   • Wear acrylic rather than cotton socks.

   • Wear a safety helmet, face mask, mouthguard, and protective pads.

   • Wear reflective clothing for walking, running, and bicycling.

   • Wear an athletic supporter and cup.

   • Wear an athletic bra when appropriate.

9. Do not participate in physical activities or sports when you have unhealed injuries.

10. Follow precautions for extreme weather conditions.

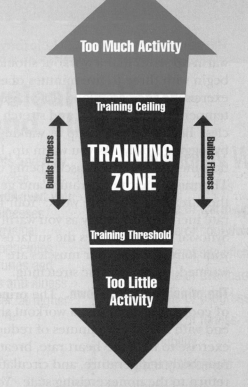

The **training threshold** is the minimum amount of overload required to obtain fitness benefits. Workouts below the training threshold do not provide fitness benefits. The **training zone** is the range of overload required to obtain fitness benefits. The **training ceiling** is the upper limit of overload required to obtain fitness benefits without risking injury or illness. Workouts that go beyond the training ceiling are dangerous to health.

Q: What is the RICE treatment?

A: The **RICE treatment** is a technique for treating musculoskeletal injuries that involves rest, compression, and elevation.

Lesson 100 will include more information about the RICE treatment.

Q: What are ten physical activity-related injuries I can avoid?

A: The ten physical activity-related injuries you can avoid are as follows:

- An overuse injury is an injury that occurs from repeated use or excessive overload. If you do too much, too fast, you may develop an overuse injury.

- A microtrauma is an injury that is not recognized or becomes worse as a person continues to workout. Microtraumas are so small that they do not show up on X-rays or during superficial examinations.

- A bruise is a discoloration of the skin caused by bleeding under the skin. Apply ice to reduce bleeding and swelling.

- A muscle cramp is the sudden tightening of a muscle. Sharp pains may signal muscle cramps. Muscle cramps can occur in any muscle. They often are caused by fatigue and dehydration. Taking precautions when exercising in hot weather and static stretching help prevent muscle cramps. Should they occur, drink plenty of fluids. Gently massage muscles that cramp.

- A muscle strain is the overstretching of a muscle that may result in tearing of a muscle or tendon. A warm-up of walking, easy jogging, and static stretching helps prevent muscle strain. Use the RICE treatment if muscle strain occurs.

- A shin splint is an overuse injury that results in pain in the front and sides of the lower leg. There may be tenderness over the shin and some swelling. To prevent shin splints, wear proper footwear and run on even surfaces. Begin your workout with static stretching of the muscles of the front of the lower leg. In most cases, shin splints clear up after a week or two of rest. Ice can be applied four times a day for 20 minutes. Check with a physician before taking aspirin or other drugs to reduce pain and inflammation.

- A side stitch is a dull, sharp pain in the side of the lower abdomen. To prevent side stitch, warm-up and follow the FITT formula. Plan your workout with appropriate frequency, intensity, and time. To relieve side stitch, bend forward while pressing your hand firmly at the point of the pain.

- A sprain is the partial or complete tearing of a ligament. A ligament is a tough fiber that connects together bones. Sprains occur from injuries in which the tissue around a joint is twisted. To prevent sprains, select shoes carefully. High-top athletic shoes can be worn to support ankles. Talk to a trainer about taping weak ankles or wearing an ankle or knee brace for extra support. Use the RICE treatment if sprain occurs.

- A stress fracture is a hairline break that results from repetitive jarring of a bone. A stress fracture usually is an overuse injury. Stress fractures can be serious. A stress fracture can be a microtrauma. It may not be detected on an X-ray or during superficial examination. To prevent stress fractures, pay attention to the FITT formula and do not overdo. The treatment for stress fractures depends on the severity and the area that is affected. Rest is important.

- Tendonitis is inflammation of a tendon. A tendon is tough tissue fiber that attaches muscles to bones. Pain and swelling occur in joints. When tendonitis is in the elbow, it is called tennis elbow. Other joints affected by tendonitis are the knees, shoulders, and backs of ankles. To prevent tendonitis, warm-up with static stretching. Choose exercises to develop muscle strength. Use the RICE treatment when tendonitis occurs. It may take as long as a month for tendonitis to heal. Check with a physician before taking aspirin or other drugs to relieve pain and inflammation.

If You Participate in Physical Activity During Extreme Weather Conditions

Q&A

Q: What precautions should I take if I work out in cold weather?

A: **Cold-temperature-related illnesses** are conditions that result from exposure to low temperatures. When you work out in very cold weather, you must protect against frostbite and hypothermia. **Frostbite** is the freezing of body parts, often the tissues of the extremities. Signs of frostbite include numbness in the affected area, waxy appearance of skin, and skin that is cold to touch and discolored. **Hypothermia** is a reduction in the body temperature so that it is lower than normal. Hypothermia results from overexposure to cool temperatures, cold water, moisture, and wind. People with hypothermia will shiver and feel cold. The pulse rate slows down and becomes irregular as the temperature drops. A person can become unconscious and die without treatment.

To prevent cold-temperature-related illnesses:

1. **Check the wind-chill before exercising in cold weather.**

2. **Postpone exercise if the wind-chill puts health status at risk.**

3. **Postpone exercise if it is icy and wet.**

4. **Wear several layers of lightweight clothing.** Dressing too warmly causes sweating that can cause chilling. The first layer of clothing should be made of polypropylene or thermax, which takes moisture away from the skin. Over this layer, wear a layer of dacron or fleeced polyester, which serves as a good insulator. The top layer should be a windbreaker of waterproof material that keeps out moisture but allows perspiration to filter out.

5. **Wear gloves, a hat, and ski mask to protect the fingers, ears, and nose.**

6. **Wear two pairs of socks or thermal socks to protect the toes.**

To determine wind chill, find the outside air temperature on the top row. Then read down the left-hand column to the measured wind speed. This is measured in MPH (miles per hour). The wind chill is the number in the box where these meet.

Wind Chill Temperatures

Wind Speed MPH	\multicolumn{19}{c}{Temperature (°F)}
	45	40	35	30	25	20	15	10	5	0	-5	-10	-15	-20	-25	-30	-35	-40	-45
0	45	40	35	30	25	20	15	10	5	0	-5	-10	-15	-20	-25	-30	-35	-40	-45
5	43	37	32	27	22	16	11	6	1	-5	-10	-16	-21	-26	-31	-37	-42	-47	-53
10	34	28	22	16	10	4	-3	-9	-15	-22	-28	-34	-40	-46	-52	-59	-65	-71	-77
15	29	22	16	9	6	-5	-12	-19	-25	-32	-39	-45	-52	-59	-66	-72	-79	-86	-93
20	25	18	11	4	-3	-11	-18	-25	-32	-39	-47	-54	-61	-68	-75	-82	-89	-96	-104
25	23	15	8	1	-7	-15	-22	-30	-37	-45	-52	-60	-67	-74	-82	-89	-97	-104	-112
30	21	13	6	-3	-11	-18	-26	-33	-41	-49	-56	-64	-72	-79	-87	-95	-102	-110	-117
35	19	11	4	-5	-13	-20	-28	-36	-44	-52	-59	-67	-75	-83	-91	-98	-106	-114	-122
40	18	10	3	-6	-14	-22	-30	-38	-46	-54	-61	-69	-77	-85	-93	-101	-109	-117	-124
45	17	9	2	-7	-15	-23	-31	-39	-47	-55	-63	-71	-79	-87	-95	-103	-111	-119	-127

Little Danger

Increasing Danger (where flesh may freeze within one minute)

Great Danger (where flesh may freeze within 30 seconds)

Q: What precautions should I take if I work out in hot weather?

A: **Heat-related illnesses** are conditions that result from exposure to temperatures higher than normal. When you work out during hot weather, you must protect against heat cramps, heat exhaustion, and heat stroke. **Heat cramps** are painful muscle spasms in the legs and arms due to excessive fluid loss through sweating. **Heat exhaustion** is extreme tiredness due to the body's inability to regulate its temperature. Signs of heat exhaustion include a very low body temperature; cool, moist, pale, and red skin; nausea and headache; dizziness and weakness; and fast pulse.

Heat stroke is an overheating of the body that is life-threatening. Sweating ceases so that the body cannot regulate its temperature. Signs of heat stroke include high body temperature; rapid pulse; rapid respiration; hot, wet, and dry skin; weakness; dizziness; and headache.

Lesson 100 will include more information about first aid procedures for heat cramps, heat exhaustion, and heat stroke.

To prevent heat-related illnesses:

1. Check the heat index before exercising in hot weather.
2. Postpone exercise if the heat index puts health status at risk.
3. Plan your workout at the time of day when the temperature is lowest.
4. Drink plenty of fluids before and during your workout.
5. Avoid vigorous workouts on extremely hot and humid days.
6. Wear porous clothing that allows air to pass through it.
7. Wear light colored clothing that reflects the sun.
8. Avoid wearing rubberized and plastic clothing. They trap heat and perspiration. They cause fluid loss and increased body temperature.
9. Wear a hat, sunglasses, and sunscreen.

To determine heat index, find the dew point on the top row. Dew point is the measure of moisture in the atmosphere. Then read down the left-hand column to the measured temperature. The heat index is the number in the box where these meet.

Heat Index

Temperature (°F)	Dew Point (°F) 50.0	55.0	60.0	65.0	70.0	75.0	80.0	85.0
65:	62.7	63.8	65.0	66.6				
70:	67.8	68.7	69.8	71.1	72.6			
75:	73.1	73.9	74.8	75.9	79.2	80.7		
80:	79.8	80.6	81.6	82.8	84.4	86.9	90.9	
85:	83.5	84.7	86.1	88.0	90.5	94.0	99.0	106.6
90:	87.9	89.4	91.2	93.6	96.9	101.2	107.2	115.6
95:	92.9	94.5	96.7	99.6	103.4	108.4	115.2	124.3
100:	98.1	99.9	102.4	105.6	109.8	115.3	122.7	132.3
105:	103.4	105.4	108.1	111.6	116.1	122.0	129.7	139.7
110:	108.7	110.9	113.8	117.5	122.3	128.4	136.3	146.5

Comfortable

Extreme

Hazardous

Dangerous

Q: How does air pollution affect my workouts?

A: Air pollution influences the safety and effectiveness of workouts. When air is polluted, you have to breath more often to deliver oxygen to body cells. Air pollution can cause shortness of breath. The media issues warnings when the PSI is high. The **pollution standard index (PSI)** is a measure of air quality based on the sum of the levels of five different pollutants. It is best not to work out outdoors when the PSI is high.

Q: How will being in a high altitude affect my workouts?

A: Being in a high altitude places extra demands on the body. Think of the extra demands of the high altitude as being a form of overload. Your body must adjust to these extra demands. Shorten the length of your workouts at first. For example, if you take a trip to the mountains to snow ski avoid hard skiing for the first two days. People who work out too much at first may develop altitude sickness. Signs of altitude sickness are shortness of breath, chest pain, and nausea.

Activity

Rate Your Athletic Shoes

Life Skill: I will prevent physical activity-related injuries and illnesses.

Materials: pencil and paper; list of questions; athletic socks

Directions: Rate your athletic shoes before you buy them. On a separate sheet of paper, copy the chart. Visit a store that sells athletic shoes and try on two pairs. Fill out a chart for each pair. Write the brand name of each pair in the chart. Check YES or NO for each question. Write a paragraph explaining which pair of shoes you would buy and why. DO NOT WRITE IN THIS BOOK.

Brand of Athletic Shoe: _____

Questions to Rate the Athletic Shoe	YES	NO
Is there adequate cushioning for shock absorption under the ball of my foot?		
Does the heel feel snug next to my foot?		
Is the heel slightly elevated to lessen strain on the back of my legs?		
Is there just enough room in the shoe to wiggle my toes?		
Is there about half an inch from my longest toe to the tip of the shoe?		
Is the tongue and upper shoe well padded and designed to stay in place?		
Does the sole of the shoe flex and bend too easily?		
Is the shoe designed to allow moisture and perspiration to escape?		
Does the shoe provide good traction so I will not slide or slip and fall?		
Does the shoe appeal to me?		

Lesson 48

Review

Vocabulary Words

Write a separate sentence using each of the vocabulary words listed on page 378.

Objectives

1. How do warm-up, cool-down, specificity, overload, progression, and fitness reversibility help you obtain maximum fitness benefits? **Objective 1**

2. What are ten guidelines to follow to prevent physical activity-related injuries? **Objective 2**

3. What is the Training Fitness Zone? **Objective 3**

4. What are ten common physical activity-related injuries? **Objective 4**

5. What precautions can you take to prevent cold-temperature-related illnesses when you work out? Heat-related illnesses? Altitude sickness? Shortness of breath from air pollution? **Objective 5**

Responsible Decision-Making

You wake up on Saturday with very sore muscles from yesterday's volleyball practice. Team tryouts are Monday. Some friends urge you to come with them now to practice. You want to practice, but your muscles are aching. Your friends tell you that what you need is a couple of hours of serious volleyball to get rid of the soreness. Write a response to this situation.

1. Describe the situation that requires you to make a decision.
2. List possible decisions you might make.
3. Name two responsible adults with whom you might discuss your decisions.
4. Evaluate the possible consequences of your decisions. Determine if each decision will lead to actions that:
   - promote health,
   - protect safety,
   - follow laws,
   - show respect for yourself and others,
   - follow the guidelines of your parents and of other responsible adults,
   - demonstrate good character.
5. Decide which decision is most responsible and appropriate.
6. Tell two results you expect if you make this decision.

 Effective Communication

Make a poster that shows how to dress properly for exercise in cold weather. Indicate the best types of material to wear and how to protect the nose, ears, fingers, and toes.

 Self-Directed Learning

Arrange an interview with your school's athletic trainer. Ask the following questions: What injuries do you see most often? What can students do to prevent these injuries? How do you treat these injuries?

 Critical Thinking

Your friend is on the wrestling team. To lose the pounds (s)he must in order to "make weight," (s)he has begun to run in a rubberized sweat suit. What are the health risks associated with wearing a rubberized sweat suit for vigorous physical activity? What would you say to your friend?

 Responsible Citizenship

Fluid intake is very important in athletic competitions. Volunteer to make water or sport drinks available to athletes during competition. You also may volunteer to work locations during a race or during track practice to monitor the safety and well-being of the athletes.

Lesson 49

You Can Follow a Physical Fitness Plan

Life Skill I will follow a physical fitness plan.

Physical fitness is the ability to perform physical activity and to meet the demands of daily living while being energetic and alert. To become physically fit, you must participate in physical activities that develop each of the components of health-related and skill-related fitness. A **physical fitness plan** is a written plan of physical activities to develop each of the components of fitness and a schedule for doing them. This lesson outlines six steps to follow when you design an individualized plan for health-related fitness. You will learn ten ways to stay motivated after you make your plan. This lesson includes a sample health behavior contract for health-related fitness. You can individualize this health behavior contract for your use.

The Lesson Outline
How to Design a Physical Fitness Plan
How to Follow a Physical FITT-ness Plan

Objectives
1. Outline six steps to follow to design an individualized plan for health-related fitness. **page 387**
2. List the four parts of the FITT formula. **page 387**
3. Identify ten ways to stay motivated to follow a physical fitness plan. **page 387**
4. Design and follow a health behavior contract to develop health-related fitness. **page 388**

Vocabulary Words
physical fitness
physical fitness plan
FITT formula

How to Design a Physical Fitness Plan

You should work to develop both health-related and skill-related fitness. There are six steps to follow when you design an individualized plan for health-related fitness.

1. **Design a physical fitness plan in the form of a health behavior contract.** The life skill you want to follow is "I will follow a physical fitness plan." Examine the sample health behavior contract on the next page.

2. **Use the FITT formula.** The **FITT formula** is a formula in which each letter represents a factor for determining how to obtain fitness benefits from physical activity: F-Frequency, I-Intensity, T-Time, and T-Type.

3. **Include a warm-up and cool-down.** A warm-up consists of three to five minutes of easy physical activity to prepare the muscles to do more work. A cool-down consists of five to ten minutes of reduced physical activity to help the body return to the nonexercising state. A warm-up and cool-down reduce the risk of physical activity-related injuries.

4. **Include aerobic exercises to develop cardiorespiratory endurance and a healthful body composition.** Aerobic exercises must be performed three to five days a week at your target heart rate. You must use 1.8 calories for each pound of your body weight. This helps you calculate how long you must work out.

5. **Include resistance exercises to develop muscular strength and muscular endurance.** Lift your own weight, lift free weights, or work with weights on a weight machine. Resistance exercises should be performed two to four days a week with a day of rest in between each workout. Record on a card the amount of resistance and the repetitions you do. Increase resistance gradually. Perform three sets of 8–12 repetitions of each exercise with free weights or weight machines. Perform additional exercises when using your body for resistance, such as when doing push-ups or sit-ups.

6. **Include static stretching exercises to develop flexibility.** Perform static stretching exercises two to three days a week. Hold each stretch for 30 seconds. Rest for 30–60 seconds between stretches. Repeat each stretch three to five times. Your flexibility workout should last for 15–30 minutes. Also include static stretching exercises as part of your warm-up and cool-down to reduce the risk of injuries.

Top Ten List of Ways to Stay Motivated to Follow a Physical Fitness Plan

1. Select a variety of physical activities.
2. Work out with a friend.
3. Work out with family members.
4. Reward yourself when you reach goals.
5. Record your progress so you can feel a sense of accomplishment.
6. Listen to energetic music while you work out.
7. Have a backup plan for bad weather.
8. Organize your day so it is easy to work out.
9. Join a sports club or team.
10. Take lessons to improve a fitness skill.

How to Follow a Physical FITT-ness Plan

The health behavior contract below is based on the FITT formula. Copy and complete the following health behavior contract. **DO NOT WRITE IN THIS BOOK.**

Health Behavior Contract

 1. **Name**_____ **Date**_____

2. **Life Skill:** I will follow a physical fitness plan.

3. **Effects on Health Status:** Regular physical activity: reduces the risk of premature death; reduces the risk of developing some cancers and non-insulin-dependent diabetes mellitus; reduces feelings of depression; helps control weight; helps build and maintain healthy bones, muscles and joints; helps older adults become stronger and better able to move about without falling; promotes psychological well-being.

 4. **Plan and Method to Record Progress:** I will complete the chart below. I will circle the days of the week I will perform exercises. I will determine my target heart rate. I will calculate the number of calories I need to use during aerobic exercises. I will select the types of exercises I want to do to develop each health-related fitness component. I will include a warm-up and a cool-down.

FITT Formula	Cardiorespiratory Endurance Body Composition	Muscular Strength Muscular Endurance	Flexibility
Frequency	• 3–5 days a week M T W Th F S S	• 2–4 days a week • A day of rest in between M T W Th F S S	• 2–3 days a week • During warm-up and cool-down M T W Th F S S
Intensity	• I must perform at my target heart rate. • My target heart rate is _____.	• I will attach a card to record the amount of resistance and number of repetitions I do.	• I will hold each stretch for 30 seconds. • I will rest 30–60 seconds between stretches. • I will repeat each stretch 3–5 times.
Time	• I will use 1.8 calories for each pound of my body weight. • I will use _____ calories.	• I will perform three sets of 8–12 repetitions of each exercise.	• 15–30 minutes
Type	• I will choose the following aerobic exercises _____ _____ _____.	• The resistance exercises I will perform with free weights or weight machines are _____. • The body exercises I will do are _____ _____.	• I will choose exercises to stretch the muscles that work each of the major joints in the body. • The static stretching exercises I will perform are _____ _____

5. **Evaluation:** _____
_____
_____

Lesson 49

Review

Vocabulary Words

Write a separate sentence using each of the vocabulary words listed on page 386.

Objectives

1. What are six steps to follow to design and individualized plan for health-related fitness? **Objective 1**

2. What are the four parts of the FITT formula? **Objective 2**

3. What are ten ways to stay motivated to follow a physical fitness plan? **Objective 3**

4. What would you use for designing a physical fitness plan to follow? **Objective 4**

5. What would you include in a sample physical fitness plan for health-related fitness? **Objective 4**

Responsible Decision-Making

A few weeks ago you made a physical fitness plan for health-related fitness. As part of your plan, you decided to get up early and walk two miles (3.2 kilometers) before school. Every morning for two weeks, you have done this. Lately, you are not motivated to get up early and walk. Write a response to this situation.

1. Describe the situation that requires you to make a decision.
2. List possible decisions you might make.
3. Name two responsible adults with whom you might discuss your decisions.
4. Evaluate the possible consequences of your decisions. Determine if each decision will lead to actions that:
   - promote health,
   - protect safety,
   - follow laws,
   - show respect for yourself and others,
   - follow the guidelines of your parents and of other responsible adults,
   - demonstrate good character.
5. Decide which decision is most responsible and appropriate.
6. Tell two results you expect if you make this decision.

 ## Effective Communication

You and a classmate each list five excuses a teen might give for not having a physical fitness plan. Read your lists to each other. Offer a convincing counterstatement for each excuse on one another's list.

 ## Self-Directed Learning

Make a map of this country. Design logos for ten sports you enjoy. Place these logos on the map to indicate geographical locations where you might participate in each of the ten sports. You can use the same logo more than once.

 ## Critical Thinking

A sedentary lifestyle is a lifestyle in which a person does not engage in much activity. For example, a person may take an elevator rather than climb stairs. What are five other examples of a sedentary lifestyle? How might a person change from being sedentary to being active?

 ## Responsible Citizenship

The President's Council on Physical Fitness and Sports provides badges that can be earned for participation in different physical activities. Write to the Council to obtain more information. Select a physical activity that family members can participate in together to earn badges.

Lesson 50

You Can Be a Responsible Spectator and Participant in Sports

Life Skill I will be a responsible spectator and participant in sports.

Sports can be an enjoyable part of your life. You can play on school or community sports teams. You might attend sports events at your school. There may be college or professional sports teams you follow. Perhaps your goal is to play college or professional sports. This lesson explains how to behave in a responsible manner when you are a spectator or participant in sports. This lesson also explains how to prepare to play sports at a college or university. You will learn about eligibility requirements, college admission, athletic scholarships, player agents, and recruitment procedures.

The Lesson Outline

How to Be a Responsible Sports Spectator

How to Be a Responsible Sports Participant

How to Prepare for Sports at a College or University

Objectives

1. Identify ten behaviors demonstrated by a responsible sports spectator. **page 391**

2. Discuss ten characteristics of a responsible sports participant. **pages 392**

3. Discuss procedures that are followed during drug testing for banned substances. **page 392**

4. Discuss ways to prepare for sports at a college or university including eligibility requirements, college admission, athletic scholarships, player agents, and recruitment procedures. **pages 393–394**

Vocabulary Words

sports spectator

fan

sports participant

drug metabolites

eligibility requirements

National Collegiate Athletic Association (NCAA)

Division I school

core course

Division II school

Division III school

Division I or II qualifier

Division I partial qualifier

Division II partial qualifier

athletic scholarship

player agent

recruitment

redshirt year

How to Be a Responsible Sports Spectator

A **sports spectator** or **fan** is a person who watches and supports sports without actively participating in them. You can behave in a responsible way when you are a sports spectator or fan.

1. I will recognize that I represent my school when I attend sports events.

2. I will learn the rules for the sports events I follow.

3. I will not boo or hiss officials, referees, players, coaches, or other fans.

4. I will show respect for officials and referees and their decisions.

5. I will respect the decisions of the coaches.

6. I will applaud the good play and sportsmanship of players for both teams.

7. I will respond with enthusiasm when cheerleaders ask me to participate.

8. I will express disapproval for rough play and poor sportsmanship.

9. I will not say or yell critical comments.

10. I will stay in control of my emotions.

11. I will not instigate or participate in any confrontations or fights.

12. I will not damage property at the opposing team's school.

13. I will not attend sports events under the influence of alcohol or other drugs.

14. I will not bet or gamble on sports events.

15. I will consider ways to support sports teams, such as being a cheerleader or a member of the band.

16. I will make encouraging remarks to participants when they lose or do not play well.

17. I will be a loyal and supportive fan during a losing as well as a winning season.

18. I will not throw paper, soda pop, or anything else at the officials when I do not agree with a call.

19. I will not make unkind remarks about any member of the opposing team.

20. I will not run onto the court or field before or immediately after the play is completed.

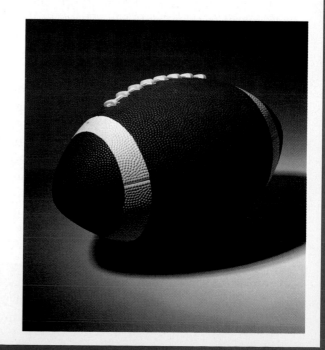

How to Be a Responsible Sports Participant

A **sports participant** is a person who plays sports. A responsible sports participant:

1. Puts forth maximum effort.
2. Has realistic expectations.
3. Keeps grades a priority.
4. Manages time effectively.
5. Avoids the use of alcohol and other drugs.
6. Does not bet on sports events.
7. Has a healthful attitude toward winning and losing.
8. Does not instigate or participate in fights.
9. Shows respect for officials, referees, coaches, and other players.
10. Cooperates with teammates.

Presently, few high schools require sports participants to take drug tests. However, drug testing is common at the college, professional, and Olympic levels. Sports participants who undergo drug testing are asked for a urine sample. The urine sample is sent to a lab for an analysis to detect drug metabolites. **Drug metabolites** are chemicals that when present in urine indicate that a person has used a banned substance. Drug tests indicate whether or not a sports participant has used a banned substance such as steroids, cocaine, or marijuana. A sports participant guilty of using one or more banned substances may be dropped from an athletic team and suspended from school.

The Winning Combination— Sports and Good Grades!

Always put forth your best effort when you play sports. At the same time, work hard to get good grades. You may not make it to the next level of sports, but you will make it to the next level of your life where you will use academic skills.

Think about these facts...

● The odds of making it to the pros for a high school male athlete are 6,000 to 1.

● The odds of making it to the NBA for a high school male are an even longer shot—10,000 to 1.

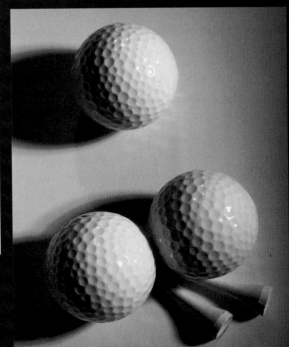

How to Prepare for Sports at a College or University

If you are very good in sports during high school, you may have the opportunity to compete at a college or university. You need to plan ahead if you are interested in playing a sport at a college or university.

Eligibility Requirements. **Eligibility requirements** are criteria that must be met to be qualified to participate on a sports team. The **National Collegiate Athletic Association (NCAA)** is the organization that regulates athletics at the college level and sets eligibility requirements. The NCAA divides colleges into three divisions for competition. A **Division I school** is a college that competes in the first or top level of NCAA competition. To be eligible to compete in sports at a Division I school, you must:

• graduate from high school,

• have a passing grade in 13 academic or core courses,

• meet grade-point and college admission test standards for the ACT or SAT.

A **core course** is a recognized academic course that offers training in English, math, social science, natural or physical science, foreign language, computer science, philosophy, or comparative religion. Vocational and personal service courses do not qualify as core courses. Neither do remedial, special education, or compensatory courses. Courses that are graded on a pass-fail basis do not count as core courses. At Division I school, only courses completed in grades nine through twelve can be counted as core courses.

A **Division II school** is a college that competes in the second level of NCAA competition. To be eligible to compete in sports at a Division II school, you must:

• be a high school graduate,

• have at least a 2.0 grade-point average on a 4.0 scale,

• have a passing grade for 13 core courses,

• have a combined score higher than 820 on the SAT or 68 sum score on the ACT.

These eligibility requirements do not apply to Division III schools. A **Division III school** is a college that competes in the third level of NCAA competition.

Suppose you meet the eligibility requirements for a Division I or a Division II school. Then you are listed as a qualifier. A **Division I or II qualifier** is a student who can practice, compete, and receive an athletic scholarship as a freshman. You will be considered a partial qualifier if you do not meet the eligibility requirements for a Division I or Division II school. A **Division I partial qualifier** is a student who cannot compete the freshman year but can practice at the home facility and can receive an athletic scholarship. A Division I partial qualifier is limited to three seasons of eligibility. A **Division II partial qualifier** is a student who cannot practice or compete during the freshman year and can receive an athletic scholarship. A Division II partial qualifier has four years of eligibility.

If you intend to play sports at a Division I or II school, you must register and be certified by the NCAA Clearinghouse. Your high school counselor and coach can give you information about registration. If you do not qualify to play in a Division I or II school, you may qualify to play at a junior college. Or, you may attend a school that belongs to the National Association of Intercollegiate Athletics (NAIA).

College Admission. Just because you meet the requirements for NCAA eligibility does not mean that you will qualify for admission at a particular college. College admission requirements often are stricter than the NCAA eligibility. Check the admission requirements for the colleges that interest you.

Athletic Scholarships. If you have special athletic talents, you may be offered an athletic scholarship by a college. An **athletic scholarship** is a grant of money given to a student athlete to cover some of the costs of attending college. You can work toward a degree in any field. Athletic scholarships:

* usually are offered on a year-by-year basis,

* can be renewed for up to four years (the amount of time to complete an undergraduate degree),

* are not guaranteed past one year, even if you are injured.

If you are offered an athletic scholarship, ask if the college has a commitment to assist student athletes for more than one year if they become injured. To keep your scholarship, you need to focus on your grades. If your grade-point average drops below the required level, you will no longer be eligible to participate. You can lose your scholarship.

Player Agents. A **player agent** is a person who represents athletes in contract negotiations with professional teams and with companies who want endorsements. A player agent may contact you while you are in high school. (S)he may want to get an advantage over other player agents who wait until an athlete's college eligibility ends. The NCAA rules prohibit any student from receiving benefits or gifts from player agents. If you accept gifts or benefits, you can lose your eligibility. You also can lose your eligibility if you agree in writing or orally to be represented by a player agent while you are in high school or college. Protect your eligibility. Tell your parents or guardian and contact the NCAA and your high school coach if a player agent approaches you.

Recruitment Procedures. **Recruitment** is contact by a coach or representative of a college athletic department about enrolling and playing sports at a college. You may be contacted by telephone or a coach or other official from the college may visit you and your family. You may be requested to make an official visit to a college campus for recruiting purposes. If you are recruited, involve your parents or guardian. Be prepared to ask questions about the college, the degrees offered, the admission requirements, the style of coaching, and playing opportunities for you. You may want to ask if the coach will "redshirt" you. A **redshirt year** is a year in which an athlete practices with the team without competing to keep an extra year of eligibility.

Lesson 50

Review

Vocabulary Words

Write a separate sentence using each of the vocabulary words listed on page 390.

Objectives

1. What are ten behaviors demonstrated by a responsible sports spectator? **Objective 1**

2. What are ten characteristics of a responsible sports participant? **Objective 2**

3. What procedures are followed during drug testing for banned substances? **Objective 3**

4. How can a high school athlete prepare for sports at a college or university? **Objective 4**

5. What is the difference in eligibility requirements for a Division I and Division II school? **Objective 4**

Responsible Decision-Making

Imagine that you are a high school senior. Your team has won the state tournament and you were named MVP. Next year, you will start college with a full scholarship. A player agent calls and tells you that you are good enough to skip college and go straight to the pros. The player agent suggests that you meet to have a serious discussion about your future. Write a response to this situation.

1. Describe the situation that requires you to make a decision.
2. List possible decisions you might make.
3. Name two responsible adults with whom you might discuss your decisions.
4. Evaluate the possible consequences of your decisions. Determine if each decision will lead to actions that:
   - promote health,
   - protect safety,
   - follow laws,
   - show respect for yourself and others,
   - follow the guidelines of your parents and of other responsible adults,
   - demonstrate good character.
5. Decide which decision is most responsible and appropriate.
6. Tell two results you expect if you make this decision.

 ## Effective Communication

Select one of your school teams. Make up a cheer that demonstrates good sportsmanship. Share the cheer with at least two classmates.

 ## Self-Directed Learning

Check the library or Internet for information released by the National Collegiate Athletic Association (NCAA). Review the eligibility requirements for Division I and Division II schools.

 ## Critical Thinking

You have been recruited by three schools to play your favorite sport. What ten questions can you ask each school to evaluate the schools to help you decide which offer to accept?

 ## Responsible Citizenship

Consider the win-loss record of the sports teams at your school. Attend a sports event for a team that does not have a winning record. Find ways to encourage members of the team.

Review Questions

Prepare for the unit test. Review your answers for each Lesson Review in this unit. Then write answers to each of the following questions:

1. What information is included in a health history? **Lesson 41**
2. How are sunglasses that protect the eyes from UV radiation labelled? **Lesson 41**
3. What are nine causes of hearing loss? **Lesson 41**
4. How often should you get a dental examination? **Lesson 42**
5. What causes periodontal disease? **Lesson 42**
6. Why should you wear a mouthguard when playing certain sports? **Lesson 42**
7. What causes dandruff and how can it be controlled? **Lesson 43**
8. Why should you avoid sunbathing or using tanning booths? **Lesson 43**
9. What are eight ways to make acne worse? **Lesson 43**
10. What happens during REM sleep? **Lesson 44**
11. Why might drinking cola beverages keep you awake at night? **Lesson 44**
12. Why do some people drink a glass of milk before going to bed? **Lesson 44**
13. How does regular physical activity affect coronary collateral circulation? **Lesson 45**
14. How does regular physical activity alter the body's response to stress? **Lesson 45**
15. What are ten ways you might obtain a moderate amount of physical activity? **Lesson 45**
16. What is the difference between isometric exercises and isotonic exercises? **Lesson 46**

17. What are nine benefits of muscular strength and endurance? **Lesson 46**
18. What are six benefits of flexibility? **Lesson 46**
19. What kind of exercises develop cardiorespiratory endurance and a healthful body composition? **Lesson 46**
20. What kind of exercises develop muscular strength and muscular endurance? **Lesson 46**
21. What kind of exercises develop flexibility? **Lesson 46**
22. What are two advantages of participating right now in lifetime sports and physical activities? **Lesson 47**
23. What health-related and skill-related fitness benefits can you get from playing golf? **Lesson 47**
24. What health-related and skill-related fitness benefits can you get from running or jogging? **Lesson 47**
25. What is the difference between the training threshold and the training ceiling? **Lesson 48**
26. What happens to fitness benefits if you stop working out for two months? **Lesson 48**
27. How can you prevent cold-temperature related illnesses? **Lesson 48**
28. Why should aerobic exercises be included in a physical fitness plan? **Lesson 49**
29. What are three examples of banned substances that can be detected from drug testing? **Lesson 50**
30. What are the eligibility requirements for a Division I school? **Lesson 50**

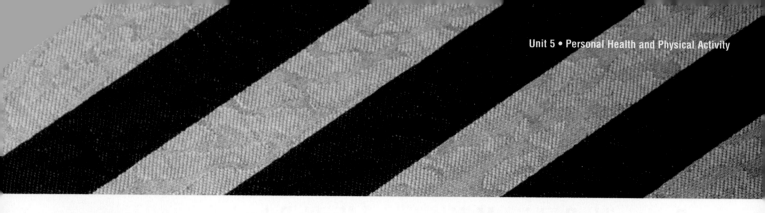

Vocabulary Words

Number a sheet of paper from 1–10. Select the correct vocabulary word and write it next to the corresponding number. DO NOT WRITE IN THIS BOOK.

dental plaque	physical activity
grooming	physical fitness
health care	skill-related fitness
health-related fitness	fan
insomnia	training principles

1. _____ is an invisible, sticky film of bacteria on teeth, especially near the gum line. **Lesson 42**

2. _____ is the ability of the heart, lungs, muscles, and joints to function at optimal capacity. **Lesson 46**

3. _____ is the professional medical and dental help that promotes a person's health. **Lesson 41**

4. _____ is the ability to perform physical activity and to meet the demands of daily living while being energetic and alert. **Lesson 49**

5. _____ is keeping the body clean and having a neat appearance. **Lesson 43**

6. _____ are guidelines to follow to obtain maximum fitness benefits and reduce the risk of injuries and illnesses. **Lesson 48**

7. _____ is the capacity to perform well in sports and physical activities. **Lesson 47**

8. _____ is the prolonged inability to fall asleep, stay asleep, or get back to sleep once a person is awakened during the night. **Lesson 44**

9. _____ is a person who watches and supports sports without actively participating in them. **Lesson 50**

10. _____ is any bodily movement produced by skeletal muscles that results in energy expenditure. **Lesson 45**

Health Literacy

Effective Communication

Design a logo for health-related fitness. Include the five components of health-related fitness. Share your logo with classmates. Observe the logos created by your classmates. Send the three best logos to the President's Council on Physical Fitness and Sports.

Self-Directed Learning

Suppose you select an aerobic exercise to develop cardiorespiratory endurance. This exercise uses 300 calories per hour. How many minutes do you need to participate in this exercise? (Remember, you need to use 1.8 calories for each pound of body weight).

Critical Thinking

Suppose you are rollerblading and fall and sprain an ankle. How would you treat this injury?

Responsible Citizenship

Help a member of your family make a health behavior contract with the following life skill: "I will follow a physical fitness plan."

Responsible Decision-Making

A friend invites you to a health club to work out. You want to run on the treadmill, but your friend suggests that you use the weight machines. You have never used weight machines before. Your friend says (s)he has been working out with weight machines for about a year. (S)he says you can lift the same weight (s)he does because you are the same sex and body weight. Write a response to this situation.

1. Describe the situation that requires you to make a decision.
2. List possible decisions you might make.
3. Name two responsible adults with whom you might discuss your decisions.
4. Evaluate the possible consequences of your decisions. Determine if each decision will lead to actions that:
   • promote health,
   • protect safety,
   • follow laws,
   • show respect for yourself and others,
   • follow the guidelines of your parents and of other responsible adults,
   • demonstrate good character.
5. Decide which decision is most responsible and appropriate.
6. Tell two results you expect if you make this decision.

Health Behavior Inventory of Life Skills

Number from 1 to 10 on a sheet of paper. Read each life skill carefully. Write YES or NO next to the same number on your paper. Each YES response indicates a life skill you practice to promote your health status. Each NO response indicates a life skill you do not practice. Plan to begin practicing these life skills.

1. I will have regular examinations.
2. I will follow a dental health plan.
3. I will be well-groomed.
4. I will get adequate rest and sleep.
5. I will participate in regular physical activity.
6. I will develop and maintain health-related fitness.
7. I will develop and maintain skill-related fitness.
8. I will prevent physical activity-related injuries and illnesses.
9. I will follow a physical fitness plan.
10. I will be a responsible spectator and participant in sports.

Multicultural Health

Countries throughout the world send athletes to participate in the Olympics. The Olympic rings were developed as symbols of the Olympic spirit. Find out what the Olympic rings mean. Why is this symbol embraced by people of different cultures?

Family Involvement

Review with members of your family A Guide to Lifetime Sports and Physical Activities. Select one lifetime sport or physical activity in which members of your family can participate together. Plan a time to enjoy this lifetime sport or physical activity.

Health Behavior Contract

Copy and complete the following health behavior contract. Evaluate your progress. Share the results with your family.

Health Behavior Contract

1. Name_____ Date_____

2. **Life Skill:** I will develop and maintain skill-related fitness.

3. **Effects on Health Status:** Skill-related fitness helps me perform well in sports and physical activities. Agility helps me rapidly change the position of my body. Balance keeps me from falling. Coordination helps me use body senses together with body parts as I move. Reaction time helps me respond quickly when I hear, see, feel, or touch, a stimulus. Speed helps me move quickly. Power helps me combine speed with strength.

4. **Plan and Method to Record Progress:** The six fitness skills are listed below. In the space provided, I will write a sport or physical activity that develops the fitness skill.

Agility _____

Balance _____

Coordination _____

Reaction Time _____

Speed _____

Power _____

I will participate in these two sports during the next week: _____

_____

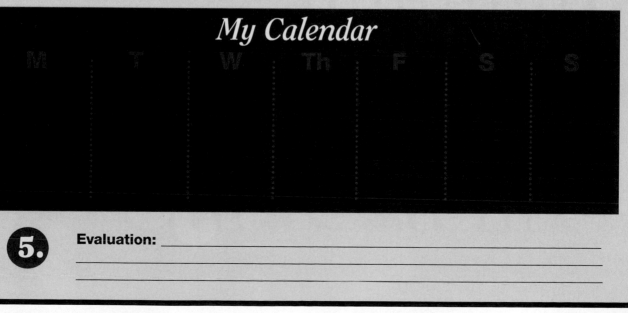

My Calendar

M	T	W	Th	F	S	S

5. **Evaluation:** _____

_____

_____

Unit 6

Alcohol, Tobacco, and Other Drugs

You Can Follow Guidelines for the Safe Use of Prescription and OTC Drugs

Life Skill **I will follow guidelines for the safe use of prescription and OTC drugs.**

A **drug** is a substance other than food that changes the way the body or mind functions. Some drugs harm health. These drugs include alcohol, tobacco, cocaine, and marijuana. Other drugs promote health. These drugs include prescription drugs and over-the-counter (OTC) drugs. For example, a teen who has diabetes may need insulin. Drugs intended to promote health can harm your health if you do not follow guidelines for their safe use. This lesson includes information that will help you use drugs in a safe way. You will learn guidelines for the safe use of prescription drugs and OTC drugs.

The Lesson Outline

What to Know About Drugs

What to Know About Prescription Drugs

What to Know About Over-the-Counter Drugs

Objectives

1. List and explain factors that influence the effects a drug will have on a person. **pages 403–404**
2. Identify the information that appears on a prescription drug label. **page 405**
3. List ten guidelines for the safe use of prescription drugs. **page 405**
4. Identify the information that appears on an OTC drug label. **page 406**
5. List ten guidelines for the safe use of OTC drugs. **page 406**

Vocabulary Words

drug
responsible drug use
drug misuse
drug abuse
snorting
skin patch
suppository
buccal absorption
sublingual absorption
dose
medicine
prescription drug
prescription
pharmacist
pharmacy
brand-name drug
generic-name drug
therapeutical equivalence
over-the-counter (OTC) drug
indication for use
contraindication for use
tamper-resistant package
side effect

What to Know About
Drugs

People use drugs in responsible and irresponsible ways. **Responsible drug use** is the correct use of legal drugs to promote health and well-being. An example of responsible drug use is taking a prescription drug for its intended purpose according to a physician's instructions.

Drugs may be misused and abused. **Drug misuse** is the incorrect use of a prescription or OTC drug. Examples of drug misuse include taking medicine leftover from a previous illness and using another person's prescription drug.

Other examples include mixing medications without consulting a physician and driving or drinking alcohol after taking certain medications. **Drug abuse** is the intentional use of a drug without medical or health reasons. Taking an illegal drug is drug abuse. So is taking a drug when there is no medical reason. Both legal and illegal drugs are abused. Responsible drug use can promote health and well-being. Drug misuse and abuse can destroy both health and relationships.

Ways Drugs Enter the Body

To produce an effect, a drug has to enter the body. Drugs can be taken by mouth, injection, inhalation, absorption, or implantation.

By mouth. The most common way of taking a drug is swallowing. A drug in the form of a pill, capsule, or liquid may be swallowed. After being swallowed, a drug travels to the stomach and small intestine. Then it is absorbed into the bloodstream. Not all drugs can be taken by mouth. Digestive juices in the stomach destroy certain drugs or make them ineffective.

By injection. Some drugs are injected using a syringe and needle. A drug that is injected goes directly under the skin into a muscle or blood vessel. Drugs must be dissolved into liquid before they can be injected into the body.

A drug that is injected into a blood vessel produces effects very quickly. Injecting drugs without medical supervision is a risk factor for infection with HIV and hepatitis B.

By inhalation. Some drugs are inhaled through the nose or mouth. A drug enters the bloodstream in the lungs. Drugs that are inhaled produce effects very quickly. People with asthma may inhale drugs that open their air passages. Some drugs that are inhaled, such as the nicotine from cigarette smoke, harm health. They irritate the tissues that line the lungs and throat. Long-term inhalation of harmful drugs can cause respiratory diseases. Snorting is a type of inhalation. **Snorting** is sniffing drugs through the nose so that they can be absorbed through the mucous membranes of the nasal passages. Snorting drugs may cause damage to the nose and nasal passages.

Lesson 58 will include more information about drugs and HIV.

By absorption. A drug that is absorbed enters the bloodstream through the skin or mucous membranes. Ointments, creams, lotions, sprays, and patches contain drugs that are absorbed. They may be applied to the skin or mucous membranes of the eyes, nose, mouth, or anus. A **skin patch** is a patch worn on the body that contains a drug that is absorbed through the skin. A **suppository** is a wax-coated form of a drug that is inserted into the anus. When the wax melts, the drug is absorbed into the bloodstream. **Buccal absorption** is the absorption of a drug between the cheek and gum. Nicotine is absorbed into the bloodstream when chewing tobacco is placed in the mouth. **Sublingual absorption** is the absorption of a drug when it is placed under the tongue.

By implantation. Some drugs are implanted, or placed, under the skin where they can be released into the bloodstream. For example, some forms of cancer therapy involve implanting drugs under the skin.

Other factors besides the ways a drug enters the body also determine the effects of a drug. The **dose** is the amount of a drug that is taken at one time. The larger the dose, the greater the effect of the drug. How a person feels is another factor. If a person is depressed, taking a drug that slows body functions can make the person more depressed. Weight, age, and health also influence the effects a drug will have. A drug will have an increased effect on a person who is young or who has a low body weight or poor health status. The reactions of more than one drug in the body can alter the effects of a drug. The effects of drugs may counteract one another. The reactions of the drugs may increase the effects.

Proven Safe and Effective

Ingredients in legal drugs must be listed as safe and effective by the Federal Drug Administration (FDA). The FDA is a federal agency that monitors the safety of cosmetics and food and the safety and effectiveness of new drugs, medical devices, and prescription and OTC drugs. The FDA must approve any new drug before it is distributed legally. It tests the drug to learn about drug effects and side effects before it can be used by people.

What to Know About
Prescription Drugs

A **medicine** is a drug that is used to treat, prevent, or diagnose illness. A **prescription drug** is a medicine that can be obtained only with a written order from a licensed health professional. A **prescription** is a written order from a physician or other licensed health professional. A prescription contains: patient's name; name of the drug; form of the drug, such as pills or liquid; dosage level; directions for use; physician's name, address, phone number, and signature; Drug Enforcement Agency registration; refill instructions. Prescription drugs are intended to be used only according to the directions on the prescription.

Obtaining or using prescription drugs without a prescription is illegal. By law, prescription drugs must be prepared and sold by licensed pharmacists. A **pharmacist** is an allied health professional who dispenses medications that are prescribed by certain licensed health professionals. Prescription drugs are obtained from a pharmacy. A **pharmacy** is a place where prescription drugs are legally dispensed.

A pharmacist fills a prescription with either a brand-name or a generic-name drug. The prescription states whether the pharmacist can substitute a generic-name drug for a brand-name drug. A **brand-name drug** is a drug with a registered name or trademark given to a drug by a pharmaceutical company. A **generic-name drug** is a drug that contains the same active ingredients as a brand-name drug. Generic-name drugs usually are less expensive. Generic and brand names of a particular drug usually have therapeutical equivalence. **Therapeutical equivalence** is when two drugs are chemically the same and produce the same medical effects.

Guidelines for the Safe Use of Prescription Drugs

1. Contact your physician if the drug does not seem to be producing the desired effects.
2. Report new or unexpected symptoms to your physician.
3. Do not stop taking the drug if you start feeling better.
4. Carefully follow the instructions on the label.
5. Follow instructions for storing the prescription drug.
6. Keep all prescription drugs out of the reach of children.
7. Never take prescription drugs that have been prescribed for another person.
8. Keep prescription drugs in their original containers.
9. Flush down the toilet prescription drugs that no longer are needed.
10. Never take prescription drugs that appear to have been tampered with, are discolored, or have a suspicious odor.

Prescription Drug Label

Prescription number · Name of the person for whom the drug was prescribed · Directions for use · Name of the drug · Date the prescription was filled · Initials of the pharmacist · Pharmacy name, address, and phone number · Name of licensed health professional · Form of the drug · Dosage level · Amount of drug contained in the container · Number of refills · Expiration date · Warnings

Smith Drugs
00055 North Steet
Anytown, USA
(000) 005-0005
R: 001450   Dr. M. Jones
Ryan Smith
Take one tablet 3 times daily
Finish all medication
Take before meals
Brythomycin Tab 500 mg.
04/23/98 JWA Qty. 35 Refills: 1
Discard after 6/23/02
May cause drowsiness

You Can Avoid Drug Dependence

Life Skill **I will not misuse or abuse drugs.**

If you ask people who are drug-dependent if they ever thought they would become hooked on drugs, most would answer "no." When people first try a drug, they may believe they can control their use of it. However, people who experiment by taking harmful drugs risk becoming hooked. This lesson will explain why harmful drug use is risky. You will learn how people become dependent on drugs. You also will learn how the behavior of people who are drug-dependent affects friends and family members.

The Lesson Outline

Why Using Drugs Is Risky

What to Know About Drug Dependence

How Family Members with Codependence Respond

Objectives

1. List and explain seven reasons why drug use is risky. **page 409**
2. Discuss drug dependence, including physical dependence and psychological dependence. **page 410**
3. Outline the five stages of drug use that can progress to drug dependence. **page 411**
4. Discuss roles played by family members who are codependent: chief enabler, family hero, scapegoat, mascot, and lost child. **page 412**

Vocabulary Words

drug dependence

overdose

dopamine

physical dependence

tolerance

withdrawal symptoms

psychological dependence

codependence

codependent

enabler

Why Using Drugs Is Risky

Drug dependence is the continued use of a drug even though it harms the body, mind, and relationships. Chemical dependence and chemical addiction are other terms for drug dependence. Drug dependence affects judgment and common sense. Using drugs becomes more important than school, work, family, and relationships. People who are drug-dependent often try to quit using drugs, but they usually are not successful.

There are many risks involved in using drugs such as alcohol, marijuana, cocaine, and amphetamines. Even experimenting with a drug "just once" can have consequences.

1. **Using drugs can lead to overdose.** People who use drugs can overdose on drugs. To **overdose** is to take an excessive amount. A drug overdose can cause serious injury or death. Both people who have taken a drug for a long time and those who take a drug for the first time can overdose. An overdose often is the result of taking more than one drug at a time. Drugs have different effects on people. Two people may take the same amount of a drug. One may feel few effects; the other may overdose.

2. **Using drugs can cause accidents.** Drugs slow reaction time, impair coordination, and affect judgment. People under the influence of drugs often think they can perform tasks they cannot, such as drive safely. Most deaths caused by motor vehicle accidents involve a person under the influence of alcohol. Many people under the influence of drugs are struck by motor vehicles as well.

3. **Using drugs increases the risk of HIV infection, sexually transmitted diseases (STDs), and unwanted pregnancy.** Drugs affect people's ability to make responsible decisions. Sexual feelings may increase when people use drugs. Teens who have been sexually active often were under the influence of drugs. This increases the likelihood of unwanted pregnancy and of having sex with a person infected with HIV or another STD. People who share needles to inject drugs are at risk for infection with HIV and hepatitis B.

4. **Using drugs can harm relationships.** People who use drugs often harm relationships with friends and family members. They may say and do things when under the influence of drugs that later they regret. They may think what they are saying or doing is appropriate even though it is not. This may cause misunderstandings and conflict.

5. **Using drugs can prevent people from developing social skills.** People who are uncomfortable in a social situation may use drugs to relax. They rely on drugs to "get through" social situations. They will not develop the social skills needed for healthful relationships.

6. **Using drugs can lead to violence and illegal behaviors.** Drugs change the way people think and act. People who use drugs often become angry and aggressive and may harm other people. Most homicides, suicides, and episodes of abuse occur when people are using drugs. People who have been using drugs also are more likely to be involved in illegal behaviors such as damaging property and shoplifting.

7. **Using drugs can lead to drug dependence.** Using drugs may stimulate the pleasure center of the brain. The pleasure center of the brain is the part of the brain that contains specialized nerve cells that release dopamine. **Dopamine** is a chemical that triggers feelings of pleasure. Certain drugs activate the pleasure center of the brain. This is the major reason why people repeatedly use drugs and become drug-dependent.

* The term drug use in this lesson refers to drug misuse and abuse.

What to Know About
Drug Dependence

People who use drugs may become physically and psychologically dependent on them. The body of people who use a drug may become used to having it. **Physical dependence** is a condition in which a person develops tolerance to a drug and the drug becomes necessary or the person has withdrawal symptoms. **Tolerance** is a condition in which the body becomes used to a substance. People with a high tolerance to a drug need a greater amount of the drug to produce the same effect as people with a low tolerance. For example, people may feel certain effects from drinking one can of beer. After repeated drinking, they may need to drink two cans of beer to achieve the same effect. Later on, they may need three cans of beer.

Withdrawal symptoms are unpleasant reactions that occur when a person who is physically dependent on a drug no longer takes it. Withdrawal symptoms include chills, muscular twitching, fever, nausea, vomiting, and cramps. People who are physically dependent on a drug must continue taking the drug in order to avoid withdrawal symptoms.

Psychological dependence is a strong desire to continue using a drug for emotional reasons. People with psychological dependence may or may not be physically dependent. It is sometimes described as a strong craving for drugs. For example, the pleasurable feelings that a drug produces may be desired again and again. Or, people may rely on a particular drug that they believe helps reduce stress or anxiety. If they stop taking the drug for a short time, they crave the drug but do not go through physical withdrawal. Psychological dependence can become so severe that people become obsessed with the drug and may center their life around buying and taking it.

According to the *Diagnostic and Statistical Manual of Mental Disorders*, people are drug-dependent if they have had three or more of the following symptoms in the past year.

1. Developing tolerance to a drug
2. Experiencing withdrawal symptoms when stopping the use of a drug
3. Taking large amounts of a drug or taking a drug for a long period of time
4. Trying to quit taking a drug with no success
5. Spending lots of time obtaining a drug, using a drug, or recovering from the effects of drug use
6. Giving up important activities, such as work or school, because of drug use
7. Continuing to use a drug even though it is causing problems, such as physical illness and injury

Adapted from the *Diagnostic and Statistical Manual of Mental Disorders*, 4th edition. Washington, DC: American Psychiatric Association.

Progression to Drug Dependency

Stages of Progression

For Example...

STAGE 1 Experimentation

"I'll just try it."

A person is tempted to experiment with a drug. (S)he tries the drug.

A teen is with friends. The friends are drinking beer. They are having fun. The teen does not want to feel left out. (S)he decides to drink just this once to see what it is like.

STAGE 2 Desired Effect

"I like the feeling."

A person enjoys the feeling (s)he gets from trying the drug. (S)he continues to use the drug.

The teen drinks the beer. (S)he feels "cool" and relaxed. The friends comment on how great it is that (s)he is drinking with them. The teen feels like (s)he fits in. The next times the teen is with these friends, (s)he drinks.

STAGE 3 Tolerance

"I need more of the drug to feel good."

A person develops a tolerance to the drug. The drug may no longer have the same pleasurable effects. The person may suffer from withdrawal symptoms when (s)he stops using the drug.

The teen has been drinking with friends several times. (S)he needs several beers to feel any effect and is able to drink large amounts at one time. (S)he is proud of winning drinking games. The teen has a headache, throws up, and has body tremors the morning after drinking.

STAGE 4 Denial

"I don't have a drug problem."

A person is in denial. (S)he does not admit that drug use is causing problems. (S)he claims that (s)he can stop using the drug at any time.

The teen does not think the drinking is a big deal since his/her friends drink. The teen misses classes due to hangovers. (S)he gets into fights with friends because (s)he says things (s)he later regrets. (S)he forgets what (s)he said and did. The teen is sexually active when drunk. The teen gets into trouble with his/her parents or guardian because (s)he breaks curfew. (S)he steals beer from his/her parents or guardian.

STAGE 5 Drug Dependence

"I have to have the drug."

A person has become drug-dependent.

The teen drinks at every social event. (S)he drinks a lot of beer at one time. (S)he brings his/her own alcohol to events and sneaks drinks. The teen decides to quit drinking, but (s)he cannot stick with the decision.

You Can Practice Protective Factors for Drug Misuse and Abuse

Life Skill I will avoid risk factors and practice protective factors for drug misuse and abuse.

Why do some teens use drugs? Why do other teens avoid drugs? There are risk factors and protective factors for drug use. A **risk factor** is something that increases the likelihood of a negative outcome. There are certain risk factors that put some teens more at risk than other teens for harmful drug use. A **protective factor** is something that increases the likelihood of a positive outcome. A protective factor is a "shield" that helps a teen resist the temptation to use drugs and behave in other harmful ways. This lesson identifies risk factors for drug misuse and abuse. You can avoid these risk factors. This lesson also identifies protective factors for drug misuse and abuse. You can practice these protective factors and stay safe and drug-free.

Vocabulary Words

risk factor

protective factor

delayed gratification

instant gratification

genetic predisposition

adverse environment

mentor

The Lesson Outline

What to Know About Risk Factors

What to Know About Protective Factors

Objectives

1. List and discuss 13 risk factors for drug use. **pages 415–416**
2. List and discuss 13 protective factors for drug use. **pages 417–418**

What to Know About
Risk Factors

Research has identified risk factors that increase a teen's risk of drug misuse and abuse. Some of these risk factors may describe your behavior or the environment in which you live. If so, you are at risk for using harmful drugs and need to recognize this risk. You have varying degrees of control over the risk factors for drug misuse and abuse. For example, you do not have control over living in a neighborhood in which drugs are easy to buy. But you do have control over whom you choose as friends. Risk factors only refer to the statistical likelihood that you might use harmful drugs. Having certain risk factors for drug use does not mean you have an excuse to use harmful drugs. You have control.

Thirteen Risk Factors for Drug Use

1. **Lacking self-respect.** Teens who lack self-respect believe they are unworthy of love and respect. They are at risk because they believe drugs will numb the negative feelings they have about themselves. They may not have enough confidence to say "no" to negative peer pressure.

2. **Being unable to express emotions in healthful ways.** Teens who have difficulty expressing emotions are more likely than other teens to use harmful drugs. Teens who cannot cope with stress, anger, and depression may think that drugs will help numb these feelings. They may use drugs instead of expressing feelings honestly.

3. **Having friends who use drugs.** One of the strongest risk factors for drug use is having friends who use drugs. They may pressure you to use drugs with them. They want you to support their unsafe and illegal habits. They may continue to pressure you when you say "no."

4. **Being unable to delay gratification.** **Delayed gratification** is voluntarily postponing an immediate reward in order to complete a task before enjoying a reward. Drug use is a form of instant gratification. **Instant gratification** is choosing an immediate reward regardless of potential harmful effects. Immediate pleasure is more important to people who use drugs than maintaining good health and staying safe.

5. **Having access to drugs.** The temptation to use drugs is greater when drugs are easily available. Having access to drugs includes living in a neighborhood where drugs are sold, going to a school where people sell drugs, and knowing people who sell drugs.

6. **Being rejected by peers.** Teens who feel rejected by peers may use drugs to try to numb feelings of loneliness or to fit in. They often are not interested in another teen's personality. They are friends with any teen who can supply them with drugs or will use drugs with them.

7. **Having a biological family member(s) who is drug-dependent.** Certain individuals may inherit a genetic predisposition to drug abuse. A **genetic predisposition** is the inheritance of genes that increase the likelihood of developing a condition. Children born to parents who have alcoholism are more likely to have alcoholism than children born to other parents.

8. **Having difficult family relationships.** Teens who live in families that do not manage conflict healthfully often have difficult family relationships. These teens have an increased risk of drug use. They may not follow family guidelines. They may not have a responsible adult with whom they can share feelings. Difficult family relationships often create a stressful atmosphere. These teens may turn to drugs to cope with stress and numb their feelings.

9. **Having role models who use drugs.** A role model may be someone a teen knows, such as a friend or family member. Or, a role model may be a celebrity, such as a sports star or entertainer. Some teens have role models who use drugs and act like it is sexy, macho, or "cool." Teens who admire role models who use drugs may use drugs to be like their role models.

10. **Using drugs early in life.** The use of drugs during early childhood and adolescence is a risk factor for harmful drug use. Teens who begin drug use at an early age are more likely to become drug-dependent when they are adults.

11. **Doing poorly in school and/or having a learning disability.** Teens who get poor grades in school are more at risk for drug use than their peers who have better grades. Teens who have learning disabilities are at special risk. They may become frustrated and feel inadequate if they compare themselves to peers who do not have learning disabilities. They may use drugs to numb these feelings.

12. **Being uninvolved in school activities and athletics.** Teens who do not participate in school activities and athletics are more likely to use harmful drugs. They are more likely to be bored and to have more time to spend using drugs.

13. **Lacking respect for authority and laws.** Teens who lack respect for authority and laws are more at risk for drug use. They disregard the guidelines of parents or guardians and other responsible adults. They disregard community laws and may not care that using drugs is against the law.

Warning Signs. . .

Recognize these warning signs of drug use in peers.

- Having slurred speech
- Having reddened eyes and using eyedrops
- Having glassy eyes and a blank stare
- Having a sloppy appearance
- Using breath fresheners
- Having a long-term runny nose and sniffing
- Having friends who use drugs
- Giving up friends who do not use drugs

- Joining a gang
- Skipping school
- Doing poorly in school
- Missing money or objects of value
- Changing eating habits
- Having mood swings and hostility
- Lacking energy and motivation

What to Know About
Protective Factors

The more protective factors you practice, the less the risk you will abuse drugs. Examine the protective factors listed on this page and the next one. Do they describe your behavior and the environment in which you live? If so, you already have some protection against harmful drug use. However, lacking protective factors does not give you an excuse to use drugs. You have control over whether or not you use harmful drugs.

Thirteen Protective Factors That Reduce the Risk of Drug Use

1. **Having self-respect.** Teens who have self-respect feel confident about themselves. They want to take care of their health and to stay safe. They know that using drugs harms health. Teens who have self-respect make responsible decisions. They are less likely to give in to negative peer pressure than other teens.

2. **Practicing resistance skills.** Teens who practice resistance skills do not give in to pressure to use drugs. They are able to say "no." They stand up to peers who want them to use drugs. They know that peers who pressure them are not concerned for their health and safety.

3. **Having friends who do not misuse and abuse drugs.** Teens who have friends who are drug-free have less temptation than other teens to experiment with drugs. Drug-free friends do not pressure you to use drugs. They encourage you to participate in drug-free activities.

4. **Being able to delay gratification.** When you are able to delay gratification, you use self-control. You recognize that using drugs interferes with long-term goals. You know that using drugs in an attempt to "feel good now" will have negative consequences later.

5. **Being resilient, even when living in an adverse environment.** An **adverse environment** is an environment that interferes with a person's growth, development, and success. A teen may be exposed to drugs in his/her neighborhood or at home. A teen may have a parent or guardian who is drug-dependent. However a teen who is resilient knows that drugs only lead to more problems. You can be resilient if you live in an adverse environment and recognize that you can control your own behavior and decisions.

You Can Resist Pressure to Misuse or Abuse Drugs

Life Skill I will use resistance skills if I am pressured to misuse or abuse drugs.

Peer pressure is influence that people of similar age or status place on others to behave in a certain way. Peer pressure can be negative or positive. For example, peers might pressure you to do well in school. This pressure is positive. **Positive peer pressure** is influence from peers to behave in a responsible way. Positive peer pressure helps you maintain self-respect and good character. If peers pressure you to use drugs, their influence is negative. **Negative peer pressure** is influence from peers to behave in a way that is not responsible. This lesson helps you gain skills in resisting pressure to use drugs. You will learn how to recognize peer pressure to use drugs. You will learn how to resist this pressure. You also will learn how to be a drug-free role model.

Vocabulary Words

peer pressure

positive peer pressure

negative peer pressure

character

resistance skills

drug-free role model

drug-free lifestyle

peer leader

The Lesson Outline

How to Recognize Peer Pressure to Use Drugs

How to Resist Pressure to Use Drugs

How to Be a Drug-Free Role Model

Objectives

1. Explain why teens who use drugs pressure their peers to use drugs. **page 421**

2. Give examples of direct and indirect peer pressure to use drugs. **page 422**

3. Outline eight resistance skills that can be used to resist pressure to use drugs. **pages 422–423**

4. List ten reasons to say "no" when pressured by peers to use drugs. **page 423**

5. List and discuss three ways to be a drug-free role model. **page 424**

How to Recognize Peer Pressure to Use Drugs

Character is a person's use of self-control to act on responsible values. To maintain self-respect, you need to have good character. It also is important to choose friends who have good character. Throughout life, you must sharpen your skills in noticing the difference between people who have good character and those who do not have good character. Always remember that people who do not have good character can bring you down. They can influence you in ways that cause you to lose self-respect. The following discussion explains what motivates teens who use drugs to try to bring you down to their level.

Why Teens Who Use Drugs Pressure Their Peers to Use Drugs

Have you ever wondered why there is so much peer pressure to use drugs? Think about it. Why should another person care if you use drugs? Does a teen who tells you that drugs will make you feel good really care about how you feel? Does a teen who tells you that using drugs will make you look more mature really care about your appearance? Does a teen who tells you that using drugs "just once" will not harm you really care about your health and safety?

Teens who use drugs often say they will not hang out with teens who do not use drugs. They pressure peers to use drugs. They do this because they want support for their wrong behavior. They think that if others are using drugs with them, their behavior is not wrong. Also, if they get caught, they won't be the only ones in trouble. Teens who use drugs are uncomfortable when their peers stand up to their pressure. They do not like being reminded that drug use is harmful, unsafe, and illegal.

Some teens who use drugs pressure their peers to use drugs because they want them to embarrass themselves. Some teens who use drugs get their peers to use drugs without knowing it. They might slip a drug into a peer's glass when (s)he is not looking. Teens who use drugs often do not care about the consequences or consider the harmful effects the drug may have.

They are not concerned that their behavior is disrespectful and illegal.

Some teens who use drugs pressure peers to use drugs because they know drugs impair judgment. For example, a teen male may want a teen female to have sex with him. The female may have said "no" when she was sober. The male knows that she is more likely to agree to have sex with him after drinking alcohol. She may drink so much she does not know what she is doing. He has sex with her without her consent. He does not realize or care that having sex with someone who does not give consent is rape.

What Teens Who Use Drugs Might Say to Their Peers

"You're not afraid, are you?"

"Everybody is doing it."

"Don't mess up the fun for everyone else."

"Don't be a nerd."

"Nobody will know but me and you."

"It can't hurt just this one time."

"If you won't do it, don't bother to come."

"It really is safe."

"Don't worry, we've been doing this for a long time."

"It will be fun."

"You will feel better than you ever have before."

How to Resist Pressure to Use Drugs

Some teens have a difficult time resisting peer pressure. They lack self-confidence. They may plan to say "no," but they give in when they are pressured. Negative peer pressure takes many forms. Sometimes it is direct. Teens who use drugs make persuasive statements. Sometimes it is indirect. Teens may not be pressured directly, but they choose to go along with the crowd.

You may face peer pressure to smoke cigarettes, chew tobacco, drink alcohol, sniff inhalants, smoke marijuana, use cocaine, or take other drugs. You must always resist the pressure to use drugs. **Resistance skills** are skills that help a person say "no" to an action or to leave a situation. Use resistance skills when you are pressured to use drugs.

1. **Say "no" to drug use with self-confidence.**

   - Look directly at the person to whom you are speaking.
   - Say "no" in a firm voice.
   - Be confident because you are being responsible.
   - Be proud because you are obeying laws and respecting family guidelines.

2. **Give reasons for saying "no" to drug use.**

   - Explain that drug use is harmful, unsafe, and illegal.

3. **Use the broken-record technique.**

   - Repeat the same response several times to convince the person pressuring you that you will not change your mind.

4. **Use nonverbal behavior to match verbal behavior. What you do and say should be consistent.**

   - Do not pretend to use a drug.
   - Do not pretend to sip a beer.
   - Do not hold or pass a cigarette or marijuana joint.
   - Do not touch a syringe or needle used to inject drugs.
   - Do not agree to buy a drug for someone else.
   - Do not do or say anything that indicates that you approve of harmful drug use.
   - Do not keep drugs for someone else.

5. **Avoid being in situations in which there will be pressure to use harmful drugs.**

   - Think ahead about what peers will be doing when they invite you to join them.
   - Ask if there will be drug use before you put yourself in a situation. Do not go anywhere you know there will be drug use.
   - Attend only drug-free activities.

6. **Avoid being with people who use harmful drugs.**
   - Choose friends who do not use drugs.
   - Stay away from people who use or sell drugs.

7. **Resist pressure to engage in illegal behavior.**
   - Learn the laws that apply to drug use in your community and state.
   - Do not break drug-use laws.
   - Stay away from people who break laws pertaining to drug use.
   - Stay away from areas where people use and sell drugs.

8. **Influence others to choose responsible behavior.**
   - Suggest drug-free activities.
   - Encourage those who pressure you to use drugs to change their behavior.
   - Be aware of places where teens who use drugs can get help.

Being High Is NEVER an Excuse for Wrong Behavior

Some teens use alcohol and other drugs as an excuse for something they say or do. Suppose a teen has been drinking and does something embarrassing. The teen thinks (s)he can laugh it off. (S)he thinks that it will not affect his/her reputation, because (s)he was drinking. Or, suppose a teen uses drugs. The teen then has sex. Later, the teen says, "I only had sex with the person because I was on drugs and couldn't help it." Suppose a teen does something illegal. Being high cannot be used as a defense for breaking the law. This is faulty thinking. **You are responsible for what you say and do at all times.**

Reasons for Saying "No" When Pressured by Peers to Use Drugs

- I don't want to betray the trust of my parents or guardian.
- I don't want to break the law and get arrested.
- I don't want to become violent and harm others.
- I don't want to say something I will regret later.
- I don't want to experience blackouts.
- I don't want to hallucinate.
- I don't want to become depressed and consider suicide.
- I don't want to spend time in jail.
- I don't want to become addicted.
- I don't want to risk overdosing.
- I don't want to increase my risk of developing cirrhosis of the liver, cancer, or cardiorespiratory diseases.
- I don't want to be suspended from school.
- I don't want to get kicked off my athletic team.
- I don't want to waste money.
- I want to think clearly.
- I want to stay in control and stick to my decision to choose abstinence.
- I want others to respect me.
- I want to be a role model for my younger siblings.
- I want to have social skills without relying on drugs.
- I want to be able to react quickly to prevent accidents.

How to Be a Drug-Free Role Model

A **drug-free role model** is a person who chooses a drug-free lifestyle, knows and follows laws and policies regarding drugs, and educates others about the risks of using drugs.

Choose a drug-free lifestyle. A **drug-free lifestyle** is a lifestyle in which a person does not misuse or abuse drugs. When you choose a drug-free lifestyle, you have more control over your life. You take responsibility for your behavior and decisions. You do not risk your health and safety or the health and safety of others. You follow laws and respect the guidelines of your parents or guardian and other responsible adults.

Know and follow policies regarding drug use. Know and follow the laws and school policies regarding legal and illegal drugs and drug use. Encourage others to follow these policies.

Educate others about the risks of drug use. Your school or community may have a drug prevention program for which you might volunteer. Some peer programs offer special training to become a peer leader or counselor. A **peer leader** is an older student who teaches younger students about drugs and how to resist pressure to use them.

Activity

Drug Comebacks

Life Skill: I will use resistance skills if I am pressured to misuse or abuse drugs.

Materials: paper, pen or pencil

Directions: For each pressure statement, or come-on, listed below, write a response, or comeback, on a separate sheet of paper. DO NOT WRITE IN THIS BOOK.

Come-On	Comeback
"Nobody will know but me and you."	
"It can't hurt just this one time."	
"You're not afraid, are you?"	
"Everybody is doing it."	
"Don't mess up the fun for everyone else."	
"Don't be a nerd."	
"If you won't do it, don't bother to come."	
"It really is safe."	
"Don't worry, we've been doing this for a long time."	
"It will be fun."	
"It will make you feel better than you ever have before."	

Lesson 54

Review

Vocabulary Words

Write a separate sentence using each of the vocabulary words listed on page 420.

Objectives

1. Why do teens who use drugs pressure their peers to use drugs? **Objective 1**

2. What are direct and indirect ways a teen might feel pressured to use drugs? **Objective 2**

3. What are eight resistance skills that can be used to resist pressure to use drugs? **Objective 3**

4. What are ten reasons to say "no" when pressured by peers to use drugs? **Objective 4**

5. What are three ways to be a drug-free role model? **Objective 5**

Responsible Decision-Making

Suppose you go to a party with a friend. When you get there, some teens are smoking marijuana. They invite you to join them. Your friend knows you do not use drugs. (S)he suggests that you pretend to smoke the marijuana. Write a response to this situation.

1. Describe the situation that requires you to make a decision.
2. List possible decisions you might make.
3. Name two responsible adults with whom you might discuss your decisions.
4. Evaluate the possible consequences of your decisions. Determine if each decision will lead to actions that:
   - promote health,
   - protect safety,
   - follow laws,
   - show respect for yourself and others,
   - follow the guidelines of your parents and of other responsible adults,
   - demonstrate good character.
5. Decide which decision is most responsible and appropriate.
6. Tell two results you expect if you make this decision.

 ## Effective Communication

Work with a partner. Review the Activity on page 424. Think of at least five other pressure statements teens use to convince other teens to use drugs. Have your partner give a comeback for each statement. Reverse roles and repeat the process.

 ## Self-Directed Learning

Investigate your school's drug policies. What substances are prohibited? What determines a drug violation? What are the consequences for violating school drug policies? What actions lead to suspension or expulsion?

 ## Critical Thinking

Review the list Reasons for Saying "No" When Pressured by Peers to Use Drugs. What are your top five reasons for saying "no"?

 ## Responsible Citizenship

Identify a drug prevention peer program in your school or community. Find out how a teen becomes involved in this program. Obtain permission from your parents or guardian to get involved in helping peers resist pressure to use drugs.

You Can Have an Alcohol-Free Lifestyle

Life Skill I will not drink alcohol.

Self-control is the degree to which a person regulates his/her own behavior. You must have self-control to have a healthy mind, body, and relationships. Drinking alcohol influences your self-control and causes harmful changes in your mind, body, and relationships. This lesson includes facts about alcohol. You will learn how drinking affects the body, thinking, and decision-making. You also will learn how drinking increases the risk of violence and illegal behavior. This lesson includes a discussion of alcoholism. It also includes resistance skills you can use if you are pressured to drink alcohol.

The Lesson Outline

What to Know About the Effects of Alcohol on the Body

How Drinking Affects Thinking and Decision-Making

How Drinking Increases the Risk of Violence and Illegal Behavior

What to Know About Alcoholism

How to Resist Peer Pressure to Drink Alcohol

Objectives

1. Discuss BAC and the effects of alcohol on the different body systems. **pages 427–431**

2. Explain nine ways drinking affects thinking and decision-making. **pages 432–433**

3. Explain how drinking increases the risk of violence and illegal behavior. **page 434**

4. Discuss alcoholism: cause, health problems, effects on others, treatment. **page 435**

5. Outline eight resistance skills that can be used to resist pressure to drink alcohol. **page 436**

Vocabulary Words

self-control
alcohol
fermentation
distillation
proof
blood alcohol concentration (BAC)
toxin
hazing activity
binge drinking
dementia
ulcer
alcoholic hepatitis
cirrhosis
malnutrition
cardiomyopathy
fetal alcohol syndrome (FAS)
hangover
blackout
domestic violence
rape
acquaintance rape
alcoholism
denial
alcohol withdrawal syndrome
delirium tremens
Alcoholics Anonymous (AA)
Al-Anon
Al-Ateen

What to Know About the Effects of Alcohol on the Body

Alcohol is a drug found in certain beverages that depresses the brain and nervous system. Alcohol is made by fermentation. **Fermentation** is a process in which yeast, sugar, and water are combined to produce alcohol and carbon dioxide. Alcohol is consumed in alcoholic beverages. The most common alcoholic beverages are beer, wine, and liquor.

Beer is an alcoholic beverage that is made by fermenting barley, corn, or rye. Most beers are about 4 percent alcohol. Malt liquor is beer that has a higher alcohol content than regular beer. Light beer is beer that has fewer calories than regular beer but about the same alcohol content.

Wine is an alcoholic beverage made by fermenting grapes or other fruits. Most wines are about 12 to 14 percent alcohol. A wine cooler is a carbonated, fruit-flavored alcoholic beverage that is 1.5 to 6 percent alcohol.

Liquor is an alcoholic beverage that is made by distillation. **Distillation** is a process that uses a fermented mixture to obtain an alcoholic beverage with a high alcohol content. Whiskey, bourbon, rye, rum, gin, vodka, tequila, and brandy are types of liquor. Liquor may also be called a distilled spirit. Most liquors are about 40 percent alcohol.

Proof is a measure of the amount of alcohol in a beverage. The proof of a beverage is double the percent of alcohol in the beverage. For example, a beverage with 20 percent alcohol is 40 proof.

How Alcohol Enters the Body

Alcohol enters the bloodstream within minutes. About 20 percent of the alcohol that a person drinks is absorbed into the bloodstream through the walls of the stomach. The rest of the alcohol is absorbed through the walls of the intestine. Alcohol affects the body immediately after it is swallowed. The alcohol is absorbed by the stomach and intestines. Then it moves quickly into the bloodstream. Alcohol affects every cell in the body. A small amount of the alcohol is excreted through urine, perspiration, or breath. Most of the alcohol is changed to harmless waste by the liver. The liver can only change about one drink per hour. If people have more than one drink, the excess amount builds up in the body. Eventually, all of the alcohol is excreted. The effects of alcohol intensify as the concentration of alcohol in the blood increases. **Blood alcohol concentration (BAC)** is the amount of alcohol in a person's blood. BAC is given as a percentage. The higher the BAC, the greater the effects of alcohol on the body. The alcohol in a drink goes to all the body tissues before being excreted.

An alcoholic beverage that contains about one-half ounce (14 grams) of alcohol is considered one drink of alcohol. One-half ounce (14 grams) of alcohol is about the amount of alcohol in one can of beer, 4 to 5 ounces (112 to 140 grams) of wine, or one mixed drink. Drinking more than this causes BAC to rise. Alcohol is a toxin. A **toxin** is a substance that is poisonous. If too large an amount is swallowed, the stomach will reject it. This causes a person to vomit. The body attempts to break down alcohol as quickly as possible to remove it from the body. However, a large amount of alcohol in the body takes a long time to be excreted. This is why people who drink alcohol at night may still feel its effects the next morning. Thease people may still be "drunk" the next day. There is no way to speed alcohol through the body. Coffee, showers, and fresh air do not break down alcohol.

Factors That Affect BAC

The following factors influence the way alcohol affects BAC.

1. **Amount of alcohol consumed.** The number of drinks people have affects their BAC. The alcohol content of each drink determines the effects of the alcohol.

2. **Speed at which alcohol is consumed.** Drinking at a faster rate increases BAC. Drinking alcohol quickly is dangerous and can be fatal. When people chug, slam, or down several alcoholic beverages in a short period of time, the liver does not have time to break down the alcohol. The alcohol does not leave the body. BAC can reach life-threatening levels.

3. **Body weight.** People with a higher body weight have a higher volume of blood than people with less body weight. The same amount of alcohol produces a greater effect on people with less body weight.

4. **Percentage of body fat.** Body fat does not absorb as much alcohol as lean body tissue. For example, suppose two people of the same weight have a drink. One person has a higher percentage of body fat than the other. The person with the higher percentage of body fat will have a higher BAC after one drink than the person with a lower percentage of body fat.

5. **Gender.** BAC rises faster in females than in males. Females usually have a higher percentage of body fat than males. Certain hormones make females more sensitive to the effects of alcohol than males. Females also have less than males of a certain stomach enzyme that breaks down alcohol before it enters the bloodstream.

6. **Feelings.** Feelings such as stress, anger, and fear can affect BAC by speeding up the time it takes alcohol to pass into the bloodstream.

7. **Amount of food eaten.** Alcohol passes more quickly into the bloodstream when the stomach is empty than when it is full.

8. **Presence of other drugs in the bloodstream.** The presence of certain drugs in the bloodstream increases the effects of alcohol. For example, tranquilizers and pain killers increase the depressant effects of alcohol.

9. **Age.** Elderly people are more sensitive to the effects of alcohol than are younger people. The bodies of elderly people contain a lower volume of blood than the bodies of younger people.

10. **Drinking carbonated alcoholic beverages.** The alcohol in carbonated beverages passes into the bloodstream more quickly than the alcohol in non-carbonated drinks. Carbonated alcoholic beverages include beer, sparkling wine, champagne, and liquor mixed with carbonated beverages.

What Happens as BAC Increases

The effects of alcohol on people intensify as BAC increases.

BAC of .02 (About one drink in an hour) People feel relaxed. They may have increased social confidence and become talkative. Thinking and decision-making abilities may be impaired.

BAC of .05 (About two drinks in an hour) Areas of the brain that control reasoning and judgment are impaired. Others may be able to tell that people have been drinking. People feel warm, relaxed, and confident. Speech may be slurred. People may say or do things they usually would not say or do. They may not realize that what they are saying or doing is not appropriate. There is a decrease in muscular coordination and reaction time is slowed.

BAC of .10 (About five drinks in an hour) Reasoning, judgment, self-control, muscular coordination, and reaction time are seriously impaired. People no longer can make responsible decisions. However, they may claim not to be affected by the alcohol. They have slurred speech and walk with a stagger. They may have unpredictable emotions. In most states, they are considered legally drunk.

BAC of .12 People usually become confused and disoriented. Their vision may be blurred. They may lose control of coordination and balance, become nauseous, and vomit.

BAC of .20 Emotions are unpredictable and may change rapidly. For example, people may quickly switch from crying to laughing. They may pass out.

BAC of .30 People whose BAC have reached this level have little or no control over their mind and body. Most people cannot stay awake to reach this BAC.

BAC of .40 People whose BAC has reached this level are likely to be unconscious. Their breathing and heartbeat slow down. They may die.

BAC of .50 People whose BAC has reached this level may enter a deep coma and die.

Drinking Can Be a Hazing Activity

Drinking often is used as a hazing activity. A **hazing activity** is an activity in which a person is forced to participate in a dangerous or demeaning act to become a member of a club or group. Some teens have been forced to drink large quantities of alcohol during hazing activities. Some teens have died from these hazing activities. Do not participate in hazing activities. Hazing activities are against the law in most states. Hazing activities violate the rules of most schools. Report incidences of hazing activities to a parent, guardian, or other responsible adult.

Drinking Games Can Be Life-Threatening

Drinking alcohol quickly—chugging, downing, doing shots, funneling, or gulping—is especially dangerous. Binge drinking also is extremely dangerous. **Binge drinking** is consuming large amounts of alcohol in a short amount of time. Binge drinking and drinking quickly can cause BAC to rise to dangerous levels very rapidly. People may become unconscious or dangerously drunk.

Some teens drink quickly playing drinking games. Some drinking games are races to finish large quantities of alcohol. Others involve drinking as a punishment for losing the game. Teens have died from playing drinking games.

How Alcohol Affects the Body

Alcohol is a leading cause of death. Almost every part of the body is harmed when people drink large quantities of alcohol. People who drink regularly usually require more health care than other people. Heavy drinking harms most of the body systems.

Nervous System

Drinking impairs the brain and other parts of the nervous system. It can destroy nerve cells. Drinking alcohol can cause blackouts and seizures. People who drink heavily may develop dementia. **Dementia** is a general decline in all areas of mental functioning. People with dementia caused by alcohol can recover from dementia if they stop drinking.

Digestive System

Drinking increases the risk of developing cancers of the mouth, esophagus, and stomach. When people drink alcohol, their mouth, esophagus, and stomach are directly exposed to alcohol. The cells in the linings of these organs change and may become cancerous. Drinking alcohol also stimulates the secretion of stomach acids. This may injure the inner lining of the stomach and cause ulcers. An **ulcer** is an open sore on the skin or on a mucous membrane. Ulcers usually are inflamed and painful.

Drinking also increases the risk of developing liver disease. As alcohol is oxidized in the liver, it poisons the liver. When the liver is poisoned by alcohol it goes through three stages of disease. The first stage occurs when the liver becomes enlarged with fatty tissue. People with a fatty liver usually do not feel sick. In the second stage, they develop alcoholic hepatitis. **Alcoholic hepatitis** is a condition in which the liver swells due to alcohol. People with this condition may have yellowing of the skin and eyes, abdominal pain, and fever. Alcoholic hepatitis can cause serious illness or death. The third stage is cirrhosis. **Cirrhosis** is a disease of the liver caused by chronic damage to liver cells. Cirrhosis can cause liver failure and death. A liver transplant is the only effective treatment for people with advanced cirrhosis.

Heavy drinking increases the risk of developing pancreatitis. Pancreatitis is inflammation of the pancreas. People with pancreatitis are at risk for developing diabetes mellitus. Diabetes mellitus, or diabetes, is a disease in which the body produces little or no insulin. Heavy drinking also may lead to pancreatic cancer.

Heavy drinking also can cause malnutrition. **Malnutrition** is a condition in which the body does not get the nutrients required for optimal health. People who drink usually eat less food and eat a poorly balanced diet. Drinking also interferes with the digestion and absorption of nutrients. Thiamin, folate, vitamin A, and zinc are commonly deficient in people who drink alcohol. Alcohol-related nutritional deficiencies can cause anemia.

Immune System

Drinking depresses the function of the immune system. This increases the risk of developing certain illnesses, such as respiratory infections, tuberculosis, and certain cancers. Long-term drinking lowers the number of infection-fighting cells in the body. It decreases the ability of these cells to fight pathogens.

Cardiovascular System

Drinking can damage the organs of the cardiovascular system. People who drink are at increased risk for developing cardiovascular diseases, high blood pressure, and stroke. Heavy drinking increases the risk of cardiomyopathy. **Cardiomyopathy** is a disease in which the heart muscles weaken and enlarge, and blood cannot be pumped effectively. Drinking also causes blood vessels to widen, giving a false feeling of warmth. People can lose body heat and get frostbite or hypothermia in cold weather.

Skeletal System

Drinking causes the body to lose calcium. Calcium is necessary for proper development of the skeletal system and bones. Frequent, long-term use of alcohol is a risk factor for developing osteoporosis. Osteoporosis is a condition in which the bones become thin and brittle. People who have osteoporosis are at high risk for breaking bones.

Urinary System

Alcohol increases urine flow. Long-term, heavy drinking can cause kidney failure.

Reproductive System

Drinking can have significant effects on the reproductive system during puberty. In females, it can delay the first menstrual cycle and cause irregular periods. It also can affect breast development. Females who drink as teens may have an increased risk of developing breast cancer later in life. In males, drinking can affect the size of the testes and the development of muscle mass. It can affect the age at which the voice deepens and the amount of body and facial hair.

Warning: Drinking Alcohol During Pregnancy Can Cause FAS

Drinking alcohol at any time during pregnancy is harmful to a developing baby. When a female who is pregnant drinks, the alcohol quickly reaches the developing baby through the bloodstream. Drinking is especially harmful during the early months of pregnancy when the body systems are being formed.

Drinking alcohol during pregnancy can cause miscarriage and stillbirth. A miscarriage is the natural ending of a pregnancy before a baby is developed enough to survive on its own. A stillbirth is a baby that is born dead. Drinking during pregnancy also increases the risk of bleeding, premature separation of the placenta, and several other complications of pregnancy.

Babies exposed to alcohol during pregnancy may be shorter and smaller than other babies. Pregnant females who have been drinking heavily during the last three months of pregnancy are more likely to have a low birth weight infant. A low birth weight infant is an infant that weighs less than five pounds (2.2 kilograms) at the time of birth. Low birth weight infants are at risk for respiratory problems, feeding problems, infections, and long-term developmental problems.

Newborn babies with mothers who are alcohol-dependent may have symptoms of alcohol withdrawal shortly after they are born. Babies born to females who drink alcohol during the later part of pregnancy may have alcohol withdrawal. These babies may have sleeping problems, abnormal muscle tension, shakes, and abnormal reflexes. They cry more frequently than other babies.

Babies of mothers who drink alcohol during pregnancy may be born with fetal alcohol syndrome. **Fetal alcohol syndrome (FAS)** is the presence of severe birth defects in babies born to mothers who drink alcohol during pregnancy. Babies with FAS may have small eye slits, a small head, and retarded physical and mental growth. FAS is a leading cause of mental retardation.

How Drinking Affects Thinking and Decision-Making

- **Drinking alcohol can cause you to make wrong decisions.** If you drink alcohol, you may not use the guidelines for making responsible decisions. You might make a choice that you would not make if you were not under the influence of alcohol. The choice may risk your health and safety. It may cause you to break the law and family guidelines, lose your self-respect and the respect of others, and ruin your reputation.

- **Drinking alcohol can give you a false sense of self-confidence in social situations.** If you are shy and insecure you should never use a drink to be more social. If you do, you are using alcohol as a crutch. Because alcohol affects communication and reasoning, you may find out later that you did or said things that were not appropriate or were out of character. For example, you may drink and suddenly have the courage to talk to someone you really like. You talk to this person and believe you had a good conversation. However, you find out later that you slurred your words.

- **Drinking alcohol can interfere with your judgment.** You may say or do things you usually would not say or do. For example, you may insult someone or share a secret you were supposed to keep. The next day you may find out that you lost a friend.

- **Drinking alcohol can make you feel invincible.** You may do something daring or dangerous. You might injure yourself or someone else. For example, teens who have been drinking alcohol have been known to jump from rooftop to rooftop. Several teens have misjudged the distance and were seriously injured.

- **Drinking alcohol can increase the likelihood that you will give in to negative peer pressure.** If you have been drinking, you are more likely to be persuaded by peers to do things you would not normally do. Suppose you drink too much alcohol and are talked into experimenting with marijuana. You have engaged in two risk behaviors that are harmful and illegal.

- **Drinking alcohol can intensify your sexual feelings and dull your reasoning.** If you drink, your sexual feelings are difficult to control. Your reasoning is dulled, and you might participate in unplanned sexual activity. Most teens who have been sexually active were drinking before they had sex. More than one-half of teen females who become pregnant report that they were under the influence of alcohol when they had sex. Many teens are infected with sexually transmitted diseases (STDs) and HIV when they are drinking alcohol.

- **Drinking alcohol slows your reaction time and affects your coordination.** If you drink, you cannot respond as quickly as usual. For example, you may be a responsible pedestrian. After a few drinks, you might cross the street as the light turns yellow rather than waiting. You might be struck by a car.

- **Drinking alcohol can cause you to have aggressive behavior.** If you drink, you are more likely to argue and get into fights. Many acts of violence, such as physical abuse and murder, occur after someone has been drinking. For example, a teen male who has been drinking alcohol at a party may have a drink spilled on him accidentally by another teen. He usually would resolve conflict without violence. However, because he has been drinking alcohol, he becomes angry and beats up the other teen.

- **Drinking alcohol intensifies your emotions.** If you drink, you will have more intense feelings than usual. You may feel extremely sad, depressed, desperate, jealous, or angry. Drinking to numb depressed feelings is very dangerous. Most suicide attempts in teens involve alcohol or other drugs.

Hangovers

A **hangover** is an aftereffect of using alcohol and other drugs. A hangover may involve a headache, increased sensitivity to sounds, nausea, vomiting, tiredness, and irritability. Hangovers may interfere with responsibilities, such as school, jobs, physical activity, and family activities. Some teens think that it is not dangerous for people in high school and college to drink and get drunk now and then. They believe faulty statements, such as "Everybody parties when they are in school" or "Drinking is OK to celebrate prom night." They say they will stop this behavior when they are older. However, drinking alcohol one time can have serious consequences. Drinking now and then can lead to drug dependence. Some experts claim that teens who drink are more at risk for developing alcoholism than adults who drink.

Blackouts

People who drink alcohol may have blackouts. A **blackout** is a period in which a person cannot remember what has happened. People who have been drinking may do something risky, embarrassing, or violent and not remember this behavior later. People who have blackouts may find themselves in a place and not remember how they got there. These people may have participated in sexual behavior and not remember. Other people may not be able to tell that a person is having a blackout. They may later tell the person what (s)he did while drinking, and the person may find it difficult to believe.

How Drinking Increases the Risk of Violence and Illegal Behavior

Alcohol and Violence

Alcohol, more than any other drug, has been linked with violence. People who drink alcohol often have a false sense of confidence and little regard for the feelings and safety of others. They may act on angry or aggressive feelings and harm others. Teens who drink or spend time with people who do are at risk for fighting, abuse, and murder. They also are more likely to engage in illegal behaviors, such as shoplifting, damaging property, and selling drugs.

Alcohol and Domestic Violence

A leading cause of divorce and broken families is domestic violence. **Domestic violence** is violence that occurs within a family. Most acts of domestic violence occur after a family member has been drinking alcohol. Each year, many children are seriously abused by a parent or guardian who uses alcohol.

Alcohol and Rape

Drinking alcohol is a risk factor for rape. **Rape** is the threatened or actual use of physical force to get someone to have sex without giving consent. **Acquaintance rape** is rape in which the rapist is known to the person who is raped. Teens who have been drinking may become victims of acquaintance rape.

People who have been drinking are more likely to commit rape. Inhibitions are reduced, thinking is impaired, and sexual feelings are increased. A person may not acknowledge the other person saying "no." People who rape someone after drinking are accountable in a court of law. People who get someone drunk in order to have sex also can be charged with rape.

Alcohol and Suicide

Drinking can intensify feelings of sadness and depression. Alcohol is a factor in many teen suicide attempts. The teens were not thinking clearly and could not see another way of coping with their problems.

Alcohol and the Law

Drinking and buying alcohol is against the law for teens. In most states, people must be 21 years old to purchase alcohol. A minor is a person who is under the legal age. Minors who drink or purchase alcohol risk being arrested, fined, and jailed. Asking someone who is over the legal age to buy alcohol is illegal. So is using fake identification to buy alcohol.

Alcohol and School Policies

Teens who drink alcohol during school hours or bring alcohol to school are breaking school policies. Most schools suspend or expel students who break school alcohol policies. Teens who drink are more likely than other teens to drop out of school and to have lower grades. Teens who drink may skip school to drink or to recover from hangovers.

Alcohol and Driving

People who drink alcohol and drive may be injured or killed. They also may injure or kill passengers, other motorists, and pedestrians. Alcohol-related motor vehicle accidents are a leading cause of death and spinal injury in young people. Many teens who have been involved in alcohol-related accidents later report they did not realize at the time that they were not able to drive.

What to Know About
Alcoholism

Alcoholism is a disease in which there is physical and psychological dependence on alcohol. Alcohol dependence is another term for alcoholism. Alcohol dependence can destroy the life of an individual and the lives of those around him/her. Alcoholism is a factor in automobile accidents, injuries, suicide, violence, job loss, divorce, serious illness, and death. Alcoholism often causes family dysfunction and relationship difficulties.

People with alcoholism have difficulty controlling their drinking. They often feel overwhelmed by the desire for another drink. Some people with alcoholism do not drink often, but they are out of control when they do.

Alcoholism causes people's personalities to change. Moods and emotions change rapidly and behavior becomes unpredictable and irresponsible. Feelings of anger, paranoia, and depression can increase.

The Family Connection

Alcoholism affects entire families. People with alcoholism often have difficulties with relationships. They experience problems with money and jobs. They may have accidents or become ill as a result of drinking. They may neglect or injure family members. Family members may not bring friends home because they fear the person with alcoholism will embarrass them or become violent. Family members of people with alcoholism often are codependent. They may blame themselves for the drinking problem.

People with alcoholism continue to drink alcohol even though it causes many problems. They are in denial. **Denial** is refusing to admit a problem. Many alcoholics deny that there is a connection between their problems and their drinking.

People with alcoholism may go through several stages. They may try to stop drinking. This often occurs after they do something they regret, such as abuse a family member. They promise to quit drinking, but they usually do not. When they do, they may suffer from alcohol withdrawal syndrome. **Alcohol withdrawal syndrome** is the reaction of the body to the sudden stopping of drinking. People with alcohol withdrawal syndrome feel nauseous, anxious, and agitated. They may vomit, have tremors ("the shakes"), trouble sleeping, and delirium tremens. **Delirium tremens** is a severe form of alcohol withdrawal syndrome in which there are hallucinations and muscle convulsions.

Children whose parents abuse alcohol are more likely to have problems with alcohol. Alcohol abuse is lower in families in which parents or guardians clearly disapprove of drinking.

Treatment for Alcoholism

People with alcoholism need treatment. This involves treatment for people with the disease as well as counseling for family members and friends. Treatment usually involves short or long-term stays at a recovery facility and may involve recovery programs. **Alcoholics Anonymous (AA)** is a recovery program for people who have alcoholism. **Al-Anon** is a recovery program for people who have friends or family members with alcoholism. **Al-Ateen** is a recovery program for teens who have a family member or friend with alcoholism. Adult Children of Alcoholics (ACOA) is a recovery program for children who have one or more parents, a guardian, or a caregiver with alcoholism. After completing a recovery program, people with alcoholism need support.

How to Resist Peer Pressure to Drink Alcohol

Peer pressure is the most important factor identified by teens who drink alcohol. Despite the fact that drinking is illegal for teens, most teens can get alcoholic beverages. You may be pressured to drink and buy alcohol. Use resistance skills to avoid drinking and buying alcohol.

1. **Use assertive behavior.** Stand tall and look directly at the person. Say "no" in a firm and confident voice.

2. **Give reasons for saying "no" to alcohol.** Explain that drinking is harmful, unsafe, and illegal for teens. Drinking does not show respect for you and others. Drinking is against the law for minors and against family guidelines. Drinking interferes with good character.

3. **Use nonverbal behavior to match verbal behavior.**
   - Do not pretend to drink alcoholic beverages.
   - Do not agree to buy alcohol.
   - Do not laugh at comedy that shows drunk people as humorous.
   - Do not behave in ways that indicate that you approve of drinking.

4. **Avoid being in situations in which there will be pressure to drink alcohol.**
   - If there will be alcohol in a situation, do not go.
   - Attend only alcohol-free activities.
   - Do not go into bars.

5. **Avoid being with people who drink alcohol.**
   - Choose friends who do not drink alcohol.
   - Stay away from gang members.
   - Stay away from minors who try to buy alcohol.
   - Stay away from people over the legal age who buy alcohol or give alcohol to minors.
   - Stay away from people who use fake ID's to buy alcohol and get into bars.

6. **Resist pressure to engage in illegal behavior.**
   - Learn the laws that apply to alcohol use in your community and state.
   - Stay away from people who break laws.
   - Stay away from parties where minors are drinking alcohol.

7. **Influence others to choose responsible behavior.**
   - Suggest alcohol-free activities.
   - Encourage those who pressure you to use alcohol to change their behavior.
   - Encourage people who drink alcohol to stop. Ask a responsible adult or trained counselor how you might help a person who has a drinking problem get treatment.
   - Know signs that indicate people have a drinking problem.

8. **Avoid being influenced by advertisements for alcohol.**
   - Do not be fooled by advertisements.
   - Realize that advertisements may portray the use of alcohol as sexy, sophisticated, adventurous, healthful, or fun.
   - Be aware that alcohol companies pay enormous amounts of money to advertise during major sporting events.
   - Be aware that alcohol companies use the Internet to advertise their products to young people.
   - Do not wear clothing that displays beer logos or logos of other alcoholic beverages.

Review

Vocabulary Words

Write a separate sentence using each of the vocabulary words listed on page 426.

Objectives

1. How does drinking affect a person's health status? **Objective 1**

2. What are nine ways drinking affects thinking and decision-making? **Objective 2**

3. How does drinking increase the risk of violence and illegal behavior? **Objective 3**

4. What are the facts about alcoholism: cause, health problems, effects on others, treatment? **Objective 4**

5. What are eight resistance skills that can be used to resist pressure to drink alcohol? **Objective 5**

Responsible Decision-Making

A friend is trying to decide whether (s)he should attend a party at which there will be drinking. Some classmates encourage the friend to go, while others do not. Your friend does not know how to make up his/her mind. Write a response to this situation.

1. Describe the situation that requires your friend to make a decision.

2. List possible decisions your friend might make.

3. Name two responsible adults with whom your friend might discuss his/her decisions.

4. Evaluate the possible consequences of your friend's decisions. Determine if each decision will lead to actions that:
   - promote health,
   - protect safety,
   - follow laws,
   - show respect for your friend and others,
   - follow the guidelines of your friend's parents and of other responsible adults,
   - demonstrate good character.

5. Decide which decision is most responsible and appropriate for your friend.

6. Tell two results your friend can expect if (s)he makes this decision.

 ### Effective Communication

Create a poster showing the effect of alcohol at increasing levels of blood alcohol concentration (BAC). For each level of BAC, draw a picture showing the effects of the alcohol. Share your poster with classmates.

 ### Self-Directed Learning

Research the laws in your state and community that regulate the use of alcohol. What is the legal drinking age? What are the penalties for underage drinking? What are the penalties for drinking and driving?

 ### Critical Thinking

A group of your friends has gotten two six-packs of beer. One of the group suggests playing drinking games. Why is it dangerous to play drinking games? What might you say to the friend who suggested this activity?

 ### Responsible Citizenship

Some schools have programs in which students sign pledges not to drink alcohol during the prom or other school activities. If your school has this type of program, sign the pledge and show it to your parents or guardian. If your school does not have this type of program, talk to your teacher or a school administrator about starting one.

You Can Have a Tobacco-Free Lifestyle

Life Skill **I will avoid tobacco use and secondhand smoke.**

Tobacco products contain a drug called nicotine. You are more likely to become addicted to nicotine after using a tobacco product once than you are to heroin injected into a vein one time. This lesson explains why you must avoid tobacco use and secondhand smoke. You will learn techniques used to convince people to use tobacco products and skills to resist pressure to use them. This lesson also includes suggestions for teens who have used tobacco products and need to quit.

The Lesson Outline

What to Know About Nicotine

How Smoking Harms Health

How Breathing Secondhand Smoke Harms Health

How Smokeless Tobacco Harms Health

How Tobacco Companies Try to Influence Teens and Young Children to Use Tobacco

How to Resist Pressure to Use Tobacco Products

How to Quit Using Tobacco Products

Objectives

1. Discuss the harmful effects of nicotine. **page 439**
2. Explain how smoking, breathing secondhand smoke, and using smokeless tobacco harm health. **pages 440–443**
3. Discuss ways tobacco companies try to get teens and young children to use tobacco products. **pages 444–445**
4. Outline eight resistance skills that can be used to resist pressure to use tobacco products. **page 446**
5. Outline 13 steps to take to quit using tobacco products. **pages 447–448**

Vocabulary Words

nicotine
tobacco
clove cigarette
eugenol
smokeless tobacco
chewing tobacco
snuff
nicotine withdrawal syndrome
carcinogen
tar
carbon monoxide
asthma
chronic obstructive pulmonary disease (COPD)
emphysema
heart attack
aortic aneurysm
secondhand smoke
environmental tobacco smoke
sidestream smoke
mainstream smoke
Group A carcinogen
leukoplakia
nicotine patch
nicotine chewing gum
tobacco cessation program

What to Know About
Nicotine

Nicotine is a stimulant drug found in tobacco products, including cigarettes and chewing tobacco. Nicotine stimulates the nervous system and is highly addictive. It dulls the taste buds, constricts the blood vessels, and increases heart rate and blood pressure. When tobacco smoke is inhaled into the lungs, nicotine is absorbed into the bloodstream and quickly reaches the brain. Nicotine also can be absorbed into the bloodstream from smokeless tobacco that is placed in the mouth. When the "pick-me-up" effect of nicotine wears off, a user is motivated to use more tobacco.

Tobacco Products That Contain Nicotine

Tobacco is a plant that contains nicotine. Tobacco can be smoked in the form of cigarettes and cigars and in pipes. A cigarette is dried and shredded tobacco wrapped in paper. A **clove cigarette** is a cigarette that has a mixture of ground cloves and tobacco. Clove cigarettes contain higher amounts of tar, nicotine, and carbon monoxide than regular cigarettes. They also contain eugenol. **Eugenol** is a chemical that numbs the back of the throat and reduces the ability to cough. A cigar is dried and rolled tobacco leaves. Pipe tobacco is shredded tobacco that is smoked in a pipe. **Smokeless tobacco** is tobacco that is chewed or snorted but not smoked. Chewing tobacco and snuff are forms of smokeless tobacco. **Chewing tobacco** is a tobacco product made from chopped tobacco leaves that is placed between the gums and cheek. **Snuff** is a tobacco product made from powdered tobacco leaves and stems that is snorted or placed between the gums and cheek.

Nicotine Dependence

Many health experts and health organizations have declared that nicotine is as addictive as heroin, cocaine, and alcohol. Nicotine dependence causes more premature death and disease than all other forms of drug dependence combined. People who regularly use tobacco develop a tolerance to nicotine. They need more and more to produce the desired effect. At first, the desired effect is to feel the stimulation that nicotine causes. Later, it is to lessen the craving for nicotine. People develop a physical dependence on nicotine when the body becomes used to its effects. Psychological dependence develops when people feel the need to smoke or chew tobacco at certain times or for specific reasons.

People who try to quit using tobacco often have nicotine withdrawal syndrome. **Nicotine withdrawal syndrome** is the body's reaction to quitting tobacco products. People with nicotine withdrawal syndrome: feel a craving for tobacco; may be anxious, irritable, restless, have headaches, and have difficulty concentrating; can become frustrated and angry; and have heart palpitations and increased appetite.

Why Experimenting with Tobacco Is Risky

Experimenting with tobacco puts you at risk for nicotine dependence. According to the Surgeon General, the probability of becoming addicted to nicotine after one exposure is higher than for other addictive substances such as heroin, cocaine, and alcohol. Teens have a harder time quitting smoking than people who start smoking when they are older. They also are more likely to become heavy smokers and to die of a disease caused by smoking.

How Smoking Harms Health

Tobacco smoke contains many harmful chemicals in addition to nicotine. Scientists estimate there are more than 4,000 different chemicals in tobacco smoke. Several carcinogens have been found in tobacco smoke. A **carcinogen** is a chemical that is known to cause cancer. Most of the carcinogens in tobacco smoke are found in tar. **Tar** is a sticky, thick fluid that is formed when tobacco is burned. Tar irritates respiratory tissues and is a major cause of lung cancer. Another dangerous substance that forms when tobacco is burned is carbon monoxide. **Carbon monoxide** is an odorless, tasteless gas. It interferes with the ability of blood to carry oxygen.

Smoking Causes Cancer

Smoking causes lung cancer and increases the risk of many other types of cancer. Lung cancer kills more people that any other cancer. According to the American Cancer Society, more females used to die of breast cancer than any other cancer. Now more females die of lung cancer than breast cancer. This is due to higher rates of smoking among females. It is rare for someone who has never smoked to develop lung cancer. Lung cancer almost always causes death. Most people with lung cancer die within five years of learning that they have cancer.

Smoking also is a major risk factor for cancer of the throat, mouth, esophagus, pancreas, and bladder. The American Cancer Society reports that one-third of all cancer deaths are due to tobacco use. They also report that nine out of every ten lung-cancer cases are caused by smoking cigarettes.

Lesson 67 will include more information on cancer.

Smoking Harms the Respiratory System

Smoking prevents the lungs from working effectively. When a person smokes, tar lines the lungs and air passages. Tobacco also harms the cilia in the nose, throat, and bronchial tubes. Cilia are hair-like structures that remove dust and other particles from the air and prevent harmful substances from reaching the lungs. Cilia are destroyed after a person has smoked for several years. This increases the risk of respiratory infection. Smoking aggravates asthma. **Asthma** is a condition in which the bronchial tubes become inflamed and constrict, making breathing difficult.

Smoking is a risk factor for chronic obstructive pulmonary disease (COPD). **Chronic obstructive pulmonary disease (COPD)** is a disease that interferes with breathing. Examples of COPDs are chronic bronchitis and emphysema. Chronic bronchitis is a recurring inflammation of the bronchial tubes that causes mucus to line the bronchial tubes. People must cough often to remove the mucus. Coughing cannot remove all the harmful matter from the air passages. This increases risk of lung infection and interferes with the ability to breathe.

Emphysema is a condition in which the alveoli lose most of their ability to function. The lungs lose their ability to properly inflate and hold air. As a result, it is difficult for oxygen to be absorbed into the bloodstream. Carbon dioxide builds up in the body because it cannot be removed from the bloodstream. It becomes increasingly difficult for people with emphysema to be active. Some people with emphysema must remain in bed and use special equipment to get an adequate amount of oxygen. Emphysema cannot be cured.

Smoking Causes Cardiovascular Diseases

The ingredients in tobacco smoke affect the cardiovascular system. Smoking is a major cause of death from heart and blood vessel diseases and of blood clots and stroke. Smoking speeds up the development of fat deposits on the arteries and damages the inner lining of arteries. Fat deposits reduce the space in the artery through which blood can flow. The risk of developing blood clots increases.

A clot in an artery in the heart can cause a heart attack. A **heart attack** is the death of cardiac muscle caused by a lack of blood flow to the heart. A clot in the brain can result in a stroke. A stroke is a condition caused by a blocked or broken blood vessel in the brain. When someone has a stroke, body parts can be paralyzed. A stroke can be fatal. Smoking also is a risk factor for aortic aneurysm. An **aortic aneurysm** is a bulging in the aorta. The aorta is the main artery in the body. An aneurysm is the result of a weakening in an artery wall.

The nicotine in tobacco smoke raises a person's resting heart rate close to 20 beats per minute. This and inhaled carbon monoxide place extra strain on the heart. Carbon monoxide replaces oxygen in some red blood cells, but body cells still need enough oxygen to survive. The heart must pump faster to deliver the oxygen. The combination of nicotine and carbon monoxide in tobacco smoke may be responsible for the large numbers of smokers who develop heart disease.

Smoking Causes Accidents

Cigarette smoking is a leading cause of fires. Many fires start when a smoldering cigarette ignites bedding, mattresses, and other household furniture. People of all ages often are seriously injured or die when a lit cigarette causes a fire. Explosions often are ignited by a lit cigarette as well. Cigarette smoking also is a factor in many motor vehicle accidents. Accidents have happened when a driver was distracted by trying to light a cigarette or by dropping a lit cigarette. Eye irritation caused by tobacco smoke may distract a driver, reduce vision, and contribute to fatigue.

Smoking Causes Other Health Problems

Smoking can harm other areas of the body in addition to the ones discussed earlier. Smokers are more likely to develop gum disease and to lose teeth and supporting gum tissues. Smoking may cause or worsen ulcers in the stomach and small intestine. Smoking causes ulcers to become inflamed and painful.

Smoking during pregnancy harms the developing baby. Studies show that quitting smoking during pregnancy could prevent 5 percent of infant deaths, 20 percent of low birth-weight babies, and 8 percent of premature deliveries.

Teens Who Smoke May Convince Themselves. . .	vs. The Truth
"I look cool when I smoke."	People who smoke have yellow teeth and dirty and stained fingernails. Their clothes stink of smoke.
"It is 'in' to smoke."	Many people will not hang out with people who smoke. They will not date a person who smokes. Many people do not want to be around people who smoke. This is one reason people choose nonsmoking sections in restaurants.
"My smoking doesn't bother anyone."	Many people do not want people to smoke around their children. Many employers do not hire people who smoke.
"My favorite TV and movie stars use tobacco products."	Most celebrities and athletes do not use tobacco products. The celebrities and athletes who use tobacco products are negative role models. They face the same risks from tobacco use as teens do. Many have developed oral cancer or have died from lung cancer.

How Breathing Secondhand Smoke Harms Health

A lit cigarette burns for about 12 minutes. During those 12 minutes, people who are near the smoker will breathe in secondhand smoke. **Secondhand smoke**, or **environmental tobacco smoke**, is exhaled smoke and sidestream smoke. **Sidestream smoke** is smoke that enters the air from a burning cigarette, cigar, or pipe. Passive smoking and involuntary smoking are other terms used to describe breathing in secondhand smoke. Sidestream smoke has more tar, nicotine, carbon monoxide, ammonia, and benzene than mainstream smoke. **Mainstream smoke** is smoke that is inhaled into the smoker's mouth and lungs.

Secondhand smoke is more than just an annoyance. Even if you do not smoke, your health is harmed by breathing in secondhand smoke. Secondhand smoke is the most hazardous form of indoor air pollution. It can cause lung cancer in nonsmokers and increase their risk of developing heart disease and respiratory problems. People who already have heart disease or respiratory problems are especially affected. Secondhand smoke is a major health risk for children with parents who smoke. The children are at increased risk for ear infection, bronchitis, and pneumonia. The lungs of children exposed to secondhand smoke may not develop properly. Secondhand smoke is an irritant. It causes the eyes to burn. It also can irritate the nose, throat, and airways. Many people report having headaches after breathing secondhand smoke.

There are many places that people can be exposed to secondhand smoke. Children are most likely to be exposed at home. Adults who do not smoke are most likely to be exposed at work. People also are exposed to secondhand smoke in social situations such as parties and in public places such as restaurants.

It is not always easy to avoid secondhand smoke. Five actions you can take to avoid secondhand smoke are:

- Speak up to the person who is smoking, but be polite. Let people know that you are concerned about your health.
- Ask smokers not to smoke in indoor areas that you share.
- Encourage your family to have a nonsmoking policy for your home.
- Encourage family members who smoke to quit smoking and to go outside if they must smoke.
- Request seating in nonsmoking sections of restaurants or in public areas.

Many steps are being taken to protect nonsmokers from secondhand smoke. Laws are being passed to prevent smoking inside public buildings and schools and in the workplace. Airlines have restricted smoking during flights. Many businesses no longer allow smoking in their office buildings or factories. People are showing greater concern for their health and the health of others.

Secondhand Smoke:
A Group A Carcinogen
The Environmental Protection Agency (EPA) classified secondhand smoke as a Group A carcinogen. A **Group A carcinogen** is a substance that causes cancer in humans.

How Smokeless Tobacco Harms Health

Smokeless tobacco is manufactured and sold in two forms. Chewing tobacco is a tobacco product made from chopped tobacco leaves that is placed between the gums and cheek. Snuff is a tobacco product made from powdered tobacco leaves and stems that is snorted or placed between the gums and cheek. Nicotine is released from smokeless tobacco, absorbed through the linings of the mouth or nose, and carried to the brain in the bloodstream. The effects of the nicotine can last for several hours if the tobacco is kept in the mouth. Smokeless tobacco has most of the same harmful ingredients as other tobacco products.

Smokeless tobacco causes nicotine dependence. Every time people use smokeless tobacco they feel the "pick-me-up" effects of nicotine. The body becomes used to these effects. People crave them and use the tobacco again and again. The body develops a tolerance to the effects. Craving and tolerance both are signs of nicotine dependence.

Smokeless tobacco contains many chemicals that harm health. Smokeless tobacco contains formaldehyde, lead, nitrosamines, cadmium, and polonium. All forms of smokeless tobacco contain carcinogens.

Smokeless tobacco increases the risk of developing cancer. When people use smokeless tobacco, the tobacco and its irritating juices are in contact with the gums, cheeks, and lips for long periods of time. This causes a changes in the cells of the mouth called leukoplakia. **Leukoplakia** are abnormal cells in the mouth that appear as white patches of tissue. The abnormal cells can develop into cancer. Using smokeless tobacco also increases the risk of cancer of the larynx, the pharynx, and the esophagus.

Smokeless tobacco causes problems with the gums and teeth. Smokeless tobacco permanently stains teeth and causes bad breath. Tiny particles of tobacco may be visible on the teeth and cause a poor appearance. Chewing tobacco includes particles that scratch and wear away teeth. The sugar in smokeless tobacco mixes with dental plaque to form acids that cause tooth decay. Smokeless tobacco also can cause the gums to pull away from the teeth, exposing the roots. The teeth become more sensitive and are more likely to fall out.

Smokeless tobacco dulls the senses of smell and taste. As a result, people who use smokeless tobacco often eat more salty and sweet foods than do other people. These foods are harmful if eaten in large amounts.

Actions Teens Who Have Used Smokeless Tobacco Must Take

- Quit using smokeless tobacco immediately. Talk to a physician, dentist, or other responsible adult about ways to quit.

- Check your gums and teeth for early signs of oral cancer. These include having a sore in the mouth that does not heal, having a lump or white patch in the mouth, having a sore throat that does not go away, having difficulty chewing and moving the tongue or jaw, and feeling as though something is stuck in the throat. Pull down your lips and check the area where you put the tobacco for leukoplakia.

- Contact a physician or dentist immediately and have an oral examination. You may need a special test to see if you have cancer. If you do have cancer, it must be treated right away. Have your mouth checked by a physician or dentist every three months.

How Tobacco Companies Try to Influence Teens and Young Children to Use Tobacco

An advertisement (ad) is a paid announcement about a product or service. Tobacco manufacturers are not allowed by law to put tobacco ads on TV or radio. Advertising in stores and on billboards and signs inside and outside of buses no longer can have photos or artwork and cannot be in color. The same rule applies to advertising in publications read by a significant number of people under the age of 18.

Tobacco manufacturers have promoted their products in many ways. One way was by distributing clothing and other items that displayed their logos and symbols. People wearing or using these items were a "walking ad" for the tobacco company. However, in 1997 the FDA prohibited the sale or giveaway of products such as caps or gym bags that carry tobacco product brand names or logos.

Tobacco companies also promote their products by offering merchandise in exchange for coupons found on cigarette packs or smokeless tobacco containers. They may have promoted their products by sponsoring sporting events and rock concerts. They wanted people to associate their product and their logo with excitement and glamour. This was a way to advertise their products on TV as advertising tobacco products on TV was banned. Now brand-name sponsorship of these events can be done in the corporate name only.

In 1997, the Food and Drug Administration (FDA) provided that within six months to two years these changes must happen:

- Anyone under the age of 27 must show a photo ID to buy tobacco products.
- Vending machines and self-service displays are banned except in facilities where children are not allowed.

Only the automobile industry spends more money than tobacco companies on advertising.

Required Warnings on Tobacco Products

Tobacco manufacturers are required by law to include warnings on their packages and in their ads to educate people about the dangers of using tobacco products. Tobacco companies must rotate the following warnings on their cigarette packages:

SURGEON GENERAL'S WARNING: Smoking Causes Lung Cancer, Heart Disease, Emphysema, and May Complicate Pregnancy.

SURGEON GENERAL'S WARNING: Quitting Smoking Now Greatly Reduces Serious Risks to Your Health.

SURGEON GENERAL'S WARNING: Smoking by Pregnant Females May Result in Fetal Injury, Premature Birth, and Low-Birth Weight.

SURGEON GENERAL'S WARNING: Cigarette Smoke Contains Carbon Monoxide.

Smokeless tobacco manufacturers are required by law to place the following three warnings on their packages and in their ads:

- This product is not a safe alternative to cigarettes.
- This product may cause gum disease.
- This product may cause mouth cancer.

What Tobacco Ads Do Not Tell You

Tobacco companies spend billions of dollars each year to convince people to use tobacco. They want you to think tobacco use is "in" and to take your attention away from the warnings. Many tobacco ads are designed to appeal to teens. People in the ads are models who are attractive, healthy looking, and well-dressed. They are having fun and are very appealing to members of the opposite sex.

Don't be fooled by these ads. What they fail to tell you is that smoking cigarettes does not help you to look attractive, healthy, or well-dressed. People are likely to be turned off by your behavior, your breath, and your stained teeth. Tobacco ads also do not tell you that more than 400,000 people die each year from smoking. They do not show people dying of lung disease or restricted to bed because of emphysema. They do not show family members grieving the death of loved ones who used tobacco.

How Tobacco Companies Hook Young Children

Tobacco companies claim they do not design ads that target children. However, ads use cartoon characters that appeal to children. On the Internet, tobacco companies appeal to children by using interactive games, giveaways, and chats to promote their products. They promote the idea that using tobacco products makes a person seem more grownup and "cool."

Cigarette companies hooked children by placing "kiddy packs" and "loosies" in stores. A kiddy pack is a package of cigarettes containing fewer than the standard 20 cigarettes in a pack. A loosie is a single cigarette that is available for purchase. However, a 1997 FDA rule banned the sale of kiddy packs and loosies. It also banned free samples of tobacco products.

Activity

Don't Be Fooled by Ads

Life Skill: I will avoid tobacco use and secondhand smoke.

Materials: ads for tobacco products, markers, colored pens, tape

Directions: Follow the steps below to complete the activity and learn more about tobacco ads.

 Find two different ads for tobacco products. Identify how each ad is designed to make tobacco appear appealing to teens.

 Write a story about the scene in each ad that tells the truth about using tobacco products. For example, the ad may show attractive people playing volleyball on a beach. Your story might explain that these people really have yellow teeth, their clothing smells, and they would not be able to play volleyball without stopping to cough and wheeze.

 Attach each story to the appropriate ad. Share the stories with your classmates.

How to Resist Pressure to Use Tobacco Products

Even though an increasing number of teens use tobacco, the majority of teens do not. You may be pressured to use tobacco. Think ahead of ways you might be pressured to use tobacco. Be ready to use resistance skills, when someone pressures you to use tobacco products.

1. **Use assertive behavior.** Stand tall and look directly at the person with whom you are speaking. Say "no" in a firm and confident voice.

2. **Give reasons for saying "no" to tobacco.** Explain that tobacco use is harmful, unsafe, and illegal for minors. Using tobacco does not show respect for you and others. Using tobacco is against the guidelines of your family and school. Buying tobacco is against the law for minors.

3. **Use nonverbal behavior to match verbal behavior.**
   - Do not send mixed messages to others.
   - Do not hold a cigarette or pretend to smoke.
   - Do not use or carry candy cigarettes or shredded gum that is designed to look like smokeless tobacco.
   - Do not agree to get tobacco for a minor.
   - Do not keep tobacco products in your possession for someone else.
   - Do not behave in ways that indicate that you approve of tobacco use.

4. **Avoid being in situations in which there will be pressure to use tobacco.**
   - Avoid situations in which there will be tobacco.
   - Think ahead about what to say or do if your peers are using tobacco.

5. **Avoid being with people who use tobacco.**
   - Choose friends who do not use tobacco.
   - Stay away from secondhand smoke.

6. **Resist pressure to engage in illegal behavior.**
   - Learn the laws that apply to tobacco use in your community and state.
   - Do not lie about your age to buy tobacco products.
   - Do not purchase tobacco products from vending machines.

7. **Influence others to choose responsible behavior.**
   - Encourage people who pressure you to use tobacco to change their behavior.
   - Encourage people who use tobacco to quit.
   - Suggest tobacco cessation programs to people who smoke or use smokeless tobacco.
   - Be a role model for a tobacco-free lifestyle.
   - Tell others who smoke not to light up around you.

8. **Avoid being influenced by tobacco ads.**
   - Recognize that ads are designed to convince people to use a product and make profit for the company.
   - Recognize that tobacco use is NOT sexy, sophisticated, adventurous, healthful, or fun.
   - Do not attend or view sporting events or concerts sponsored by tobacco companies.
   - Pay attention to the warnings on tobacco ads.
   - Make complaints to city officials if billboards for tobacco are placed in your neighborhood or near your school.
   - Do not wear clothing that displays tobacco logos.
   - Do not accept free samples of cigarettes.

How to Quit Using Tobacco Products

There are many reasons to quit using tobacco. People who quit using tobacco live longer than those who continue to use tobacco. They reduce their risk of heart disease, stroke, emphysema, chronic bronchitis, and some forms of cancer.

There are even more immediate rewards to quitting smoking. Within a day after people stop smoking, the body begins to heal itself from the damages caused by tobacoo. Breathing is easier and a smoker's cough is not as frequent. The sense of taste and smell improve.

How to Quit Using Tobacco

Quitting tobacco use takes planning and effort. Suppose you know someone who uses tobacco and wants to quit. Share the following steps with the person.

1. **List the reasons you want to quit.** Focus on all the things that you do not like about using tobacco. For example, you might think about the mess, the inconvenience, wasting money, the way it makes you smell, the cravings, and the dangers. Ask family members and friends to contribute to reasons.

2. **Decide when you want to quit.** Set a target date to quit. Know what to expect. Understand that nicotine withdrawal symptoms are temporary. Understand that quitting is not easy, but it is possible. Expect to experience pressures to use tobacco when you feel stress.

3. **Make a health behavior contract.** Make a health behavior contract with the life skill "I will stop using smokeless tobacco" or "I will stop smoking." Describe the effect that the life skill will have on your well-being. Design a plan to quit using tobacco. Determine how you will evaluate your progress.

4. **Consider situations in which you usually have a cigarette or use smokeless tobacco.** Change your daily routines to avoid situations in which you used to use tobacco. For example, go for a walk instead of participating in activities that make you want to smoke. Stay busy and active.

5. **Get help from a health care professional.** Make an appointment with a school nurse or a physician to help you with your plan. A physician might prescribe a low-dose nicotine patch or nicotine chewing gum. A **nicotine patch** is a patch worn on the skin of the upper body or arms that releases nicotine into the bloodstream at a slow rate. **Nicotine chewing gum** is chewing gum that releases nicotine when chewed. Nicotine patches and chewing gum release nicotine into the bloodstream without the cancer-causing chemicals from tobacco. They help people cope with cravings for tobacco and withdrawal from nicotine. They can gradually eliminate the need for nicotine. However, there can be side effects. Using nicotine gum can result in sore jaws, upset stomach, nausea, heartburn, loosened dental fillings and problems with dentures. Nicotine patches can cause redness, itching, swelling, nervousness, dry mouth, and inability to sleep.

6. **Join a tobacco cessation program.** A **tobacco cessation program** is a program to help a person stop smoking or using smokeless tobacco. Tobacco cessation programs are offered by local chapters of the American Cancer Society, the American Lung Society, and the American Heart Association; health departments; schools; and hospitals.

7. **Get help from others.** Tell family members and friends that you are quitting. Ask for encouragement and support. If you have a friend or family member who uses tobacco, ask this person to quit with you.

8. **Throw away all tobacco products.** Get rid of items associated with tobacco use, such as ashtrays, lighters, and matches.

9. **Be prepared for temptation.** For the first few weeks or longer after quitting, you may have the urge to use tobacco. These cravings will be strongest during situations in which you used to use tobacco the most. Try to stay away from people who use tobacco. Substitute the urge to use tobacco with another activity.

10. **Participate in activities that keep your mind off of using tobacco.** Try vigorous exercise to release beta-endorphins. Beta-endorphins may help relieve tension caused by quitting. Participating in other activities, such as working on a hobby or going to a movie, also may help.

11. **Avoid weight gain.** Eat a healthful diet with the proper amount of protein, carbohydrates, and fat. Eat plenty of fruits and vegetables. Have low-fat and low-calorie snacks. Participate in physical activity regularly. Do not overeat.

12. **Keep your guard up.** The urge to use tobacco often comes at predictable times. Continue to plan ahead for these situations. Find ways to cope with urges to use tobacco.

13. **If you slip up and use tobacco, keep trying to quit.** Do not feel discouraged. Slipping up does not have to mean failure. Think of it as a setback. Figure out why you slipped up and how to avoid it the next time.

Every day, almost 3,000 teens in the United States—1 million a year—become smokers. One-third of these teens will eventually die from smoking.

About 90 percent of all smokers began smoking before the age of 18.

Smokers who die of smoking-related diseases would have lived about 12 to 15 years longer if they had not smoked

More than 400,000 people die each year—about 1,100 a day—from smoking-related diseases.

Cigarette smoking kills more people each year than illegal drugs, alcohol, homicides, suicides, AIDS, car accidents, and fires combined.

More than one in every six deaths are caused by smoking.

Smoking just two cigarettes a day doubles a person's risk of lung cancer.

Lesson 56

Review

Vocabulary Words

Write a separate sentence using each of the vocabulary words listed on page 438.

Objectives

1. What are the harmful effects of nicotine? **Objective 1**
2. How do smoking, breathing secondhand smoke, and using smokeless tobacco harm health? **Objective 2**
3. What are ways tobacco companies try to get teens and young children to use tobacco products? **Objective 3**
4. What are eight resistance skills that can be used to resist pressure to use tobacco products? **Objective 4**
5. What are 13 steps to take to quit using tobacco products? **Objective 5**

Responsible Decision-Making

Suppose your friend offers you a cigarette. You have never smoked before. Your friend tells you that trying one cigarette won't do any harm. Write a response to this situation.

1. Describe the situation that requires you to make a decision.
2. List possible decisions you might make.
3. Name two responsible adults with whom you might discuss your decisions.
4. Evaluate the possible consequences of your decisions. Determine if each decision will lead to actions that:
   • promote health,
   • protect safety,
   • follow laws,
   • show respect for yourself and others,
   • follow the guidelines of your parents and of other responsible adults,
   • demonstrate good character.
5. Decide which decision is most responsible and appropriate.
6. Tell two results you expect if you make this decision.

Effective Communication

Design a warning label for a pack of cigarettes. Include information about the effects of smoking on health and appearance.

Self-Directed Learning

Find out the average price of a pack of cigarettes. Calculate the cost of smoking one pack of cigarettes per day for a month, a year, and ten years. How much money would smoking cost for each period of time?

Critical Thinking

Refer to the chart on page 441 about teens who smoke. Write three new items for each column of the chart.

Responsible Citizenship

Identify ten restaurants and other businesses in your community that are smoke-free. Select one of these businesses. Write a letter to the business showing appreciation for its smoke-free policy.

You Can Avoid Illegal Drug Use

Life Skill I will not be involved in illegal drug use.

A **controlled drug** is a drug whose possession, manufacture, distribution, and sale are controlled by law. A prescription is needed to obtain controlled drugs. **Illegal drug use** is the use of a controlled drug without a prescription. It is illegal to buy or sell controlled drugs on the street. This lesson discusses controlled drugs. You will learn the powerful effects that controlled drugs have on the mind and body. You will learn how to resist pressure to be involved in illegal drug use.

Vocabulary Words

See the Word Search Activity on page 459 for the vocabulary words in this lesson.

Objectives

1. Explain how the illegal use of stimulants harms health. **pages 451–452**

2. Explain how the illegal use of sedative-hypnotics harms health. **page 453**

3. Explain how the illegal use of narcotics harms health. **page 454**

4. Explain how the illegal use of hallucinogens harms health. **page 455**

5. Explain how the illegal use of marijuana harms health. **page 456**

6. Explain how the illegal use of anabolic-androgenic steroids harms health. **page 457**

7. Explain how the illegal use of inhalants harms health. **page 458**

8. Outline seven resistance skills that can be used to resist pressure to use illegal drugs. **page 460**

The Lesson Outline

How Stimulants Affect Health Status

How Sedative-Hypnotics Affect Health Status

How Narcotics Affect Health Status

How Hallucinogens Affect Health Status

How Marijuana Affects Health Status

How Anabolic-Androgenic Steroids Affect Health Status

How Inhalants Affect Health Status

How to Resist Pressure to Use Illegal Drugs

How Stimulants Affect Health Status

Stimulants are a group of drugs that speed up the activities of the central nervous system. Stimulants are sometimes called "uppers" because they make people feel alert, awake, and active. They increase blood pressure, heart rate, and breathing rate. Teens use legal and illegal stimulants to get a high, stay awake, and to lose weight.

The use of stimulants is always followed by a "crash." A crash is the intense down period that follows a stimulant "high." People who crash feel fatigued, weak, sleepy, very sad, and depressed. People who use stimulants often take larger amounts of stimulants to avoid the crash. They develop physical and psychological dependence.

Kind of Stimulants

Cocaine is a highly addictive stimulant that is obtained from the leaves of the coca bush. It can be snorted, injected, or smoked. It takes about three minutes for cocaine to reach the brain when it is snorted, about fifteen seconds when it is injected into a vein, and seven seconds when it is smoked. Cocaine stimulates the stress response and may cause death by heart attack, stroke, or seizure. Trying cocaine even once can be fatal.

Cocaine Is Illegal.
Cocaine also is known as:
- Coke
- White Lady
- Snow
- Blow
- Bernies
- Charlie
- Gold Dust

Crack is purified cocaine that is smoked to produce a rapid and intense reaction. It is named for the sound it produces when smoked. Crack is even more addictive than regular cocaine. Crack is a type of cocaine that is known as freebase cocaine. The effects of crack and freebase cocaine are ten times greater than those of snorted cocaine. People who use crack may become rapidly addicted. Trying crack even once can be fatal.

Crack Is Illegal.
Crack also is known as:
- Rock

Amphetamines are chemically manufactured stimulants that are highly addictive. They used to be taken as diet pills. They no longer are sold for this purpose because of possible harmful effects.

A **look-alike drug** is a drug manufactured to resemble another drug and mimic its effects. Look-alike drugs often are made for amphetamines. Look-alike amphetamines contain large amounts of legal, nonprescription stimulants such as caffeine.

Methamphetamines are a group of stimulant drugs that fall within the amphetamine family. The effects are similar to those of cocaine. Methamphetamines are swallowed, snorted, injected, or smoked. **Ice** is a smokable form of pure methamphetamine.

Methamphetamines Are Illegal.
Methamphetamines also are known as:
- Meth
- Crystal Meth
- Crystal
- Crank
- Crystal Tea
- Ice

Methcathinone is a stimulant that has effects similar to those of methamphetamine. It is swallowed, snorted, injected, or smoked. The abuse of methcathinone is increasing.

Methcathinone Is Illegal.
Methacathinone also is known as:
- Cat
- Wildcat
- Bathtub Speed
- Goob

Ephedrine is a stimulant that is found naturally in the ephedra plant. It is a common ingredient in decongestants, bronchodilators, and diet pills. A **decongestant** is a drug used to relieve a stuffed-up nose. A **bronchodilator** is a drug that is taken to make breathing easier. Ephedrine is prescribed to relieve asthma. It may be used for cooking methamphetamine and methcathinone. The Food and Drug Administration (FDA) banned the over-the-counter sale of decongestants and bronchodilators that contain ephedrine.

Ephedrine Is Illegal Without a Prescription.
Ephedrine also is known as:
- Effies
- White Cross

Methylphenidate is a stimulant that is used to treat Attention Deficit Hyperactivity Disorder. **Attention Deficit Hyperactivity Disorder (ADHD)** is a learning disability in which a person is easily distracted and also is hyperactive. Methylphenidate stimulates a portion of the brain that helps a person pay attention and reduces hyperactivity.

Caffeine is a stimulant found in chocolate, coffee, tea, some soda pops, and some prescription and over-the-counter drugs. It is the most widely used stimulant and is not a controlled substance. Caffeine produces a quick "pick-me-up" effect. It increases the likelihood of having irregular heartbeats, irritates the stomach, and increases urine production. Some people develop caffeinism. **Caffeinism** is poisoning due to heavy caffeine intake.

How the Illegal Use of Stimulants Can Harm Health

By causing immediate death. Within minutes, people who have taken a stimulant may have seizures, stop breathing, and die. Some people lack a chemical in the liver needed to break down cocaine. They can have an immediate fatal reaction. Mixing other drugs with stimulants increases the risk of overdose and possible death.

By harming the body. People who use stimulants may experience body tremors, vomiting, a racing heart, increased alertness, and quickened movements. Stimulants raise heart rate and blood pressure, which can lead to the breaking of a blood vessel in the brain. This can cause a stroke. Snorting stimulants causes sores and burns in and around the nose. People who snort large amounts may develop holes between their nostrils and have a running nose, sore throat, and hoarse voice.

By harming the mind. People who use stimulants can become confused, anxious, aggressive, and paranoid. Their emotions change. They may have hallucinations. A **hallucination** is an imagined sight, sound, or feeling.

By causing dependence. The body builds up tolerance to stimulants very quickly. Some people who use stimulants increase their doses rapidly and become physically dependent. This can occur after using stimulants only one time.

By increasing the risk of becoming infected with HIV and hepatitis B. People infected with HIV or hepatitis B may leave infected blood on a needle after injecting themselves with stimulants. If the needle is used by other people, the infected blood may enter their bodies and infect them.

By increasing the risk of accidents, violence, and crime. Stimulants impair reasoning and judgment, often resulting in accidents. They increase feelings of anger and aggressiveness and can lead to violence. Selling and buying cocaine and other stimulants often is associated with gangs and violence. Laboratories that produce illegal stimulants may explode and emit toxic gases.

How Sedative-Hypnotics Affect Health Status

Sedative-hypnotics are a group of drugs that depress the activities of the central nervous system. A **sedative** is a drug that has a calming effect on a person's behavior. A **hypnotic** is a drug that produces drowsiness and sleep. Sedative-hypnotics include tranquilizers and sleeping pills. They are highly addictive and are illegal when used without a prescription.

The two major types of sedative-hypnotics are barbiturates and benzodiazepines. A **barbiturate** is a type of sedative-hypnotic that used to be prescribed to help people sleep and to relieve tension. Today, physicians rarely prescribe barbiturates because they are very addictive and

dangerous. **Benzodiazepines** are sedative-hypnotics. They often are prescribed by physicians to treat anxiety. They are commonly known as tranquilizers. Benzodiazepines also are prescribed to relax muscles and as anticonvulsants. An **anticonvulsant** is a drug that is taken to prevent or relieve epileptic seizures. Benzodiazepines are dangerous unless used under medical supervision. An example is flunitrazepam, the "date rape drug."

Sedative-Hypnotics Are Illegal Without a Prescription.

Sedative-Hypnotics also are known as:
- Roofies
- Bank Bandits
- Reds
- Barbs
- Ludes
- Blockbusters

How the Illegal Use of Sedative-Hypnotics Can Harm Health

By causing immediate death. Combining sedative-hypnotics with alcohol is extremely risky and can be fatal. Alcohol multiplies the depressive effects of sedative-hypnotics on the central nervous system. This combination of drugs slows respiration and can cause coma and death.

By harming the body. Sedative-hypnotics slow body functions. People who take sedative-hypnotics may have slurred speech, lack of coordination, clammy skin, dilated pupils, and an inability to stay awake.

By harming the mind. People who take sedative-hypnotics cannot use reasoning and judgment to make responsible decisions. They may be lazy and constantly tired. Some people who take sedative-hypnotics develop depression.

By causing dependence. The use of barbituates and benzodiazepines can lead to physical dependence. People physically dependent on barbituatcs or benzodiazepines have withdrawal

if they stop taking the drug. Withdrawal symptoms include anxiety, sweating, difficulty sleeping, restlessness, agitation, and muscle tremors. People who are physically dependent can have seizures, hallucinations, and elevated blood pressure and heart rate. Withdrawal from sedative-hypnotics can be fatal.

By increasing the risk of becoming infected with HIV and hepatitis B. People who use sedative-hypnotics cannot make responsible decisions. They may have sex with a person infected with HIV or hepatitis B and become infected themselves.

By increasing the risk of accidents, violence, and crime. Sedative-hypnotics impair reasoning and judgment, cause confusion, reduce muscular coordination, and slow reaction time. It is risky to use sedative-hypnotics when driving a car, riding a bicycle, or operating machinery. Sedative-hypnotics also cause feelings of anger and aggressiveness and can lead to violence. Selling and buying sedative-hypnotics is illegal.

How Narcotics Affect Health Status

Narcotics are a group of drugs that slow down the central nervous system and relieve pain. They slow down body functions, such as breathing and heart rate. Narcotics often are prescribed by physicians as analgesics. An **analgesic** is a drug that relieves pain. Narcotics also are used to suppress coughs and control diarrhea. Narcotics should be used only with the supervision of a physician.

Some narcotics are made from opium and morphine. **Opium** is a white, milky fluid from the seedpod of the poppy plant. **Morphine** is a narcotic found naturally in opium that is used to control pain. Morphine is one of the strongest pain relievers used in medicine. It causes addiction and severe withdrawal symptoms. **Codeine** is a painkiller produced from morphine. **Heroin** is an illegal narcotic derived from morphine. It often is injected, snorted, smoked, and taken as a pill. People who inject heroin are at high risk for infection with HIV and hepatitis B.

Morphine Is Illegal Without a Prescription.
Morphine also is known as:
- Morph
- Miss Emma

Heroin Is Illegal.
Heroin also is known as:
- Smack
- Junk
- Brother
- Garbage

How the Illegal Use of Narcotics Can Harm Health

By causing immediate death. Narcotic drugs suppress the central nervous system. Large doses of narcotic drugs slow down breathing and can cause coma and even death.

By harming the body. People who use narcotics may experience euphoria, drowsiness, nausea, rapid heartbeat, and clammy skin. Large doses can induce sleep and may cause vomiting. Narcotics can be especially dangerous to people who have respiratory problems. Narcotics interfere with breathing and coughing. People allergic to narcotics may develop a skin rash.

By harming the mind. People who use narcotics cannot use reasoning and judgment to make responsible decisions. They may become depressed and lazy. Their emotions may change and they may have mood swings.

By causing dependence. Repeated use of narcotics results in increasing tolerance. This leads to physical dependence. People physically dependent on narcotics have withdrawal if they stop taking the drug. They may become deeply depressed, have mood swings, and be very sensitive to pain. Narcotics also cause psychological dependence. People who use narcotics become preoccupied with taking and obtaining the drug. They often lack energy and motivation and neglect themselves and their responsibilities. They may suffer from malnutrition, infection, illness, or injury. They may rob or steal to get narcotics.

By increasing the risk of becoming infected with HIV and hepatitis B. People who are infected with HIV or hepatitis B may leave blood on a needle after injecting themselves with narcotics. If the needle is used by other people, the infected blood may enter their bodies and infect them. Heroin and morphine are narcotics that usually are injected.

By increasing the risk of accidents, violence, and crime. People who use narcotics may fall in and out of sleep. This is called "nodding out." Nodding out can cause an accident if a person is driving a car, riding a bicycle, or operating machinery. When people who smoke nod out, they can suffer burns or start a fire.

How Hallucinogens Affect Health Status

Hallucinogens are a group of drugs that interfere with the senses and cause hallucinations. A hallucination is an imagined sight, sound, or feeling. Hallucinogens also are called psychedelic drugs. The effects of hallucinogens may last for several hours or days.

LSD is an illegal hallucinogen sold in the form of powder, tablets, liquid, or capsules. LSD also is taken in the form of blotter acid. **Blotter acid** is a small paper square that contains LSD. LSD causes the pupils to dilate, skin to become flushed, and heart rate and body temperature to increase. People who take LSD may have terrifying hallucinations known as a "bad trip." They often believe they are invincible.

LSD Is Illegal.
LSD also is known as:
- Acid
- Beast
- Diamonds
- Trips
- Doses
- Lucy
- Tabs

PCP (angel dust) is a hallucinogen that can act as a stimulant, sedative-hypnotic, or painkiller. It is sold illegally in the form of liquid, powder, or pills and is swallowed, smoked, and sniffed. People who use PCP feel restless, disoriented, anxious, isolated, angry, aggressive, and invincible.

PCP Is Illegal.
PCP also is known as:
- Dust

Mescaline is an illegal hallucinogen made from the peyote cactus. It causes many of the same effects as LSD.

Mescaline Is Illegal.
Mescaline also is known as:
- Mesc
- Microdots
- Peyote
- Buttons

Psilocybin is an illegal hallucinogen made from a specific type of mushroom. The effects of psilocybin are similar to LSD and mescaline.

Psilocybin Is Illegal.
Psilocybin also is known as:
- Magic Mushrooms
- Mushrooms
- Shrooms

MDMA is a hallucinogen that also acts a stimulant. It has many of the same harmful effects as LSD. It also may damage chemicals in the brain.

MDMA Is Illegal.
MDMA also is known as:
- Ecstasy
- XTC

How the Illegal Use of Hallucinogens Can Harm Health

By harming the body. Hallucinogens cause vomiting, nausea, loss of muscle control, chills, sweating, stomach cramps, an increase or decrease in heart rate, body temperature, blood sugar level, and blood pressure.

By harming the mind. Hallucinogens impair short-term memory and affect perception of time. People who take hallucinogens may believe something is real when it is not. They cannot control their emotions, may have mood swings, and may take unnecessary risks that can harm health. They also can have flashbacks.

A **flashback** is a sudden hallucination a person has long after having used a drug.

By causing dependence. People who regularly use hallucinogens may develop tolerance. The people need to take more and more of the drug to get the same effects.

By increasing the risk of accidents, violence, and crime. Hallucinogens impair reasoning and judgment, slow reaction time, and a person's ability to judge distances. Some hallucinogens increase feelings of anger and aggressiveness and can lead to violence.

How Marijuana Affects Health Status

Marijuana is the dried leaves and tops of the cannabis plant, which contains THC. **THC** is a drug found in the cannabis plant that produces psychoactive effects. THC is a fat-soluble drug that settles and builds up in the fatty parts of the body, including the brain, heart, and liver. Marijuana usually is smoked or eaten. A marijuana cigarette is called a joint. The effects of smoking or eating marijuana depend on the amount of THC. Marijuana used to contain between 1 and 5 percent THC. Today's marijuana is much more potent. It usually contains between 8 and 15 percent THC.

Hashish is a drug that is made from marijuana. It is smoked alone, mixed with tobacco, or eaten in cookies or candies. **Hashish oil** is the liquid resin from the cannabis plant. Hashish oil is placed on cigarettes and then smoked. Hashish and hashish oil are stronger than marijuana. Marijuana, hashish, and hashish oil are considered gateway drugs. A **gateway drug** is a drug whose use increases the likelihood that a person will use other harmful drugs.

Marijuana Is Illegal Without a Prescription.
Marijuana also is known as:

- Chronic
- Ganja
- Grass
- Herb
- Mary Jane
- Pot
- Reefer
- Tea
- Weed

How the Illegal Use of Marijuana Can Harm Health

By harming the body. People who use marijuana feel relaxed, euphoric, drowsy, and have an increased appetite. Eating marijuana brownies can causes nausea and vomiting. Smoking marijuana damages the lungs and respiratory system. Marijuana smoke contains many of the same carcinogens as tobacco smoke. Long-term use of marijuana can affect the reproductive system. A pregnant female who uses marijuana may harm the developing baby.

By harming the mind. Marijuana causes short-term memory loss and impairs concentration. People who smoke marijuana often lose their train of thought. They may say and do things they later regret. They may take unnecessary risks that harm health.

Marijuana causes amotivational syndrome. **Amotivational syndrome** is a persistent loss of ambition and motivation. Marijuana can cause drowsiness and sleep and loss of interest in daily activities, such as school and work. People who use marijuana may not pursue goals. They may not maintain a nice appearance.

People who use marijuana can have flashbacks weeks or months after using it. Marijuana has been known to cause ones similar to the ones experienced by people who have used hallucinogens.

By causing dependence. People who use marijuana develop tolerance after high doses and long-term use. They can develop psychological dependence. They become preoccupied with using and obtaining marijuana. They may feel they have to use marijuana to enjoy other activities. It is not clear if marijuana causes physical dependence and withdrawal symptoms.

By increasing the risk of becoming infected with HIV and hepatitis B. People who use marijuana cannot make responsible decisions. A person who has smoked marijuana may have sex with a person who is infected with HIV or hepatitis B; and become infected.

By increasing the risk of accidents, violence, and crime. Marijuana impairs a person's ability to judge distances and slows a person's reaction time. A person under the influence of marijuana is more likely to cause a motor vehicle accident or have an accident operating machinery.

How Anabolic-Androgenic Steroids Affect Health Status

Steroids are a group of drugs that are made from hormones. One type of steroid is an anabolic-androgenic steroids. An **anabolic-androgenic steroid** is a steroid made from the male hormone testosterone. Many people refer to anabolic-androgenic steroids as steroids. Steroids are injected or taken by mouth. Their effects include deepening of the voice, growth of facial and body hair, increase in muscle size, and increase in aggressiveness. Physicians prescribe anabolic-androgenic steroids to treat certain medical conditions. Using anabolic-androgenic steroids without the supervision of a physician is illegal. Steroids are taken to improve athletic performance and strength. The use of steroids is banned in most sports. Many people use steroids to build muscles and improve their appearance.

Corticosteroids are drugs that are similar to cortisol. **Cortisol** is a natural hormone produced by the adrenal glands. Corticosteroids are used to treat allergic conditions, arthritis, multiple sclerosis, and other diseases. They cause many side effects, including weight increase, mood swings, and headaches.

How the Illegal Use of Steroid Can Harm Health

By harming the body. Many teens believe that steroids only improve a person's appearance. However, taking steroids causes acne, oily skin, rashes, purple and red spots, and bad breath. Steroids increase the risk of heart disease and stroke. Steroids cause fluid to build up in the body, which leads to high blood pressure. Steroids also lower the level of high-density lipoproteins (HDLs) in the blood. This increases the risk of heart disease and stroke.

Steroids harm the reproductive system. In males, using steroids causes reduced sperm count, sterility, baldness, painful urination, swelling of the prostate gland, and testicles to shrink. Males who use steroids may develop large breasts. In females, using steroids causes missed menstrual periods, shrinking of the uterus, hair growth on the face and body, and deepened voice. The breasts of females who use steroids may become smaller.

Steroid use is particularly risky for teens because they are still growing. Using steroids may cause bone growth to stop. Teens who use steroids may have large muscles, but their growth is permanently stunted. People who use steroids often injure their tendons because their muscles grow but their tendons do not become stronger.

By harming the mind. Using steroids often causes severe emotional changes. People who use steroids may become angry and aggressive, and have roid rages that result in violence. A **roid rage** is an outburst of anger and hostility caused by using steroids.

By causing dependence. People who regularly use steroids may develop physical or psychological dependence. When they stop using steroids, they become very depressed, anxious, and restless. They may be tired, have frequent headaches, feel nauseous, and become sick. If they start using steroids again, these symptoms disappear.

By increasing the risk of becoming infected with HIV and hepatitis B. People who are infected with HIV or hepatitis B may leave blood on a needle after injecting themselves with steroids. If the needle is used by another person, the infected blood may enter this person's body and (s)he becomes infected.

By increasing the risk of accidents, violence, and crime. People who use steroids may have roid rages that result in violence. Many people illegally buy and sell steroids. They are breaking the law and can spend time in jail.

How Inhalants Affect Health Status

Inhalants are chemicals that affect mood and behavior when inhaled. Inhalants are not controlled drugs. Most inhalants are chemicals that are not produced to be inhaled or used as drugs. Inhalants often are the first drug that a young person used because they are easily accessible. Inhalants produce a very quick "high" because they are inhaled. However, the high usually lasts only a few minutes. There are several ways to use inhalants. **Huffing,** or **sniffing** is inhaling fumes to get high. **Bagging** is inhaling fumes from a bag to get high. Inhalants also are inhaled from balloons, aerosol cans, and other containers.

Examples of Inhalants
There are many kinds of inhalants. The following are just some of them:

- Amyl nitrite and butyl nitrite
- Fingernail polish remover
- Furniture polish
- Gasoline
- Glue
- Hairspray
- Laughing gas (nitrous oxide)
- Lighter fluid
- Liquid wax
- Marker fluid
- Paint thinner
- Paper correction fluid
- Rubber cement
- Shoe polish
- Spray paint
- Transmission fluid

How the Illegal Use of Inhalants Can Harm Health

By causing immediate death. Inhalants can cause heart failure and instant death. They also cause the central nervous system to slow down. This interferes with breathing and may cause suffocation. People who use inhalants may become unconscious and have seizures. They could choke on their own vomit if they get sick.

By harming the body. People who use inhalants may experience euphoria, nausea, vomiting, headache, dizziness, and uncontrollable laughter. Inhalants reduce the flow of oxygen to the brain and can cause permanent brain damage. People who use inhalants may have an irregular heartbeat, difficulty breathing, and headaches. Inhalants damage the immune system, heart, kidneys, blood, and bone marrow. Some inhalants can cause leukemia and lead poisoning.

By harming the mind. People who use inhalants cannot make responsible decisions because reasoning and judgment are impaired. They can have hallucinations that may cause them to harm themselves or others.

By causing dependence. People who use inhalants can develop psychological or physical dependence. They need to take more and more of the inhalant to get the desired effects.

By increasing the risk of accidents, violence, and crime. Inhalants affect reasoning and judgment. They also affect vision, coordination and reaction time. Inhalants can cause disorientation and confusion. People who use inhalants do not have the skills needed to drive and make responsible decisions.

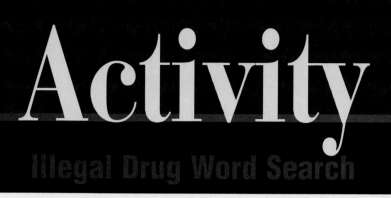

Activity

Illegal Drug Word Search

Life Skill: I will not be involved in illegal drug use.

Materials: paper, ruler, pencil or pen

Directions: The vocabulary words for this lesson are listed below. Each word is defined in this lesson as well as in the Glossary. Use the vocabulary words to design a word search like the sample below. Hide the words horizontally, vertically, diagonally, backwards, or forwards. As clues, list the definitions of the words at the bottom of the page. Exchange your word search with a classmate.

Sample Word Search

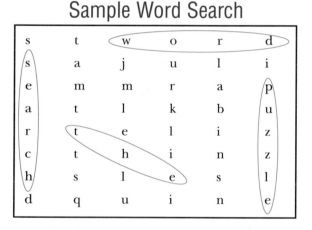

s	t	w	o	r	d
s	a	j	u	l	i
e	m	m	r	a	p
a	t	l	k	b	u
r	t	e	l	i	z
c	t	h	i	n	z
h	s	l	e	s	l
d	q	u	i	n	e

controlled drug

illegal drug use

stimulants

cocaine

crack

amphetamines

look-alike drug

methamphetamine

ice

methcathinone

ephedrine

decongestant

bronchodilator

methylphenidate

Attention Deficit
Hyperactivity Disorder
(ADHD)

caffeine

caffeinism

hallucination

sedative-hypnotic

sedative

hypnotic

barbiturate

benzodiazepines

anticonvulsant

narcotics

analgesic

opium

morphine

codeine

heroin

hallucinogens

LSD

blotter acid

PCP (angel dust)

mescaline

psilocybin

MDMA

flashback

marijuana

THC

hashish

hashish oil

gateway drug

amotivational
syndrome

steroids

anabolic-androgenic
steroid

corticosteroids

cortisol

roid rage

inhalants

huffing

sniffing

bagging

resistance skills

How to Resist Pressure to Use Illegal Drugs

You can resist pressure to use illegal drugs. Review resistance skills outlined in Lesson 54.

Resistance skills are skills that help a person say "no" to an action or to leave a situation.

1. **Use assertive behavior.** Stand tall and look directly at the person with whom you are speaking. Say "no" in a firm and confident voice. Be confident because you are being responsible. Be proud because you are obeying laws and following the guidelines of your parents or guardian.

2. **Give reasons for saying "no" to drug use.** Explain that you could be arrested for using, selling, carrying, or buying illegal drugs. There is no way of knowing what a drug actually contains. You could overdose on illegal drugs. Illegal drugs lead to violence and accidents.

3. **Use nonverbal behavior to match verbal behavior.**
   - Do not try to fit in by using illegal drugs.
   - Do not buy or carry materials or objects associated with drug use.
   - Do not listen to music that promotes illegal drug use.
   - Do not keep illegal drugs in your possession for someone else.
   - Do not attend parties where illegal drugs are being used.

4. **Avoid being in situations in which there will be pressure to use illegal drugs.**
   - Think ahead about whether peers will be using illegal drugs. Avoid any situation in which they will be.
   - Always tell your parents or guardian where you will be.

5. **Avoid being with people who use illegal drugs.**
   - Choose friends who are drug-free.
   - Stay away from people who buy and sell illegal drugs.

6. **Resist pressure to engage in illegal drug use.**
   - Learn the laws that apply to illegal drug use in your community and state.
   - Do not buy or sell drugs.
   - Do not attempt to grow or make illegal drugs.

7. **Influence others to choose responsible behavior.**
   - Encourage people who pressure you to use illegal drugs to change their behavior.
   - Encourage people who use illegal drugs to talk to their parents, guardian, or other responsible adults about their drug use.
   - Encourage people who use illegal drugs to seek treatment for drug dependency.
   - Be a role model for a drug-free lifestyle.
   - Volunteer to participate in a drug prevention program as a peer leader.

Drugs in the Media

Some movies and TV programs promote illegal drug use. They show people using drugs, living a glamorous life, and staying safe and healthy. Some music entertainers record songs that promote illegal drug use. Do not be fooled. Know that illegal drugs cannot improve the quality of your life. They can damage your health and safety. Avoid forms of media that promote illegal drug use. Do not purchase music that promotes illegal drug use. Remember, if you are influenced by the media, you are giving in to pressure.

Lesson 57

Review

Vocabulary Words

Write a separate sentence using 15 of the vocabulary words listed on page 459.

Objectives

1. How can the illegal use of stimulants harm health? **Objective 1**

2. How can the illegal use of sedative-hypnotics harm health? **Objective 2**

3. How can the illegal use of narcotics harm health? **Objective 3**

4. How can the illegal use of hallucinogens harm health? **Objective 4**

5. How can the illegal use of marijuana harm health? **Objective 5**

6. How can the illegal use of anabolic-androgenic steroids harm health? **Objective 6**

7. How can the illegal use of inhalants harm health? **Objective 7**

8. What are seven resistance skills that can be used to resist pressure to use illegal drugs? **Objective 8**

Responsible Decision-Making

Suppose you are tired in class one day. Your friend tells you she has been working late at night all week. She has stayed up by using OTC caffeine pills. She says taking these pills is the same as drinking a soda pop and that the pills will help you stay up. Write a response to this situation.

1. Describe the situation that requires you to make a decision.

2. List possible decisions you might make.

3. Name two responsible adults with whom you might discuss your decisions.

4. Evaluate the possible consequences of your decisions. Determine if each decision will lead to actions that:
   • promote health,
   • protect safety,
   • follow laws,
   • show respect for yourself and others,
   • follow the guidelines of your parents and of other responsible adults,
   • demonstrate good character.

5. Decide which decision is most responsible and appropriate.

6. Tell two results you expect if you make this decision.

Effective Communication

Write a brief essay that explains how using illegal drugs can interfere with effective communication.

Self-Directed Learning

Check the library or Internet for recent statistics about teens and illegal drug use. Which drugs do teens most commonly use? Which drugs are not as popular? What reasons do teens give for using these drugs? For not using them?

Critical Thinking

Suppose your younger sibling tells you his/her classmates are sniffing glue during art class. The classmates think it's fun and want him/her to try it. Write a short essay explaining to your younger sibling the risks involved in using inhalants.

Responsible Citizenship

Select one of the drugs discussed in the lesson. Design a poster warning about the harmful effects of this drug. Obtain permission from your teacher or principal to hang the poster in a school hallway.

You Can Choose a Drug-Free Lifestyle to Reduce the Risk of HIV Infection and Unwanted Pregnancy

Life Skill I will choose a drug-free lifestyle to reduce the risk of HIV infection and unwanted pregnancy.

A **drug-free lifestyle** is a lifestyle in which a person does not misuse or abuse drugs. When you choose a drug-free lifestyle, you protect yourself from the harmful effects of drugs. There are other ways you protect yourself when you have a drug-free lifestyle. You stay in control of your reasoning and judgment and avoid risk behaviors. This lesson explains why drug use increases the risk of HIV infection. You will learn why drug use increases the risk of unwanted pregnancy.

Vocabulary Words

drug-free lifestyle

human immunodeficiency virus (HIV)

Acquired Immunodeficiency Syndrome (AIDS)

abstinence from sex

rape

prostitution

injection drug use

sexual feelings

The Lesson Outline

How a Drug-Free Lifestyle Reduces the Risk of HIV Infection

How a Drug-Free Lifestyle Reduces the Risk of Unwanted Pregnancy

Objectives

1. List and explain four reasons why teens who use drugs increase their risk of HIV infection. **page 463**
2. List and explain four reasons why teens who use drugs increase their risk of unwanted pregnancy. **page 464**

How a Drug-Free Lifestyle Reduces the Risk of HIV Infection

Human immunodeficiency virus (HIV) is a pathogen that destroys infection-fighting T cells in the body. People who are infected with HIV develop AIDS. **Acquired Immunodeficiency** **Syndrome (AIDS)** is a condition that results in a breakdown of the body's ability to fight infection. There are at least four reasons why teens who use drugs increase their risk of HIV infection.

1. **Teens who use drugs may not stick to their decision to practice abstinence from sex.** **Abstinence from sex** is voluntarily choosing not to be sexually active. HIV is transmitted from one person to another during intimate sexual contact. Teens who drink alcohol or use marijuana or other drugs that change reasoning and judgment do not think clearly. During drug use, they are not clear as to the consequences of their behavior. Most teens who have been sexually active were under the influence of alcohol during their first sexual experience. Remember, one sexual contact can cause HIV infection and change your life.

2. **Teens who use drugs increase their risk for being in situations in which rape occurs.** **Rape** is the threatened or actual use of physical force to get someone to have sex without giving consent. When teens use drugs, they are less likely to think about the consequences of their behaviors. Females under the influence of drugs may take risks they usually would not take. For example, they might leave a party with a male they do not know well. They might agree to go into a male's bedroom. Males under the influence of drugs may not control their sexual advances. They may disregard a female's disapproval of sexual advances. Rape is illegal and increases the risk of HIV infection.

3. **Teens who are drug-dependent may have sex as a way of getting drugs.** Teens who are drug-dependent have a compelling need for drugs. Suppose they are not able to support their drug habit. They may engage in prostitution to get money to buy drugs. **Prostitution** is sexual activity for pay. Some teens who are drug-dependent exchange sex for drugs. Prostitution and the exchange of sex for drugs is illegal and increases the risk of HIV infection.

4. **Teens who are involved in injection drug use may share a needle with infected blood on it.** **Injection drug use** is drug use that involves injecting drugs into the body. When people inject drugs, the needle or syringe they use will have droplets of their blood on it. Suppose a needle or syringe has been used by a person infected with HIV. A teen uses this same needle or syringe to inject drugs. The droplets of blood infected with HIV will enter the teen's body and (s)he will be infected with HIV. Injection drug use is illegal and increases the risk of HIV infection.

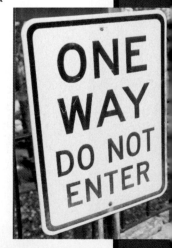

How a Drug-Free Lifestyle Reduces the Risk of Unwanted Pregnancy

Fact: Teens who use drugs are four times more likely to have an unwanted pregnancy than teens who do not use drugs.

Two people are involved in every unwanted teen pregnancy—a male and a female. For this reason, teen males as well as teen females must examine why unwanted pregnancies occur. There are at least four reasons why teens who use drugs increase their risk of having an unwanted pregnancy.

1. **Teens who use drugs are less likely to be in control of their sexual feelings.** **Sexual feelings** are feelings that result from a strong physical and emotional attraction to another person. To control sexual feelings, teens must set limits for expressing affection. However, these limits are easy to surpass when teens are under the influence of drugs. Drugs can intensify sexual feelings very quickly.

2. **Teens who use drugs may not stick to their decision to practice abstinence from sex.** Teens who drink alcohol or use marijuana or other drugs do not think clearly. While under the influence of drugs, they are not as clear as to the consequences of their behavior. Most teens who have been sexually active were under the influence of alcohol or another drug during their first sexual experience. Remember, one sexual contact can result in an unwanted pregnancy.

3. **Teens who use drugs are more at risk for being in situations in which rape occurs.** When teens use drugs, they are less likely to think about the consequences of their behaviors. Females under the influence of drugs may take risks they usually would not take. For example, they might spend time with a male of whom their parents or guardian do not approve. They might agree to go to a party where no adults are at home. They might leave a party at night and walk home alone. They might drink too much, pass out, and not even know that they had sex. Males under the influence of drugs can become more aggressive. Their judgment is impaired, and they may not respect their own or a female's limits for expressing affection. Rape can result in unwanted pregnancy. Using drugs is never a defense for rape.

4. **Teens who use drugs are more likely to justify their wrong sexual behavior with the fact they were under the influence of drugs at the time.** Some teens plan ahead to use drugs so they will have an excuse for wrong sexual behavior. For example, they may drink too much, have sex, and later say they would not have had sex if they had not been drinking. They do not think ahead as to other consequences for their actions, such as unwanted pregnancy.

Lesson 58

Review

Vocabulary Words

Write a separate sentence using each of the vocabulary words listed on page 462.

Objectives

1. What are four reasons why teens who use drugs increase their risk of HIV infection? **Objective 1**

2. Why might teens who are drug-dependent become involved in prostitution? **Objective 1**

3. What are four reasons why teens who use drugs increase their risk of unwanted pregnancy? **Objective 2**

4. What are three examples of risk situations in which females who have been drinking are vulnerable to being raped? **Objective 2**

5. Why are males who are using drugs more likely to continue with unwelcome sexual advances? **Objective 2**

Responsible Decision-Making

A classmate tells you that she is considering having sex with her boyfriend. She says she does not want to appear too easy. She plans to drink a lot. That way she can say that she would not have had sex if she had not been drinking. Write a response to this situation.

1. Describe the situation that requires your friend to make a decision.
2. List possible decisions your friend might make.
3. Name two responsible adults with whom your friend might discuss his/her decisions.
4. Evaluate the possible consequences of your friend's decisions. Determine if each decision will lead to actions that:
    - promote health,
    - protect safety,
    - follow laws,
    - show respect for your friend and others,
    - follow the guidelines of your friend's parents and of other responsible adults,
    - demonstrate good character.
5. Decide which decision is most responsible and appropriate for your friend.
6. Tell two results your friend can expect if (s)he makes this decision.

Effective Communication

Write a short story about a teen who has sex only once and becomes infected with HIV. Describe the teen's reaction when (s)he is told (s)he is HIV positive.

Self-Directed Learning

At the library find a book, video, or tape that deals with drugs and HIV or drugs and unwanted pregnancy. Write a review of the book, video, or tape to share with classmates.

Critical Thinking

Character is a person's use of self-control to act on responsible values. Teens who have good character protect their health and the health of others. Consider the facts in this chapter. How can drug use alter a teen's character?

Responsible Citizenship

Write an editorial for the school or local newspaper. The editorial should explain why teens who use drugs increase their risk of HIV infection and unwanted pregnancy.

Why Drug Use Increases the Risk of Accidents

Drug use increases the risk of accidents for a number of reasons. People who have been using drugs are not able to think clearly and use wise judgment. They may take risks that they normally would not take. They may engage in foolish behavior. For example, they may play driving games such as "chicken" or accept a dare to walk along a train track.

People who have been using drugs have a slower reaction time and have less coordination and balance. As a result, they do not respond quickly to prevent accidents. For example, they may be driving and are unable to turn the wheel in time to avoid hitting another motor vehicle. People who use drugs cannot judge the distance of an oncoming car. They may be hit by an oncoming vehicle because they are not be able to hear the vehicle when they are walking.

People who have been using drugs have dulled senses. Their senses of hearing, smell, touch, and sight are not sharp. They may not respond quickly to sounds that warn them of danger. They may not smell smoke or fire. They may not experience hot, cold, or pain as they should. Their vision is blurry and their depth perception can be affected.

Activity

Drug-Related Accidents

Life Skill: I will choose a drug-free lifestyle to reduce the risk of violence and accidents.

Materials: newspapers, magazines, computer (optional)

Directions: Many injuries and deaths are due to accidents involving drug use. Complete the steps below to identify situations in which people were injured or killed due to drug use.

 Review the kinds of accidents that often are related to drug use. These include traffic accidents, pedestrian accidents, boating accidents, drownings, fires, and falls.

 Your teacher will divide the class into eight groups. Each group will be assigned one of the items on the list. The group will check the library or Internet to find articles about its assigned type of accident. These articles should be about a person or people being injured or killed in that type of accident.

 **The group will prepare a five-minute presentation based on its findings.** The presentation should be in the form of a TV news report. Each group member should have a role in the presentation.

 The presentation should include the following information about each accident: what occurred, who was injured or killed, the injuries that resulted, and how the accident was related to drug use. Each group will give its presentation to the class.

Lesson 59

Review

Vocabulary Words

Write a separate sentence using each of the vocabulary words listed on page 466.

Objectives

1. Why does alcohol use increase the risk of violence? The use of stimulants? The use of marijuana and hallucinogens? The use of PCP? The use of anabolic-androgenic steroids? **Objective 1**

2. How does drug trafficking contribute to violence? **Objective 2**

3. What are six ways to protect yourself from violence associated with drug use? **Objective 3**

4. How does a safe and drug-free school zone decrease the risk of drug trafficking? **Objective 4**

5. How does drug use increase the risk of accidents? **Objective 5**

Responsible Decision-Making

A group of classmates plan to go downhill skiing. When you arrive at the slopes, you smell beer on one classmate's breath. You are concerned that your classmate may have a slower reaction time and less balance on the slopes. When you mention this to your classmate, everyone laughs. They say drinking a few beers relaxes a person. They say a person is not as likely to be injured in a fall and will stay warm. They suggest that you have a few beers. Write a response to this situation.

1. **Describe the situation that requires you to make a decision.**

2. **List possible decisions you might make.**

3. **Name two responsible adults with whom you might discuss your decisions.**

4. **Evaluate the possible consequences of your decisions. Determine if each decision will lead to actions that:**
   - **promote health,**
   - **protect safety,**
   - **follow laws,**
   - **show respect for yourself and others,**
   - **follow the guidelines of your parents and of other responsible adults,**
   - **demonstrate good character.**

5. **Decide which decision is most responsible and appropriate.**

6. **Tell two results you expect if you make this decision.**

 ### Effective Communication

Write a short story in which a person who has used drugs causes another person to be injured.

 ### Self-Directed Learning

Find a newspaper article about an incidence of violence in your community that was associated with drug use. Explain how drug use was involved in the violence.

 ### Critical Thinking

How does marijuana use increase the risk of violence? Cocaine use? PCP use? Narcotics use?

 ### Responsible Citizenship

Obtain permission from your parents or guardian and your teacher. Write a letter to the editor of the local newspaper. Explain the importance of having safe and drug-free school zones in your community.

You Can Be Aware of Resources for the Treatment of Drug Misuse and Abuse

Life Skill I will be aware of resources for the treatment of drug misuse and abuse.

Most people who are drug-dependent are in a state of denial. **Denial** is refusing to admit a problem. They do not admit that they are dependent on drugs. They do not recognize the effects their behavior is having on others. They may even blame others for the consequences of their behavior. Because people who are drug-dependent are in a state of denial, they usually do not seek treatment. Other people must intervene. This lesson discusses intervention and treatment for people who misuse and abuse drugs. You will learn steps to take if you are part of a formal intervention. You will learn the different forms of treatment available for people who are drug-dependent and the people who care about them.

The Lesson Outline

What to Know About Formal Intervention

What to Know About Treatment

Objectives

1. List and explain four steps teens can take to get help for someone who misuses or abuses drugs. **page 471**
2. Discuss what happens during a formal intervention. **page 471**
3. Explain what happens during detoxification. **page 472**
4. Discuss different kinds of treatment for people who are drug-dependent. **page 472**
5. Explain why the family members and friends of people who are drug-dependent may need treatment. **page 472**

Vocabulary Words

denial

formal intervention

honest talk

I-message

relapse

detoxification

withdrawal symptoms

inpatient care

outpatient care

halfway house

student assistance program

What to Know About
Formal Intervention

Suppose you know someone who misuses or abuses drugs. This person could be a family member, a close friend, or someone on a school team. Do not participate in denial. Be straightforward. There are four steps to take when you want to get help for someone who is misusing or abusing drugs.

1. **List the person's specific behaviors and signs of drug abuse.** Write out a detailed list that describes specific situations and dates.

2. **Share the list with a responsible adult.** The adult can review what you have written and decide appropriate steps to take. If the adult with whom you share the list does not respond, share the list with another responsible adult.

3. **Know that you have made a responsible decision by sharing the list with an adult.** Recognize that people who look the other way or make excuses for a person who abuses drugs are enablers. Be proud that you have made a responsible decision.

4. **Follow the advice of the adult who takes action.** The adult may choose to contact a trained counselor or other health care professional. There may be a formal intervention.

How a Formal Intervention Helps

A **formal intervention** is an action by people, such as family members, who want a person to get treatment. The goal is to help drug-dependent people recognize the effects of their drug misuse or abuse. A trained counselor guides people through the formal intervention process.

A formal intervention should be carefully planned with a trained counselor. The counselor usually holds a planning session before the intervention. The people who will be involved discuss the person's drug use and its consequences. The formal intervention is practiced and rehearsed. The trained counselor will make sure that a treatment program is selected ahead of time and that the appropriate arrangements are made.

During a formal intervention, family members, friends, and other significant people describe the behavior of the person who is drug-dependent and explain how it affects them. Specific situations in which the person's behavior caused negative consequences are discussed. The people involved in the intervention explain that they want the person who is drug-dependent to get treatment.

It is best for a person who is drug-dependent to enter treatment immediately after the formal intervention. A person who is drug-dependent is likely to come up with excuses not to enter treatment if (s)he has time to think about it. Family members often have packed a suitcase and made plans to take the person to a treatment facility immediately following the formal intervention.

How Honest Talk Helps

Family members, friends, and employers who use honest talk and I-messages often are successful at convincing a person who is drug-dependent to agree to treatment. **Honest talk** is the straightforward sharing of feelings. An **I-message** is a statement that contains a specific behavior or event, the effect of the behavior or event on a person, and the emotions that result. People who are healthy recognize when other people are drug-dependent. They use honest talk and I-messages to express their feelings. For example, a teen might say:

● I feel that I cannot trust you when you lie about your drug use, and this stresses me.

● I cannot bring friends over because I don't know if you have been drinking; this makes me sad.

● I cannot relax when you are out drinking with your friends because I worry that you might have an accident.

What to Know About
Treatment

People who are drug-dependent need help to discontinue drug use. It is important to make sure that a person uses the treatment approach that will work best for him/her.

Treatment programs do not only focus on getting people off of drugs. They also try to teach people to live more effectively than before. This helps people avoid having a relapse. A **relapse** is a return to a previous behavior or condition.

Detoxification

Detoxification usually is the first stage of treatment programs. **Detoxification** is the process in which an addictive substance is withdrawn from the body. Detoxification often causes people to suffer from withdrawal symptoms. **Withdrawal symptoms** are unpleasant reactions that occur when a person who is physically dependent on a drug no longer takes it. Physicians give some people in detoxification medications to ease withdrawal symptoms.

Inpatient Care

Inpatient care is treatment that requires a person to stay overnight at a facility. The facility may be a hospital or drug treatment center. The main advantages of inpatient care are the medical supervision and the drug-free setting. Inpatient care may last from a few weeks to a year. However, most inpatient drug treatment programs last for 28 days.

Outpatient Care

Outpatient care is treatment that does not require a person to stay overnight at a facility. Outpatient care is offered by many hospitals and community treatment centers. People in outpatient drug treatment programs can work or attend school while recovering from drug dependence.

Halfway Houses

A **halfway house** is a live-in facility that helps a person who is drug-dependent gradually adjust to living independently in the community. Halfway houses provide food, shelter, and drug treatment. They provide a supportive, drug-free environment for living. Halfway house residents often learn job skills and receive counseling about ways to live responsibly.

Recovery Programs

There are many recovery programs available for people who are drug-dependent. In these programs, people recovering from drug dependence give one another feedback and support. Narcotics Anonymous is a recovery program that helps people deal with narcotics dependence. Cocaine Anonymous is a recovery program that helps people deal with cocaine abuse. There also are recovery programs for other drug dependencies.

School Resources

Many schools offer resources to help students with drug problems. Your school may participate in a student assistance program. A **student assistance program** is a school-based program to help prevent and treat alcoholism and other drug dependencies. Some schools also have recovery groups for students.

Others May Need Treatment, Too

Treatment programs are available for people affected by other people's drug dependence. These programs often focus on helping people who are codependent and enablers. It is difficult for people to stop being codependent and enablers because they do not want to let the person who is drug-dependent suffer the consequences of his/her drug use. People who are drug-dependent may become angry when people who are codependent try to stop being an enabler.

Lesson 60

Review

Vocabulary Words

Write a separate sentence using each of the vocabulary words listed on page 470.

Objectives

1. What are four steps teens can take to get help for someone who misuses or abuses drugs? **Objective 1**

2. What usually happens during a formal intervention? **Objective 2**

3. What happens during detoxification? **Objective 3**

4. What are different kinds of treatment for people who are drug-dependent? **Objective 4**

5. Why might the family members and friends of people who are drug-dependent need treatment? **Objective 5**

Responsible Decision-Making

Suppose you have a sibling who is drug-dependent. Your sibling causes many problems for your family. You are concerned for his/her safety and the safety of other family members. You suggest to your sibling that (s)he stops using drugs and gets help from your parents or guardian. Your sibling tells you that (s)he does not have a problem and to mind your own business. Write a response to this situation.

1. Describe the situation that requires you to make a decision.
2. List possible decisions you might make.
3. Name two responsible adults with whom you might discuss your decisions.
4. Evaluate the possible consequences of your decisions. Determine if each decision will lead to actions that:
   - promote health,
   - protect safety,
   - follow laws,
   - show respect for yourself and others,
   - follow the guidelines of your parents and of other responsible adults,
   - demonstrate good character.
5. Decide which decision is most responsible and appropriate.
6. Tell two results you expect if you make this decision.

Effective Communication

Suppose your friend is drug-dependent. Write five I-messages you might use to tell your friend about his/her behavior when (s)he uses drugs.

Self-Directed Learning

Obtain permission from a parent or guardian to contact a facility in your community that has a treatment program for people who are drug-dependent. Call the facility and request a brochure or information sheet describing its drug treatment program. Share the information with your classmates.

Critical Thinking

Why might a person who uses drugs become angry or anxious if a person who has acted as his/her enabler seeks treatment?

Responsible Citizenship

Make a phone directory of drug treatment facilities and services in your community. Identify the treatment approach used by each facility or service in your directory. What is the approach? Who is eligible for treatment? Does the program involve inpatient or outpatient care? What is the cost? Share your directory with your family.

Unit Review

Review Questions

Prepare for the unit test. Review your answers for each Lesson Review in this unit. Then write answers to each of the following questions:

1. What are five ways drugs enter the body? **Lesson 51**

2. What federal agency must approve a drug before it can be distributed? **Lesson 51**

3. What is the difference between a brand-name drug and a generic drug? **Lesson 51**

4. How can drug use prevent a teen from developing social skills? **Lesson 52**

5. What is the difference between physical dependence and psychological dependence? **Lesson 52**

6. How does a scapegoat cope with drug dependence in the family? **Lesson 52**

7. How does having a biological parent who has alcoholism affect a person's risk of developing alcoholism? **Lesson 53**

8. What are eight warning signs of drug use in peers? **Lesson 53**

9. How do protective factors influence the likelihood that you will be tempted to use drugs? **Lesson 53**

10. Why might teens who use drugs avoid being friends with teens who do not use drugs? **Lesson 54**

11. What are five nonverbal behaviors that send a message that you will not use drugs? **Lesson 54**

12. Will a teen who breaks the law while under the influence of drugs be held accountable? **Lesson 54**

13. Why are drinking games and hazing activities dangerous? **Lesson 55**

14. Why is it dangerous for a female who is pregnant to drink alcoholic beverages? **Lesson 55**

15. How does drinking alcohol increase the risk of acquaintance rape? **Lesson 55**

16. What are five ways to avoid secondhand smoke? **Lesson 56**

17. What are the four warnings that tobacco companies must rotate on cigarette packages? **Lesson 56**

18. Why are tobacco products addictive? **Lesson 56**

19. What are five examples of controlled drugs? **Lesson 57**

20. Why is marijuana potent? **Lesson 57**

21. What is a gateway drug? **Lesson 57**

22. How does being involved in injection drug use increase the risk of HIV infection? **Lesson 58**

23. Why does drinking alcohol increase a teen's risks of being sexually active? **Lesson 58**

24. Why does passing out increase the risk of being raped? **Lesson 58**

25. Why do people who are drug-dependent rarely seek help on their own? **Lesson 59**

26. What should you do if you tell an adult that a person abuses drugs and the adult does not take action? **Lesson 59**

27. Why are people who are going through detoxification usually admitted to a treatment facility? **Lesson 59**

28. Why is the use of anabolic-androgenic steroids associated with an increased risk of violence? **Lesson 60**

29. What is a safe and drug-free school zone? **Lesson 60**

30. Why is drug use responsible for so many traffic fatalities? **Lesson 60**

Vocabulary Words

Number a sheet of paper from 1–10. Select the correct vocabulary word and write it next to the corresponding number. DO NOT WRITE IN THIS BOOK.

tolerance	drug-free lifestyle
alcoholism	relapse
instant gratification	hallucination
side effect	drug trafficking
FAS	nicotine

1. _____ is a disease in which there is physical and psychological dependence on alcohol. **Lesson 55**

2. _____ is an unwanted body change that is not related to the main purpose of a drug. **Lesson 51**

3. _____ is the presence of birth defects in babies born to mothers who drink alcohol during pregnancy. **Lesson 58**

4. _____ is to fall back into a former condition. **Lesson 59**

5. _____ is a condition in which the body becomes used to a substance. **Lesson 52**

6. _____ is an imagined sight, sound, or feeling. **Lesson 57**

7. _____ is choosing an immediate reward regardless of potential harmful effects. **Lesson 53**

8. _____ is a drug in tobacco that stimulates the nervous system and is highly addictive. **Lesson 56**

9. _____ is a lifestyle in which a person does nor misuse or abuse drugs. **Lesson 54**

10. _____ is the production, distribution, transportation, buying, and selling of illegal drugs. **Lesson 60**

Health Literacy

Effective Communication

Obtain permission from your parent or guardian. Interview a professional who works with drug-dependent teens, such as a drug counselor from a hospital or drug treatment center. Ask the person about the effects of drugs on teens they have seen. Write an essay about your answers.

Self-Directed Learning

Identify three of your long-term goals, such as going to college or becoming a responsible parent. Write an essay about how using drugs might interfere with these goals.

Critical Thinking

Review the reasons on pages 436, 446, and 460 for saying "no" to alcohol, to tobacco, and to illegal drugs. On a sheet of paper, add five new reasons to say "no" to alcohol, tobacco, and illegal drugs.

Responsible Citizenship

Identify an organization, such as SADD, that works to prevent drug use. Write down the address, telephone number, and a brief description of the goals of the progam. Combine your information with your classmates to create a Directory of Programs to Promote a Drug-Free Lifestyle.

Responsible Decision-Making

Suppose you live in a neighborhood where many people use drugs. You often are pressured to use drugs. Your friend tells you that you might as well use drugs. Other friends tell you that if you don't use drugs, you might have no friends. Write a response to this situation.

1. **Describe the situation that requires you to make a decision.**
2. **List possible decisions you might make.**
3. **Name two responsible adults with whom you might discuss your decisions.**
4. **Evaluate the possible consequences of your decisions. Determine if each decision will lead to actions that:**
   - **promote health,**
   - **protect safety,**
   - **follow laws,**
   - **show respect for yourself and others,**
   - **follow the guidelines of your parents and of other responsible adults,**
   - **demonstrate good character.**
5. **Decide which decision is most responsible and appropriate.**
6. **Tell two results you expect if you make this decision.**

Health Behavior Inventory of Life Skills

Number from 1 to 10 on a sheet of paper. Read each life skill carefully. Write YES or NO next to the same number on your paper. Each YES response indicates a life skill you practice to promote your health status. Each NO response indicates a life skill you do not practice. Plan to begin practicing these life skills.

1. **I will follow guidelines for the safe use of prescription and OTC drugs.**
2. **I will not misuse or abuse drugs.**
3. **I will avoid risk factors and practice protective factors for drug misuse and abuse.**
4. **I will use resistance skills if I am pressured to misuse or abuse drugs.**
5. **I will not drink alcohol.**
6. **I will avoid tobacco use and secondhand smoke.**
7. **I will not be involved in illegal drug use.**
8. **I will choose a drug-free lifestyle to reduce the risk of HIV infection and unwanted pregnancy.**
9. **I will choose a drug-free lifestyle to reduce the risk of violence and accidents.**
10. **I will be aware of resources for the treatment of drug misuse and abuse.**

Multicultural Health

Identify another country in which drug use is a problem. The problem might be an increase in drug use or drug trafficking. Write an essay describing the problems this country is having with drugs and what is being done to resolve the problem.

Family Involvement

Write a list of "Top Ten Drug-Free Activities" you enjoy. Choose one of the items on your list that you can do with family members. Do the activity with one or more of your family members. Share the list with them.

Health Behavior Contract

Copy and complete the following health behavior contract. Evaluate your progress.
Share the results with your family.

Health Behavior Contract

1. Name_____ Date_____

2. **Life Skill:** I will not misuse or abuse drugs.

3. **Effects on Health Status:** Misusing and abusing drugs is harmful to my health status. Drugs increase the risk of illness and disease. They increase the risk of being a victim of and participant in violence. Misusing and abusing drugs leads to actions that do not show respect for myself or others or family guidelines. Participating in drug-free activities allows me to have fun without the risks of using drugs.

4. **Plan and Method to Record Progress:** I will participate in drug-free activities that I enjoy. I will identify ten drug-free activities I enjoy and in which I can participate. When I participate in one of these activities, I will write each of the activities in the space provided for the day of the week. I will list ways that I benefited from participating in drug-free activities in the Evaluation.

My Calendar

M	T	W	Th	F	S	S

5. **Evaluation:** _____
_____
_____

Unit 7

Communicable and Chronic Diseases

Lesson 61

You Can Reduce Your Risk of Infection with Communicable Diseases

Life Skill **I will choose behaviors to reduce my risk of infection with communicable diseases.**

Most teens have two to three colds a year. The cold virus is spread through both direct and indirect contact. You can become infected by breathing air into which someone who has a cold has sneezed. You might become infected if you drink from the glass of someone who has a cold. Perhaps you borrow a pencil from a classmate and put the pencil into your mouth. You can become infected with the cold virus in this way too. This lesson explains ways to reduce your risk of infection with communicable diseases, such as the common cold. You will learn how to prevent the spread of pathogens. This lesson also explains how the immune system protects you when a pathogen enters your body.

The Lesson Outline

How to Prevent the Spread of Pathogens
How the Immune System Protects the Body

Objectives

1. Identify six types of pathogens that cause disease. **page 481**
2. Discuss five ways pathogens are spread. **page 481**
3. Identify ten ways to reduce the risk of infection with communicable diseases. **page 481**
4. Explain how the immune system responds when a pathogen enters the body. **page 482**
5. Discuss ways to develop active and passive immunity. **page 482**

Vocabulary Words

pathogen
communicable disease
infectious disease
bacteria
toxin
rickettsia
virus
fungi
protozoa
helminth
immune system
lymphocytes
B cell
antibody
helper T cell
macrophage
immunity
active immunity
vaccine
immunization
passive immunity

How to Prevent the Spread of Pathogens

A **pathogen** is a germ that causes disease. A **communicable disease**, or **infectious disease**, is an illness caused by pathogens that can be spread from one living thing to another. There are many types of pathogens that cause disease.

Bacteria are single-celled microorganisms. There are more than 1,000 types of bacteria. Most bacteria are beneficial, but close to 100 types are known to cause disease. Bacteria cause disease by releasing toxins. A **toxin** is a substance that is poisonous. Some diseases caused by bacteria are syphilis, gonorrhea, strep throat, tuberculosis, tetanus, diphtheria, and Lyme disease. **Rickettsia** (ri·KET·see·uh) are pathogens that grow inside living cells and resemble bacteria. Two diseases caused by rickettsia are typhus and Rocky Mountain spotted fever.

A **virus** is the smallest known pathogen. When a virus enters a cell, it takes over the cell and causes it to make more viruses. Newly produced viruses then are released and take over other cells. In this way, viruses spread rapidly. Some viral diseases are the common cold, mumps, hepatitis, mononucleosis, chicken-pox, HIV, and influenza.

Fungi are single- or multi-celled parasitic organisms. Fungi obtain their food from organic materials, such as plant, animal, or human tissue. Fungi can live on the skin, mucous membranes, and lungs and cause disease in the process. Some diseases caused by fungi are athlete's foot, ringworm, jock itch, nail infections, and thrush.

Protozoa are tiny, single-celled organisms that produce toxins that cause disease. Malaria, African sleeping sickness, and dysentery are diseases caused by protozoa. A **helminth** is a parasitic worm. People can become infected with helminths when they eat undercooked pork or fish or practice poor hygiene. Some helminths, such as tapeworms, pinworms, and hookworms, can infect the human digestive tract. Other helminths can infect muscle tissue and blood.

How Pathogens Are Spread

Pathogens are spread in different ways. They may be spread through direct contact with an infected person, such as shaking hands, intimate kissing, sexual intercourse, receiving a transfusion of the person's blood, touching ulcers or sores, or handling body fluids such as blood or urine. They may be spread through the air by coughing or sneezing. Contact with contaminated objects spreads pathogens. This includes sharing a needle with an infected person to inject drugs or get a tattoo and using objects such as combs, toothbrushes, razors, or eating utensils touched by an infected person. Contact with animals and insects, such as handling or being bitten by an infected insect or animal, also spreads pathogens. So does contact with contaminated food and water by drinking infected water, eating infected food, undercooking meats and other foods, improperly canning or preparing foods, and not washing hands after using the restroom.

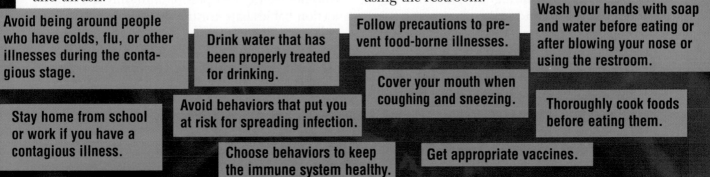

Avoid being around people who have colds, flu, or other illnesses during the contagious stage.

Drink water that has been properly treated for drinking.

Follow precautions to prevent food-borne illnesses.

Wash your hands with soap and water before eating or after blowing your nose or using the restroom.

Cover your mouth when coughing and sneezing.

Stay home from school or work if you have a contagious illness.

Avoid behaviors that put you at risk for spreading infection.

Thoroughly cook foods before eating them.

Choose behaviors to keep the immune system healthy.

Get appropriate vaccines.

How the Immune System Protects the Body

The **immune system** removes harmful organisms from the blood and combats pathogens. The immune system is composed of body organs, tissues, cells, and chemicals. The skin is the first line of defense. Unbroken skin acts as a barrier to prevent pathogens from entering the body. Perspiration and oils on skin kill pathogens. Tears also contain chemicals that kill pathogens and prevent them from entering the eyes. Mucus and hairs that line the inside of the nose trap and destroy pathogens, and many are killed by saliva in the mouth. Other pathogens that are swallowed are destroyed by stomach acids.

Lymphocytes are white blood cells that help the body fight pathogens. When a pathogen enters the body, lymphocytes multiply in lymph tissue to fight infection. Two types of lymphocytes are B cells and helper T cells. A **B cell** is a white blood cell that produces antibodies. An **antibody** is a special protein that helps fight infection. A **helper T cell** is a white blood cell that signals B cells to produce antibodies.

Soon after a pathogen invades the body, helper T cells send signals to B cells to produce antibodies. B cells enter the lymph nodes and other lymph tissues. Antibodies then travel through the blood to destroy the pathogen. Antibodies can make pathogens ineffective and sensitive to macrophages. A **macrophage** (MAK·roh·fahj) is a white blood cell that surrounds and destroys pathogens. Antibodies attach to pathogens and make them easier for macrophages to destroy. Destroyed pathogens enter lymph, are filtered in lymph nodes, and removed by the spleen.

The immune system helps people develop immunity. **Immunity** is the body's resistance to disease-causing agents. **Active immunity** is resistance to disease due to the presence of antibodies. For example, suppose a person comes into contact with the chickenpox virus. The chickenpox antibody remains in the body after the person has recovered and protects him/her from developing chickenpox. Active immunity also can result from being given a vaccine. A **vaccine**, or **immunization**, is a substance containing dead or weakened pathogens that is introduced into the body to give more immunity. Vaccines are given by injection and orally. Vaccines cause the body to make antibodies for a specific pathogen. If these pathogens enter the body again, the antibodies destroy them. People should be immunized against diphtheria, pertussis (whooping cough), tetanus, measles, mumps, rubella (German measles), polio, hepatitis A, hepatitis B, and chickenpox.

Another type of immunity is passive immunity. **Passive immunity** is immunity that results from introducing antibodies into a person's bloodstream. The antibodies may be from another person's blood. This type of immunity is short-term and is used when the risk of developing a disease is immediate. For example, a person who has not had hepatitis B immunizations and travels to a country where it is widespread may be given an injection with hepatitis B antibodies. Another example of passive immunity is the protection babies have for the first few months of life because of the antibodies received before birth from their mothers. Babies who are breast fed also receive some antibodies from breast milk.

Lesson 61

Review

Vocabulary Words

Write a separate sentence using each of the vocabulary words listed on page 480.

Objectives

1. What are six types of pathogens that cause disease? **Objective 1**

2. What are five ways that pathogens are spread? **Objective 2**

3. What are ten ways to reduce the risk of infection with communicable diseases? **Objective 3**

4. How does the immune system respond when a pathogen enters the body? **Objective 4**

5. How does a person develop active and passive immunity? **Objective 5**

Responsible Decision-Making

You have a cold. You may have the flu. Your classmate had planned to come to your house to study with you for a big test. Write a response to this situation.

1. **Describe the situation that requires your classmate to make a decision.**
2. **List possible decisions your classmate might make.**
3. **Name two responsible adults with whom your classmate might discuss his/her decisions.**
4. **Evaluate the possible consequences of your classmate's decisions. Determine if each decision will lead to actions that:**
   • **promote health,**
   • **protect safety,**
   • **follow laws,**
   • **show respect for your classmate and others,**
   • **follow the guidelines of your classmates's parents and of other responsible adults,**
   • **demonstrate good character.**
5. **Decide which decision is most responsible and appropriate for your classmate.**
6. **Tell two results your classmate can expect if (s)he makes this decision.**

Effective Communication

Prepare a 30-second public service announcement explaining ten ways to reduce the risk of infection with communicable diseases. Record your announcement and send the tape to a local radio station.

Self-Directed Learning

Contact your local public health department. Find out what immunizations are recommended by the Centers for Disease Control and Prevention (CDC). When should these immunizations be received? What should a teen who has not received all of these immunizations do?

Critical Thinking

Suppose one of your family members has a severe cold. Write a short essay describing the actions you could take to reduce your risk of catching the cold?

Responsible Citizenship

Talk to your parents or guardian about the immunizations you have received. Find out what immunizations you have had and when. If you still need certain immunizations, make an appointment with your physician or the local public health department to get these immunizations.

You Can Reduce Your Risk of Infection with Respiratory Diseases

Life Skill **I will choose behaviors to reduce my risk of infection with respiratory diseases.**

Many diseases affect your respiratory system. Some of these are infectious, while others are not. An infectious disease is a communicable disease. It can be spread from one person to another. This lesson includes A Guide to Infectious Respiratory Diseases. The guide includes five infectious respiratory diseases: the common cold, influenza, pneumonia, strep throat, and tuberculosis. You will learn these facts for each disease: the cause, methods of transmission, symptoms, diagnosis and treatment, and prevention.

The Lesson Outline

A Guide to Infectious Respiratory Diseases

Objectives

1. Discuss the cause, methods of transmission, symptoms, diagnosis and treatment, and prevention of the common cold. **page 485**

2. Discuss the cause, methods of transmission, symptoms, diagnosis and treatment, and prevention of influenza. **page 485**

3. Discuss the cause, methods of transmission, symptoms, diagnosis and treatment, and prevention of pneumonia. **page 486**

4. Discuss the cause, methods of transmission, symptoms, diagnosis and treatment, and prevention of strep throat. **page 486**

5. Discuss the cause, methods of transmission, symptoms, diagnosis and treatment, and prevention of tuberculosis. **page 486**

Vocabulary Words

common cold

rhinovirus

influenza

flu

Reye's syndrome

pneumonia

strep throat

rheumatic fever

tuberculosis

tuberculin skin test

isoniazid

A Guide to Infectious Respiratory Diseases

Basic information about some of the most common infectious respiratory diseases follows.

The Common Cold

The **common cold** is a respiratory infection caused by more than 200 different viruses. One-third of all colds are caused by rhinoviruses. A **rhinovirus** is a virus that infects the nose. High levels of stress can increase a person's chances of catching a cold. Being exposed to cold weather or getting chilled does not cause a cold.

Methods of Transmission. Cold viruses are released into the air when an infected person coughs or sneezes. Since the viruses can remain in the air for a while, people can inhale them and become infected. They also can become infected by shaking hands with an infected person or by touching contaminated objects. The viruses spread from the hands when people touch their eyes or nose.

Symptoms. Symptoms include runny nose, watery eyes, difficulty in breathing, sneezing, sore throat, cough, and headache and can last from 2 to 14 days.

Diagnosis and Treatment. People with colds need to get plenty of rest and drink plenty of fluids. OTC medicines may help relieve some symptoms, but they will not cure or shorten the length of a cold. Gargling with warm salt water may bring relief to a sore throat. Applying petroleum jelly to the nose may help an irritated nose.

Prevention. The most effective way to keep from getting a cold is to wash the hands frequently and not touch the nose or eyes. Sneeze or cough into a facial tissue. Whenever possible, avoid close contact with anyone who has a cold. To keep colds from spreading in a family, wash dishes and other objects separately that have been used by the family member who has a cold.

Influenza

Influenza, or the **flu**, is a highly contagious viral infection of the respiratory tract. Most people recover within a week or two, but it can be life-threatening for elderly people, newborn babies, and people with chronic diseases. The flu can lead to pneumonia. Flu viruses are constantly changing, making it difficult for the immune system to form antibodies to new variations of the flu virus. The illness that people often call "stomach flu" is not influenza.

Methods of Transmission. Flu viruses spread primarily from person to person as they enter the air when people cough and sneeze. They can enter the body through the mucous membranes of the eyes, nose, or mouth. Flu can spread rapidly in crowded places. The infected person who spreads it often does not show symptoms yet. An infected person is particularly contagious during the first three days of infection.

Symptoms. Symptoms include headache, chills, sneezing, stuffy nose, sore throat, and dry cough, followed by body aches and fever.

Diagnosis and Treatment. A physician usually determines if people have the flu by their symptoms and by whether the flu is present in the community. Treatment consists of bed rest and drinking lots of fluids. Aspirin or acetaminophen may relieve fever and discomfort. Children and teens should not take aspirin to relieve symptoms as it may increase the chances of developing Reye's syndrome. **Reye's syndrome** is a disease that causes swelling of the brain and deterioration of liver function. Antibiotics are not effective against flu viruses but may help prevent the pneumonia that sometimes follows it.

Lesson 63

You Can Reduce Your Risk of Infection with Sexually Transmitted Diseases

Life Skill **I will choose behaviors to reduce my risk of infection with sexually transmitted diseases.**

A **sexually transmitted disease (STD)** is a disease caused by pathogens that are transmitted from an infected person to an uninfected person during intimate sexual contact. This lesson includes A Guide to Sexually Transmitted Diseases. The guide includes information about chlamydia, genital herpes, genital warts, gonorrhea, pubic lice, syphilis, trichomoniasis, and viral hepatitis. You will learn these facts about each STD: the cause, methods of transmission, symptoms, diagnosis, treatment, and complications. This lesson also includes a discussion of how to prevent STDs. You will learn the importance of abstinence, monogamous marriage, and a drug-free lifestyle.

The Lesson Outline

A Guide to Sexually Transmitted Diseases

How Abstinence, Monogamous Marriage, and a Drug-Free Lifestyle Reduce the Risk of STDs

Objectives

1. Discuss the cause, methods of transmission, symptoms, diagnosis, treatment, and complications for these STDs: chlamydia, gonorrhea, syphilis, genital herpes, genital warts, trichomoniasis, pubic lice, and viral hepatitis. **pages 489–493**
2. Discuss ways to reduce the risk of STDs. **page 494**

Vocabulary Words

sexually transmitted disease (STD)
chlamydia
pelvic inflammatory disease (PID)
ectopic pregnancy
tubal pregnancy
genital herpes
herpes simplex virus type 1 (HSV-1
herpes simplex virus type 2 (HSV-2
acyclovir
genital warts
gonorrhea
pubic lice
lice
nits
syphilis
spirochete
primary syphilis
chancre
secondary syphilis
latent syphilis
late syphilis
tertiary syphilis
trichomoniasis
viral hepatitis
jaundice
monogamous marriage
universal precautions

A Guide to
Sexually Transmitted Diseases

Chlamydia

Cause. **Chlamydia** (kluh·MID·ee·uh) is an STD that is caused by the bacterium *Chlamydia trachomatis* that produces inflammation of the reproductive organs. It is the most common STD in the United States.

Methods of Transmission. Chlamydia is spread by intimate sexual contact with an infected partner. A pregnant female may pass the infection to her newborn baby during delivery. During delivery the *Chlamydia* bacteria can enter the baby's eyes or lungs. If not treated, the baby can become blind or develop pneumonia.

Symptoms. In males: One fourth of infected males have no symptoms. *Chlamydia* bacteria can continue to multiply in a male who does not know he is infected. Males with symptoms may have painful urination, a discharge from the penis, inflammation of the urethra, and pain or swelling in the scrotum. Symptoms usually appear within one to three weeks after exposure. Some males never have symptoms but still can infect a sexual partner. In females: One-half of infected females have no symptoms. A female may not know she has chlamydia until complications develop. Symptoms include inflammation of the vagina and cervix, a burning sensation during urination, and an unusual discharge from the vagina.

Diagnosis and Treatment. A physician uses a cotton swab to collect a sample of the discharge, which is examined in a laboratory for the presence of the *Chlamydia* bacteria. Antibiotics are used to treat chlamydia. Infected persons must take all the prescribed antibiotics,even after the symptoms disappear. A follow-up visit to a physician is necessary to be sure that the infection is cured. All sex partners of persons infected with chlamydia should be checked and treated.

Complications. **Pelvic inflammatory disease (PID)** is a serious infection of the internal female reproductive organs. Many cases occur in females infected with chlamydia but who had no symptoms. PID can cause a scarring of the Fallopian tubes, which can block the tubes and cause sterility. To be sterile means that a person is unable to produce children. Ectopic pregnancy is also linked to PID. An **ectopic pregnancy**, or **tubal pregnancy**, occurs when a fertilized egg implants in a Fallopian tube instead of in the uterus. This condition results in the death of the fetus and can be fatal for the pregnant female. If left untreated, chlamydia can cause sterility in males. A baby born to a mother with chlamydia may develop pneumonia or a serious eye infection that can lead to blindness if not treated promptly. Babies infected with chlamydia usually develop pneumonia within three to six weeks after birth.

Genital Herpes

Cause. **Genital herpes** is an STD caused by the herpes simplex virus (HSV) that produces cold sores or fever blisters in the genital area and mouth. **Herpes simplex virus type 1 (HSV-1)** is a virus that causes cold sores or fever blisters in the mouth or on the lips. HSV-1 also may cause genital sores. **Herpes simplex virus type 2 (HSV-2)** is a virus that causes genital sores but also may cause sores in the mouth. The viruses remain in the body for life.

Methods of Transmission. Genital herpes is spread by intimate sexual contact with an infected person. Infected people are highly contagious when blisters break and form red, painful open sores. Through touch, they can spread them to other areas of the body. If they have lesions in the mouth and place their fingers there and then touch the genitals or eyes, the virus is spread.

Symptoms. Symptoms of genital herpes occur within a week after contact with an infected partner. Early symptoms can include an itching or burning sensation; pain in the legs, buttocks, or genital area; vaginal discharge; or a feeling of pressure in the abdominal area. Clusters of small, painful blisters that may develop into open sores appear in the genital area. Other symptoms that accompany the outbreak of the blisters can be fever, headache, muscle aches, painful or difficult urination, vaginal discharge, and swollen glands in the groin area. The symptoms may last from two to four weeks and then disappear. In some people, these symptoms may reappear during times of stress or illness.

Diagnosis and Treatment. The sores of genital herpes usually are visible. Diagnosis is made by growing the virus from a swab of the ulcers. Blood tests can be given to detect the presence of antibodies to HSV in the blood. They can distinguish whether people have HSV-1 or HSV-2. There is no known cure for genital herpes. **Acyclovir** (ay·SEE·kloh·vir) is an antiviral drug approved for the treatment of herpes simplex infections. It relieves symptoms and prevents some recurrences of genital herpes. Sores need to be kept clean and dry, hands need to be washed after contact with the sores.

Complications. Genital herpes sores are painful and disrupt people's lives. People with genital herpes fear recurrences and spreading the infection to others. Genital herpes increases the risk of infection with HIV. HIV can easily enter the body through broken blisters if people infected with herpes have intimate contact with a person who has HIV. Episodes of genital herpes can be long-lasting and severe in people with weak immune systems. An infected pregnant female can infect her baby during vaginal delivery.

Genital Warts

Cause. **Genital warts** is an STD caused by certain types of the human papilloma virus (HPV) that produces wart-like growth on the genitals. More than 60 different types of HPV have been discovered, several of which can cause genital warts.

Methods of Transmission. Genital warts are very contagious and are spread during intimate sexual contact and by direct contact with infected bed linens, towels, and clothing. They can be spread from a pregnant female to her baby during vaginal delivery of the baby.

Symptoms. Genital warts appear three to eight months after infection. They usually are soft, red, or pink, and resemble a cauliflower. Sometimes they are hard and yellow-gray. In addition to appearing on or near the genitals, they may develop in the mouth. In males: Genital warts usually appear on the tip of the penis. They also may be found on the shaft of the penis, on the scrotum, or in the anus. In females: Genital warts may appear on the vulva, labia, inside the vagina, on the cervix, or around the anus.

Diagnosis and Treatment. A physician inspects the warts to make a diagnosis. Several new laboratory tests can identify specific types of HPV. These tests may be helpful in determining whether or not the infection is likely to progress to cancer and be spread from a pregnant female to a newborn. A Pap smear also may be given to females who are sexually active because of the increased risk of cervical cancer. No treatment is available that will completely get rid of the virus causing genital warts. Once infected, people will always have the virus in their bodies. Medication can be placed on genital warts and laser surgery used to remove them. Genital warts may be frozen and removed by using liquid nitrogen but may reappear after removal.

Complications. Besides being an embarrassment, several types of HPV increase the risk of cancers of the cervix, vulva, anus, and penis. Genital warts often enlarge during pregnancy and make urination difficult for a pregnant female. If genital warts are on the vaginal wall, delivery of the baby is very difficult. Babies born to a mother with genital warts can develop warts in their throats. To prevent the blocking of the airway, an infected baby may need laser surgery to remove the warts from the throat.

Gonorrhea

Cause. **Gonorrhea** is a highly contagious STD caused by the gonococcus bacterium *Niesseria gonorrhoeae.* Gonorrhea infects the linings of the genital and urinary tracts of males and females.

Methods of Transmission. Gonorrhea is spread by intimate sexual contact with an infected person. A baby born to an infected female can become infected during childbirth if the bacteria enter the baby's eyes.

Symptoms. In males: Males usually have a white, milky discharge from the penis and a burning sensation during urination. They may experience pain and increased urination within two to ten days after infection. They may not have symptoms but still may be contagious. In females: Many infected females have no symptoms. If symptoms appear, they include a burning sensation when urinating and a discharge from the vagina that usually appear within two to ten days after sexual contact with an infected partner. Severe symptoms, such as abdominal pain, bleeding between menstrual periods, vomiting, or fever, can occur if gonorrhea is not treated.

Diagnosis and Treatment. Diagnosis of gonorrhea is made by a microscopic examination of the discharge. The gram stain is a test that involves placing a smear of the discharge on a slide stained with a dye. The test is accurate for males but not for females. The preferred method for females is the culture test, which involves placing a sample of the discharge on a culture plate and letting it grow for up to two days. Antibiotics are used to treat gonorrhea. Some strains are resistant to some antibiotics, making treatment difficult. People with gonorrhea should take the full course of prescribed medication. A follow-up visit to a physician is necessary. All sex partners of infected people should be tested even if they have no symptoms. Most states require that the eyes of newborn babies be treated with silver nitrate or other medication immediately after birth to prevent gonococcal infection of the eyes in case the mother was infected.

Complications. The bacteria can spread to the bloodstream and infect the joints, heart valves, and the brain. Gonorrhea in both males and females can cause permanent sterility. It is a major cause of pelvic inflammatory disease (PID). In newborns, gonococcal infection can lead to blindness.

Pubic Lice

Cause. **Pubic lice** is infestation of the pubic hair by pubic or crab lice that survive by feeding on human blood. **Lice** are insects that pierce the skin and secrete a substance that causes itching and swelling.

Methods of Transmission. Lice can be spread from one person to another through intimate sexual contact. Because lice can live outside the body for as long as a day, people can become infected by sleeping on infested sheets, wearing infested clothing, sharing infested towels, and sitting on a toilet seat that has been used by a person who has lice.

Symptoms. The main symptom is itching in the pubic area. The lice may be visible as little black spots on body parts that have dense hair growth.

Diagnosis and Treatment. A physician examines the body to find the lice. Pubic lice and their nits are easily diagnosed because they are visible by the naked eye or through a magnifying glass. **Nits** are tiny white lice eggs that attach to body hair. A prescription drug is used as a shampoo to kill the lice. OTC preparations also are used. After the lice are killed, itching may continue because the skin has been irritated and requires time to heal. Certain medications can stop the itching.

Complications. The major health problem is the discomfort from itching and irritation.

Syphilis

Cause. **Syphilis** is an STD caused by the spirochete bacterium *Treponema pallidum.* A **spirochete** (SPY·roh·keet) is a spiral-shaped bacterium. Syphilis spirochetes enter the body through tiny breaks in the mucous membranes and then burrow their way into the bloodstream.

Methods of Transmission. Syphilis is spread by intimate sexual contact with an infected person. The spirochete also can be transmitted from a pregnant female to her fetus.

Symptoms. **Primary syphilis** is the first stage of syphilis. The first symptom of syphilis is a chancre. A **chancre** (SHAN·ker) is a painless, open sore that appears at the site where the spirochetes entered the body. This might be on the genitals or in the mouth. Chancres appear within ten days to three months after exposure to syphilis. Because a chancre is painless and sometimes occurs inside the body, it may not be noticed. Chancres contain spirochetes so syphilis can spread to people who have contact with a chancre. The chancre will disappear within a few weeks whether or not a person is treated. However, the pathogens for syphilis remain in the body and the disease progresses to secondary syphilis.

Secondary syphilis is the stage of syphilis characterized by a skin rash and begins anywhere from three to six weeks after the chancre appears. The skin rash may cover the whole body or appear in only a few areas, such as the hands or soles of the feet. People are very contagious during secondary syphilis. The rash heals within several weeks or months. Other symptoms, such as fever, tiredness, headache, sore throat, swollen lymph glands, and loss of weight and hair, may occur during this stage. The symptoms will disappear without treatment and may come and go during the next one or two years.

Diagnosis and Treatment. People with a suspicious skin rash or sore in the genital area should be checked by a physician. A blood test will detect the presence of the spirochetes that cause syphilis in any stage of the disease. Syphilis is treated with antibiotic drugs. People being treated for syphilis need to have regular blood tests to check that the pathogens are no longer present. Treatment in the later stages cannot reverse the damage done to body organs in the early stages of the disease.

Complications. If secondary syphilis is not treated it may become latent syphilis. **Latent syphilis** is a stage of syphilis in which there are no symptoms but the spirochetes are still present and may damage tissues and organs. Latent syphilis can last for years and even for decades. Some people with latent syphilis will not suffer any further damage from the disease. However, people who are infected will develop late syphilis. **Late syphilis**, or **tertiary syphilis**, is the final stage of syphilis in which spirochetes damage body organs. The spirochetes damage the heart, eyes, brain, nervous system, bones, joints, or other body parts. Mental illness, blindness, paralysis, heart disease, liver damage, and death may occur. The damage to body organs cannot be reversed. If a pregnant female has syphilis, the fetus is at risk. The pregnancy may result in a miscarriage, stillbirth, or fetal death. More than two out of three babies born to a mother with syphilis are born with syphilis. Babies with syphilis may have skin sores, rashes, fever, hoarse crying, a swollen liver and spleen, yellowish skin, and anemia and are at high risk for being born with mental retardation and other birth defects.

Trichomoniasis

Cause. **Trichomoniasis** (trik·oh·moh·NY·uh·sis) is an STD caused by the single-celled protozoan *Trichomonas vaginalis.* The most common site of infection in males is the urethra. In females, the most common site of infection is the vagina.

Methods of Transmission. Trichomoniasis is spread during intimate sexual contact with an infected person. It can be transmitted even when no symptoms are present and without sexual contact. The protozoa may survive for up to 24 hours on damp towels. Sharing infected towels is a means of transmission. Females who use vaginal sprays and douches may change the natural condition of their vagina enough to create a favorable environment for the protozoa to multiply.

Symptoms. In males: Symptoms include a thin, whitish discharge from the penis and painful or difficult urination. Most males do not experience any symptoms. In females: About half of all infected females have no symptoms. There may be a yellow-green or gray vaginal discharge that has an odor, painful urination, irritation and itching in the genital area, and, on rare occasions, pain in the abdomen.

Diagnosis and Treatment. A smear of the discharge is examined under a microscope. The drug Metronidazole is used to treat trichomoniasis. People taking this drug should not drink alcohol. Mixing the two drugs can cause severe nausea and vomiting.

Complications. Trichomoniasis may cause pregnant females to deliver low birth weight or premature babies.

Viral Hepatitis

Cause. **Viral hepatitis** is a viral infection of the liver. There are several different viruses that cause hepatitis, including hepatitis A (HAV), hepatitis B (HBV), hepatitis C (HCV), delta hepatitis (HDV), and hepatitis E (HEV).

Methods of Transmission. All types of viral hepatitis, except infection by HEV, are known to be spread through intimate sexual contact. HBV, HCV, and HDV also are spread through sharing contaminated drug needles. HAV is most commonly spread by contaminated food and water. HEV is spread mainly through contaminated water in areas with poor sanitation. HBV can be spread from a pregnant female to her baby.

Symptoms. Many infected people have no symptoms. When symptoms are present, they may be mild or severe. The most common early symptoms are mild fever, headache, muscle aches, tiredness, loss of appetite, nausea, vomiting, or diarrhea. Later symptoms may include dark and foamy urine, pale-colored feces, abdominal pain, and jaundice. **Jaundice** is yellowing of the skin and whites of the eyes. Infection with each type of virus can produce different symptoms.

Diagnosis and Treatment. Blood tests confirm viral hepatitis. A physician also can observe symptoms. Treatment consists of bed rest, a healthful diet, and avoidance of alcoholic beverages. Drugs may be prescribed to improve liver function. Vaccines are now available for life-long immunity to hepatitis A and hepatitis B. Immune globulin also is available to provide immediate and short-term protection against hepatitis B.

Complications. Many cases of hepatitis are not a serious threat to health. Others are long-lasting and can lead to liver failure and death. Viral hepatitis increases the risk of developing liver cancer.

You Can Reduce Your Risk of HIV Infection

Life Skill **I will choose behaviors to reduce my risk of HIV infection.**

Any person regardless of gender, age, race, or sexual orientation, can become infected with HIV by engaging in specific risk behaviors. This lesson explains how to reduce your risk of being infected with HIV and how HIV infection progresses to AIDS. You will learn about the risk behaviors and risk situations through which HIV is transmitted. You also will learn ways HIV is not transmitted. The lesson describes the latest HIV tests and treatments and outlines ways you can reduce your risk of being infected with HIV.

The Lesson Outline

What to Know About HIV Infection and AIDS

What to Know About HIV Transmission

What to Know About HIV Tests

What to Know About Treatment for HIV Infection and AIDS

How to Reduce the Risk of HIV Infection

Objectives

1. Discuss the progression of HIV infection to AIDS. **page 498**
2. List and discuss ways HIV is and is not transmitted. **pages 500–501**
3. List and discuss tests used to determine HIV status. **page 502**
4. Discuss treatment approaches for HIV and AIDS. **page 503**
5. List and discuss ten ways to reduce the risk of HIV infection. **page 504**

Vocabulary Words

lymphocytes
B cell
helper T cell
antibody
macrophages
human immunodeficiency virus (HIV)
opportunistic infection
thrush
oral hairy leukoplakia
pneumocystis carinii pneumonia (PCP)
Kaposi's sarcoma (KS)
AIDS dementia complex
HIV wasting syndrome
injecting drug user
perinatal transmission
ELISA
Western blot
home collection kit for HIV testing
HIV positive
HIV negative
Orasure Western blot
Amplicor HIV-1 Monitor Test
monogamous marriage
universal precautions
autoclave

Activity

An AIDS Compassion Quilt

Life Skill: I will choose behaviors to reduce my risk of HIV infection.

Materials: posterboard, scissors, felt tip pens or markers, tape

Directions: Several years ago, people made an AIDS quilt to show compassion for people who had died of AIDS. The quilt contained thousands of patches or sections, each containing information and symbols to honor a particular person who had died of AIDS. The quilt is used as a memorial. Follow the steps in this activity to make an AIDS compassion quilt from posterboard.

 Cut a 6-inch by 6-inch (15-centimeter by 15-centimeter) square from posterboard to represent a piece of quilt.

 Select the name of a person you know who has died of AIDS.

 Design your piece of posterboard to represent qualities, interests, accomplishments, and special characteristics of the person you selected.

 Tape your piece of posterboard to those of classmates to make a large posterboard quilt.

 Look closely at each separate piece of posterboard that makes up the completed quilt. Note the qualities, interests, accomplishments, and special characteristics of all the people represented on the quilt.

 Write a one-page paper based on your observations of the entire quilt. Describe how the quilt makes you feel. Explain the great loss to society that the quilt represents.

What to Know About
HIV Infection and AIDS

Lymphocytes are white blood cells that help the body fight pathogens. When a pathogen enters the body, lymphocytes multiply in lymph tissue to fight infection. A **B cell** is a white blood cell that produces antibodies. A **helper T cell** is a white blood cell that signals B cells to produce antibodies. An **antibody** is a special protein that helps fight infection.

In most cases, your B cells produce antibodies in your blood soon after a pathogen enters the body. B cells enter the lymph nodes and other lymph tissues. Antibodies then travel through lymph vessels to destroy the pathogen. Antibodies can make pathogens ineffective and susceptible to macrophages. **Macrophages** are white blood cells that surround and destroy pathogens. Antibodies help macrophages by attaching to pathogens and making them easier to be engulfed and digested. Digested pathogens enter lymph and are destroyed in lymph nodes. They also are removed by the spleen.

The **human immunodeficiency virus (HIV)** is a pathogen that destroys infection-fighting T cells in the body. When HIV enters the body, it attaches to a molecule called CD4 on helper T cells. HIV then takes control of the helper T cells and reproduces more HIV. As HIV reproduces and makes more HIV, it attacks the other helper T cells and takes control of them. Some signs of HIV infection may include flu-like symptoms, such as fever, sore throat, skin rash, diarrhea, swollen glands, loss of appetite, and night sweats. These signs may come and go as the helper T cell count fluctuates.

People are susceptible to many opportunistic infections when they are infected with HIV. An **opportunistic infection** is an infection that develops in a person with a weak immune system. The pathogens that cause opportunistic infections already are present in the bodies of most people but usually are harmless unless a person has HIV or some other disease that weakens the immune system. There are many opportunistic infections. **Thrush** is a fungal infection of the mucous membranes of the tongue and mouth. White spots and ulcers cover the infection. Infections of the skin and mucous membranes also appear. There may be sores around the anus, genital area, and mouth. **Oral hairy leukoplakia** is an infection with fuzzy white patches found on the tongue. **Pneumocystis carinii pneumonia (PCP)** is a form of pneumonia that may affect people infected with HIV.

People who are infected with HIV are at risk for developing tuberculosis. They also are at risk for developing cancers. **Kaposi's sarcoma (KS)** is a type of cancer that affects people who are infected with HIV. KS causes purplish lesions and tumors on the skin and in the linings of the internal organs. These lesions spread to most of the linings of the body.

HIV destroys brain and nerve cells. **AIDS dementia complex** is a loss of brain function caused by HIV infection. There is gradual loss of a person's ability to think and move, personality change, and loss of coordination. As AIDS dementia complex progresses, confusion increases and memory loss becomes severe.

People who have AIDS may develop HIV wasting syndrome. **HIV wasting syndrome** is a substantial loss in body weight that is accompanied by high fevers, sweating, and diarrhea.

To date, half of all people infected with HIV have developed AIDS within ten years. According to the Centers for Disease Control and Prevention, a person infected with HIV who has 200 or fewer helper T cells per microliter of blood or an opportunistic infection has AIDS.

When HIV Enters the Body

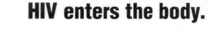 HIV enters the body.

HIV attaches to and takes
control of helper T cells.

HIV reproduces itself and
destroys helper T cells.

HIV continues to reproduce,
and to attack and destroy other
helper T cells. This weakens the
body's ability to fight infection.

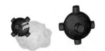

According to the Centers for Disease
Control and Prevention, a person infected
with HIV has AIDS when (s)he has 200
or fewer helper T cells per microliter of
blood or an opportunistic infection.

What to Know About
HIV Transmission

People who are infected with HIV have HIV in most of their body fluids. HIV is spread from infected persons to others by contact with certain body fluids. These body fluids are blood, semen, vaginal secretions and, in a few cases, breast milk. Minute traces of HIV have been found in saliva, sweat, and tears. To date, there have been no documented cases of HIV transmission through saliva and tears. HIV is transmitted when a person engages in specific risk behaviors or is involved in risk situations.

Having Sexual Contact with an Infected Person

During sexual contact, HIV from an infected person may enter the body of an uninfected partner through exposed blood vessels in small cuts or tiny cracks in mucous membranes. HIV can spread from male to male, male to female, female to male, or female to female. HIV transmission can occur if the male ejaculates or if he withdraws before ejaculation. This is because HIV is present in the preejaculatory fluid.

Increased risks from sexual contact include:

1. **Having multiple sex partners.** The greater the number of sex partners people have, the more likely they will have sex with someone who is infected with HIV.

2. **Having sex with a prostitute.** Because male and female prostitutes have a large number of sexual partners, people who have sex with them are at an increased risk for being infected with HIV. Prostitutes also are known to use injecting drugs.

3. **Having other sexually transmitted diseases.** STDs that produce sores or lead to bleeding or discharge provide body openings through which HIV can spread more easily. Genital sores provide an exit point for infected people and an entry point for uninfected people for transmission of HIV in blood, semen, and vaginal secretions.

Open-Mouth Kissing

The Centers for Disease Control and Prevention warns against open-mouth kissing with a person infected with HIV because of the possibility of contact with infected blood.

Sharing Needles, Syringes, or Other Injection Equipment for Injecting Drugs

An **injecting drug user** is a person who injects illegal drugs into the body with syringes, needles, and other injection equipment. When an infected person injects drugs, droplets of HIV-infected blood remain on the needle, syringe, or other injection equipment. A second person who shares a needle, syringe, or other injection equipment to inject drugs will get the HIV-infected blood into his/her body. Then this person will be infected with HIV.

Sharing Needles to Make Tattoos and to Pierce Ears and Other Body Parts

Droplets of HIV-infected blood remain on the needle when an infected person uses a needle to make a tattoo or to pierce ears or other body parts. A second person who shares the needle will get the HIV-infected blood into his/her body and could become infected.

Having Contact with the Blood or Other Body Fluids, Mucous Membranes, or Broken Skin of an Infected Person

People who handle the body fluids of a person who is infected with HIV risk having HIV enter their bodies through small cuts or tears on the skin or through splash in the eyes. People who use something such as a razor or toothbrush that may have droplets of infected blood on it risk having the infected blood enter their bodies through small cuts or tears in the mucous membranes or skin. Touching the mucous membranes or broken skin of an HIV-infected person may result in contact with exposed blood vessels. HIV-infected blood can enter the body through small cuts or tears on the skin.

Having a Blood Transfusion with Infected Blood or Blood Products

In the United States, the FDA controls blood donations, blood donor centers, and blood labs. All donors are screened. After donation, blood is tested for HIV, hepatitis B, and syphilis. People traveling to countries other than the United States should inquire about the safety of the blood supply. You cannot become infected with HIV from donating blood.

Having a Tissue Transplant (Organ Donation)

In the United States, screening and testing procedures have reduced the risk of being infected by human tissue transplants. Potential donors for all human tissues must be tested for HIV, hepatitis B, and hepatitis C. They also must be screened for risk behaviors and symptoms of AIDS and hepatitis. Imported tissues must be accompanied by records showing that the tissues were screened and tested. If no records are available, tissues are shipped under quarantine to the United States. People having tissue transplants outside the United States should check screening and testing procedures.

Being Born to a Mother Infected with HIV

A pregnant female infected with HIV can transmit HIV through the umbilical cord to her developing embryo or fetus. A baby also can be infected while passing through the mother's vagina at birth. Infected blood in the vagina can enter the baby's blood through a cut on the baby's body. A nursing baby can become infected with HIV through the breast milk of an infected mother. From 15 to 30 percent of all pregnant females infected with HIV infect their babies with HIV through perinatal transmission. **Perinatal transmission** is the transfer of an infection to a baby during pregnancy, during delivery, or after birth through breast milk.

Ways HIV Is Not Transmitted

To date, there have been no documented cases of HIV transmission through saliva, sweat, or tears. According to the Centers for Disease Control and Prevention, HIV is not spread through casual contact, such as:

- closed-mouth kissing;
- hugging;
- touching, holding, or shaking hands;
- coughing or sneezing;
- sharing food or eating utensils;
- sharing towels or combs;
- having casual contact with friends;
- sharing bathroom facilities or water fountains;
- sharing a pen or pencil;
- being bitten by insects;
- donating blood;
- eating food prepared or served by someone else;
- attending school;
- using a telephone or computer used by someone else;
- swimming in a pool;
- using sports and gym equipment.

What to Know About
HIV Tests

You cannot tell if people are infected with HIV by the way they look. They may look and feel healthy and not have symptoms and still spread the virus to others. Therefore, anyone who has engaged in a risk behavior or been in a risk situation for HIV transmission should be tested for HIV.

An HIV-antibody test is the only way to tell whether or not a person is infected with HIV. When HIV enters the body, the immune system responds by making antibodies. The HIV-antibody test detects HIV antibodies in the blood and tells whether people are infected. HIV antibodies usually show up in the blood within three months after infection, but could take up to six months. The test will detect antibodies in most people infected within six months. It does not tell if people have AIDS or when they will get AIDS. HIV antibodies do not protect from disease or prevent someone from infecting others with HIV.

ELISA is a blood test used to check for antibodies for HIV. If an ELISA test is positive, it is repeated to confirm the result. If two or more positive ELISA tests are positive, a Western blot test is given. **Western blot** is a blood test used to check for antibodies for HIV and to confirm an ELISA test. It is more specific and takes longer to perform. Used together, ELISA and Western blot are correct more than 99.9 percent of the time.

The FDA has approved use of a few home collection kits for HIV antibody testing. A **home collection kit for HIV testing** is a kit that allows a person to take a blood sample at home, place drops of blood on a test card, mail the card to a lab, and call a toll-free number to get HIV results. The blood sample contains a personal identification number that the caller gives when using the toll-free number for the test results. The tests usually are available within a week. If the test is positive, a counselor usually comes on the telephone. Many health care professionals are concerned about people being told over the telephone that they are HIV positive. Teens who need to be tested for HIV should talk to their parents or guardian and decide together where to have testing and get results.

A positive test result means a person is HIV positive. **HIV positive** is a term used to describe a person who has antibodies for HIV present in the blood. **HIV negative** is a term used to describe a person who does not have antibodies for HIV present in the blood. A teen who engaged in a risk behavior this past week might test HIV negative today. However, (s)he would have to be tested again in a few months because antibodies for HIV do not show up in the blood right away.

Tests for HIV Approved by the FDA in 1996

Orasure Western blot is a test for HIV in which a tissue sample is collected by using a cotton swab between the gum and cheek. Because many people do not like to get their finger pricked or have a blood sample drawn, more people may agree to be tested with this newer test.

Amplicor HIV-1 Monitor Test is a test that measures the level of HIV in the blood. Higher levels of HIV in the blood can be correlated with an increased risk that the disease will progress to AIDS.

What to Know About Treatment for HIV Infection and AIDS

There is no cure for HIV infection or AIDS. Treatment focuses on slowing the progression of the virus by taking drugs and practicing healthful habits. Early treatment is critical in slowing the rate at which HIV multiplies. This, in turn, delays the progression of HIV to AIDS. As of June 1996, the FDA had approved 22 drugs for HIV and AIDS-related conditions.

FDA-Approved Drugs for HIV and AIDS-Related Conditions

- **ddi** is a drug that slows down the rate at which HIV multiplies.

- **AZT** (zidovudine) is a drug that slows down the rate at which HIV multiplies.

- **Aerosolized pentamidine isethionate** is a drug to prevent pneumocystis carinii pneumonia (PCP). PCP is the most life-threatening infection of people with AIDS.

- **Interferon alfa-2a** and **Interferon alfa-2b** are drugs to treat Kaposi's sarcoma (KS).

- **Protease inhibitors** are antiviral drugs that decrease the amount of HIV in the blood and increase the helper T cell count.

Protease inhibitors are newer and more effective against HIV than some other drugs. However, researchers are not sure how long protease inhibitors will work in people infected with HIV or how well they will work in different people. They are hopeful that people who take these drugs will live longer, healthier lives. Some people have had the amount of HIV in the blood drop to a level where it cannot be detected. However, physicians believe HIV is still in their bodies and will reproduce quickly if they stop taking the protease inhibitors. Clinical trials are being conducted to help answer where HIV "hides" and why people have different results with protease inhibitors.

People who are infected with HIV or who have developed AIDS should practice healthful habits. They should eat healthful foods, get enough rest and sleep, exercise, and avoid alcohol, tobacco, and other drugs. People who have HIV wasting syndrome need to follow food safety practices. Their weakened immune system leaves them vulnerable to illnesses that are spread in contaminated food. They should avoid eating nonpasteurized dairy products, raw eggs, and raw seafood. They should cook food thoroughly before eating it. They should wash their hands and eating utensils with soap and water.

Scientists have made progress in the treatment of HIV and AIDS. They continue to test vaccines and research ways to keep people with HIV and AIDS as healthy as long as possible. Some people may import for their personal use unapproved, but promising, drugs for HIV and life-threatening AIDS-related diseases. Because there are many scams, the FDA initiated an AIDS Health Fraud Task Force to explain how to identify phony health products and to distribute general information about HIV infection.

You Can Reduce Your Risk of Cardiovascular Diseases

Life Skill I will choose behaviors to reduce my risk of cardiovascular diseases.

A **cardiovascular disease** is a disease of the heart and blood vessels. Cardiovascular diseases account for almost half of all deaths in the United States. They also disable millions of people each year. This lesson includes A Guide to Cardiovascular Diseases. It also includes a discussion of risk factors for cardiovascular disease. You will learn about the risk factors you cannot control and the risk factors you can control.

The Lesson Outline

A Guide to Cardiovascular Diseases

How to Reduce Your Risk of Cardiovascular Diseases

Objectives

1. List and discuss eight cardiovascular diseases. **pages 507–508**
2. Identify four cardiovascular disease risk factors that cannot be controlled. **page 509**
3. Identify seven cardiovascular disease risk factors that can be controlled. **pages 509–510**

Vocabulary Words

cardiovascular disease
angina pectoris
nitroglycerin
arteriosclerosis
atherosclerosis
plaque
congestive heart failure
coronary heart disease (CHD)
coronary artery
arrhythmia
pacemaker
heart attack
myocardial infarction (MI)
rheumatic fever
rheumatic heart disease
stroke
cerebrovascular accident
aneurysm
cardiovascular disease risk factors
premature heart attack
cholesterol
lipoprotein analysis
low density lipoproteins (LDLs)
high density lipoproteins (HDLs)
saturated fat
heart-healthy diet
antioxidant
high blood pressure
antihypertensives
stress management skills

A Guide to
Cardiovascular Diseases

Angina Pectoris

Angina pectoris (an·JY·nuh PEK·tuh·ris) is chest pain that results from narrowed coronary arteries. The pain occurs because the heart is not getting an adequate amount of oxygen. Sudden physical exertion, vigorous exercise, or excessive stress can cause angina pectoris in people with coronary heart disease. Many people with coronary heart disease take nitroglycerin pills to relieve chest pains. **Nitroglycerin** is a drug that widens the coronary arteries allowing more oxygen to get to cardiac muscle. Angina pectoris is a warning sign for a heart attack. A heart attack may occur if the narrowing that causes angina pectoris is very severe.

Congestive Heart Failure

Congestive heart failure is a condition that occurs when the heart's pumping ability is below normal capacity and fluid accumulates in the lungs and other areas of the body. Causes of congestive heart failure are heart attack, atherosclerosis, birth defects, high blood pressure, and rheumatic fever. Drugs that improve the heart's pumping ability and get rid of excess fluids are used to treat congestive heart failure. Reducing the amount of sodium in the diet is helpful.

Arteriosclerosis and Atherosclerosis

Arteriosclerosis (ahr·tee·ree·oh·skluh·ROH·sis) is a general term to describe several conditions that cause hardening and thickening of the arteries. Some arteriosclerosis occurs naturally as people age. One type of arteriosclerosis is atherosclerosis. **Atherosclerosis** is a disease in which fat deposits on artery walls. The fatty deposits may harden and form plaque. **Plaque** is hardened deposits. Medical scientists believe that high blood cholesterol levels, a high-fat diet, high blood pressure, and smoking can cause injury to the lining of arteries and contribute to plaque buildup. The buildup of plaque in artery walls may begin as early as two years of age. It does not develop suddenly in later life.

Coronary Heart Disease

Coronary heart disease (CHD) is a disease in which the coronary arteries are narrowed or blocked. A **coronary artery** is a blood vessel that carries blood to the heart muscles. The coronary arteries encircle the heart and continuously nourish it with blood. Plaque buildup in the coronary arteries causes coronary heart disease, which can cause a heart attack.

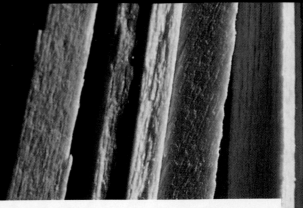

Heart Rhythm Abnormalities

The heart must beat in rhythm to effectively pump blood throughout the body. **Arrhythmia** (ay·RITH·mee·uh) is a heart condition in which the heart may beat very slowly or very fast for no obvious reason. The heart may skip beats or beat irregularly. Various drugs are available to treat arrhythmia. People who do not improve after taking drugs may need to have surgery to implant a pacemaker. A **pacemaker** is a device that is implanted in the heart to stimulate normal heart contractions.

Rheumatic Fever

Rheumatic fever is an auto-immune action in the heart that can cause fever, weakness, and damage to the valves in the heart. **Rheumatic heart disease** is permanent heart damage that results from rheumatic fever. The symptoms of rheumatic fever are painful, swollen joints and skin rashes. Rheumatic fever is most common in children and teens. Prevention of rheumatic fever involves getting prompt treatment for strep throat.

Heart Attack

A **heart attack** is the death of cardiac muscle caused by a lack of blood flow to the heart. **Myocardial infarction** (my·oh·KAR·dee·uhl in·FARK·shun) **(MI)** is the medical term for heart attack. A coronary artery that is narrowed by plaque might become clogged by a blood clot. If this happens, blood flow to the heart muscle is blocked. A heart attack may result in disability or death. The warning signs include uncomfortable pressure or pain in the center of the chest; pain that spreads to the shoulders, neck, jaw, or back; lightheadedness; fainting; sweating, nausea; and shortness of breath. The American Heart Association (AHA) warns that not all of these signs occur in every heart attack. AHA advises that people get medical help immediately when some of these symptoms occur.

Stroke

A **stroke**, or **cerebrovascular** (se·ree·broh·VAS·cue·luhr) **accident**, is a condition caused by a blocked or broken blood vessel in the brain. Brain cells in the area of the blocked or broken blood vessel are deprived of the oxygen they need. The brain cells die within minutes, and the affected area of the brain and the parts of the body controlled by those brain cells cannot function. One of the most common causes of a stroke is a blood clot in an artery in the brain. Strokes also can be caused if an aneurysm in the brain bursts. An **aneurysm** (AN·yuh·RIZ·uhm) is a weakened area of a blood vessel. Strokes also can be caused by a head injury. A stroke may result in paralysis, disability, or death. High blood pressure, cigarette smoking, high blood cholesterol, and having heart disease or diabetes are major risk factors for having a stroke.

How to Reduce Your Risk of Cardiovascular Diseases

Scientific studies have identified several cardiovascular disease risk factors. **Cardiovascular disease risk factors** are characteristics of people and ways they might behave that increase the possibility of cardiovascular disease. The greater the number of cardiovascular disease risk factors people have, the greater their risk of cardiovascular disease. The severity of a risk factor also determines its importance. For example, if two people have high blood cholesterol levels, the one with the higher level is more at risk for cardiovascular disease.

Some cardiovascular disease risk factors cannot be controlled. These include age, gender, race, and having blood relatives with cardiovascular disease. The risk of cardiovascular disease increases with age. Four out of five people who die of heart attack are over the age of 65. Males have a higher incidence of cardiovascular disease than females. However, after menopause, the incidence of cardiovascular disease increases in females. People whose family members and other close relatives have suffered a premature heart attack also have an increased risk. A **premature heart attack** is a heart attack that occurs before age 55 in males and age 65 in females.

Some cardiovascular disease risk factors can be controlled. The seven actions that follow can help control cardiovascular disease risk factors.

Maintain a Healthy Blood Cholesterol Level. The risk of a heart attack rises as blood cholesterol level increases. **Cholesterol** is a fat-like substance made by the body and found in certain foods. It is a normal part of your blood and causes problems when the level is too high. People can check their blood cholesterol level by having a small amount of their blood analyzed and, if cholesterol is high, a lipoprotein analysis. A **lipoprotein analysis** is a measure of two main types of lipoproteins in the blood. **Low density lipoproteins (LDLs)** are substances in the blood that carry cholesterol to body cells. **High density lipoproteins (HDLs)** are substances in the blood that carry cholesterol to the liver for breakdown and excretion. The higher the HDL level in the blood, the lower the risk of developing heart disease. Saturated fat raises blood cholesterol level. **Saturated fat** is a type of fat from dairy products, solid vegetable fat, and meat and poultry. Reducing the amount of saturated fat in the diet can help lower blood cholesterol level. People who are overweight can lower blood cholesterol level by losing excess weight. Physical activity and quitting smoking also helps increase the level of HDLs.

Choose a Heart-Healthy Diet. A **heart-healthy diet** is a low-fat diet rich in fruits, vegetables, whole grains, nonfat and low-fat milk products, lean meats, poultry, and fish. Sugars, sweets, fats, oils, and salt are limited. Choosing a heart-healthy diet can help control factors that influence the risk of cardiovascular disease, such as blood cholesterol level, blood pressure, and weight. A heart-healthy diet includes foods that contain antioxidants. An **antioxidant** is a substance that protects cells from being damaged by oxidation. A balanced diet that includes antioxidants may lower the risk of heart disease. Vitamins C and E, beta-carotene, and selenium are antioxidants. Fruits and vegetables are good sources of antioxidants.

You Can Reduce Your Risk of Diabetes

Life Skill I will choose behaviors to reduce my risk of diabetes.

The American Diabetes Association reports that 16 million people in the United States have diabetes. Half of these people do not yet know they have diabetes because their symptoms seem minor and they do not have medical checkups. As a result, they are not being treated. This lesson includes information on three types of diabetes. You will learn the symptoms for each type. You also will learn how people who have diabetes manage their disease. Finally, you will learn how you can reduce your risk of diabetes.

The Lesson Outline

What to Know About Diabetes

How to Manage Diabetes

How to Reduce the Risk of Diabetes

Objectives

1. Explain the three types of diabetes. **page 513**
2. Discuss ways that people who have diabetes can manage their disease. **page 514**
3. List five complications from diabetes. **page 514**
4. Identify four risk factors for diabetes. **page 514**
5. List and discuss ways to reduce the risk of diabetes. **page 514**

Vocabulary Words

diabetes

diabetes mellitus

insulin

metabolism

glucose

insulin-dependent diabetes mellitus (IDDM)

Type I diabetes

autoimmune disease

non-insulin-dependent diabetes mellitus (NIDDM)

Type II diabetes

gestational diabetes

What to Know About
Diabetes

Diabetes, or **diabetes mellitus**, is a disease in which the body produces little or no insulin. **Insulin** is a hormone that regulates the blood sugar level. If the pancreas fails to produce enough insulin, a person develops diabetes. Diabetes disrupts metabolism. **Metabolism** is the rate at which food is converted into energy in body cells. **Glucose** is a simple sugar that is the main source of energy for the body. Normally, insulin regulates the amount of glucose in the blood and the delivery of glucose into body cells. If there is not enough insulin, or if the body does not use the insulin, glucose levels build up in the blood. This causes the excess glucose to overflow into urine and pass out of the body. Since glucose is the main source of energy, the body loses its source of fuel even though the blood contains large amounts of glucose.

There are three types of diabetes: insulin-dependent, non-insulin-dependent, and gestational diabetes. **Insulin-dependent diabetes mellitus (IDDM)**, or **Type I diabetes**, is a type of diabetes in which the body produces little or no insulin. It is considered to be an autoimmune disease. An **autoimmune disease** is a disease that results when the immune system produces antibodies that turn against the body's own cells. In IDDM, the immune system attacks and destroys cells that produce insulin. Genetic factors and viruses are thought to trigger the body's immune system to attack these cells.

Between 5 and 10 percent of people who have diabetes have IDDM. IDDM used to be called juvenile-onset diabetes because it appears most often in children and young adults. However, this term was not appropriate because a lot of adults have IDDM from when they were very young. IDDM usually appears suddenly and progresses quickly. Symptoms of IDDM include increased thirst, frequent urination, constant hunger, weight loss, blurred vision, and extreme tiredness. These symptoms are caused by the buildup of sugar in the blood and the loss of sugar in the urine. People who have IDDM need daily injections of insulin to stay alive. They also need to follow a special diet.

Non-insulin-dependent diabetes mellitus (NIDDM), or **Type II diabetes**, is a type of diabetes in which the body produces insulin but it cannot be used by cells. NIDDM is the most common type of diabetes. About 90 to 95 percent of people who have diabetes have NIDDM. NIDDM used to be called adult-onset diabetes because it appears most often in adults over age 40. However, this term was not appropriate because NIDDM can occur in people of any age. The onset of NIDDM is usually gradual and the symptoms are not as noticeable as those of IDDM. As a result, NIDDM may go undetected for many years. Symptoms include feeling tired, frequent urination, unusual thirst, weight loss, blurred vision, frequent infections, and slow healing of sores. About 80 percent of people who have NIDDM are overweight. NIDDM often can be treated through weight loss, diet, physical activity, and oral medications.

Gestational diabetes is diabetes that occurs in some females during pregnancy. Insulin is produced, but the body does not respond to it. The resistance to insulin is caused by hormones the placenta produces during pregnancy. Gestational diabetes usually is treated with diet, not with oral medications. Oral medications might harm the baby. Gestational diabetes usually disappears after the birth of the baby. Women who have had gestational diabetes are at higher risk of developing non-insulin-dependent diabetes.

You Can Reduce Your Risk of Cancer

Life Skill **I will choose behaviors to reduce my risk of cancer.**

People of all ages get cancer. However, nearly all types of cancer are more common in middle-aged and elderly people than they are in young people. The most common type of cancer for both males and females is skin cancer. The next most common type among males is prostate cancer. Among females, it is breast cancer. Lung cancer is the leading cause of cancer deaths in both males and females. This lesson discusses facts about cancer. It includes A Guide to the Most Common Cancers. You will learn the risk factors, signs and symptoms, and ways to detect each type of common cancer. You also will learn about the treatments for cancer and ways to reduce your risk of cancer.

The Lesson Outline

What to Know About Cancer

A Guide to the Most Common Cancers

What to Know About Treatment Approaches

How to Reduce Your Risk of Developing Cancer

Objectives

1. Discuss the growth and spread of cancerous cells. **page 517**
2. Outline facts about 14 common cancers: risk factors, signs and symptoms, and early detection. **pages 518–519**
3. Discuss different treatment approaches to cancer. **page 520**
4. List and discuss ten ways to reduce the risk of cancer. **pages 521–522**

Vocabulary Words

cancer

tumor

benign tumor

malignant tumor

metastasis

radiation therapy

chemotherapy

immunotherapy

carcinogen

ultraviolet (UV) radiation

malignant melanoma

radon

What to Know About
Cancer

All cells in a person's body usually divide in an orderly pattern to produce more cells. This enables the body to grow and repair itself. Normal cell division is under precise control. Sometimes there are problems, and cells do not divide in the usual way. **Cancer** is a group of diseases in which cells divide in an uncontrolled manner. These cells can form a tumor. A **tumor** is an abnormal growth of tissue. Tumors can be benign or malignant. A **benign tumor** is a tumor that is not cancerous and does not spread to other parts of the body. Benign tumors rarely are life-threatening. They usually can be removed and do not grow back. A **malignant tumor** is a tumor that is cancerous and may spread to other parts of the body. **Metastasis** (muh·TAS·tuh·suhs) is the spread of cancer. Cancer cells can break away from a malignant tumor and enter the bloodstream or lymphatic system. They can form new tumors in other parts of the body.

Cancer is not contagious. You cannot get cancer from another person. Cancer also is not caused by an injury, such as a bump or bruise. Although the causes of cancer are not completely understood, many risk factors for cancer have been identified. These risk factors increase people's chances of getting cancer.

Some people are fearful of cancer. They do not realize that many types of cancer can be prevented or successfully treated when detected early. They can improve the chance that cancer will be detected early if they have regular physical examinations, perform certain self-examinations, and are aware of risk factors for and signs and symptoms of cancer. A Guide to the Most Common Cancers contains information on risk factors, signs and symptoms, and early detection of several types of cancer.

A Guide to the
Most Common Cancers

Type of Cancer	Risk Factors	Signs and Symptoms	Early Detection
Bladder	• Cigarette smoking • Air pollution • Exposure to industrial chemicals	• Blood in urine • Increased frequency of urination • Weight loss and loss of appetite	• Examination of the bladder by a physician
Breast	• Family history of breast cancer • Early start of menstruation • Late menopause • Never having children • Late age when first having children	• Breast tenderness • Lumps or thickenings in the breast • Dimpling or puckering of the skin on a breast • Changes in a nipple • Discharge from a nipple	• Monthly breast self-examination • Physical exams by a physician every 3 years for women 20 to 40 • Mammogram beginning at age 40
Cervical	• Early age at first sexual intercourse • Having multiple sexual partners • Cigarette smoking • Infection with human papilloma virus (HPV)	• Abnormal bleeding from the uterus or spotting • Abnormal vaginal discharge • Pain	• Annual Pap smear for women who are sexually active or after age 18 to check if cells of the cervix are abnormal • Regular pelvic examinations
Colon and Rectal	• Family history of colo-rectal cancer • Polyps in the colon or rectum • Inflammatory bowel disease • High-fat and low-fiber diet • Physical inactivity	• Changes in bowel habits (such as constipation or diarrhea) • Bleeding in the rectum • Blood in the stool • Unexplained weight loss	• Annual digital rectal examination after age 40 • Annual stool blood test after age 50 • Examination of the colon and rectum by a physician
Endometrial	• Obesity • Early start of menstruation • Late menopause • Family history of infertility • Failure to ovulate • Use of estrogen drugs	• Abnormal vaginal bleeding after menopause • Irregular menstrual cycles • Pain • Weight loss	• Annual pelvic exam by a physician after age 40 • Regular Pap smears (only partially effective)
Lymphoma: Hodgkin's Disease	• Largely unknown • Reduced immune function • Exposure to certain infectious agents	• Enlarged lymph nodes • Unexplained fever • Unexplained weight loss • Fatigue • Night sweats • Itching	• No early detection tests available
Lymphoma: Non-Hodgkin's Disease	• Largely unknown • Reduced immune function • Exposure to certain infectious agents • Exposure to chemicals	• Enlarged lymph nodes • Unexplained weight loss and fever • Anemia • Buildup of fluid in the membranes lining the chest or abdominal cavities	• No early detection tests available

Type of Cancer	Risk Factors	Signs and Symptoms	Early Detection
Leukemia	• Down's syndrome • Exposure to radiation • Exposure to certain chemicals • Infection with human T-lymphotropic virus, Type I • Cigarette smoking	• Fever • Weight loss • Fatigue • Easy bleeding • Repeated infections • Enlarged lymph nodes • Swelling of liver and spleen	• No early detection tests available • Early detection is difficult because symptoms often appear late in the disease.
Lung	• Cigarette smoking • Exposure to secondhand smoke • Air pollution • Exposure to asbestos • Exposure to radon • Family history of lung cancer • Exposure to industrial chemicals • Exposure to radiation	• Chronic coughing • Blood in sputum • Wheezing • Chest pain • Recurring pneumonia or bronchitis • Weight loss • Hoarseness • Shortness of breath	• Early detection is difficult because symptoms often appear late in the disease. • Chest X-ray • Examination of sputum • Examination of bronchial tubes
Oral	• Tobacco use • Heavy alcohol use • Smoking and using drugs multiplies risk	• Lump or thickening in the mouth • Leukoplakia • A sore that bleeds easily and doesn't heal in the mouth • Difficulty chewing and swallowing • Bad breath • Loose teeth • Pain	• Regular dental checkups • Regular physical checkups • Looking for signs and symptoms
Ovarian	• Never having children • Family history of ovarian cancer • Increased risk with age	• Enlarged abdomen • Abdominal pain and discomfort • Abnormal vaginal bleeding	• Very difficult to detect early • Regular pelvic examinations • Signs or symptoms do not appear until late in the disease.
Pancreatic	• Cigarette smoking • Chronic pancreatitis • Diabetes • Cirrhosis of the liver • High-fat diet	• Weight loss • Pain • Change in bowel habits	• Ultrasound imaging • CT scans • Signs and symptoms often do not appear until late in the disease.
Prostate	• Risk increases with age • High-fat diet • Family history of prostate cancer • African Americans have the highest rate of incidence in the world	• Weak or interrupted urine flow • Frequent urination • Painful or burning urination • Bloody urine • Persistent pain in the back, hips, or pelvis	• Annual digital rectal examination after age 40 • Annual blood test after age 50
Skin	• Exposure to UV radiation from the sun and tanning booths and sunlamps • Repeated sunburn • Fair complexion • Family history of skin cancer • Exposure to coal, tar, pitch, creosote, arsenic, or radium	• Changes in the size, shape, color, thickness, or number of moles • Skin sores that do not heal • Pain, tenderness, or itchiness of the skin • Changes in skin pigmentation	• Recognition of changes in skin and moles • Monthly skin self-examination

What to Know About Treatment Approaches

Many people who have cancer are treated successfully. In some cases, the cancer is cured. In other cases, the progress of the cancer is slowed, life is prolonged, and quality of life is improved. Common treatment approaches for cancer include surgery, radiation therapy, chemotherapy, and immunotherapy.

Surgery is the most common treatment for cancer. If tumors are confined to a particular site, physicians can remove the cancerous tissue from the body. If tumors are spread out, surgery is more difficult to perform. Surgery often is combined with radiation therapy and chemotherapy.

Radiation therapy is treatment of cancer with high-energy radiation to kill or damage cancer cells. Radiation therapy usually is performed using a machine that generates radiation. It also is performed by placing radioactive materials in or near the cancer. Radiation therapy may produce side effects, such as fatigue, nausea, and vomiting. The skin also may become red and blistered in the areas that are treated. Radiation therapy does not make patients radioactive.

Chemotherapy is treatment with anti-cancer drugs. These drugs kill cancer inside the body. Chemotherapy works mainly on cancer cells. However, healthy cells can be harmed as well. Almost all people taking chemotherapy experience unwanted side effects, such as nausea, vomiting, hair loss, and fatigue. Most of these side effects do not last long and will gradually go away. Nausea and vomiting usually stop a day or two after each treatment. If hair is lost, it usually grows back after the treatment has stopped. Many people wear wigs, caps, or scarves until their hair grows back. Fatigue may last several months.

Immunotherapy is a process in which the immune system is stimulated to fight cancer cells. One type of immunotherapy involves injecting patients with cancer cells that have been made harmless by radiation. The immune system responds by producing antibodies that attack cancer cells in the body. Other types of immunotherapy involve injecting patients with other substances that stimulate the immune system.

How to Reduce Your Risk of Cancer

Some risk factors for cancer cannot be controlled. For example, people cannot control their heredity. However, almost all cancers are associated with choices over which people do have control. There are things people can do to help reduce their risk of developing cancer.

Ten Things You Can Do to Help Reduce Your Risk of Developing Cancer

1. Know the warning signs of cancer.
Detecting cancer in the early stages increases the chances that it can be treated successfully. The American Cancer Society recommends that people learn seven early warning signs of cancer. The beginning letter of each warning sign corresponds to a letter in the word CAUTION.

- **C**hange in bowel or bladder habits
- **A** sore that does not heal
- **U**nusual bleeding or discharge
- **T**hickening or lump in a breast or elsewhere
- **I**ndigestion or difficulty in swallowing
- **O**bvious change in a wart or mole
- **N**agging cough or hoarseness

2. Choose a tobacco-free lifestyle.
Tobacco use is the most preventable cause of cancer death. Tobacco products contain many carcinogens. A **carcinogen** is a chemical that is known to cause cancer. Using tobacco products and being exposed to secondhand smoke are leading causes of cancer death. Cases of lung cancer would be greatly reduced if people would never begin to smoke. People who smoke one pack of cigarettes a day are ten times more likely than nonsmokers to get lung cancer. Exposure to secondhand smoke increases the risk of lung cancer for nonsmokers. Smokeless tobacco increases the risk of cancers of the mouth, gums, and throat. If you use tobacco products, quit today. Lesson 56 includes more information on tobacco cessation programs.

3. **Protect yourself from the sun and avoid tanning booths and sunlamps.** **Ultraviolet (UV) radiation** is a type of radiation that comes from the sun and also is emitted by sunlamps and tanning booths. Repeated exposure to UV radiation increases the risk of skin cancer, including malignant melanoma. **Malignant melanoma** is the form of skin cancer that is most often fatal. The sun's harmful UV rays are strongest during the summer between 10 a.m. and 3 p.m. Avoid exposure to the sun during these hours. If you are in the sun, wear protective clothing. Use sunscreen lotions that have a sun protective factor (SPF) of at least 15. Never use a tanning booth or sunlamp. Check your skin regularly. If you notice any abnormal growths, consult your physician.

4. **Follow dietary guidelines to reduce cancer risk.** Eat a variety of foods so that your body has a combination of nutrients. Eat several servings and a variety of fruits and vegetables each day. Fruits and vegetables contain antioxidants that help prevent cancer. Eat several servings of fiber-rich foods, such as whole-grain cereals, legumes, vegetables, and fruits. Avoid fatty foods. Limit consumption of foods that are smoked, salted, or nitrite-cured. Lesson 34 contains more information on dietary guidelines to reduce cancer risk.

5. **Maintain your desirable weight and a healthful body composition.** People who are overweight and have a high percentage of body fat are more at risk for developing cancer. Exercise regularly and manage your weight. Lesson 39 contains more information on weight management.

6. **Avoid drinking alcohol.** Drinking alcohol may cause changes in body cells. Alcohol also takes vitamins needed for optimal health away from your body. Drinking alcohol increases the risk of cancer of the liver, throat, mouth, breast, and stomach. Chances of developing cancer are multiplied further if you drink alcohol and smoke tobacco or marijuana.

7. **Avoid exposure to dangerous chemicals and airborne fibers.** The following have been found to increase risk of cancer: benzene, benzidene, vinyl chloride, uranium, radon, nickel, cadmium, asbestos, and pesticides. Wear rubber gloves and a mask when exposed to dangerous chemicals. Wear protective clothing if you will be exposed to airborne fibers.

8. **Avoid air pollution.** Polluted air contains many carcinogens. Avoid the exhaust from cars, buses, and trucks. Have your home tested for radon. **Radon** is an odorless, colorless radioactive gas that is released by rocks and soil. It can collect and be trapped in basements and crawl spaces. Inhaling radon can increase the risk of lung cancer.

9. **Avoid infection with HIV and sexually transmitted diseases (STDs).** Many people who are infected with HIV develop Kaposi's sarcoma and other cancers. People who have genital warts are at increased risk for cervical cancer. Choose abstinence to reduce your risk of cancer. Do not inject drugs, such as steroids and heroin. Discuss ear-piercing or getting a tattoo with a parent or guardian. Avoid contact with blood and body fluids.

10. **Know your family's cancer history.** Some cancers, such as breast, colon, and ovarian cancers, occur more frequently in certain families. This may be due to heredity or the family's environment and lifestyle habits. Be aware of family members and other relatives who have had cancer. If a family member or other relative has had cancer, have regular cancer checkups and keep your physician informed.

Lesson 67

Review

Vocabulary Words

Write a separate sentence using each of the vocabulary words listed on page 516.

Objectives

1. How do cancer cells originate and spread in the body? **Objective 1**
2. What are the risk factors, signs and symptoms, and early detection and ways to detect cancer early? **Objective 2**
3. What are different treatment approaches for cancer? **Objective 3**
4. What are ten ways to reduce the risk of developing cancer? **Objective 4**
5. What are the warning signs of cancer? **Objective 4**

Responsible Decision-Making

One of your friends works at the tanning salon and gives you three free sessions in the tanning booth. (S)he says that it will make you look great. Write a response to this situation.

1. Describe the situation that requires you to make a decision.
2. List possible decisions you might make.
3. Name two responsible adults with whom you might discuss your decisions.
4. Evaluate the possible consequences of your decisions. Determine if each decision will lead to actions that:
   - promote health,
   - protect safety,
   - follow laws,
   - show respect for yourself and others,
   - follow the guidelines of your parents and of other responsible adults,
   - demonstrate good character.
5. Decide which decision is most responsible and appropriate.
6. Tell two results you expect if you make this decision.

 ### Effective Communication

Write a newspaper article with the headline "Teens Can Reduce Their Risk of Developing Cancer." Include a list of ten ways teens can reduce their risk of developing cancer. Submit your article to the school newspaper.

 ### Self-Directed Learning

Contact the local chapter of the American Cancer Society. Find out what services are offered to people who have cancer and to their families.

 ### Critical Thinking

Suppose some of your classmates smoke cigarettes and chew tobacco. They say using tobacco right now does not affect their bodies and that they will quit later. List reasons why these classmates are wrong. Include information on how tobacco use increases people's risk of developing several types of cancer.

 ### Responsible Citizenship

Plan a three-day menu of foods known to prevent cancer. Choose menu items that are high in fiber. Include several servings of fruits and vegetables each day. Avoid fatty foods. Avoid foods that are smoked, salted, or nitrite-cured.

You Can Recognize Ways to Manage Asthma and Allergies

Life Skill **I will recognize ways to manage asthma and allergies.**

Asthma is a condition in which the bronchial tubes become inflamed and constrict, making breathing difficult. Asthma is a serious condition that is common in children, teens, and adults. It is the leading cause of school absence and hospitalization for children under the age of 15. An **allergy** is an overreaction of the body to a substance that, in most people, causes no response. Many people are allergic to substances such as pollen, animal dander, feathers, and mites. This lesson discusses ways to manage asthma and allergies. You will learn about asthma triggers and how to prevent and manage an asthma attack. You also will learn about different kinds of allergies.

The Lesson Outline

What to Know About Asthma
How to Manage Asthma
What to Know About Allergies

Objectives

1. Discuss asthma including asthma triggers, symptoms, and ways to prevent asthma attacks. **page 525**
2. List 12 ways to manage asthma. **page 526**
3. Identify four common airborne allergens and explain what people can do about them. **page 526**

Vocabulary Words

asthma
allergy
asthma triggers
asthma attack
exercise-induced asthma (EIA)
peak flow meter
allergen
animal dander
pollen
hay fever
mites
skin patch test
wheal

What to Know About
Asthma

Asthma is a chronic disease that cannot be cured. Symptoms of asthma include coughing, wheezing, and shortness of breath. People with asthma have sensitive lungs that react to certain asthma triggers. **Asthma triggers** are substances that cause the airways to tighten, swell, and fill with mucus. The airways become narrow and blocked, and it is difficult to breathe. Asthma triggers include pollen from trees; grasses and weeds; dust and mold; dogs, cats or other animals; cigarette smoke; air pollution; having a cold or the flu; aspirin or other OTC drugs; perfumes and fragrances; odors from sprays and paints; insecticides; certain foods; and smoke from burning wood, paper, or other items. Asthma also can be triggered by emotional stress, especially during childhood and adolescence. Asthma attacks can be very serious. An **asthma attack** is an episode of coughing, wheezing, and shortness of breath experienced by a person who has asthma. Some people may become extremely sick from asthma attacks and need to be hospitalized. Some people have died from them.

Most children who suffer from asthma continue to have asthma as adults. However, for about one-fourth of children with asthma, the symptoms decrease significantly as they get older. Sometimes asthma does not develop until a person is an adult.

Exercise-induced asthma (EIA) is a condition in which a person has difficulty breathing during or shortly after strenuous physical activity. The symptoms of EIA can be mild or severe and include coughing, wheezing, shortness of breath, and chest pain. Some people with EIA suffer an asthma attack only with exercise. A high percentage of people with EIA suffer asthma from allergies to airborne substances such as air pollutants, dust, and animal dander. Exposure to cold, dry air during physical activity is a major trigger.

EIA can be prevented by avoiding exercise. However, since regular physical activity improves health status, learning to manage EIA is important. Proper medication allows most people who have EIA to participate in regular physical activity. EIA often can be reduced and prevented by improving physical fitness. Breathing warm, moist air usually helps the condition. Swimming and other indoor water sports provide an ideal environment for people who have EIA. People with EIA frequently breathe in puffs of medication from an inhaler before they exercise to prevent the EIA from starting.

Ways to Prevent Asthma Attacks

People who have asthma can prevent asthma attacks by avoiding asthma triggers, by recognizing warning signs, and by taking certain medication. If they fail to recognize these signs, their symptoms may get worse. If you have asthma, make a plan with your parents or guardian and your physician about what to do when you notice warning signs and symptoms of asthma.

Six Warning Signs and Symptoms of Asthma

- **Coughing**
- **Wheezing**
- **Shortness of breath**
- **Tightness in the chest**
- **Rapid breathing**
- **Itchy or sore throat**

How to Manage Asthma

Most people who have asthma can live a normal life that includes participation in physical activity and sports. They can become free of symptoms by learning how to manage their asthma.

Twelve Ways to Manage Asthma

1. **Get medical treatment and advice from a physician who treats people with asthma.**

2. **Make a daily management plan and an emergency plan with your physician.**

3. **Avoid asthma triggers.**

4. **Use your peak flow meter every day if your physician recommends one.** A **peak flow meter** is a small device that measures how well a person is breathing.

5. **Know warning signs and symptoms of asthma attacks.**

6. **Take medications as directed by a physician.**

7. **Keep with you the medications required for emergencies.**

8. **Know when and how to get medical help for severe asthma attacks.**

9. **Avoid taking sleeping pills or sedatives if unable to sleep because of asthma.** They slow down breathing and can make it more difficult.

10. **Avoid smoking and breathing secondhand smoke.**

11. **Practice stress management skills.**

12. **Participate in regular physical activity if recommended by a physician.**

What to Know About Allergies

An allergy is an overreaction of the body to a substance that, in most people, causes no response. An **allergen** is a substance that produces an allergic response. Most allergens are harmless substances. They come into contact with the skin, respiratory airways, the eye's surface, or stomach.

The most common airborne allergens are animal dander, feathers, pollens, and mites. **Animal dander** is flakes of dead skin or dander from an animal. People who have allergy symptoms such as dizziness, nausea, skin rash, drops in blood pressure, or difficulty in breathing when they are near cats, dogs, horses, or other animals are allergic to animal dander. Many people believe it is the hair of the animal to which they are allergic, but it actually is the flakes of dead skin.

Pollen is a yellowish powder made in flowers and grass. Pollen from flowers, flowering trees and plants, and grass may become airborne and trigger an allergic response. The most common response is hay fever. **Hay fever** is a common term for seasonal respiratory allergies. Symptoms include coughing, sneezing, and inflammation of the nasal mucous membranes. Hay fever occurs most often in the spring and fall. People who have hay fever may take medicine or have shots to lessen their response to pollen.

Some people are allergic to feathers in bedding and pillows. They can use pillows and quilts with synthetic stuffing. Some people are allergic to house dust because it usually contains small fragments of mites and their feces. **Mites** are tiny, eight-legged animals that resemble spiders.

Skin tests can be used to identify allergens that produce allergic reactions. A **skin patch test** is putting allergens on a patch, taping the patch to the skin, and observing the reaction. A **wheal** is a round skin lump that indicates sensitivity to a particular allergen. Another test involves using a needle to place allergens under the skin and observing the reaction. A wheal indicates sensitivity to a particular allergen.

Lesson 68

Review

Vocabulary Words

Write a separate sentence using each of the vocabulary words listed on page 524.

Objectives

1. What are ten examples of asthma triggers? **Objective 1**

2. How can people with exercise-induced asthma (EIA) manage their condition? **Objective 1**

3. What are 12 ways to manage asthma? **Objective 2**

4. What are four common airborne allergens? **Objective 3**

5. What causes hay fever and how can it be treated? **Objective 3**

Responsible Decision-Making

Suppose you suffer from exercise-induced asthma and usually use an inhaler to manage asthma attacks. Today you forgot your inhaler, and you have athletic practice after school. Your teammates say that you can practice and that it will be OK for just this one day. Write a response to this situation.

1. Describe the situation that requires you to make a decision.
2. List possible decisions you might make.
3. Name two responsible adults with whom you might discuss your decisions.
4. Evaluate the possible consequences of your decisions. Determine if each decision will lead to actions that:
   • promote health,
   • protect safety,
   • follow laws,
   • show respect for yourself and others,
   • follow the guidelines of your parents and of other responsible adults,
   • demonstrate good character.
5. Decide which decision is most responsible and appropriate.
6. Tell two results you expect if you make this decision.

 ### Effective Communication

Check the library or the Internet for information on hay fever. Write a pamphlet on hay fever using the information you find. Include causes, signs and symptoms, and treatment. Make an illustration for the cover of your pamphlet.

 ### Self-Directed Learning

Many radio and television stations issue statements about the pollen count. Research information on pollen count. When are warnings issued? Where and when is the pollen count the highest? The lowest?

 ### Critical Thinking

Suppose you have a family pet, such as a cat or dog. Your closest friend is highly allergic to animal dander. You would like to ask your friend to a party you are having at your home. How might you handle this situation?

 ### Responsible Citizenship

Suppose a person who has asthma is going to visit your home. Make a list of three things you can do in your home to reduce the risk of this person having an asthma attack as a result of the visit.

Lesson 69

You Can Recognize Ways to Manage Chronic Health Conditions

Life Skill **I will recognize ways to manage chronic health conditions.**

It is estimated that 5 to 15 percent of young people have chronic health conditions. **Chronic health conditions** are recurring or persistent conditions. Chronic health conditions can cause great suffering and, in some cases, death. People who have chronic health conditions have to cope with changes in their health status over long periods of time. They need to take care of themselves and may take medications or have special diets to follow. They may need surgery or other medical care. They may require assistance with daily activities. Often, they must work through feelings of anxiety, fear, and isolation. This lesson includes A Guide to Chronic Health Conditions. You will learn the description, characteristics, and ways to manage and treat each chronic health condition listed in the guide.

The Lesson Outline

A Guide to Chronic Health Conditions

Objectives

1. Identify the incidence of chronic health conditions in young people. **page 528**

2. Discuss some of the adjustments people who have chronic health conditions must make. **page 528**

3. Discuss the following chronic health conditions: arthritis, cerebral palsy, chronic fatigue syndrome (CFS), cystic fibrosis, Down's syndrome, epilepsy, hemophilia, migraine headaches, multiple sclerosis (MS), muscular dystrophy, narcolepsy, Parkinson's disease, peptic ulcer, sickle cell anemia, systemic lupus erythematosus (SLE). **pages 529–531**

Vocabulary Words

See the Chronic Health Conditions Crossword Puzzle Activity on page 532 for the vocabulary words in th lesson.

A Guide to
Chronic Health Conditions

Chronic Health Condition	Description and Characteristics	Management and Treatment
Arthritis is the painful inflammation of the joints.	Arthritis affects the muscles, tendons, and ligaments that surround joints. There are two major types of arthritis. **Osteoarthritis** is the wearing down of the moving parts of joints. **Rheumatoid arthritis** is a condition in which joints become deformed and may lose function.	• Medications, such as aspirin, to reduce inflammation • Physical therapy and physical activity to improve movement of joints and prevent loss of joint function • Adequate rest • Crutches or walker • Surgery to improve movement in joints or implant new joints
Cerebral palsy is a disorder of the nervous system that interferes with muscle coordination.	Possible causes include too much pressure on the head during childbirth, head injury, lead poisoning, accidental injury, and certain illnesses. People with cerebral palsy may stand and walk in an awkward manner and have difficulty speaking, hearing, and seeing. They may be mentally retarded, although a portion have normal or high intelligence.	• Physical therapy and physical activity to improve range of motion • Speech therapy • Braces or other special devices • Support of family members and friends • Medications • Surgery
Chronic fatigue syndrome (CFS) is a condition in which recurring tiredness makes it difficult for people to function in normal ways.	Symptoms include headache, sore throat, low-grade fever, fatigue, and weakness. People with CFS also may have tender lymph glands, muscle and joint aches, and inability to concentrate. CFS symptoms may recur for more than six months. CFS may begin during periods of high stress. CFS may develop after mononucleosis in teens. There is no cure.	• Balanced diet • Adequate rest and sleep • Regular physical activity • Stress management • Medications
Cystic fibrosis is a condition in which large amounts of abnormally thick mucus are produced, particularly in the lungs and pancreas.	Body organs, such as the lungs and pancreas, may be damaged by accumulations of this mucus. Signs and symptoms of cystic fibrosis include coughing, wheezing, difficulty breathing, vomiting, and constipation. The sweat of people with cystic fibrosis contains an excessive amount of salt. Physicians use a sweat test to diagnose cystic fibrosis. Many people who have cystic fibrosis survive into adulthood. Cystic fibrosis is caused by an abnormal gene.	• Physical therapy • Dietary changes • Vitamins • Medications • Oxygen to help breathing • Loosening and removal of mucus secretions • Support of family members and friends

Chronic Health Condition	Description and Characteristics	Management and Treatment
Down's syndrome is a genetic disorder in which a child is born with an extra chromosome in each cell.	Children born with Down's syndrome have mental retardation, short arms and legs, and a flattened face with upward slanting, almond-shaped eyes. The heart and other organs also may be affected.	• Surgery to correct heart defects and other problems • Antibiotics for recurring infections • Special education • Support of family members and friends
Epilepsy is a disorder in which abnormal electrical activity in the brain causes a temporary loss of control of the mind and body.	A **seizure** is a period in which a person loses control over mind and body. **Petit mal** is a small seizure in which a person loses consciousness for a few seconds. **Grand mal** is a major seizure in which a person may have convulsions. During a convulsion, the body stiffens and twitching may occur. People who are having major seizures can be helped by removal of objects that may injure them. Do not place anything in the mouth. Although people of any age can get epilepsy, it primarily affects children, teens, and young adults. Epilepsy can be caused by head injury, brain tumor, stroke, poisoning, or infection. Heredity also plays a role in some cases of epilepsy.	• Medication to control seizures • Adequate rest and sleep • Regular physical activity • Awareness of school personnel to a person who has epilepsy • Surgery
Hemophilia is an inherited condition in which blood does not clot normally.	A minor injury to a person with hemophilia can lead to uncontrolled bleeding. Spontaneous bleeding also occurs. Hemophilia occurs almost exclusively in males. A defective gene is passed from the father to his offspring. To inherit hemophilia, a female must get the defective gene from both parents.	• Avoidance of injuries that can cause bleeding • Learning how to manage bleeding when cut or scraped • Learning how to recognize emergency situations • Receipt of clotting factors and blood transfusions
Migraine headache is severe head pain that is caused by dilation of blood vessels in the brain.	The symptoms may include severe throbbing, blurred vision, nausea, and vomiting. In some cases, the pain is so severe that people cannot attend school or work.	• Medications to reduce pain • Rest and relaxation • Stress management • Management of conditions that lead to headaches, such as high blood pressure and colds
Multiple sclerosis (MS) is a disease in which the protective covering of nerve fibers in the brain and spinal cord are destroyed.	It is believed that the immune system attacks this protective covering, resulting in scarring of nerve fibers. People who have MS experience tingling and numbness in the body and may feel tired and dizzy. They may have these symptoms for several weeks to several months. Relapses may follow illness or periods of stress. Some people who have MS are not able to walk or care for themselves. There is no cure for MS. MS is more common in young adults.	• Physical therapy to strengthen muscles • Medications • Avoidance of stress and extreme temperatures • Psychological counseling • Support of family members and friends

Table 17.2 Common Physical and Chronic Diseases

Chronic Health Condition	Description and Characteristics	Management and Treatment
Muscular dystrophy is a genetic disease in which the muscles progressively deteriorate.	There is gradual loss of muscle function. Muscular dystrophy is rare. The most common type affects males. There is no cure.	• Physical therapy and physical activity to keep muscles in good condition • Weight management • Surgery in some cases • Wheelchairs to improve mobility
Narcolepsy is a chronic sleep disorder in which people are excessively sleepy even after adequate nighttime sleep.	People who have narcolepsy often become drowsy and fall asleep in inappropriate situations. They may fall asleep without warning several times each day. This often interrupts their daily lives and interferes with school or work. The cause of narcolepsy is unknown. Symptoms usually appear in the teen years. Although there is no cure, there is treatment.	• Medication to control sleepiness • Adequate rest and sleep • Support of family members and friends • Support groups to help people with the condition and their families
Parkinson's disease is a brain disorder that causes muscle tremors, stiffness, and weakness.	Parkinson's disease usually affects people over the age of 50. Signs and symptoms include rigid posture, slow movement, fixed facial expression, and a shuffling walk. Symptoms may become worse when a person is tired or emotionally distressed. The intellect is not affected until late in the disease, although speech is slow.	• Medications to control symptoms • Physical therapy • Support of family members and friends • Surgery to reduce tremors and rigid posture
Peptic ulcer is an open sore on the lining of the esophagus, stomach, or first part of the small intestine.	The most common symptom is a burning pain in the abdomen. There may be upset stomach, back pain, and bleeding. Peptic ulcers can be fatal if they are not treated. Peptic ulcer is caused by a bacterial infection, which is treated with antibiotic.	• Antibiotics • Medications to reduce inflammation • Bleeding ulcers require emergency treatment • Avoidance of cigarettes, alcohol, aspirin, and caffeinated beverages
Sickle cell anemia is an inherited blood disease in which the red blood cells carry less oxygen.	Sickle cell anemia occurs primarily in African Americans. The red blood cells of people who have sickle cell anemia are sickle-shaped and are fragile and easily destroyed. The sickle-shaped cells do not easily pass through tiny blood vessels. Symptoms appear after six months of age and include fatigue, headache, and shortness of breath. Children who have sickle cell anemia are at increased risk for developing pneumonia and other infections. There is no cure.	• Immunization against communicable diseases • Oxygen therapy • Antibiotics to protect against blood poisoning • Medications to reduce pain • Fluids to prevent dehydration during physical activity, sickness, and hot weather • Regular checkups
Systemic lupus erythematosus (SLE) is a condition in which connective tissue becomes inflamed.	SLE affects the skin, kidneys, joints, muscles, and central nervous system. There may be bleeding in the central nervous system, kidney failure, or heart failure. Symptoms include fatigue, fever, loss of appetite, nausea, joint pain, and weight loss. A red, blotchy rash may develop on the cheeks and nose. SLE occurs most often during the teen years and is more common in females than males.	• Varied treatment depending on body tissues affected • Medications to reduce inflammation and fever • Medications to relieve skin rashes • Support of family members and friends

Activity

Chronic Health Conditions Crossword Puzzle

Life Skill: I will recognize ways to manage chronic health conditions.
Materials: paper, pen or pencil
Directions: Complete the steps to create a Chronic Health Conditions Crossword Puzzle.

1. Use the vocabulary words below from this lesson to make a crossword puzzle.

2. Design the puzzle using at least 15 words.

3. Exchange your crossword puzzle with a classmate.

Chronic Health Conditions Crossword Puzzle

chronic health conditions
arthritis
osteoarthritis
rheumatoid arthritis
cerebral palsy
chronic fatigue syndrome (CFS)
cystic fibrosis
Down's syndrome
epilepsy
seizure
petit mal

grand mal
hemophilia
migraine headaches
multiple sclerosis (MS)
muscular dystrophy
narcolepsy
Parkinson's disease
peptic ulcer
sickle cell anemia
systemic lupus erythematosus (SLE)

Lesson 69

Review

Vocabulary Words

Write a separate sentence using 15 of the vocabulary words listed on page 532.

Objectives

1. What is the incidence of chronic health conditions in young people? **Objective 1**

2. What adjustments must be made by people who have chronic health conditions? **Objective 2**

3. What is chronic fatigue syndrome and how is it managed and treated? **Objective 3**

4. What is cystic fibrosis and how is it managed and treated? **Objective 3**

5. What is epilepsy and how is it managed and treated? **Objective 3**

Responsible Decision-Making

A classmate has hemophilia and cannot participate in certain school activities. However, (s)he wants to "fit in." Other students are playing football after school, and they invite this classmate to join in the game with them. Write a response to this situation.

1. Describe the situation that requires your classmate to make a decision.

2. List possible decisions your classmate might make.

3. Name two responsible adults with whom your classmate might discuss his/her decisions.

4. Evaluate the possible consequences of your classmate's decisions. Determine if each decision will lead to actions that:
   • promote health,
   • protect safety,
   • follow laws,
   • show respect for your classmate and others,
   • follow the guidelines of your classmates's parents and of other responsible adults,
   • demonstrate good character.

5. Decide which decision is most responsible and appropriate for your classmate.

6. Tell two results your classmate can expect if (s)he makes this decision.

Effective Communication

Design a pamphlet that describes a chronic health condition. Include information about the symptoms of the condition and ways that it can be managed and treated.

Self-Directed Learning

Choose one of the chronic health conditions in A Guide to Chronic Health Conditions. Find an article about the condition in a medical journal or other periodical. Read the article and write a short summary.

Critical Thinking

Suppose you have a family member who has epilepsy. What special challenges would this person face? How would epilepsy affect his/her life? How would epilepsy affect your life and the lives of other family members? What could you do to help your family member?

Responsible Citizenship

There are many agencies that help children who have chronic health conditions such as cerebral palsy, cystic fibrosis, and muscular dystrophy. Find out what agencies are in your community. Ask your parents or guardian for permission to volunteer at one of the agencies.

You Can Keep a Personal Health Record

Life Skill **I will keep a personal health record.**

You might keep a personal diary or journal in which you write about your experiences and record the important events in your life along with details and the dates they took place. Have you ever thought about keeping a personal health record? A **personal health record** is documentation of information pertaining to a person's health, health care, and health care providers. When you keep a personal health record, you have important information about your health collected in one place. You can obtain information quickly when it is needed. This lesson includes information that will help you make a personal health record. You will learn why you need to include a detailed family health history in your personal health record.

Vocabulary Words

personal health record

family health history

heredity

genetic predisposition

risk factor

The Lesson Outline

How to Keep a Personal Health Record

Why Keep a Detailed Family Health History

Objectives

1. List and discuss ten kinds of information to include in a personal health record. **page 535**

2. Explain why a person should keep a detailed family health history. **page 536**

How to Keep a
Personal Health Record

A personal health record should include the following information.

1. **Vital statistics regarding your birth.** Record the date of your birth and your birth weight. Include information such as the name and address of the hospital in which you were born, your biological father, and your biological mother. Also include any pertinent information regarding your health status at birth. Obtain a copy of your birth certificate.

2. **Detailed family health history.** A **family health history** is information about the health of a person's blood relatives. Close blood relatives might include parents, brothers, sisters, aunts, uncles, and grandparents. Record information pertaining to alcoholism, allergies, anemia, asthma, cancer (breast, colon, uterine, prostate), diabetes type II, gastric reflux, hay fever, heart disease, hemophilia, high blood pressure, kidney disease, liver disease, lupus, migraine headaches, multiple sclerosis, muscular dystrophy, obesity, osteoporosis, rheumatic fever, seizures, sickle cell anemia, stroke, thyroid disease, ulcers, vision problems. Include the age of onset for these conditions. Record the age at time of death.

3. **Record of immunizations.** Keep a record of the dates that you have had immunizations or boosters for: polio, diphtheria-tetanus-pertussis (DTP), measles-mumps-rubella (MMR), *Haemophilus influenza* type b (Hib), hepatitis B (HBV), and chickenpox (VZV).

4. **Personal health information.** Keep pertinent information about your health status, including height, weight, blood pressure, blood cholesterol, blood lipids, vision, hearing, and allergies.

5. **Health habits.** Keep details about your health habits. Health care providers may ask whether or not you have ever drunk alcohol or smoked; how much you exercise; how well you handle stress; what kind of eating patterns you have; the amount of sleep you get; the quality of your relationships with family; the quality of your relationships with friends; your success at school; your extracurricular activities.

6. **Medical history.** Keep a record of your visits to a physician and other health care providers. Record the date, the professional whom you saw, the reason for the visit, the findings, and the health care provider's recommendations.

7. **Dental history.** Keep a record of your visits to a dentist/dental hygienist. Record the date, the professional whom you saw, the reason for the visit, the findings, and the recommendations of the dentist/dental hygienist.

8. **Medications.** Keep a record of all medications you have taken. Include: the date, name of medication, prescription number, physician who prescribed the medication, pharmacy, side effects. Keep copies of information on prescription drugs given to you by a pharmacy.

9. **Health insurance information.** Record the following: name, address, and telephone number of insurance company; policy holder's name; and policy number. Keep copies of your health insurance policies with your personal health record.

10. **Health care professionals.** Keep a list of the health care professionals you have seen. Include name, specialty, telephone number, and address.

Why Keep a Detailed Family Health History

Your family health history provides information about heredity and genetic predisposition. **Heredity** is the passing of characteristics from biological parents to their children. **Genetic predisposition** is the inheritance of genes that increase the likelihood of developing a condition. Heredity and genetic predisposition are risk factors for many diseases and conditions. A **risk factor** is something that increases the likelihood of a negative outcome. If you have a genetic predisposition for a disease or condition, you cannot change the risk factor. However, there may be actions you can take to offset it. For example, suppose you have biological relatives who have type II diabetes. There are four risk factors for type II diabetes: being overfat and overweight, being 40 years of age or older, being female, and having family members with diabetes. You know that you can control at least one risk factor—your weight. You can maintain a healthful weight and participate in regular physical activity. A detailed family health history provides information that your physician can use in diagnosing and treating conditions and diseases. It helps you and your physician make a plan to offset risk factors.

Diseases and Conditions for Which a Person Might Have a Genetic Predisposition

- Alcoholism
- Allergies
- Asthma
- Cancer (breast, colon, uterine, prostate)
- Diabetes type II
- Hay fever

- Hay fever
- Heart disease
- Hemophilia
- High blood pressure
- Kidney disease
- Liver disease

- Lupus
- Migraine headaches
- Multiple sclerosis
- Muscular dystrophy
- Obesity
- Osteoporosis

- Seizures
- Sickle cell anemia
- Stroke
- Thyroid disease
- Ulcers
- Vision problems

Activity

Your Personal Health Record

Life Skill: I will keep a personal health record.

Materials: paper, pen or pencil

Directions: Complete this activity to make a personal health record. Refer to the ten kinds of information that should be included in a personal health record. These are discussed on page 535.

 1. Create a personal health record that includes the ten kinds of information identified. Check with your parents or guardian if you do not have all the necessary information.

2. Share your personal health record with your parents or guardian, physician, dentist, and other health care professionals.

Lesson 70

Review

Vocabulary Words

Write a separate sentence using each of the vocabulary words listed on page 534.

Objectives

1. What are ten kinds of information to include in a personal health record? **Objective 1**

2. What immunizations should a person keep a record of having had? **Objective 1**

3. What personal habits of a person are of interest to his/her physician? **Objective 1**

4. Why should a person keep a detailed family health history? **Objective 2**

5. What are five examples of conditions and diseases for which a person might have a genetic predisposition? **Objective 2**

Responsible Decision–Making

Your grandfather died of a premature heart attack at age 57. Your father has high blood pressure and had a heart attack two years ago. At times, you feel it is in the cards that you will die of a premature heart attack at an early age. Write a response to this situation.

1. Describe the situation that requires you to make a decision.
2. List possible decisions you might make.
3. Name two responsible adults with whom you might discuss your decisions.
4. Evaluate the possible consequences of your decisions. Determine if each decision will lead to actions that:
   • promote health,
   • protect safety,
   • follow laws,
   • show respect for yourself and others,
   • follow the guidelines of your parents and of other responsible adults,
   • demonstrate good character.
5. Decide which decision is most responsible and appropriate.
6. Tell two results you expect if you make this decision.

 Effective Communication

Create a logo or design that depicts a healthful lifestyle to use on the cover of your personal health record.

 Self-Directed Learning

Call a physician's office, a hospital, or a health care clinic. Find out what screening tests are recommended for people with a family history of heart disease.

 Critical Thinking

Suppose you have several blood relatives who suffer from hay fever. When you work in the yard, you notice that your eyes itch and you begin to cough and sneeze. What actions might you take?

 Responsible Citizenship

Have a family meeting to discuss the completion of your personal health record. Obtain information for your family health history. Check with your family physician or other health care professional to determine if (s)he has additional categories for you to add to the ten identified in the lesson. Remember, your personal health record must be readily available if you or your parent or guardian need it.

Unit Review

Review Questions

Prepare for the unit test. Review your answers for each Lesson Review in this unit. Then write answers to each of the following questions:

1. What are three ways pathogens are spread by direct contact? **Lesson 61**

2. What are two types of lymphocytes that respond when pathogens enter the body? **Lesson 61**

3. What are five ways to keep the immune system healthy? **Lesson 61**

4. How can you reduce your risk of getting colds? **Lesson 62**

5. How do you know if you have strep throat versus a sore throat? **Lesson 62**

6. Why should you avoid taking aspirin if you have flu symptoms? **Lesson 62**

7. How might sharing a needle to pierce ears result in infection with viral hepatitis? **Lesson 63**

8. Why is it important to commit to monogamous marriage to prevent STDs? **Lesson 63**

9. What are ten reasons to avoid infection with STDs? **Lesson 63**

10. What are early symptoms of HIV infection? **Lesson 64**

11. How does sharing a needle to pierce one's ears put a person at risk for HIV infection? **Lesson 64**

12. How can protease inhibitors help treat HIV? **Lesson 64**

13. What are the signs that a person may be having a heart attack? **Lesson 65**

14. How does the distribution of body weight influence a person's risk of developing cardiovascular disease? **Lesson 65**

15. What is an ex-smoker's risk of having a heart attack one year after quitting smoking? **Lesson 65**

16. Why is type I diabetes considered an autoimmune disease? **Lesson 66**

17. What are the symptoms for type II diabetes? **Lesson 66**

18. What are four risk factors for diabetes? **Lesson 66**

19. What is the leading cause of cancer death for both males and females and how can it be prevented? **Lesson 67**

20. What is the difference between a benign and a malignant tumor? **Lesson 67**

21. What kinds of foods might be included in your diet to reduce the risk of cancer? **Lesson 67**

22. Why do some people cough and sneeze around animals? **Lesson 68**

23. What should a person do if (s)he is allergic to pillows or quilts made with feathers? **Lesson 68**

24. Should people with exercise-induced asthma participate in physical activity? Why or why not? **Lesson 68**

25. What are ways to manage and treat hemophilia? **Lesson 69**

26. What causes migraine headaches? **Lesson 69**

27. What is the difference between multiple sclerosis and muscular dystrophy? **Lesson 69**

28. Why is it important to keep a personal health record? **Lesson 70**

29. Why might a physician ask if one of your biological relatives has been treated for alcoholism? **Lesson 70**

30. What are two purposes of a family health history? **Lesson 70**

Vocabulary Words

Number a sheet of paper from 1–10. Select the correct vocabulary word and write it next to the corresponding number. DO NOT WRITE IN THIS BOOK.

communicable disease	gonorrhea
human immunodeficiency virus (HIV)	heart-healthy diet
	cancer
personal health record	autoimmune disease
flu	allergen
chronic health condition	

1. A _____ is an illness caused by pathogens that can be spread from one living thing to another. **Lesson 61**

2. The _____ is a highly contagious viral infection of the respiratory tract. **Lesson 62**

3. _____ is a group of diseases in which there is uncontrolled multiplication of abnormal cells in the body. **Lesson 67**

4. A _____ is documentation of information pertaining to a person's health, health care, and health care providers. **Lesson 70**

5. _____ is a highly contagious STD caused by the gonococcus bacterium *Niesseria gonorrhoeae*. **Lesson 63**

6. A _____ is a low-fat diet rich in fruits, vegetables, whole grains, non-fat and low-fat milk products, lean meats, poultry, and fish. **Lesson 65**

7. An _____ is a substance that produces an allergic response. **Lesson 68**

8. An _____ is a disease that results when the immune system produces antibodies that turn against the body's own cells. **Lesson 66**

9. _____ are recurring or persistent conditions. **Lesson 69**

10. _____ is a pathogen that destroys infection-fighting T cells in the body. **Lesson 64**

Health Literacy

Effective Communication

Design a pamphlet on ways to reduce the risk of infection with HIV. Explain why abstinence from sex reduces your risk of infection with HIV. Discuss how a monogamous marriage can help you avoid infection with HIV. Discuss how drug use can lead to infection with HIV. Explain how universal precautions can prevent infection with HIV.

Self-Directed Learning

Obtain permission from your parents or guardian to interview a community member who works with cancer patients, such as a doctor who specializes in cancer or a nurse who cares for cancer patients. Ask about risk factors and about new trends in treatment. Write a short report to share with your classmates.

Critical Thinking

Suppose a family member has high blood cholesterol and high blood pressure. What can (s)he do to reduce blood cholesterol? To reduce blood pressure? To reduce the risk of cardiovascular disease?

Responsible Citizenship

Ask your parents or guardian for permission to volunteer for a community organization that helps people who have communicable or chronic diseases. You might volunteer at a hospital that specializes in treating people who have cancer or an organization that works with children who have Down's syndrome.

Responsible Decision-Making

Suppose your classmate is dating an older person who is pressuring him/her to become sexually active. The person says that to have a strong relationship, you must have sex. This person tells your classmate that (s)he doesn't understand because (s)he is so young and has threatened to end the relationship if they do not have sex. Write a response to this situation.

1. Describe the situation that requires your classmate to make a decision.
2. List possible decisions your classmate might make.
3. Name two responsible adults with whom your classmate might discuss his/her decisions.
4. Evaluate the possible consequences of your classmate's decisions. Determine if each decision will lead to actions that:
   - promote health,
   - protect safety,
   - follow laws,
   - show respect for your classmate and others,
   - follow the guidelines of your classmates's parents and of other responsible adults,
   - demonstrate good character.
5. Decide which decision is most responsible and appropriate for your classmate.
6. Tell two results your classmate can expect if (s)he makes this decision.

Multicultural Health

Different cultures and countries are more at risk than others for certain diseases and health conditions because of differences in diet, climate, and other factors. Find an article in a medical journal or other periodical that talks about a disease or health condition that is more common in a certain culture or country. Write a summary of this article and share the information with your classmates.

Health Behavior Inventory of Life Skills

Number from 1 to 10 on a sheet of paper. Read each life skill carefully. Write YES or NO next to the same number on your paper. Each YES response indicates a life skill you practice to promote your health status. Each NO response indicates a life skill you do not practice. Plan to begin practicing these life skills.

1. I will choose behaviors to reduce my risk of infection with communicable diseases.
2. I will choose behaviors to reduce my risk of infection with respiratory diseases.
3. I will choose behaviors to reduce my risk of infection with sexually transmitted diseases.
4. I will choose behaviors to reduce my risk of HIV infection.
5. I will choose behaviors to reduce my risk of cardiovascular diseases.
6. I will choose behaviors to reduce my risk of diabetes.
7. I will choose behaviors to reduce my risk of cancer.
8. I will recognize ways to manage asthma and allergies.
9. I will recognize ways to manage chronic health conditions.
10. I will keep a personal health record.

Family Involvement

Make an information sheet on ways to reduce the risk of developing cancer. Include a brief explanation of the warning signs of cancer. Share the information sheet with your family. Discuss ways you and other family members can improve your behavior to reduce your risk of developing cancer. For example, your family might decide to follow dietary guidelines to reduce the risk of developing cancer.

Health Behavior Contract

Copy and complete the following health behavior contract. Evaluate your progress.
Share the results with your family.

Health Behavior Contract

1. Name_____Date_____

2. **Life Skill:** I will choose behaviors to reduce my risk of infection with communicable diseases.

3. **Effects on Health Status:** Communicable diseases are illnesses caused by pathogens that can be spread from one living thing to anther. Certain behaviors reduce the risk that I will become infected with communicable diseases. When I choose these behaviors, I will be less likely to develop certain diseases. If I have a communicable disease, I will be less likely to give the disease to another person.

4. **Plan and Method to Record Progress:** I will always choose behaviors to reduce my risk of infection with communicable diseases, especially when I am with people who have communicable diseases.

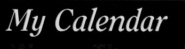

My Calendar

M   T   W   Th   F   S

5. **Evaluation:** _____
_____
_____

Unit 8

Consumer and Community Health

You Can Choose Sources of Health Information Wisely

Life Skill **I will choose sources of health information wisely.**

Open the newspaper and you are likely to find health-related stories. You might read magazines that contain health-related stories and advertise health products. Turn on the TV or radio. A health issue surely will be discussed on the news, on a program, or in a commercial. Visit a bookstore and you will find an entire section devoted to books that contain health information. Log on to the Internet and you will find a huge variety of health-related web sites. This lesson discusses how to choose sources of health information wisely. The lesson includes A Guide to Sources of Health Information.

The Lesson Outline

A Guide to Sources of Health Information

How to Check the Reliability of Health Information

Objectives

1. Discuss the kinds of health information that can be obtained from the mass media, books, on-line communication, health care professionals, and community agents. **page 545**

2. List and discuss eight questions that can be used to evaluate sources of health information. **page 546**

Vocabulary Words

mass media

infomercial

on-line

local health department

state health department

National Health Information Center (NHIC)

A Guide to Sources of
Health Information

Mass Media

Mass media are sources of mass communication that reach large audiences of people. Forms of mass media include TV, radio, magazines, and newspapers. All health information appearing in the mass media should be critically evaluated. A mass media source can only exist if it makes money by selling lots of magazines or newspapers or has many people watching or listening. To attract a large audience, mass media sources may exaggerate stories, use misleading or sensational headlines, or use unreliable sources of information.

Television often uses infomercials to attract audiences. Companies often purchase TV time for infomercials. An **infomercial** is a TV program meant to sell products or services. The intent of the infomercial is to persuade a person to buy something, not to provide accurate health information.

Books

Thousands of books are published each year about health topics. Some books are written by reliable authors and contain accurate health information. However, many popular and best-selling books contain unreliable information about health. Select books written by health professionals with proven credentials.

Alert. . . . Expert Opinions

TV and radio programs often interview "experts" about a health topic. Some of these experts are very reliable sources. However, some experts are selected more for their ability to attract an audience than for their reliability.

Lesson 3 included more information on using technology as a source of health information.

On-line Communication

You can gain health-related information by going on-line. **On-line** is the interactive use of computers using telecommunication technology. Many sources of health information are available on-line and on the World Wide Web (WWW).

Health Care Professionals

Talking to health care professionals such as physicians often is a good way to get reliable health information. Many physicians' and dentists' offices offer pamphlets on health topics in their waiting rooms.

Local and State Health Departments

A **local health department** is an official agency that has responsibility for providing health services and programs for people living within a community. A **state health department** is an official agency that has responsibility for providing health services and programs for people living within a state. Health departments are good sources of health-related information.

Federal Government Agencies

Several federal government agencies provide reliable health information. One source of health information is the National Health Information Center (NHIC). The **National Health Information Center (NHIC)** is an agency that refers consumers to organizations that can provide health-related information.

Community Agencies

Many community agencies provide health-related information on the World Wide Web (WWW) and through information sheets, pamphlets, videos, and public service announcements on radio and TV. An example of a community agency that provides reliable health information is the American Cancer Society.

How to Check the Reliability of Health Information

It is important to choose sources of health information wisely. You can check the accuracy of health information and avoid becoming misinformed. Reliable health information is based solely on scientific research and information. It does not attempt to influence your decisions about what to buy. You can evaluate health information by asking questions. Use the following questions to evaluate sources of health information.

How to Evaluate Sources of Health Information

1. **What is the source of the information?** Reliable sources include health care professionals, government agencies, and community agencies.

2. **Is the information based on current research and scientific evidence?** It should not be opinion. You should be able to get copies of the research.

3. **Have reputable physicians, dentists, and other health care professionals evaluated and accepted the information?** A good test of the accuracy of the information is if health professionals agree with the information. Does the health information agree with accepted medical knowledge? If it goes against current medical knowledge, it is less likely to be accurate.

4. **What is the purpose of the information?** If the information is meant to convince you that you need to buy a specific product or service, it probably is not reliable. The purpose of reliable health information is to inform, not to sell or make money.

5. **Is the information presented in a way to appeal to your emotions?** Health information that is accurate does not have to appeal to your emotions. The information should be presented in a way that educates without arousing emotions such as fear or anxiety.

6. **Does the information make realistic claims?** You can often judge the accuracy of health information by the claims that are made. For example, be very wary of claims of curing diseases that scientists do not know how to cure or food supplements that burn body fat.

7. **Are you able to get more information if you request it?** Sources of reliable information will give you additional sources to check the information.

8. **Does the health information use testimonials or the opinions of only a few individuals?** Reliable health information does not rely upon opinions of celebrities or only a few individuals. These individuals often have been paid or will make a profit from sales of a product.

Lesson 71

Review

Vocabulary Words

Write a separate sentence using each of the vocabulary words listed on page 544.

Objectives

1. What are five sources of health information? **Objective 1**

2. Why might health information in the media be exaggerated? **Objective 1**

3. Why should people be cautious of the health information obtained from an infomercial? **Objective 1**

4. What is the purpose of the National Health Information Center? **Objective 1**

5. What are eight questions to ask to check the reliability of health information? **Objective 2**

Responsible Decision-Making

You are watching a TV program with a friend. A physician is interviewed about a new acne cream (s)he discovered. Then a celebrity is interviewed who says (s)he tried the cream and it worked instantly. The physician gives a phone number to order the cream. Your friend says that it must work since a physician invented it and a celebrity endorsed it. You have acne. Your friend tells you to order the product. Write a response to this situation.

1. **Describe the situation that requires you to make a decision.**

2. **List possible decisions you might make.**

3. **Name two responsible adults with whom you might discuss your decisions.**

4. **Evaluate the possible consequences of your decisions. Determine if each decision will lead to actions that:**
   - **promote health,**
   - **protect safety,**
   - **follow laws,**
   - **show respect for yourself and others,**
   - **follow the guidelines of your parents and of other responsible adults,**
   - **demonstrate good character.**

5. **Decide which decision is most responsible and appropriate.**

6. **Tell two results you expect if you make this decision.**

 ### Effective Communication

Obtain permission from a parent or guardian. Call a physician's office or a local hospital. Ask for the titles of three pamphlets or information sheets they offer to patients.

 ### Self-Directed Learning

Read a magazine article on a health topic. Evaluate the article by using the information in How to Check the Reliability of Health Information.

 ### Critical Thinking

You have read two articles about the same health issue. Which is the more accurate? Explain how you determined this.

 ### Responsible Citizenship

Identify three community agencies that provide health-related information in your area. Many of these agencies use volunteers to help distribute health information. Obtain permission from your parent or guardian. Call the agencies and ask if they use volunteers and what the volunteers do. Share the information with classmates.

Lesson 72

You Can Be Aware of Consumer Rights

Life Skill **I will recognize my rights as a consumer.**

A **consumer** is a person who chooses sources of health-related information and buys or uses health products and services. **Products** are material goods, such as food, medicine, and clothing, that are made for consumers to purchase. **Services** are work that is provided. **Consumerism** is the practice of obtaining reliable and tested products, services, and information. This lesson provides skills that will help you to be a responsible consumer. The lesson includes "The Consumer Bill of Rights." You can use these rights to your advantage. The lesson also includes information on health fraud and quackery. You will learn how to protect yourself when you purchase products and services.

The Lesson Outline

What to Know About Consumer Rights

What to Know About Health Fraud

Objectives

1. List and discuss the four rights of a consumer. **page 549**
2. Discuss three reasons why people must protect themselves from health fraud. **page 549**
3. Explain why health fraud is targeted at teens and elderly people. **page 549**
4. List questions that can be asked to uncover health fraud. **page 550**
5. List five steps to take before purchasing products and services if health fraud is suspected. **page 550**

Vocabulary Words

consumer

products

services

consumerism

consumer rights

health fraud

quack

What to Know About
Consumer Rights

Consumer rights are the privileges that a consumer is guaranteed. There are four consumer rights that often are called "The Consumer Bill of Rights." By exercising your consumer rights, you become an intelligent consumer. You can avoid being misled by inaccurate information. You can protect your health and the health of others.

The Consumer Bill of Rights

1. **The right to choose.** You have the right to have access to a variety of products and services at a competitive price whenever possible.

2. **The right to be heard.** You have the right to make a complaint when you are not satisfied.

3. **The right to be safe.** You have a right to be protected against the marketing of goods and services that are hazardous to your health.

4. **The right to be informed.** You have the right to be protected against deception, fraud, and misleading information so that you can be given the information to make informed choices.

What to Know About
Health Fraud

Health fraud is the advertising, promotion, and sale of products and services that have not been scientifically proven safe and effective. A **quack** is a person or company who is involved in health fraud.

The Food and Drug Administration (FDA) identified categories in which health fraud is most frequent. The categories include:

- instant weight-loss schemes,
- AIDS cures,
- arthritis products,
- cancer treatments,
- baldness treatments,
- nutritional supplements.

There are several reasons you must protect yourself from health fraud.

1. You don't want to waste money on products or services that do not do what has been claimed.

2. You don't want to use products or services that cause harmful reactions or injuries.

3. You don't want to delay valuable medical treatment.

Health fraud often is targeted at teens and elderly people. Teens who are overly concerned about their looks are vulnerable. They may buy useless products to clear up acne, build muscles, or lose weight quickly. Elderly people with chronic health problems and life-threatening diseases are vulnerable. They may buy useless products and medicines. They hope these will provide quick cures or recapture their youth.

Questions to Uncover Health Fraud

Quacks often use the same methods to sell products and services. If the answer to any of the questions is "yes," quackery may be indicated.

1. Is there a promise of cure for a condition for which medical scientists do not have a cure?

2. Is there a promise of quick and/or painless results?

3. Is there a claim that a product or treatment works by a secret formula or in a mysterious way?

4. Is the product or treatment sold over the telephone, door-to-door, or by mail-order?

5. Is the product available only through a P.O. box address?

6. Is the product or service promoted by a little-known person or group?

7. Is the product or service promoted on the back pages of magazines?

8. Is the product or service promoted through infomercials or in newspaper ads that look like articles?

9. Are testimonials from people who claim that they were cured by the product or service?

10. Are celebrity endorsements used to promote the product or service?

11. Does the seller claim that the medical profession does not recognize the product or service?

12. Are tactics that play on emotions used to sell the product or service?

13. Are there claims that the product or service is effective for many unrelated disorders?

14. Does the seller say it is not necessary to talk to a physician about using the product or service?

15. Does the product fail to have labels that provide directions for use or cautions about use?

16. Does the seller claim that traditional medical treatment is more harmful than healthful?

17. Does a seller make claims that a product is "all-natural?"

18. Do providers of a treatment lack credentials from accredited schools?

Steps to Take Before You Buy a Product If You Suspect Health Fraud

Before you buy a product that may be phony:

● Contact the Better Business Bureau or a consumer protection office to check for complaints against the company.

● Ask about the refund or exchange policy.

● Read the warranty to find out what you must do if there is a problem.

● Check to see if you can trace a P.O. box address.

● Do not respond to any prize or gift offer that requires you to pay any money.

Lesson 72

Review

Vocabulary Words

Write a separate sentence using each of the vocabulary words listed on page 548.

Objectives

1. What are the four rights in The Consumer Bill of Rights? **Objective 1**

2. What are three reasons why people must protect themselves from health fraud? **Objective 2**

3. Why do quacks target teens and elderly people? **Objective 3**

4. What are ten examples of questions that can be asked to uncover health fraud? **Objective 4**

5. What are five steps to take before purchasing products and services if health fraud is suspected? **Objective 5**

Responsible Decision-Making

You are reading a magazine. You find an advertisement for a weight-loss product. You recognize the television star in the advertisement. (S)he claims to have lost weight quickly using the product. You would like to lose weight. Write a response to this situation.

1. Describe the situation that requires you to make a decision.
2. List possible decisions you might make.
3. Name two responsible adults with whom you might discuss your decisions.
4. Evaluate the possible consequences of your decisions. Determine if each decision will lead to actions that:
   - promote health,
   - protect safety,
   - follow laws,
   - show respect for yourself and others,
   - follow the guidelines of your parents and of other responsible adults,
   - demonstrate good character.
5. Decide which decision is most responsible and appropriate.
6. Tell two results you expect if you make this decision.

 ### Effective Communication

Design an advertisement that would be considered quackery. Include at least six methods identified on page 550 in Questions to Uncover Health Fraud. Share your advertisement with a classmate. Have the classmate identify the methods you used in the advertisement.

 ### Self-Directed Learning

Find a magazine advertisement that appears to be an example of quackery. Use the Questions to Uncover Health Fraud on page 550 to evaluate the advertisement.

 ### Critical Thinking

Why is it important to be an intelligent consumer?

Responsible Citizenship

Some people do not realize that they have rights as a consumer. Design a poster about the four consumer rights. Obtain permission to display your poster in a public place.

Lesson 73

You Can Take Action If Your Consumer Rights Are Violated

Life Skill I will take action if my consumer rights are violated.

Suppose you purchase a product and it is defective. Suppose you purchase a product and parts are missing. Suppose you purchase a service and the provider does not provide what you expected. You would not be satisfied and you would have every right to take action. This lesson explains what to do if your consumer rights are violated. The lesson discusses the role of federal agencies, state and local agencies, and private organizations in consumer protection. You will learn ten actions you can take if your consumer rights are violated.

The Lesson Outline

What to Know About Consumer Protection

What to Do If Your Consumer Rights Are Violated

Objectives

1. List and discuss federal government agencies that play a role in consumer protection. **page 553**
2. Explain why some products are recalled. **page 553**
3. Explain how state and local agencies help consumers. **page 553**
4. List and discuss private organizations that provide assistance to consumers. **page 554**
5. Outline ten actions a consumer can take when his/her rights have been violated. **page 554**

Vocabulary Words

Consumer Information Center

Consumer Product Safety Commission (CPSC)

recall

Federal Bureau of Investigation (FBI)

Federal Trade Commission (FTC)

Food and Drug Administration (FDA)

National Health Information Center (NHIC)

United States Department of Agriculture (USDA)

United States Postal Service (USPS)

local health department

state health department

Council of Better Business Bureaus

Consumer's Union (CU)

Center for Science in the Public Interest (CSPI)

National Council Against Health Fraud (NCAHF)

What to Know About
Consumer Protection

Federal, state, and local government agencies play important roles in consumer protection. Professional associations help consumers by monitoring the credentials of their members and their actions. Private organizations provide additional assistance to consumers.

Federal Government Agencies

- The **Consumer Information Center** provides free and low-cost publications on numerous consumer topics.

- The **Consumer Product Safety Commission (CPSC)** establishes and enforces product safety standards, receives consumer complaints about the safety of products, and distributes product safety information. The CPSC has authority to recall products. A **recall** is an order to take a product off the market due to safety concerns.

- The **Federal Bureau of Investigation (FBI)** is responsible for federal criminal offenses, including investigation of health fraud such as insurance scams.

- The **Federal Trade Commission (FTC)** enforces consumer protection laws and monitors trade practices and the advertising of foods, drugs, and cosmetics.

- The **Food and Drug Administration (FDA)** monitors the safety of cosmetics and food and the safety and effectiveness of new drugs, medical devices, and prescription and OTC drugs.

- The **National Health Information Center (NHIC)** is an agency that refers consumers to organizations that can provide health-related information.

- The **United States Department of Agriculture (USDA)** enforces standards to ensure the safe processing of food and oversees the distribution of food information to the public. The USDA also publishes consumer pamphlets on nutrition and food safety topics.

- The **United States Postal Service (USPS)** offers postal services and protects the public when products and services are sold through the mail.

State and Local Agencies

- The **local health department** is an official agency that has responsibility for providing health services and programs for people living within a community. Responsibilities include investigating consumer complaints, collecting health statistics, and offering maternal and child care programs, alcohol and other drug abuse programs, health education, and communicable disease control.

- The **state health department** is an official agency that has responsibility for providing health services and programs for people living within a state. Responsibilities include investigating consumer complaints, collecting and distributing health information, and preventing and controlling disease.

Private Organizations

- The **Council of Better Business Bureaus** is a nonprofit organization that monitors consumer complaints and advertising and selling practices. It provides listings of businesses that have received consumer complaints and publishes materials to help educate consumers about advertising and selling practices.

- **Consumer's Union (CU)** is an organization that tests products and publishes a magazine, *Consumer Reports*, that provides ratings for consumers to compare product performance and safety. The CU publishes books and pamphlets on consumer topics.

- The **Center for Science in the Public Interest (CSPI)** is a nonprofit organization that conducts activities to improve government and industry policies regarding food, nutrition, and other health concerns. The CSPI publishes educational materials for consumers.

- The **National Council Against Health Fraud (NCAHF)** is an organization that provides legal counsel and assistance to victims of health fraud. NCAHF provides many educational materials to consumers on the topic of health fraud.

What to Do If Your Consumer Rights Are Violated

Even informed consumers may buy a product or use a service that does not meet expectations. The consumer can report his/her complaint to one of the agencies or organizations identified in this lesson. If (s)he does not know where or how to make a complaint, (s)he can contact the local health department for advice.

Ten Actions to Take When Your Consumer Rights Have Been Violated

1. **Talk to your parents or guardian and agree on a plan of action.**

2. **Save all paperwork related to the purchase in a file.**

3. **Contact the business that sold you the item or performed the service.** Describe the problem and the action you want taken. For example, do you want your money back or the product exchanged?

4. **Keep a record of your actions.** Write down the name of the person to whom you spoke and a summary of the conversation.

5. **Allow time for the person you contacted to resolve the problem.**

6. **Write a letter to the company headquarters if you are not satisfied with the actions taken to resolve the problem.** Address your letter to the consumer office or the company president. Include the following information: date and place of purchase; a description of the product or service, what went wrong, and what you want done. Include copies of all documents such as receipts or warranties. Do not send the originals. Keep a copy of the letter in your file.

7. **Send a copy of the letter to a consumer group, the state's attorney general, or the local Better Business Bureau if the company does not respond in an adequate amount of time.** Contact your local or state consumer protection agency right away if you think a law has been broken.

8. **Advise the company that you have notified groups responsible for consumer protection.**

9. **Inform the news media when you believe an ad for a product or service is deceptive or inaccurate.**

10. **Consider the legal actions your family might take.**

Lesson 73

Review

Vocabulary Words

Write a separate sentence using each of the vocabulary words listed on page 552.

Objectives

1. How does the Consumer Information Center help consumers? the CPSC? the FBI? the FTC? the FDA? the NHIC? the USDA? the USPS? **Objective 1**

2. Why are products recalled by the Consumer Product Safety Commission? **Objective 2**

3. How do state and local agencies help consumers? **Objective 3**

4. How does the Council of Better Business Bureau assist consumers? the CU? the CSPI? the NCAHF? **Objective 4**

5. What are ten actions a consumer can take when his/her rights have been violated? **Objective 5**

Responsible Decision-Making

Last month you bought an inexpensive radio through the mail. It hasn't worked right since you got it. You are really angry. Your friend says, "It was cheap. Just throw it away, and buy another one." Write a response to this situation.

1. **Describe the situation that requires you to make a decision.**
2. **List possible decisions you might make.**
3. **Name two responsible adults with whom you might discuss your decisions.**
4. **Evaluate the possible consequences of your decisions. Determine if each decision will lead to actions that:**
   - **promote health,**
   - **protect safety,**
   - **follow laws,**
   - **show respect for yourself and others,**
   - **follow the guidelines of your parents and of other responsible adults,**
   - **demonstrate good character.**
5. **Decide which decision is most responsible and appropriate.**
6. **Tell two results you expect if you make this decision.**

 Effective Communication

Suppose you have purchased a product that does not work. Make up a name of a product and a company that sells it. Write a letter to the company making a consumer complaint.

 Self-Directed Learning

Both the USDA and the FDA monitor the safety of food. Research the agencies in the library or on the Internet. List two ways their responsibilities differ.

 Critical Thinking

Suppose a baby for whom you are childsitting is playing with a new toy recommended for the baby's age group. The string on the toy gets wrapped around the baby's neck. What steps might you take to protect other babies from the toy?

 Responsible Citizenship

Select one of the federal government agencies identified in this lesson. Obtain permission from a parent or guardian. Choose a topic about which the agency distributes information. Write a letter to the agency requesting information on the topic. Share the information you receive with classmates.

Lesson 74

You Can Evaluate Advertisements

Life Skill I will evaluate advertisements.

What is your favorite brand of jeans? Favorite fast food restaurant? Favorite soda pop? Advertising might have influenced your answers. **Advertising** is a form of selling products and services. There are various kinds of advertising. An **advertisement (ad)** is a paid announcement about a product or service. Ads appear on-line; on TV, radio, and billboards; and in magazines and newspapers. A **commercial** is an advertisement on TV or radio. Companies know that teens spend lots of money on products and services each year. They have ads created especially to influence teens to spend their money on certain products. In this lesson, you will learn how advertising tries to influence people to buy products and services. You also will learn how to evaluate ads.

The Lesson Outline

What to Know About Advertisements

How to Evaluate Advertisements

Objectives

1. Discuss reasons why the advertising industry is big business. **page 557**
2. List seven questions a person should ask if (s)he is tempted to buy something seen in an ad. **page 557**
3. List and discuss ten appeals found in ads. **page 558**

Vocabulary Words

advertising

advertisement (ad)

commercial

brand loyalty appeal

false image appeal

bandwagon appeal

humor appeal

glittering generality appeal

scientific evidence appeal

progress appeal

reward appeal

sex appeal

testimonial appeal

What to Know About
Advertisements

The advertising industry is big business. Advertising agencies help companies by designing ads to influence people's choices. A lot of money, time, and effort goes into the production of ads. People who create ads carefully develop them to appeal to the wants and needs of a certain audience. Many ads are designed to influence a person's feelings as to what life will be like with a certain product. For example, ads for alcoholic beverages often show people having a good time with lots of friends. Even though the ad does not claim that the alcoholic beverage will make a person popular, it gives a strong message that it will. Most teens want to be popular. People who create ads know this and design ads to appeal to this need. Ads usually show young, healthy, vibrant, happy, and attractive people. As a result, viewers of the ad get the message that this product will make them more attractive, youthful, happy, and healthy.

Companies spend lots of money to place ads in the media. Advertisers think very carefully about when and where to place their ads. They want to place them where they will have the greatest influence. For example, commercials for children's toys often are shown during Saturday morning cartoons. Commercials for cars often appear during televised football, baseball, and basketball games. Ads for clothes for teens are placed in teen magazines and other places where teens will see them. Tobacco and beer ads often are placed in magazines read by teens and young adults. Advertisers use their logos as a form of advertising. They pay celebrities to wear their logos during sporting events and social events.

How to Evaluate Advertisements

Remember, the bottom line for a company that places an ad is profit. You can evaluate ads. You can tell whether a product is needed or whether it is waste of money. You can recognize that the purpose of advertising is to influence people to purchase a product or service. You can recognize that companies spend large amounts of money on ads to influence purchases. Use the Questions to Evaluate Ads to evaluate whether an advertisement is appealing to your emotions.

Questions to Evaluate Ads

1. What is being advertised?
2. Where and when did the ad appear?
3. Why was this particular type of media selected?
4. What appears to be the targeted audience? How do you know this?
5. What advertising appeals (page 558) are used in the ad?
6. What does the advertiser want me to believe?
7. What do I know to be fact?

How Shopping Addiction Harms Health

Shopping addiction is the compelling need to purchase things. People with shopping addiction go on shopping sprees even when they do not need anything. They get a temporary "high" from shopping that may relieve their boredom, loneliness, or insecure feelings. Shopping addiction can lead to debt.

Teens with shopping addiction often have a strong need for approval from others. Some teens think that if they purchase something new others will notice it and compliment them. Other teens purchase presents for others in the hope that they will like them. Teens with shopping addiction need treatment.

Guidelines for Comparison Shopping

Comparison shopping is evaluating products and services using the following five criteria.

- **Price:** the cost
- **Convenience:** something that saves time or effort
- **Features:** the outstanding characteristics
- **Quality:** the degree of excellence of a product or service
- **Warranty:** a written assurance that a product or service will be repaired or replaced if a problem occurs

Lesson 75

Review

Vocabulary Words

Write a separate sentence using each of the vocabulary words listed on page 560.

Objectives

1. What are three tips for staying organized? **Objective 1**

2. What are 12 priorities for which a person needs to make time? **Objective 2**

3. How does a person make a budget? **Objective 3**

4. Why should a person be cautious if (s)he uses a credit card to make purchases? **Objective 4**

5. What are five criteria that can be used when comparison shopping? **Objective 5**

Responsible Decision-Making

Suppose you are dating another teen. You really like him/her. However, (s)he seems to be losing interest in you. You see an expensive shirt in a store. You know (s)he would really like this shirt. Last time you purchased a gift (s)he became more attentive. You consider purchasing the shirt. Write a response to this situation.

1. Describe the situation that requires you to make a decision.
2. List possible decisions you might make.
3. Name two responsible adults with whom you might discuss your decisions.
4. Evaluate the possible consequences of your decisions. Determine if each decision will lead to actions that:
   - promote health,
   - protect safety,
   - follow laws,
   - show respect for yourself and others,
   - follow the guidelines of your parents and of other responsible adults,
   - demonstrate good character.
5. Decide which decision is most responsible and appropriate.
6. Tell two results you expect if you make this decision.

Effective Communication

Suppose you share a room with a sibling. Your sibling is very messy. You often are late to school because you are looking in your room for your belongings. What might you say to your sibling about being organized?

Self-Directed Learning

Determine how to make a to-do list that would help you organize your time. You might keep the list in a notebook, on a sticky note, or on an index card. Complete the list for one week. You may choose to continue keeping to-do list on a regular basis.

Critical Thinking

Suppose you purchase a product for $100 on a credit card that charges 15 percent interest. You do not pay off the monthly balance. How much interest would you have to pay after one month? One year? Ten years? What might you be able to buy with the money you spent in interest?

Responsible Citizenship

Make a budget. Use the steps on page 563 as a guide. Review your budget with your parents or guardian.

You Can Choose Healthful Entertainment

Life Skill **I will choose healthful entertainment.**

Consider the importance of choosing a healthful diet. When you eat nutritious foods, your body is well-nourished. Now consider the importance of choosing healthful entertainment. When you choose healthful entertainment, your mind is well-nourished. You feed your mind with messages that help you live in a responsible way. This lesson focuses on why you must make wise choices when choosing entertainment. You will learn how to evaluate entertainment.

The Lesson Outline

What to Know About Entertainment

How to Evaluate Entertainment

Objectives

1. Differentiate between real life and life portrayed in entertainment. **page 567**

2. Explain why television addiction is risky. **page 568**

3. Explain why computer addiction is risky. **page 568**

4. List four guidelines to follow when choosing entertainment. **page 568**

5. Discuss how a family can use television ratings and a V-chip to protect against harmful entertainment? **page 568**

Vocabulary Words

entertainment

promiscuous

television addiction

desensitization

V-chip

What to Know About
Entertainment

Consider the definition of entertainment. **Entertainment** is something that is designed to hold the interest of people. How entertaining would it be to turn on a television show and watch a teen cleaning his/her room or helping his/her father with the dishes? Would it be entertaining to watch two teens who cared about each other sharing a firm decision to abstain from sex until marriage? Would it be entertaining to see a teen trying to figure out what to do about his/her acne? Would a teen who was overweight become a television heart throb?

By now, you should recognize that entertainment often includes situations and people who differ from real life. This approach to entertainment is taken to get you "hooked" on what life might be like in another situation. The danger to becoming too involved in entertainment is that you may get real life out of perspective. Consider the following.

Teens in real life may get infected with STDs and HIV and have unwanted pregnancies if they are sexually active. Teens protect themselves by abstaining from sex. Teens in television programs and in movies often are promiscuous. To be **promiscuous** is to engage in sexual intercourse with many people. Now consider a steady diet of watching teens who are promiscuous on TV or at the movies. You would begin to fill your mind with unrealistic views. This is NOT the way to live. Being promiscuous is not a satisfying lifestyle. If you behaved in this way, you might become infected with STDs or HIV. An unwanted pregnancy might occur.

Teens in real life may get seriously injured or killed if they engage in violent or unsafe actions. Teens protect themselves by respecting authority and obeying laws. Rappers and other musical artists may perform songs and raps with violent lyrics. Now consider a steady diet of listening to these songs or raps. You might begin to believe that violence against police or other authority figures is OK. This is not OK. You are expected to obey the law and respect authority. This protects your safety and the safety of others. Also, consider the engaging car chases on the movie screen. Suppose you decided to ride with someone on a high speed chase. You would put your life in danger.

Teens in real life ruin their health and relationships and disrupt their education if they get hooked on drugs. Teens protect themselves by being drug-free. Actors and actresses in movies and in television programs often smoke and drink. They light up or pour a drink as the suspense builds. Now consider a steady diet of watching this form of coping. You may begin to believe that a cigarette or drink is the answer when life gets difficult. Programs usually do not show the misery that accompanies drug misuse and abuse.

Teens in real life have a limited wardrobe and an average appearance. Teens form a positive self-image by accepting who they are and how they look. Actors, actresses, and musical artists have a more extensive budget for clothing. They also can dress in unusual ways that would not be acceptable at your school or follow parental guidelines. Now consider a steady diet of "heart-throb" worship. You may expect yourself and others to dress and look like a star.

Set goals to be the best person you can be. Avoid getting hooked on entertainment that portrays life in an unrealistic way.

Why Television Addiction Is Risky

Television addiction is the compelling need to watch television. Teens with television addiction watch many hours of TV each day. They center their lives around their favorite TV programs. They may skip school and put off homework and chores to watch a program. They have little time to participate in physical activities and are at increased risk of being overweight.

Some teens may become "hooked" on a TV program because they are not satisfied with their lives. They become wrapped up in the lives of TV characters and copy their hairstyle, clothing, or way of speaking. These teens do not form their own identity.

Some teens substitute TV characters for friends and family members. They pretend that the family members on TV are their family members. These teens do not have opportunities to develop social skills.

Some teens get hooked on talk shows that feature people who discuss their problems. These shows often contain inappropriate content, such as discussions about violent behaviors. The people on talk shows often use offensive language and put-downs and get into fights with one another.

Some teens watch a lot of violent programs. They are at risk for being desensitized to violence. **Desensitization** is the effect of reacting less and less to the exposure of something. Teens who are exposed to lots of media violence begin to see violence as a way of life.

Why Computer Addiction Is Risky

Some teens spend large amounts of time using the computer. They play computer games for long periods of time. They form relationships on-line by e-mailing people and participating in discussion groups. They may find it easier to talk with others by computer than to have in-person relationships. These teens may pretend to be someone else when they are on-line. They may believe other people will like their computer "personality" more than their real one. These teens do not have the opportunity to have healthful friendships and develop social skills.

How to Evaluate Entertainment

Teens should follow these guidelines when choosing entertainment.

1. Entertainment should follow family guidelines.
2. Entertainment should be approved for your age group.
3. Entertainment should not show inappropriate content, such as violence or sex.
4. Entertainment should not portray harmful drug use as acceptable behavior.

The V-Chip

The **V-chip** is a small electronic device that allows television programs to be blocked. Parents or guardians can use it to block programs they feel are not appropriate for their children.

How Entertainment Is Rated

Discuss with your parents or guardian the TV programs and movies you watch.

The television rating system that went into effect in 1997 rates programs as follows:

- **TV-Y**   Suitable for All Children
- **TV-Y7**   Directed to Older Children
- **TV-G**   General Audiences
- **TV-PG**   Parental Guidance Suggested
- **TV-14**   Parents Strongly Cautioned
- **TV-M**   Mature Audiences Only

Movies shown in theaters and on video are rated by the film industry as follows:

- **G**   General Audience
- **PG**   Parental Guidance Suggested
- **PG 13**   Parental Guidance Suggested. May not be suitable for children under 13.
- **R**   Restricted to people under age 17 unless accompanied by a parent or guardian.
- **NC-17**   Adult Content. May be viewed only by people over the age of 17.
- **X**   Adults Only

Lesson 76

Review

Vocabulary Words

Write a separate sentence using each of the vocabulary words listed on page 566.

Objectives

1. Why is it dangerous to confuse real life with life portrayed in entertainment? **Objective 1**

2. Why is television addiction risky? **Objective 2**

3. Why is computer addiction risky? **Objective 3**

4. What are four guidelines to follow when choosing entertainment? **Objective 4**

5. How can a family use television ratings and a V-chip to protect against harmful entertainment? **Objective 5**

Responsible Decision-Making

Suppose you have permission from your guardian to go to a certain movie with a group of your friends. On the way to the movie, a friend suggests that you go to a different film instead of the one the group was planning to see. The movie your friend has suggested is one you know your guardian would not approve. Write a response to this situation.

1. Describe the situation that requires you to make a decision.
2. List possible decisions you might make.
3. Name two responsible adults with whom you might discuss your decisions.
4. Evaluate the possible consequences of your decisions. Determine if each decision will lead to actions that:
   - promote health,
   - protect safety,
   - follow laws,
   - show respect for yourself and others,
   - follow the guidelines of your parents and of other responsible adults,
   - demonstrate good character.
5. Decide which decision is most responsible and appropriate.
6. Tell two results you expect if you make this decision.

Effective Communication

Write a short script for a scene in a movie or a TV program. The scene should include a teen character who makes a responsible decision.

Self-Directed Learning

Check the library or Internet for two articles about products that control children's access to computers or TVs. Write a summary of the articles.

Critical Thinking

Keep a journal for five days. Record the amount of time you spend watching TV. What might you have accomplished during this time if you had not been watching TV?

Responsible Citizenship

Find a local television guide in your newspaper or library. Find the TV ratings. Identify five TV programs that would be appropriate for young children to watch. Share these with friends, neighbors, or family members who are responsible for the care of young children.

Lesson 77

You Can Make Responsible Choices About Health Care Providers and Facilities

Life Skill **I will make responsible choices about health care providers and facilities.**

The **health care system** is a system that includes health care providers, health care facilities, and payment for health care. The next lesson focuses on ways to pay for health care. This lesson focuses on how to make responsible choices about health care and facilities. You will learn about the different types of health care providers.

Questions are included that can be used to evaluate your experience after a visit to a health care provider. This lesson also includes a discussion of the different health care facilities. You will learn when to promptly go to an emergency facility. This lesson also includes the American Hospital Association's Patient Bill of Rights.

The Lesson Outline

What to Know About Health Care Providers

What to Know About Health Care Facilities

Objectives

1. Discuss the credentials of different health care providers. **page 571**
2. List questions that can be used to evaluate a health care provider after the initial visit. **page 572**
3. List and discuss various health care facilities. **page 573**
4. List symptoms that indicate prompt treatment is needed at an emergency facility. **page 574**
5. List ten rights included in the American Hospital Association's Patient's Bill of Rights. **page 574**

Vocabulary Words

health care system
health care provider
physician
medical doctor
osteopath
primary care
specialist
health care practitioner
podiatrist
dentist
optometrist
allied health professional
health care facility
hospital
inpatient care
outpatient care
private hospital
voluntary hospital
government hospital
teaching hospital
walk-in surgery center
health center
health department clinic
mental health clinic
extended care facility
home health care
hospice
emergency room
freestanding emergency center
urgent care center

What to Know About
Health Care Providers

A **health care provider** is a trained professional who provides people with health care.

Physicians, health care practitioners, and allied health professionals are health care providers.

Physicians

A **physician** is an independent health care provider who is licensed to practice medicine. Physicians obtain medical histories, perform physical examinations, give diagnoses to patients, and are licensed to prescribe medications. Some physicians are licensed to perform surgery.

There are two main types of physicians. A **medical doctor** is a physician who is trained in a medical school and has a doctor of medicine (MD) degree. An **osteopath** is a physician who

is trained in an school of osteopathy and has a doctor of osteopathy (DO) degree. Medical doctors and osteopaths can choose to work in primary care or become specialists. **Primary care** is general health care. Physicians who provide primary care often are the first health care providers that a patient consults. They can refer patients to specialists. A **specialist** is a professional who has specialized training in a particular area. Almost two-thirds of physicians are specialists.

Cardiologist	A physician who specializes in the treatment of the heart and blood vessels
Dermatologist	A physician who specializes in the care of the skin
Family Practice Physician	A physician who provides general care
Gastroenterologist	A physician who specializes in disorders of the digestive tract
Geriatrician	A physician who specializes in the treatment of the elderly
Gynecologist	A physician who specializes in female reproductive health
Internist	A physician who specializes in diagnosis and nonsurgical treatment of the internal organs
Neurologist	A physician who specializes in disorders of the nervous system
Obstetrician	A physician who specializes in the care and treatment of pregnant women and their unborn babies
Oncologist	A physician who specializes in the treatment of tumors and cancer
Ophthalmologist	A physician who specializes in medical and surgical care and treatment of the eyes
Orthopedist	A physician who specializes in the treatment of muscles, bones, and joints
Otolaryngologist (ENT)	A physician who diagnoses and treats disorders of the ears, nose, and throat
Pathologist	A physician who conducts lab studies of tissues, cells, and blood and other body fluids.
Pediatrician	A physician who specializes in the care of children and adolescents
Plastic Surgeon	A physician who specializes in surgery to correct, repair, or improve body features
Psychiatrist	A physician who specializes in the treatment of mental disorders
Radiologist	A physician who specializes in the use of radiation for the diagnosis and treatment of illness and disease
Urologist	A physician who specializes in the treatment of urinary disorders and the male reproductive system

Health Care Practitioners

A **health care practitioner** is an independent health care provider who is licensed to practice on a specific area of the body. Health care practitioners can provide general or specialized care. Podiatrists, dentists, and optometrists are health care practitioners. A **podiatrist** is a doctor of podiatric medicine (DPM) who specializes in problems of the feet. A **dentist** is a doctor of dental surgery (DDS) or a doctor of medical dentistry (DMD) who specializes in dental care. An **optometrist** is an eye care professional who is specially trained in a school of optometry.

An **allied health professional** is a trained health care provider who practices under the supervision of a physician or health care practitioner, such as nurses, audiologists, dental hygienists, pharmacists, and physical therapists.

> **Lesson 80 will include more information about health care providers.**

Choosing Health Care Providers

Some people pose as health care providers and make money treating people, but do not have reliable credentials. It is important to carefully choose reliable health care providers to protect health status. Health care providers are listed in the yellow pages of the telephone directory. Local chapters of the American Medical Association (AMA) and the American Dental Association (ADA) also keep lists of their members. Hospitals often have lists of physicians they will recommend, and a trusted physician or other health care provider may offer recommendations.

It is important to choose a primary care physician who will provide basic medical care and help prevent illness. Primary care physicians are most often family practitioners, pediatricians, or internists. The primary care physician should be familiar with the patient's medical history and health care needs. (S)he may refer a patient to a specialist if further diagnosis or treatment is needed.

Get to Know Your Health Care Provider

After you visit a health care provider for the first time, ask the questions that follow. Based on your responses, determine whether you are satisfied with your health care provider or want to find a different one.

- Am I feeling comfortable sharing my needs and concerns with the health care provider?
- Did the health care provider answer my questions?
- Did the health care provider help me make a plan for my health?
- What are the credentials of the health care provider?
- What hospital affiliations does the health care provider have?
- What arrangements can be made for care on weekends or after hours?
- Who will care for me if the health care provider is out of town or unavailable?
- Does the health care provider emphasize prevention of illness and injury?
- How much are fees?
- How are fees paid?
- Is this health care provider eligible for payment if my family has a health care plan?
- How long do I have to wait to get an appointment with the health care provider?
- How long do I have to wait in the office for an examination or visit?

What to Know About
Health Care Facilities

A **health care facility** is a place where people receive health care. People should be aware of the types and locations of health care facilities in their community. They also should know the hours the facilities are open, the services they provide, and the fees they charge.

A **hospital** is a health care facility where people can receive medical care, diagnosis, and treatment on an inpatient or outpatient basis. **Inpatient care** is treatment that requires a person to stay overnight at a facility. **Outpatient care** is treatment that does not require a person to stay overnight at a facility. There are different types of hospitals.

- A **private hospital** is a hospital that is owned by private individuals and operates as a profit-making business.

- A **voluntary hospital** is a hospital that is owned by a community or organization and does not operate for profit.

- A **government hospital** is a hospital that is run by the federal, state, or local government for the benefit of a specific population. For example, the Veteran's Administration operates hospitals for military veterans.

- A **teaching hospital** is a hospital that is associated with a medical school and/or school of nursing. Teaching hospitals provide training for health professionals in addition to the regular services of most hospitals.

A **walk-in surgery center** is a facility where surgery is performed on an outpatient basis. The cost of outpatient surgery averages less than one-third to one-half the cost of inpatient fees. Many health insurance companies encourage or require patients who need certain types of surgery to choose outpatient surgery in walk-in surgery centers. However, certain types of surgery require inpatient care.

A **health center** is a facility that provides routine health care to a special population. For example, there are health centers that provide health care to low-income families. A **health department clinic** is a facility in most state and local health departments that keeps records and performs services. A **mental health clinic** is a facility that provides services for people who have mental disorders. Many mental health clinics are open 24 hours a day, seven days a week to help people in crisis situations.

An **extended care facility** is a facility that provides nursing, personal, and residential care. Extended care facilities also provide care for people who need assistance with daily living. Nursing homes and convalescent centers are examples of extended care facilities. Home health care may be more convenient and affordable than staying in an extended care facility. **Home health care** is care provided within a patient's home. Home health care organizations offer a variety of services including nursing care, medical treatment, and therapy in the home.

Many patients receive hospice care in their home or in the home of a loved one. Others receive hospice care in hospices. **Hospice** is a facility for people who are dying and their families. Hospice services usually provide care 24 hours a day. Hospice care extends after the patient dies. Contact and support from hospice staff continues for at least a year after a family member dies.

You Can Evaluate Ways to Pay for Health Care

Life Skill **I will evaluate ways to pay for health care.**

The price of health care has soared. High-tech equipment, disease epidemics, malpractice lawsuits, and an increase in the number of tests performed on a patient are some of the reasons. As health care costs have soared, it has become much more difficult for people to pay for health care. Health care can be unexpected and expensive. Many people use health insurance to help pay for health care costs. This lesson discusses how to pay for health care. You also will learn how to evaluate health insurance.

The Lesson Outline

What to Know About Health Insurance

How to Evaluate Health Insurance

Objectives

1. Discuss two kinds of managed care programs to cover health care costs. **page 577**
2. Identify the populations who receive health care coverage through Medicare and Medicaid. **page 577**
3. Discuss the effects of malpractice insurance on health care costs. **page 577**
4. List and explain five kinds of coverage in health insurance plans. **page 578**
5. List 15 questions that can be asked to evaluate health insurance coverage. **page 578**

Vocabulary Words

health insurance

insurance policy

premium

deductible

co-payment

managed care

health maintenance organization (HMO)

preferred provider organization (PPO)

preferred provider

Medicare

Medicaid

malpractice insurance

malpractice lawsuits

covered expense

exclusion

medical insurance

major medical insurance

hospitalization insurance

surgical insurance

disability insurance

preexisting condition

What to Know About
Health Insurance

Health insurance is financial protection that provides benefits for sickness or injury. When a person purchases insurance, the insurance provider agrees to pay or reimburse for the costs of care. The insurance provider calculates that over a long period of time it will take in more money than it will pay out.

An **insurance policy** is the legal document issued to the policyholder that outlines the terms of the insurance. Insurance policies are issued by insurance companies and the federal government. Insurance policies vary greatly regarding coverage, costs, and limitations. A premium must be paid at certain periods of time. A **premium** is a specific amount of money that will guarantee that an insurance company will help pay for health services. Premiums for health insurance provided by private insurance companies are paid by the individual, by the company where the individual works, or by a combination of both.

Some insurance policies pay the entire cost of medical care. Others pay a portion. A **deductible** is an amount that insurance does not cover that must be paid by the individual. A **co-payment** is the portion of the medical fee the individual must pay.

Managed care is an organized system of health care services designed to control health care costs. Managed care insurance plans control the types of health care that insured people receive. They also limit what is paid out for specific kinds of care. Health maintenance organizations (HMOs) and preferred provider organizations are two kinds of managed care.

A **health maintenance organization (HMO)** is a business that organizes health care services for its members. HMOs try to provide care at a reduced cost. Except for emergency care, policyholders are covered only for services received directly from the HMO or with specific approval. HMOs encourage regular checkups for preventative health care.

A **preferred provider organization (PPO)** is a health insurance plan that has a contract with a group of health care providers who agree to provide health care services at a reduced rate. A **preferred provider** is a health care provider who appears on a list that has been approved by the health insurance provider. People covered under these plans must select preferred providers within the plan or pay a higher cost for health services.

Federal and state governments offer health care payment for some people. The major sources of insurance coverage include Medicare, Medicaid, coverage for veterans, and coverage for government employees. **Medicare** is a government health insurance plan for people 65 years of age and older and for people who receive Social Security disability benefits for two years. Medicare covers a portion of a person's health care costs. The rest is paid by the person, other programs such as Medicaid, or supplemental insurance programs. **Medicaid** is a health insurance plan for people with low incomes that is managed and paid for by the government. The state government and federal government divide the costs of the health care. Medicaid programs are different from state to state.

Malpractice insurance is insurance that health care providers and health care facilities purchase to provide coverage for malpractice lawsuits. **Malpractice lawsuits** are claims made by patients that a health care provider did not provide appropriate health care treatment. The great number of malpractice lawsuits is one reason health care costs have risen. Health care providers have to pay a great deal for malpractice insurance.

How to Evaluate Health Insurance

Health insurance should cover standard risks of illness and injury for family members. It also should cover special conditions family members might have that require on-going medical attention. There are two kinds of expenses. A **covered expense** is a medical expense that is paid for under the terms of a health insurance plan. An **exclusion** is a service for which a health insurance plan will not pay. Health insurance plans must be studied carefully in order to know exactly what services are covered and excluded.

Five Kinds of Coverage in Health Insurance Plans

1. **Medical insurance** is insurance that pays physician's fees, laboratory fees outside a hospital, and fees for prescription drugs.

2. **Major medical insurance** is insurance that pays for extra expenses not covered by other insurance policies. Major medical insurance might cover treatment for diseases such as cancer or AIDS.

3. **Hospitalization insurance** is insurance that pays the cost of a hospital stay.

4. **Surgical insurance** is insurance that pays for fees related to surgery.

5. **Disability insurance** is insurance that replaces lost income due to accidents or illnesses requiring a period of recovery.

Health insurance plans are not all the same. Some cost more than others, and some cover more than others. People must evaluate health insurance plans in terms of their own and their family's needs. They should take the following actions:

1. Obtain and read carefully a copy of the health insurance plan.

2. Ask representatives from the health insurance plan questions.

3. Shop around for health insurance plans. Choose plans that give the most comprehensive coverage at the most affordable price.

Some insurance providers will not sell insurance to people they consider high risks, such as people with disabilities or preexisting conditions. A **preexisting condition** is a health problem that a person had before being covered by the insurance. According to law, people must disclose all health information to the insurer. If they do not, the insurance provider may cancel the contract.

Fifteen Questions to Ask to Evaluate Health Insurance Coverage

1. Is the entire family covered?
2. Are regular checkups covered?
3. Are the services I need covered?
4. Are immunizations covered?
5. Is maternity care covered?
6. Is vision or dental care covered?
7. Are psychological services covered?
8. Is physical therapy covered?
9. Are there time limits for extended treatment?
10. What is not covered?
11. How much are the deductibles?
12. How many days in the hospital are covered?
13. Is there a waiting period before coverage begins?
14. Are there limitations on choices of health care providers or facilities?
15. Is the insurance renewable or can the company cancel it in certain situations?

Lesson 78

Review

Vocabulary Words

Write a separate sentence using each of the vocabulary words listed on page 576.

Objectives

1. What are two kinds of managed care? **Objective 1**

2. What populations receive health care coverage through Medicare or Medicaid? **Objective 2**

3. How does the cost of malpractice insurance effect health care costs? **Objective 3**

4. What are five kinds of coverage that may be included in health insurance plans? **Objective 4**

5. What are 15 questions that can be asked to evaluate health insurance coverage? **Objective 5**

Responsible Decision-Making

Your cousin and his wife have been looking at insurance policies from two different companies. They are on a very tight budget. One policy costs less than the other, but it does not have maternity coverage. Your cousin's wife is six months pregnant. Write a response to this situation.

1. Describe the situation that requires your cousin to make a decision.

2. List possible decisions your cousin might make.

3. Name two responsible adults with whom your cousin might discuss his decisions.

4. Evaluate the possible consequences of your cousin's decisions. Determine if each decision will lead to actions that:
   • promote health,
   • protect safety,
   • follow laws,
   • show respect for your cousin and others,
   • follow the guidelines of your cousin's parents and of other responsible adults,
   • demonstrate good character.

5. Decide which decision is most responsible and appropriate for your cousin.

6. Tell two results your cousin can expect if he makes this decision.

 ## Effective Communication

Write a script in which a person who is interested in purchasing insurance meets with a representative from an insurance provider. Refer to Fifteen Questions to Ask to Evaluate Health Insurance Coverage on page 578.

 ## Self-Directed Learning

Obtain permission from a parent or guardian. Call an insurance provider in your community. Obtain a copy of a sample insurance form. Identify the different parts on the form.

 ## Critical Thinking

Suppose your classmate tells you that (s)he would not tell an insurance provider about a preexisting condition. (S)he says that not telling is a way make sure the insurance provider provides coverage. What would you tell this classmate?

 ## Responsible Citizenship

Research the requirements to be eligible for Medicaid in your state. Make a poster or brochure that shows this information. Obtain permission from a parent or guardian. Offer to post or distribute the information at a local community center.

Lesson 79

You Can Be a Health Advocate by Being a Volunteer

Life Skill **I will be a health advocate by being a volunteer.**

Someone once said, "People can be divided into three groups—those who make things happen, those who watch things happen, and those who wonder what happened." You can be one of those who makes things happen by being a health advocate for the community. **Health advocacy** is taking responsibility to improve the quality of life. Health advocacy means spending time and efforts to help in your community. This lesson discusses ways that you can be a health advocate and contribute to your community as a volunteer. You also will learn guidelines for being a volunteer.

Vocabulary Words

health advocacy
volunteer
beta-endorphins
healthy helper syndrome
volunteer center
volunteer burnout

The Lesson Outline

How Being a Volunteer Affects Health Status

How to Get Involved as a Volunteer

Objectives

1. Explain the positive effects that being a volunteer has on health status. **page 581**

2. List at least ten volunteer opportunities for teens. **page 581**

3. Explain eight steps that can be taken to get involved as a volunteer. **page 582**

How Being a Volunteer Affects Health Status

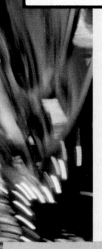

One way to be a health advocate is to volunteer to help others in the community. A **volunteer** is a person who provides a service without pay. Teens who offer their services recognize that being a volunteer contributes to their self-respect, helps them learn new skills, and provides opportunities for them to meet new people. You can be a volunteer in your community.

Being a volunteer can improve health status. The positive feelings that come from giving good deeds help boost the effectiveness of the immune system. You will have more resistance to some infections. Acts of giving stimulate the brain to release beta-endorphins. **Beta-endorphins** are substances produced in the brain that create a feeling of well-being. The release of beta-endorphins helps produce the healthy helper syndrome. The **healthy helper syndrome** is a state in which a person feels increased energy, relaxation, and improved mood as a result of giving service to others. Volunteers who experience the healthy helper syndrome are less likely to suffer from flu and colds, migraine headaches, arthritis pains, symptoms of lupus, and asthma attacks.

Hafen, B.Q., Karren, K.J., Frandsen, K.J., & Smith, N.L. (1996). *Mind Body Health: The Effects of Attitudes, Emotions, and Relationships.* Needham Heights, MA: Allyn and Bacon.

You Can Volunteer to . . .

- Work in a homeless shelter.
- Spend time with an elderly person.
- Perform chores for a person who has a physical disability.
- Tutor younger children.
- Coach a youth sports team.
- Become a peer leader.
- Form a teen coalition to counter tobacco and alcohol advertising in your community.
- Clean up a vacant lot, park, roadway, or other area in need.
- Organize a fund-raising activity for a community organization.
- Collect food or clothing for needy persons.
- Deliver meals to people are not able to leave their home.
- Childsit for parents or guardians that need a break.
- Read stories to children in a hospital.

- Make greeting cards to take to a children's hospital or nursing home.
- Organize a singing group to perform at a nursing home.
- Write letters to elected officials about a cause.
- Speak up about issues at community meetings and forums.
- Write letters to your local newspaper about issues that concern you.
- Participate in walk-a-thons and fun-runs that raise money for good causes.
- Organize a neighborhood watch for crime and drug prevention.
- Become a volunteer in a hospital or nursing home.
- Organize drug- and alcohol-free activities for peers.
- Coordinate a graffiti clean-up project.
- Plant a garden or tree.

How to Get Involved as a Volunteer

Eight Steps to Take to Be a Volunteer.

1. **Assess your interests, skills, talents, and resources.** List your skills and talents and the issues and problems in your community that concern and interest you. Determine how much time you have to spend in volunteer service.

2. **Identify organizations in your community that use or need volunteers.** Check with teachers, school counselors, parents or guardian, and clergy, or look in the phone book and local newspaper for organizations in your community that use or might need volunteers. You also might call a volunteer center. A **volunteer center** is an organization that matches people with volunteer jobs.

3. **Call or visit organizations or agencies for which you would like to volunteer.** Obtain permission from a parent or guardian. Call the organization for which you would like to volunteer, express your interest in volunteering, and arrange a visit to discuss the organization and volunteering. Explore volunteer opportunities in more than one organization. Ask questions such as the following: What does the organization do? What are the tasks and responsibilities of volunteers? What training and skills are needed? Who provides the training? Who supervises volunteers? What hours is a volunteer expected to work?

4. **Create and organize your own projects if you do not find an organization or agency where you can serve as a volunteer.** Identify how you can help your community. You can spearhead a project to meet a need or help solve a problem. Obtain permission from a parent or guardian and, if necessary, from a teacher, principal, or community organization or official. Involve others in the project, and organize needed supplies, transportation, and equipment.

5. **Make final preparations.** Obtain permission from a parent or guardian to volunteer. Determine how you will get back and forth from the location at which you will be volunteering. Keep your parents or guardian informed as to where you will be working, what your schedule will be, and what tasks you will be performing.

6. **Set high expectations for yourself.** Show up on time appropriately dressed, follow organization rules and guidelines, and complete your assigned tasks in a timely fashion. Call and inform your supervisor as far in advance as possible if you must be late or absent.

7. **Keep a journal of your volunteer experiences.** Writing about your volunteer experiences in a journal will help you to remember specifics. It also will help you to see what new skills you have learned. It will help you evaluate your effectiveness as a volunteer. Answer the following questions in your journal. Did the project help the community? What did you learn? How could the experience be improved? Would you do it again?

8. **Avoid volunteer burnout.** Be careful not to overdo your volunteer efforts. Take on responsibilities that you can handle. Overdoing can result in volunteer burnout. **Volunteer burnout** is a loss of enthusiasm about volunteering that results from feeling overwhelmed. Watch out for signs of burnout, such as feeling stressed, overwhelmed, frustrated, and exhausted.

Lesson 79

Review

Vocabulary Words

Write a separate sentence using each of the vocabulary words listed on page 580.

Objectives

1. What is the healthy helper syndrome? **Objective 1**

2. Why do people who volunteer often experience improved mood? **Objective 1**

3. What are ten examples of volunteer opportunities for teens? **Objective 2**

4. What are eight steps that can be taken to get involved as a volunteer? **Objective 3**

5. What are signs of volunteer burnout? **Objective 3**

Responsible Decision-Making

Suppose you volunteer a few hours each Saturday at a children's hospital. Your friend invites you to a sports game that is during the hours you volunteer. Your friend tells you to blow off volunteering for the day. (S)he says that since you do not get paid, not showing up one Saturday will be no big deal. Write a response to this situation.

1. Describe the situation that requires you to make a decision.
2. List possible decisions you might make.
3. Name two responsible adults with whom you might discuss your decisions.
4. Evaluate the possible consequences of your decisions. Determine if each decision will lead to actions that:
   - promote health,
   - protect safety,
   - follow laws,
   - show respect for yourself and others,
   - follow the guidelines of your parents and of other responsible adults,
   - demonstrate good character.
5. Decide which decision is most responsible and appropriate.
6. Tell two results you expect if you make this decision.

 ### Effective Communication

List ten ways teens can make a difference by being a health advocate for the community. Include examples of ways that teens have made a difference in your school or community. Share the list with your parents or guardian.

 ### Self-Directed Learning

Check your local newspaper. Identify five organizations that might use volunteers.

 ### Critical Thinking

Review You Can Volunteer to... on page 581. Add five more examples to the list. Then identify ten volunteer tasks in which you would be interested.

 ### Responsible Citizenship

Obtain permission from a parent or guardian. Volunteer for at least three hours once a week for one month. Write about the experience in a journal. Include answers to these questions: What did I learn from this experience? Will I continue to volunteer? How else might I volunteer?

You Can Investigate Health Careers

Life Skill **I will investigate health careers.**

Suppose you had to write a short paper in which you described what you will be doing ten years from today. Think about the details of your life at that point in time. Will you be in school? Will you have a career in which you work outside your home? Will you have a career inside the home? Will you have a career as a homemaker? Opportunties in the health field are increasing. This lesson includes A Guide to Health Careers to help you investigate health care careers and what they involve. This lesson also discusses the importance of being a homemaker. You will learn ways a homemaker is involved in promoting health.

The Lesson Outline

How to Investigate Health Careers

A Guide to Health Careers

What to Know About Being a Homemaker

Objectives

1. List and discuss seven ways to investigate health careers. **page 585**

2. Explain what it means to be licensed and to have certification for a health career. **page 585**

3. List ways a homemaker is involved in promoting health and why these contributions are important. **page 590**

Vocabulary Words

health career

credentials

license for a health career

certification

Certified Health Education Specialist (CHES)

shadowing

mentor

homemaker

How to
Investigate a Health Career

A **health career** is a profession or occupation in the health field for which one trains. A health career may be of interest to you. There are steps to take to investigate a health career.

1. **Review a listing of health careers that includes information about responsibilities and credentials.** A Guide to Health Careers in this lesson provides this information for you about more than 20 different health careers.

2. **Match interests and abilities with the responsibilities required of people in the health career.** Consider careers that focus on personal interests and abilities. For example, a career as a certified athletic trainer may be of interest to someone who enjoys athletics. Someone interested in reading about nutrition and who gets good grades in science courses might be interested in a career as a dietician.

3. **Examine the credentials required of people in the health career. Credentials** are the qualifications a person must have to do something. To be qualified for certain health careers, specific education and training may be needed, such as a bachelor's or master's degree in a designated area of study. A license or certification may be needed. A **license for a health career** is a document that grants a person the right to practice or use a certain title. A government agency awards a license. For example, a state will grant a physician a license to practice. **Certification** is the process a person completes to meet specific standards of professional competence. A non-governmental agency grants certification to individuals. For example, health educators may complete a process and be given the designation of CHES. A **Certified Health Education Specialist (CHES)** is a person who has completed the certification process recommended for health educators.

4. **Investigate opportunities available for obtaining the credentials including admission requirements.** Suppose a person must attend college, a vocational school, or other place that offers training to get the appropriate credentials. That person must ask: What are the options? Do I meet the admission requirements?

5. **Evaluate the resources (time and money) needed to obtain credentials.** Consider the personal resources that can be committed to getting credentials. A person must determine if (s)he is willing to commit to a certain amount of time and has the money needed for training. If (s)he does not have the money, is it possible to obtain financial support such as a scholarship or loan?

6. **Investigate employment opportunities and salaries.** What is the likelihood of being gainfully employed in the health career of choice? Choose a health career for which there are employment opportunities and a satisfactory salary.

7. **Participate in activities such as shadowing to get firsthand experience in what a health career might be like. Shadowing** is spending time with a mentor as (s)he performs work activities. A **mentor** is a responsible person who guides another person. You can shadow various professionals while you are in high school to learn more about a health career.

A Guide to Health Careers

An **audiologist** is a specialist who diagnoses and treats hearing and speech-related problems.

Responsibilities: An audiologist tests for hearing problems, prescribes hearing aids and devices, and plans hearing conversation programs. (S)he also teaches speech or lip reading.

Credentials: An audiologist must have a master's degree in audiology and a state license.

A **community health educator** is a health educator who focuses on educating people in a specific community.

Responsibilities: A community health educator identifies community health problems and needs and plans health promotion programs in a community.

Credentials: A community health educator must have a bachelor's degree in health education or a related area. (S)he may need to have certification as a Certified Health Education Specialist (CHES).

A **certified athletic trainer** is a specialist who works with athletes to maintain fitness and prevent and treat injuries.

Responsibilities: A certified athletic trainer treats emergency athletic injuries, assists with rehabilitation, and educates athletes concerning safety and injury prevention. (S)he can refer athletes for further medical treatment.

Credentials: A certified athletic trainer has a bachelor's degree and may have a master's degree. (S)he must have certification by the National Association of Athletic Trainers. Many states require certified athletic trainers to have a state license.

A **dental hygienist** is a trained dental health professional who works under the direction of a dentist to provide dental care.

Responsibilities: A dental hygienist cleans teeth, provides preventive dental care, teaches people how to practice good oral hygiene, examines patients teeth and gums, and takes and develops dental X-rays.

Credentials: A dental hygienist must have a associate's or bachelor's degree. (S)he must have certification from an accredited school of dental hygiene and a state license.

A **clinical psychologist** is a psychologist who has a Ph.D. and has had an internship in a psychiatric setting.

Responsibilities: A clinical psychologist helps people deal with mental disorders, stressors, and life crises; provides individual, group, and family psychotherapy; and plans behavioral modification programs.

Credentials: A clinical psychologist must have a doctoral degree in clinical psychology and a state license.

A **dentist** is a doctor of dental surgery (DDS) or a doctor of medical dentistry (DMD) who specializes in dental care.

Responsibilities: A dentist diagnoses, treats, and prevents problems of the teeth and mouth. (S)he examines X-rays, removes decay and fills cavities, repairs fractured teeth, removes teeth, and places protective sealants on teeth.

Credentials: A dentist must have a doctor of dental surgery (DDS) or doctor of medical dentistry (DMD) degree and a state license.

A **dietitian**, or **nutritionist**, is a specialist who counsels people about diet and nutrition.

Responsibilities: A dietitian plans nutritional programs, supervises the preparation of foods, evaluates diets, develops menus for people with health problems, and consults with other health care providers about nutrition.

Credentials: A dietitian must have a bachelor's degree in dietetics, foods and nutrition, food systems management, or a related field. (S)he may need certification as a registered dietitian (RD) and a state license.

An **emergency medical technician (EMT)** is a health care professional who gives health care to people in emergency situations before they reach the hospital.

Responsibilities: There are three types of emergency medical technicians. An EMT-basic gives immediate care to people in emergency situations and transports them to medical facilities. An EMT-intermediate has the same responsibilities as an EMT-basic, but also can administer intravenous fluids, use defibrillators to give life-saving shocks to a person with a stopped heart, and perform other intensive care procedures. An EMT-paramedic has the same responsibilities as an EMT-intermediate, but also can administer drugs orally and intravenously, read EKGs, perform endotracheal intubations, and use monitors and other complex equipment.

Credentials: An EMT-basic must be at least 18 years old, have a driver's license, and have a high school diploma or equivalent. (S)he must have basic EMT training and state certification. An EMT-intermediate must have intermediate EMT training and state certification. An EMT-paramedic must have EMT-paramedic training and state certification.

A **guidance counselor** is a specialist who assists students with personal, family, education, and career decisions and concerns.

Responsibilities: A guidance counselor helps students develop job-finding skills, provides college counseling, and helps students develop life skills needed to prevent and deal with problems.

Credentials: A guidance counselor must have a master's degree in counseling and state school counseling certification. (S)he may need a teaching certificate.

A **health education teacher** is a teacher who specializes in health education.

Responsibilities: A health education teacher promotes the development of health knowledge, life skills, and positive attitudes toward health and well-being in students. A health education teacher works with students and their family members, school principles, teachers, counselors, nurses, and community members.

Credentials: A health education teacher must have a bachelor's degree in health education and a teaching certificate with specialization in health education. Many health educators hold the title of Certified Health Education Specialist (CHES).

A **health services manager and administrator** is a professional who manages a health services organization.

Responsibilities: A health services manager and administrator plans, organizes, coordinates, and supervises a health services organization.

Credentials: A health services manager and administrator must have a bachelor's or master's degree in health services administration, business administration, public health, public administration, or another related field. Health services managers and administrators usually do not require special training or a state license. However, a nursing home administrator must have special training and a state license.

A **licensed practical nurse (LPN)**, or licensed vocational nurse (LVN), is a nurse who provides nursing care under the direction of registered nurses or physicians.

Responsibilities: A licensed practical nurse cares for people who are sick or injured.

Credentials: A licensed practical nurse must have a high school diploma or equivalent and training as a practical nurse. (S)he may need a state license.

A **medical writer** is a writer who specializes in the areas of medicine and health.

Responsibilities: A medical writer may write for the media, such as a newspaper column on medicine or an article for a medical journal. (S)he may write brochures, newsletters, and information sheets for hospitals, medical schools, health organizations, and medical companies. (S)he also may write for on-line medical services.

Credentials: A medical writer has a bachelor's degree with courses in technical writing, English, journalism, communications, and the biological sciences.

An **occupational therapist** is a health professional who helps people who have disabilities learn to make adjustments.

Responsibilities: An occupational therapist assists people who have disabilities to develop, recover, or maintain daily living and work skills.

Credentials: An occupational therapist must have a bachelor's degree in occupational therapy. (S)he may need a state license.

A **pharmacist** is an allied health professional who dispenses medications that are prescribed by certain licensed health professionals.

Responsibilities: A pharmacist prepares and dispenses drugs, provides information to patients about drugs, and consults with health care professionals about drugs.

Credentials: A pharmacist must have either a bachelor's degree or a graduate degree in pharmacy and a state license. (S)he must complete an internship under a licensed pharmacist.

A **pharmacologist** is a specialist in the composition of drugs and their effects.

Responsibilities: A pharmacologist studies the effects of drugs on the body and mind, researches the safety and effectiveness of drugs, and develops new drugs.

Credentials: A pharmacologist must have a bachelor's degree or master's degree in pharmacy, chemistry, medicine, or another related field.

A **physical therapist** is an allied health professional who helps people rehabilitate physical disabilities and injuries.

Responsibilities: A physical therapist helps improve mobility, relieves pain, and limits permanent physical disability in people who are physically disabled or injured. (S)he teaches people exercises to speed recovery and tests strength and range of motion to evaluate recovery.

Credentials: A physical therapist must have certification from an accredited program in physical therapy and a state license.

A **physician** is an independent health care provider who is licensed to practice medicine.

Responsibilities: Physicians obtain medical histories, perform physical examinations, and give diagnoses to patients. Physicians are licensed to prescribe medications to patients. Specially trained physicians are licensed to perform surgery.

Credentials: There are two main types of physicians. A medical doctor is a physician who is trained in a medical school and has a doctor of medicine (MD) degree. An osteopath is a physician who is trained in a school of osteopathy and has a doctor of osteopathy (DO) degree. Medical doctors and doctors of osteopathy must have a state license.

A **radiologic technologist** is an allied health professional who works under the direction of a radiologist.

Responsibilities: A radiologic technologist prepares patients for X-ray examination; takes and develops X-rays; and assists with other imaging procedures, such as ultrasound scanning and MRIs. Radiologic technologists also prepare radiation therapy for patients who have cancer.

Credentials: A radiologic technologist usually has an associate's or bachelor's degree in radiologic technology and a state license.

A **recreational therapist** is a health care professional who plans and directs medically approved recreational activities.

Responsibilities: A recreational therapist uses recreational activities to help patients maintain physical, emotional, and mental well-being. (S)he instructs patients in relaxation techniques to reduce stress and tension.

Credentials: A recreational therapist must have an associate's or bachelor's degree in recreational therapy. (S)he may need a state license or other certification.

A **registered nurse (RN)** is a nurse who is certified for general practice or for one or more of several nurse specialties.

Responsibilities: A registered nurse monitors patients and records symptoms, assists physicians during examinations and treatments, administers medications, and assists in the recovery and rehabilitation of patients. (S)he also provides emotional care for patients and their families.

Credentials: A registered nurse must have a degree from an accredited nursing school and both a national and state license. Nurses who want to specialize to be clinical nurse specialists, nurse practitioners, or nurse anesthetists must have additional training.

A **social worker** is a person who helps people with a wide range of social problems.

Responsibilities: A social worker investigates, treats, and gives aid to people who have social problems, such as such as mental illness, lack of job skills, serious health conditions, financial difficulties, disability, substance abuse problems, child or domestic abuse, and unwanted pregnancy.

Credentials: A social worker must have a master's degree in social work (MSW) and a state license.

A **school psychologist** is a psychologist who works with students, parents, school personnel, and teachers to solve learning and behavioral problems.

Responsibilities: A school psychologist tests students' intellectual, emotional, and behavioral skills. (S)he works with students who have disabilities or are gifted and talented. (S)he also teaches students conflict resolution skills.

Credentials: A school psychologist must have a graduate degree in psychology and a state license. (S)he must complete a one-year internship with a school psychologist.

A **speech pathologist** is an allied health professional who helps people overcome speech disorders.

Responsibilities: A speech pathologist works with people who suffer from speech and language disorders and people who have oral motor problems that cause eating and swallowing difficulties. (S)he also counsels parents or guardian and family members of these people.

Credentials: A speech pathologist must have a master's degree in speech pathology and a state license.

What to Know About
Being a Homemaker

A **homemaker** is a person who manages a home. A homemaker can be male or female, single or married, live with or without children, and have a career inside or outside the home. There often are two homemakers in a home. For example, a married couple works together to manage their home. College roommates work together to manage the space they share. At one time or another, everyone is a homemaker. How much thought have you given to the important role a homemaker plays?

Review the list of responsibilities of a homemaker. Do not blow off the role of homemaker. A homemaker plays a vital role in our society.

Match interests and abilities with the responsibilities of a homemaker. Each of a homemaker's responsibilities is extremely important. How would these responsibilities be covered if the homemaker chose not to do them? What would happen if they were left undone?

Examine the credentials of people who choose to be homemakers. What qualifications are needed to be a homemaker? For example, to plan healthful meals, a person needs to know about nutrition. To raise children, a person needs to understand how children grow and develop as well as the immunizations they require.

Investigate opportunities for obtaining credentials as a homemaker. How might a person get the skills needed to be a responsible homemaker? What high school courses are offered to help teens develop these skills? What training opportunities exist in the community? For example, the local chapter of the American Red Cross offers courses on emergency care and first aid.

Evaluate willingness and desire to be a homemaker. Not everyone enjoys being a homemaker. Different people devote different amounts of time and energy to homemaking.

Participate in activities to get firsthand experience as a homemaker. Teens should prepare to be homemakers. They can help with grocery shopping, prepare meals, and care for younger siblings. They can help their parents or guardian plan an emergency escape route from their home. Consider ways you can get firsthand experience as a homemaker.

Responsibilities of a Homemaker

- Prepare meals
- Choose family entertainment
- Provide first aid
- Purchase insurance
- Keep the home clean
- Select health care providers
- Protect against violence
- Raise children
- Plan for emergencies
- Keep family health records
- Make a budget
- Precycle and recycle
- Care for ill family members

Lesson 80

Review

Vocabulary Words

Write a separate sentence using each of the vocabulary words listed on page 584.

Objectives

1. What are seven steps to take to investigate health careers? **Objective 1**

2. What is the difference between a license for a health career and certification? **Objective 2**

3. What does it mean when a person has the designation of CHES? **Objective 2**

4. What are the responsibilities of a home-maker that promote health? **Objective 3**

5. How can teens prepare for the role of homemaker? **Objective 3**

Responsible Decision-Making

Your friend is on a diet. She tells you a dietitian recommended the number of calories and foods she should eat. She says that the dietitian's fee is low because he is not licensed or registered. You know that dietitians in your state must be licensed. Write a response to this situation.

1. Describe the situation that requires your friend to make a decision.
2. List possible decisions your friend might make.
3. Name two responsible adults with whom your friend might discuss his/her decisions.
4. Evaluate the possible consequences of your friend's decisions. Determine if each decision will lead to actions that:
   • promote health,
   • protect safety,
   • follow laws,
   • show respect for your friend and others,
   • follow the guidelines of your friend's parents and of other responsible adults,
   • demonstrate good character.
5. Decide which decision is most responsible and appropriate for your friend.
6. Tell two results your friend can expect if (s)he makes this decision.

 ## Effective Communication

Select a health career that interests you. Prepare a two-minute speech on the career that you can deliver to classmates. Include a creative opening and closing statement.

 ## Self-Directed Learning

Obtain permission from your parents or guardian to shadow a professional involved in a health career that interests you. Determine your expectations for the shadowing experi-ence. Make arrangements with a health pro-fessional in the career you selected. Complete the shadowing experience. Write a summary of the experience.

 ## Critical Thinking

What do you believe is a fair wage for a full-time homemaker with a spouse and two children? Explain how you determined this fair wage.

 ## Responsible Citizenship

With classmates, plan a Health Career Recognition Day. Invite professionals who have a health career to your class. Brainstorm ways to recognize these professionals as a group.

Unit 8

Unit Review

Review Questions

Prepare for the unit test. Review your answers for each Lesson Review in this unit. Then write answers to each of the following questions:

1. What are four forms of mass media that distribute health information? **Lesson 71**
2. Why is it important to know the credentials of people who serve as health experts on television and radio talk shows? **Lesson 71**
3. What are three community agencies that you can contact for health information? **Lesson 71**
4. What is The Consumer Bill of Rights? **Lesson 71**
5. Why are some teens vulnerable to buying useless health products? **Lesson 72**
6. Who might you call to check if there have been any past complaints about a company in your community? **Lesson 72**
7. Which federal agency recalls products that are unsafe? **Lesson 72**
8. Which federal agency should be contacted if you receive ineffective health products through the mail? **Lesson 73**
9. What kind of information is contained in Consumer Reports? **Lesson 73**
10. Why do ads for children's toys often appear during the cartoons on Saturday mornings? **Lesson 74**
11. What appeal is being used when sports figures wear clothing with a special logo? **Lesson 74**
12. Why might ads for tobacco depict people in outdoor settings? **Lesson 74**
13. What health problems are associated with being unable to manage time and money? **Lesson 75**
14. What is the purpose of time management? **Lesson 75**
15. How quickly should purchases on a credit card be paid off to avoid paying interest? **Lesson 75**
16. Why is it risky to watch violent television programs? **Lesson 76**
17. How do the lives of teens portrayed in the media differ from teens in real life? **Lesson 76**
18. What is the difference between a movie rated PG and a movie rated NC-17? **Lesson 76**
19. What services are provided by a primary care physician? **Lesson 77**
20. Where can you find a list of health care providers? **Lesson 77**
21. What is home health care? **Lesson 77**
22. Why do people buy health insurance policies? **Lesson 78**
23. Who pays the premiums for health insurance coverage provided by private insurance companies? **Lesson 78**
24. Why must people disclose information about preexisting conditions when they purchase health insurance? **Lesson 78**
25. How can you develop the healthy helper syndrome? **Lesson 79**
26. What services are provided by a volunteer center? **Lesson 79**
27. What is health advocacy? **Lesson 79**
28. What credentials does a person need to be a certified athletic trainer? **Lesson 80**
29. What credentials does a person need to be a health education teacher? **Lesson 80**
30. What are five health-related responsibilities of a homemaker? **Lesson 80**

Vocabulary Words

Number a sheet of paper from 1–10. Select the correct vocabulary word and write it next to the corresponding number. DO NOT WRITE IN THIS BOOK.

on-line	deductible
debt	credentials
volunteer	testimonial appeal
desensitization	consumer rights
walk-in surgery center	recall

1. A _____ is the condition of owing.
   Lesson 75

2. A _____ is an order to take a product off the market due to safety concerns.
   Lesson 73

3. A _____ is an advertising technique that uses a spokesperson who names the benefits of a specific product or service.
   Lesson 74

4. _____ are the qualifications a person must have to do something. **Lesson 80**

5. A _____ is a person who provides a service without pay. **Lesson 79**

6. A _____ is a facility where surgery is performed on an outpatient basis.
   Lesson 77

7. A _____ is an amount that insurance does not cover that must be paid by the individual. **Lesson 78**

8. A _____ is the effect of reacting less and less to the exposure of something.
   Lesson 76

9. _____ are the privileges that a consumer is guaranteed. **Lesson 72**

10. _____ is the interactive use of computers using telecommunication technology.
    Lesson 71

Health Literacy

Effective Communication

Write a television commercial for an imaginary product. Target the commercial to teens. Include one or more of the ten advertising appeals from Lesson 74. Share your television commercial with classmates.

Self-Directed Learning

There are many books on managing money. Choose a book from the library on money management. Review the book with a parent or guardian. Skim the book. Write a one-page summary about the contents.

Critical Thinking

Identify the television programs that have been the most popular during a certain period of time, such as the last week. What is the rating of each program? Identify the movies that have been the most popular during a certain period of time. What is the rating of each movie? How many of these TV programs and movies are rated appropriate for children and teens?

Responsible Citizenship

When a product is considered unsafe or ineffective for public use, it is recalled. Identify a product you believe should be recalled. What steps might you take to alert the manufacturer and the public about the problems with the product?

Responsible Decision-Making

You are watching a TV program on which a celebrity is being interviewed about a new weight-loss product. The celebrity claims the product represents a medical breakthrough no one else has discovered yet. You would like to lose weight. A toll-free number is shown on the screen. Write a response to this situation.

1. **Describe the situation that requires you to make a decision.**
2. **List possible decisions you might make.**
3. **Name two responsible adults with whom you might discuss your decisions.**
4. **Evaluate the possible consequences of your decisions. Determine if each decision will lead to actions that:**
   - **promote health,**
   - **protect safety,**
   - **follow laws,**
   - **show respect for yourself and others,**
   - **follow the guidelines of your parents and of other responsible adults,**
   - **demonstrate good character.**
5. **Decide which decision is most responsible and appropriate.**
6. **Tell two results you expect if you make this decision.**

Health Behavior Inventory of Life Skills

Number from 1 to 10 on a sheet of paper. Read each life skill carefully. Write YES or NO next to the same number on your paper. Each YES response indicates a life skill you practice to promote your health status. Each NO response indicates a life skill you do not practice. Plan to begin practicing these life skills.

1. **I will choose sources of health information wisely.**
2. **I will recognize my rights as a consumer.**
3. **I will take action if my consumer rights are violated.**
4. **I will evaluate advertisements.**
5. **I will make a plan to manage time and money.**
6. **I will choose healthful entertainment.**
7. **I will make responsible choices about health care providers and facilities.**
8. **I will evaluate ways to pay for health care.**
9. **I will be a health advocate by being a volunteer.**
10. **I will investigate health careers.**

Multicultural Health

Health care programs vary widely from one country to another. Select a country other than your own and research its health care system. Write a two-page summary of your findings.

Family Involvement

Watch with a parent or guardian a TV program that has characters who are teens. Afterwards, discuss with your parent or guardian how the teen characters were portrayed. Did they make responsible decisions? Did they experience negative consequences if they made wrong decisions? Did they follow family guidelines? Did they have healthful friendships?

Health Behavior Contract

Copy and complete the following health behavior contract. Evaluate your progress.
Share the results with your family.

Health Behavior Contract

1. Name_____Date_____

2. **Life Skill:** I will make a plan to manage time and money.

3. **Effects on Health Status:** Managing time wisely will help make time for family members and friends. It will help me keep from feeling stressed because I will not be over-whelmed by too many commitments. I will make time to eat healthfully and participate in physical activity. I will make time to study and to participate in school activities.

4. **Plan and Method to Record Progress:** Managing time wisely includes being organized. I will keep a calendar to organize my activities. I will design a calendar with enough space to fill in my activities. I will write down activities I have planned for the week, such as family plans and physical activities. I will write down due dates for school projects and exams. I will review my calendar with my parents or guardian.

My Calendar

5. **Evaluation:** _____
_____
_____

Environmental Health

You Can Stay Informed About Environmental Issues

Life Skill I will stay informed about environmental issues.

The **environment** is everything around a person. It includes the air people breathe, the water they drink, the food they eat, and the noise they hear. It includes Earth and everything in, on, and around Earth. Environment is an important part of people's everyday life. You need to be informed about the environment. You need to know about basic environmental issues. This lesson will make you aware of major environmental issues facing society today. You will learn about the agencies, organizations, and laws that protect the environment. You also will learn how to stay informed about environmental issues.

The Lesson Outline

What to Know About Environmental Issues

How to Stay Informed About Environmental Issues

Objectives

1. List and describe five global environmental issues.
   pages 599–600
2. Identify ways to stay informed about environmental issues.
   pages 601–602

Vocabulary Words

environment

global environmental issues

developing country

poverty

malnutrition

greenhouse effect

global warming

ozone

ozone layer

rain forest

deforestation

biodiversity

regulatory agency

Environmental Protection Agency (EPA)

pollution

Occupational Safety and Health Administration (OSHA)

National Institute for Occupational Safety and Health (NIOSH)

pollutants

extinction

habitat

What to Know About
Environmental Issues

The environment and people depend on one another. The actions that people take affect the quality of the environment. The environment affects the quality of people's lives. **Global environmental issues** are environmental concerns that can affect the quality of life of people everywhere. Four environmental issues that interest many people all over the globe are population growth, poverty and hunger, the greenhouse effect and global warming, destruction of the ozone layer, and destruction of rain forests.

Population Growth

Population growth is an important environmental issue. About 6 billion people live on Earth. Worldwide improvements in health have helped population grow. People are living longer, and fewer infants are dying. As the population grows, the demand for Earth's resources increases. Some nations that experience high population growth are not always able to produce enough food to feed all of their people. Land suitable for growing crops may be inhabited by people. Natural resources may be low. As the number of people increases, so does the demand for health services and other public services. More than two-thirds of the world's population live in developing countries in Africa, Asia, and South America. A **developing country** is a country that is working to achieve an acceptable standard of health conditions. A developed country is a country that has achieved an acceptable standard of health conditions. Most developed countries keep on working to improve conditions. Population in developing countries grows at a faster rate.

Poverty and Hunger

Poverty and hunger exist in all parts of the world. **Poverty** is a condition in which a person does not have sufficient resources to eat and live healthfully. People who are poor and hungry often have stunted growth and are more at risk for disease. Some suffer from malnutrition.

Malnutrition is a condition in which the body does not get the nutrients required for optimal health. People are more likely to be depressed, hostile, and stressed. Some scientists believe that poverty is responsible for many environmental problems faced by developing nations.

Greenhouse Effect and Global Warming

Some gases, such as carbon dioxide, trap heat near Earth's surface and prevent it from escaping into the atmosphere. The effect is similar to the warming effects of glass in a greenhouse. The glass permits light to enter but prevents heat from escaping. The **greenhouse effect** is a process by which water vapor and gases in the atmosphere absorb and reflect infrared rays and warm Earth's surfaces. Greenhouse gases such as carbon dioxide, ozone, methane, and chlorofluorocarbons (CFCs) have warmed Earth's surface during the last 100 years. **Global warming** is an increase in Earth's temperature. Global warming has caused glaciers to melt and sea levels to rise. The greenhouse effect and global warming may be affected by burning fuels that produce greenhouse gases. These fuels currently are sources of energy.

Scientists do not have all the answers yet. Some scientists are concerned that global warming will cause weather patterns to change and that flooding and droughts may become more common. Other scientists do not agree.

Destruction of the Ozone Layer

Ozone is a form of oxygen. The **ozone layer** is a protective layer of the upper atmosphere that traps ultraviolet (UV) radiation from the sun and prevents it from reaching Earth's surface. Too much UV radiation is harmful to living tissue. It can cause skin cancer, cataracts, and other health conditions and harm farms and forests. Use of certain chemicals destroys the ozone layer. These chemicals rise into the upper atmosphere when they are released into the air and destroy the ozone layer.

Chemicals That Destroy the Ozone Layer

Chlorofluorocarbons (CFCs) are a group of gases that are easy to compress and expand. CFCs are used as a propellant in aerosol sprays and as coolants in air conditioners, insulation, and refrigerators. They are a leading cause of destruction to the ozone layer.

- **Halons** are chemicals that are used in fire extinguishers.
- **Methyl chloroform** is a cleaning solvent.
- **Methyl bromide** is an agricultural pesticide.

Destruction of Rain Forests

Rain forests are located near the equator in countries of Latin America, Africa, and Asia. A **rain forest** is a hot, wet forested area that contains many species of trees, plants, and animals. Rain forests cover about 7 percent of the land on Earth. The vegetation in rain forests produces oxygen and removes carbon dioxide from the atmosphere. Rain forests provide a place for half of the world's plant and animal species to live and are a source of food, rubber, and timber. Many of the active ingredients in prescription drugs are extracted from plants in tropical rain forests.

Deforestation is the destruction of forests. Many of the world's rain forests have been destroyed in this century. In many developing countries, the forests may be cleared for agriculture. People need the land to grow food and to house their families. In some countries, people need to use the wood for fuel. Industries, such as gold mining and forestry, may take lumber and other products from the land. Change in weather patterns also has contributed to deforestation. Trees produce oxygen and absorb carbon dioxide. Deforestation causes less oxygen to be produced and less carbon dioxide to be absorbed because there are fewer trees. It can kill many species of plants and animals. This affects biodiversity. **Biodiversity** is the variety of life on Earth.

How to Stay Informed About Environmental Issues

There are many ways to stay informed about environmental issues. The media is a source of environmental information. Environmental agencies and organizations have home pages on the Internet. Radio and TV newscasts and other programs often deal with or focus on environmental issues. Many magazines and journals continually report on environmental issues.

Environmental Agencies and Organizations

Government and some nongovernment agencies and organizations are reliable sources of information about environmental issues. A number of regulatory agencies have been established to protect the environment and the general public. A **regulatory agency** is an agency that enforces laws to protect the general public.

State regulatory agencies that protect the environment often are known as departments of environmental quality or environmental protection. On the local level, a public health department is the environmental regulatory agency. Local public health departments enforce environmental standards and regulations and provide information on the environment. There also are a number of nongovernmental environmental organizations, that advocate for the environment, educate the public on environmental issues, and organize projects to improve the environment.

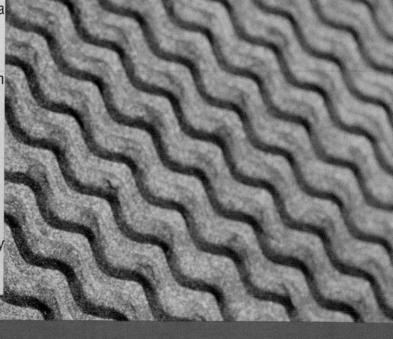

Federal Agencies That Protect the Environment

- The **Environmental Protection Agency (EPA)** is a federal regulatory agency responsible for reducing and controlling environmental pollution. **Pollution** is any change in air, water, soil, noise level, or temperature that has a negative effect on life and health. The EPA publishes information on environmental issues and regulations.

- The **Occupational Safety and Health Administration (OSHA)** is a federal regulatory agency responsible for workplace environment. It sets and enforces standards for a safe and healthy workplace.

- The **National Institute for Occupational Safety and Health (NIOSH)** is a federal regulatory agency that conducts research on health hazards in the workplace.

Eight Acts to Regulate the Environment

- The **Clean Air Act** is a law that allows the EPA to set standards for major air pollutants. **Pollutants** are harmful substances in the environment.

- The **Comprehensive Environmental Response, Compensation, and Liability Act** is a law that provides federal funding to clean up uncontrolled or hazardous waste sites and oil and chemical spills.

- The **Clean Water Act** is a law that sets regulations on wastes going into water and on the operation of waste treatment plants and makes it illegal to release pollutants into the water.

- The **Safe Drinking Water Act** is a law that protects the quality of drinking water. It also sets standards for owners and operators of public water systems.

- The **Endangered Species Act** is a law that protects animal and plant species threatened by extinction. **Extinction** is the death of all members of a species of animal or plant. The act makes it illegal to remove an endangered species from its natural habitat. A **habitat** is a place where an animal or plant normally lives.

- The **National Environmental Policy Act** is a law that requires all government agencies to consider and assess the impact on the environment before taking any action that might affect the environment.

- The **Toxic Substances Control Act** is a law that authorizes the EPA to set standards for the manufacturing, use, transportation, and disposal of toxic substances.

- The **Occupational Safety and Health Act** is a law that sets a series of minimum safety and health standards that all employers must meet.

Activity

The Earth Bank

Life Skill: I will stay informed about environmental issues.

Materials: posterboard, markers, green construction paper, scissors, pencil or pen, paper

Directions: Follow the steps to create and use an Earth Bank.

 Make a sign for an Earth Bank. Use posterboard to create a sign for a classroom Earth Bank.

 Create paper money to depict Earth's resources. Each classmate uses construction paper to make a different denomination of money to represent each of these resources: air, water, plants, animals, fossil fuels.

 Create an Earth Bank filled with paper money. Appoint a student bank president. (S)he will collect all the money to deposit in the bank.

 Decide how to use the deposited money. Each classmate lists five environmental concerns that need to be addressed.

 Decide on which resource concerns to spend money. Ask the bank president for a bill that is the denomination of money that represents the concern on which you want to spend money. Describe the action you want to take on the back of the bill.

 Return the bills to the Earth Bank president, and determine the state of the bank's resources. The bank president reads the actions to the class and determines how many of each bill were used. Brainstorm ways to conserve all the resources.

Lesson 81

Review

Vocabulary Words

Write a separate sentence using each of the vocabulary words listed on page 598.

Objectives

1. What are five global environmental issues? **Objective 1**

2. How does the ozone layer protect health? **Objective 1**

3. What are causes of deforestation? **Objective 1**

4. What are three regulatory agencies to contact to obtain environmental information? **Objective 2**

5. What are eight federal acts that regulate the environment? **Objective 2**

Responsible Decision-Making

Your classmate has just changed the oil in his/her car and does not know where to dispose of it. Another classmate suggests throwing it in the stream behind his/her house. Write a response to this situation.

1. Describe the situation that requires your classmate to make a decision.

2. List possible decisions your classmate might make.

3. Name two responsible adults with whom your classmate might discuss his/her decisions.

4. Evaluate the possible consequences of your classmate's decisions. Determine if each decision will lead to actions that:
   • promote health,
   • protect safety,
   • follow laws,
   • show respect for your classmate and others,
   • follow the guidelines of your classmates's parents and of other responsible adults,
   • demonstrate good character.

5. Decide which decision is most responsible and appropriate for your classmate.

6. Tell two results your classmate can expect if (s)he makes this decision.

 Effective Communication

Write a letter to one of the environmental agencies or organizations discussed in this lesson. Request information about the purposes and goals of the organization or agency.

 Self-Directed Learning

Locate a magazine or other periodical that contains an article on one of the environmental issues discussed in this lesson. Read the article. On an index card, write three facts that you have learned about the issue.

 Critical Thinking

Suppose you have been assigned a report on one of the major environmental issues. What sources might you go to for reliable and up-to-date information on which to base the report?

 Responsible Citizenship

Make a directory of environmental organizations in your community. List the telephone number and address of each organization. Describe the organization and its objectives. Share this directory with your classmates.

You Can Breathe Clean Air

Life Skill **I will help keep the air clean.**

Has the air outside ever smelled funny to you? Did you ever notice a haze in the sky? What you saw or smelled was probably air pollution. **Air pollution** is a contamination of the air that causes negative effects on life and health. Natural events such as dust storms, forest fires, or erupting volcanoes cause some air pollution. However, people cause most air pollution. Over the years the human population has grown. Air pollution has increased as it has grown. This lesson describes how air pollution affects your health status. You also will learn ways you can help keep the air clean.

The Lesson Outline

How Air Pollution Affects Health Status

How to Keep the Air Clean

Objectives

1. List and describe five sources of air pollution. **pages 605–607**
2. List 20 ways to help keep the air clean. **page 608**

Vocabulary Words

air pollution

atmosphere

cilia

fossil fuel

carbon monoxide

sulfur oxides

nitrogen oxides

acid rain

particulates

motor vehicle emissions

smog

thermal inversion

ozone

secondhand smoke

environmental tobacco smoke

Group A carcinogen

formaldehyde

asbestos

radon

sick building syndrome (SBS)

How Air Pollution Affects Health Status

Many things contribute to air pollution. All have an effect on health status.

How Air Pollution Harms Health Status

The quality of the air people breathe is affected when materials are released into Earth's atmosphere. The **atmosphere** is the layer of gases that surrounds Earth. Many kinds of waste substances pollute the air. These include chemicals, smoke, harmful gases, and solid particles such as soot. These harmful substances are released into the air and contribute to air pollution. Air pollution harms health status in different ways. For example, pollutants in the air can interfere with the action of cilia in the respiratory system. **Cilia** are hair-like structures that remove dust and other particles from the air. Pollutants can damage or destroy cilia. This increases the likelihood of respiratory diseases and infections such as asthma, emphysema, bronchitis, and lung cancer. Air pollution also contributes to heart disease, eye and throat irritation, and a weakened immune system. Even healthy people who exercise and stay fit can become ill in areas where air pollution is concentrated.

Sources of Air Pollution

Sources of air pollution include the following.

Fossil Fuels

A **fossil fuel** is a fuel that is formed from plant or animal remains as a result of pressure over many years. Coal, oil, gasoline, and natural gas are fossil fuels. Fossil fuels are the major sources of energy on Earth. They also are a leading source of air pollution because when they are burned they produce carbon monoxide, carbon dioxide, nitrogen oxides, sulfur oxides, and other solid substances. **Carbon monoxide** is an odorless, tasteless gas. Carbon monoxide is poisonous and reduces the ability of blood to carry oxygen to body cells. Although it is a normal part of the atmosphere, in large amounts it pollutes the air.

When fossil fuels are burned, sulfur oxides and nitrogen oxides are released into the atmosphere. **Sulfur oxides** are sulfur-containing chemicals that irritate the nose, throat, and eyes and smell like rotten eggs. **Nitrogen oxides** are nitrogen-containing chemicals that irritate the respiratory system and appear as a yellow-brown haze in the atmosphere. The combination of sulfur oxides and nitrogen oxides with water vapor in the air results in acid rain. **Acid rain** is rain or another form of precipitation that has a high acid content. Acid rain destroys plants and crops, changes the composition of water in lakes, causes fish to die, and damages buildings.

Particulates

Particulates are tiny particles in the air. Soot, ash, dirt, dust, and pollen are particulates. Particulates harm the cilia and other surfaces of the respiratory system. Very tiny particulates escape the cilia and travel deep into the lungs. This damages the lungs and can cause coughing, wheezing, asthma attacks, respiratory infections, bronchitis, and lung cancer.

Motor Vehicle Emissions

Motor vehicle emissions are substances released into the atmosphere by motor vehicles with gasoline engines. They include carbon monoxide, airborne lead, sulfur oxides, and nitrogen oxides. Inhaling motor vehicle emissions increases the risk of respiratory diseases, including lung cancer, asthma, and bronchitis.

Smog

Smog is a combination of smoke and fog. In the presence of sunlight, the water vapor in the air, motor vehicle emissions, and the smoke and particles from factories combine to form smog. Smog is a threat to the health of the elderly and to people who have respiratory illnesses. The amount of smog often is increased by thermal inversions. A **thermal inversion** is a condition that occurs when a layer of warm air forms above a layer of cool air. Air cannot circulate and pollutants are trapped in the cooler layer.

Smog contains harmful gases. Ozone is one of these gases. **Ozone** is a form of oxygen. Most ozone is found in the upper atmosphere of Earth, where it is produced naturally when sunlight reacts with oxygen. This helps protect the earth from the sun's harmful rays. However, some ozone is formed close to Earth's surface by chemical reactions between sunlight and pollutants. This ozone is a health hazard. It helps form more smog. It can irritate the eyes, lungs, and throat and produce headaches, coughing, and shortness of breath.

Indoor Air Pollution

There is air pollution indoors as well as outdoors. The concentration of pollutants may be even higher indoors because pollutants are trapped. Secondhand smoke is an indoor air pollutant. **Secondhand smoke**, or **environmental tobacco smoke**, is exhaled smoke and side-stream smoke. Secondhand smoke has been declared a Group A carcinogen by the EPA. A **Group A carcinogen** is a substance that causes cancer in humans. Breathing secondhand smoke is a major cause of lung cancer and increases the risk of respiratory infections and asthma.

Wood-burning stoves, gas appliances, unvented kerosene heaters, and poorly vented furnaces or stoves also are sources of indoor air pollution. Wood-burning stoves emit particulates, carbon monoxide, and sulfur dioxide. Faulty space heaters, furnaces, and water heaters can release carbon monoxide and cause carbon monoxide poisoning. Carbon monoxide poisoning can be fatal. Signs of carbon monoxide poisoning include headaches, nausea, vomiting, fatigue, dizziness, and unconsciousness.

Building materials can be sources of indoor air pollution. **Formaldehyde** is a colorless gas with a strong odor. Formaldehyde can be found in plywood, furniture, and other wood products. Formaldehyde also is found in insulation, cosmetics, upholstery, carpets, floor coverings, household appliances, and cigarette smoke. Breathing formaldehyde causes shortness of breath, coughing, dizziness, eye irritation, headaches, nausea, asthma attacks, and cancer.

Asbestos is a heat-resistant mineral found in many building materials. Building materials that contain asbestos may be found in many older buildings and homes, heating systems, floor and ceiling tiles, shingles, and insulation around household pipes. Asbestos fibers can get into the air. Breathing asbestos has been linked to lung and gastrointestinal cancer.

Many cleaning agents and some hobby supplies, such as glues, also release toxic fumes into the air. Inhaling toxic fumes from some cleaning agents and some types of glues can cause respiratory damage and may affect the brain.

Radon is an odorless, colorless radioactive gas that is released by rocks and soil. Radon can enter homes through cracks in the floors and basement walls and through drains and sump pumps. Many homes have unsafe radon levels. Inhaling radon increases the risk of lung cancer.

Sick building syndrome (SBS) is an illness that results from indoor air pollution. SBS is very risky for the elderly, infants, and people with asthma. Signs of SBS include headaches, irritated eyes, nausea, dizziness, drowsiness, hoarseness, and respiratory conditions. Symptoms usually disappear when people leave the building and get fresh air.

How Clean Is the Air You Breathe?

The Environmental Protection Agency (EPA) reports that six out of ten people in the United States live in areas that have excessive levels of air pollution. Almost 100 cities fail to meet air quality standards for ozone, 72 cities exceed the level for particulates, and 41 cities exceed the standard for carbon monoxide. The amount of sulfur dioxide and particulate matter in the air has decreased since 1970. However, the amount of nitrogen oxides in the air has increased.

How to Keep the Air Clean

Everyone on Earth has a responsibility to help keep the air free from pollutants and protect the atmosphere. No one should rely on others to keep the air they breathe clean.

Twenty Actions You Can Take to Keep the Air Clean

1. Do not smoke. Carbon monoxide and other chemicals from cigarette smoke pollute the air.

2. Support laws that restrict tobacco smoking in indoor areas. Make your home a smoke-free environment. If you have family members or friends who smoke, encourage them to quit.

3. Avoid driving at high speeds. Driving at high speeds burns more fuel and releases more pollutants into the atmosphere.

4. Do not leave a motor vehicle running when it is not being driven.

5. Drive a motor vehicle that gets good gas mileage and uses only unleaded gas.

6. Service your motor vehicle to keep the engine running efficiently. Keep a log book of the maintenance schedule.

7. Walk or ride a bicycle when going short distances.

8. Use public transportation whenever possible.

9. Carpool with others to school activities and other social gatherings.

10. Have your home checked for asbestos. Have any asbestos removed or sealed in place.

11. Check the radon level in your home. Home testing kits are available at hardware stores. Seal cracks in the floor and basement walls and install fans to lower the radon level.

12. Install a carbon monoxide detector in your home.

13. Check often to see that space heaters, furnaces, water heaters, or wood-burning stoves are working properly.

14. Change the filter in the furnace regularly.

15. Make sure that any wood products are sealed to eliminate formaldehyde fumes.

16. Limit the use of household cleaners that give off toxic fumes.

17. Use hobby supplies such as glues only in well-ventilated areas.

18. Use non-toxic glues and paints.

19. Do not burn trash or yard waste.

20. Plant trees whenever possible. Trees produce oxygen and absorb carbon dioxide.

Lesson 82

Review

Vocabulary Words

Write a separate sentence using each of the vocabulary words listed on page 604.

Objectives

1. What are five sources of air pollution?
   Objective 1

2. What causes outdoor air pollution?
   Objective 1

3. What causes smog? **Objective 1**

4. What are five sources of indoor air pollution? **Objective 1**

5. What are 20 actions to take to help keep the air clean? **Objective 2**

Responsible Decision-Making

You and a friend are supposed to meet to run in the park. The weather announcer on the news says that a thermal inversion has settled over your area and a cloud of smog is developing. You call your friend to tell him/her about the thermal inversion. (S)he says (s)he doesn't see any reason to cancel your plans. Write a response to this situation.

1. Describe the situation that requires your classmate to make a decision.

2. List possible decisions your classmate might make.

3. Name two responsible adults with whom your classmate might discuss his/her decisions.

4. Evaluate the possible consequences of your classmate's decisions. Determine if each decision will lead to actions that:
   - promote health,
   - protect safety,
   - follow laws,
   - show respect for your classmate and others,
   - follow the guidelines of your classmates's parents and of other responsible adults,
   - demonstrate good character.

5. Decide which decision is most responsible and appropriate for your classmate.

6. Tell two results your classmate can expect if (s)he makes this decision.

Effective Communication

Make a poster that shows different types of air pollutants. Under each type of pollutant, write a short explanation describing how it affects the environment. Ask permission to display the poster in an area where many people will see it.

Self-Directed Learning

Check the library, the Internet, or your local pharmacy to find more information on radon. What are the health effects of radon? How can it be detected? What actions can you take to avoid exposure to radon?

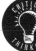

Critical Thinking

Suppose you read a newspaper editorial that says that secondhand smoke does not affect the environment. Write a response to this editorial explaining ways that secondhand smoke affects the environment.

Responsible Citizenship

Review with family members Twenty Actions You Can Take to Keep the Air Clean. Which of these suggestions does your family follow? Which of these suggestions does your family ignore? Suggest that family members follow all of the suggestions.

You Can Have Safe Water

Life Skill I will help keep the water safe.

Two-thirds of Earth is covered by water. About 97 percent of the water supply is salt water. More than 2 percent is frozen in icecaps and glaciers. Less than 1 percent of the water on Earth is fresh water. **Fresh water** is water that is not contaminated or salty. People need clean, fresh water to live. People use water to drink, prepare food, and bathe and for many other personal purposes. People also use water for industrial purposes and to generate power and irrigate crops. The fresh water we use comes from lakes, streams, rivers, reservoirs, and wells. We need to conserve this water and keep it clean and safe. This lesson focuses on how water pollution affects health status. You will learn ways to keep water clean and safe.

The Lesson Outline

How Water Pollution Affects Health Status

How to Keep Water Safe

Objectives

1. List and discuss water pollutants and ways water pollution affects health status. **pages 611–612**
2. List 15 ways to help keep the water safe. **pages 613–614**

Vocabulary Words

fresh water

water pollution

water runoff

PCBs

dioxins

eutrophication

sediments

low-level radioactive waste

thermal pollution

trihalomethanes

giardia lamblia

giardiasis

dysentery

Clean Water Act (CWA)

Safe Drinking Water Act (SDWA)

biodegradable product

How Water Pollution Affects Health Status

Water is necessary for life. You would die within a few days if you did not drink water. **Water pollution** is contamination of water that causes negative effects on life and health. Water is contaminated in many ways. Contamination may be caused by chemicals, radioactive wastes, sewage, and other substances dumped or accidentally spilled directly into or near sources of fresh water.

When pollutants are dumped near water sources, they enter the water source as water runoff. **Water runoff** is water that runs off the land into a body of water. When snow melts, it rains, or people water lawns, parks, or crops, some of the water is absorbed. The rest of the water flows along the surface of the land until it reaches a river, stream, or lake. Some of the water runoff soaks into the ground until it reaches an underground stream known as groundwater. As the water runoff flows, it picks up pollutants dumped into the environment and carries them to fresh water supplies. There are many different kinds of pollutants, including toxic chemicals, fertilizers, sediments, and radioactive waste.

Toxic Chemicals

Toxic chemicals, such as cleaning agents, paints, pesticides, weed killers, solvents, and oil often find their way into streams, rivers, and lakes. Factories and industries may dump or release them into bodies of water or they may result from water runoff. These chemicals can kill plants, fish, and other animals. Humans who eat contaminated fish may become ill.

PCBs are chemicals that contain chlorine. They are used in insulation and to manufacture products such as plastics. PCBs can be released from manufacturing plants or when electrical equipment at dumpsites breaks open. When PCBs are in the body, they collect in fatty tissues and in the liver. People who drink water that contains PCBs are at risk for birth defects, reproductive disorders, liver and kidney damage, and cancer.

Dioxins are a group of chemicals used in insecticides. Small amounts of dioxins are produced naturally by forest fires and volcanic eruptions. Paper mills also produce dioxins as a result of bleaching pulp and paper. Dioxins often are found in fish that live downstream from paper mills. People who eat these fish can become ill.

Lead can enter the water supply from lead pipes and water lines in older houses. Lead affects most body systems. The most sensitive body system is the central nervous system, particularly in children. Lead can damage nerve cells. Lead also damages the kidneys and the immune system. The effects of lead are the same whether it is breathed or swallowed.

Fertilizers

When fertilizers enter natural waterways, they cause an overgrowth of algae and other plant life. The balance between plants and animals is disrupted by eutrophication. **Eutrophication** (yoo·TROH·fik·a·shun) is the build-up of nutrients in water that causes an overgrowth of plants that use up oxygen. As a result, much of the animal life dies.

Sediments

Sediments are suspended solids that settle to the bottom of waterways. As sediments fill lakes and streams, they destroy the feeding grounds of fish and other animals. The rapid construction of homes, streets, office buildings, and malls has contributed to the problem of sediments. Large-scale construction also has caused erosion in many areas. Areas that are covered with cement and asphalt cannot absorb rainwater.

Radioactive Waste

Low-level radioactive waste is any radioactive by-product from such activities as nuclear research and the development of nuclear medicines. Low-level radioactive waste can pollute water and affect plants, fish, and other animals.

Thermal Pollution

Water is used to cool machinery in many factories, power plants, and nuclear reactors. In the cooling process, this water is heated. When it is returned to the water supply, thermal pollution can result. **Thermal pollution** is a harmful condition caused by the addition of heated water to a water supply. The temperature of the water supply is raised which can cause oxygen levels in water to decrease. As a result, many plants and animals die.

Trihalomethanes

Trihalomethanes are harmful chemicals that are produced when chlorine attacks pollutants in water. Most water treatment systems use chlorine to purify water. Drinking water that contains trihalomethanes is dangerous. Trihalomethanes increase the risk of certain cancers, birth defects, and disorders of the central nervous system.

Microorganisms

Microorganisms such as parasites and bacteria may enter water supplies from human or animal sewage. The improper operation of a septic tank or the failure of a waste treatment plant to properly treat sewage can be the source of microorganism contamination. Microorganism contamination can cause illness.

One microorganism that occasionally gets into water systems is *Giardia lamblia*. **Giardia lamblia** is a parasite that lives in the intestines of humans and other mammals and causes giardiasis. **Giardiasis** (jee·ar·dee·AH·sis) is a stomach and intestinal infection that causes abdominal cramps, nausea, gas, and diarrhea. **Dysentery** is a severe infection of the intestines, causing diarrhea and abdominal pain.

Millions of people in developing countries become sick each year from microorganisms. In many developed countries, the public is alerted at once if the water supply is found to contain microorganisms. Beaches may be closed and people advised to boil water to eliminate microorganisms. Water contamination often is the result of natural disasters, such as earthquakes and floods. Contamination also can occur when heavy rains interfere with waste treatment.

How to Keep Water Safe

Steps have been taken to reduce water pollution. The Environmental Protection Agency (EPA) requires public suppliers to notify people if water does not meet safety standards or if required monitoring has not taken place. The **Clean Water Act (CWA)** is a law that sets regulations on wastes going into water and the operation of waste treatment plants. This act makes it illegal to release pollutants into the water. The **Safe Drinking Water Act (SDWA)** is a law that protects the quality of drinking water. This law sets standards for owners and operators of public water systems. Laws enacted by local governments also help protect people from water pollution. New methods being used by manufacturers and companies have helped promote a reduction in water pollution.

Water Use at Home

The water you use in your home comes from either a ground-water souce, such as well, or from a surface-water source, such as a lake or reservoir. After water is used at home, it usually goes into a septic tank in the backyard or is returned to a sewage-treatment plant through a sewer system. The average person uses about 80–100 gallons of water per day. The average water use for one person each day is:

- Toilets   35 gallons
- Baths and showers   28 gallons
- Clothes washing   18 gallons
- Faucets   13 gallons
- Dishwashing   3 gallons

Check Your Water

Drinking water from a faucet might be contaminated if it has an unusual odor or an orange, red, or brown appearance. Contact the local public health department or water company to have it tested. Until you are assured it is safe, drink bottled water. Water treatment systems such as water filters are available. Evaluate these systems carefully to be sure they work effectively before purchasing them.

Bottled Water vs. Tap Water

Is bottled water safer than tap water? Perhaps not. The FDA sets standards for bottled waters almost identical to those for tap water. Labels on bottled water must carry a list of minerals for the water.

Caution:
Outdoor Water Safety Hazards

Water from streams or ponds may look, smell, and taste clean. However, this water may be contaminated. Do not drink water of unknown safety. Carry your own bottled water or boil water for ten minutes before using it for drinking or cooking.

Hard Water vs. Soft Water

Water is said to be "soft" if it has a low concentration of calcium and magnesium in it. Water is said to be "hard" if it has a higher concentration of calcium and magnesium. Hard water is more difficult to wash off.

Ways to Help Keep the Water Safe

You might think that personal and individual habits and activities have little impact on the quality of the water. However, each person has a great influence on the quality of the water that is available where (s)he lives. The following are ways to help keep the water safe.

Fifteen Ways to Help Keep the Water Safe

1. Do not pour toxic chemicals down the drain or in the toilet. Dispose of them at hazardous waste collection centers.

2. Do not pour toxic chemicals on the ground. These substances can contaminate ground water supplies in water runoff.

3. Use phosphate-free detergents and biodegradable soaps and shampoos. A **biodegradable product** is a product that can be broken down by living organisms into harmless and useable materials.

4. Let water run for at least 30 seconds when first turned on. Water in the pipes may collect lead. Or, boil water for ten minutes.

5. Pump out septic tanks once a year.

6. Support community efforts to clean up rivers, lakes, and streams and to preserve wetlands.

7. Support local and state legislation to control water pollution.

8. Do not dump garbage or toxic chemicals into lakes, streams, rivers, ponds, storm sewers, or ditches.

9. Do not dispose of plastics, such as plastic cups and bags, in waterways.

10. Select yard plants that require little or no fertilizer.

11. Plant trees and shrubs to discourage water runoff and soil erosion.

12. Convert yard trimmings into compost. As plant materials decay, they can be used as a soil conditioner, gradually releasing nutrients to a lawn or garden. This allows less fertilizer to be used.

13. Contact the public health department or water company if water from a faucet has an unusual appearance, smell, or taste. It could be contaminated. Use bottled water until water is tested and pronounced safe to drink.

14. Follow the recommendations of the public health department or water company in regards to drinking water.

15. Test drinking water for lead contamination if the presence of lead is suspected.

Lesson 83

Review

Vocabulary Words

Write a separate sentence using each of the vocabulary words listed on page 610.

Objectives

1. What are five ways water may be polluted? **Objective 1**

2. What are three toxic chemical that may pollute water? **Objective 1**

3. What are two acts that protect water? **Objective 2**

4. What happens to water after it is used at home? **Objective 2**

5. What are 15 ways to help keep the water safe? **Objective 2**

Responsible Decision-Making

You are mountain biking with a friend and you stop for water. Your friend dips his/her canteen into a stream and takes a drink. (S)he offers you a drink. Write a response to this situation.

1. Describe the situation that requires you to make a decision.

2. List possible decisions you might make.

3. Name two responsible adults with whom you might discuss your decisions.

4. Evaluate the possible consequences of your decisions. Determine if each decision will lead to actions that:
   • promote health,
   • protect safety,
   • follow laws,
   • show respect for yourself and others,
   • follow the guidelines of your parents and of other responsible adults,
   • demonstrate good character.

5. Decide which decision is most responsible and appropriate.

6. Tell two results you expect if you make this decision.

 ### Effective Communication

Design a pamphlet that warns about the dangers of water runoff. Explain how water runoff can carry toxic chemicals into the water supply.

 ### Self-Directed Learning

Contact your local wastewater treatment plant or water treatment facility. Find out how water is treated in your community.

 ### Critical Thinking

Suppose you go fishing in a stream near a factory. Why shouldn't you eat any fish that you catch?

 ### Responsible Citizenship

Review the list of ways to help keep the water safe. Which of these suggestions does your family follow? Which of these suggestions does your family ignore? Make a copy of the list and give it to your family members. Suggest that family members try to follow all suggestions in the list.

You Can Keep Noise at a Safe Level

Life Skill **I will help keep noise at a safe level.**

Do you like to play your stereo or boombox? How do family members react to the volume of your stereo or boombox? Stereos and boomboxes fill the air with sounds. Sounds can be a source of relaxation and pleasure. Sounds also can be a source of noise. **Noise** is a sound that produces discomfort or annoyance. Noise can cause health problems and is a leading pollutant of the environment. This lesson explains ways to recognize how noise affects health status. You will learn clues that alert you that a sound may be too loud. You also will learn what actions you can take to keep noise at a safe level.

The Lesson Outline

How Noise Affects Health Status

How to Keep Noise at a Safe Level

Objectives

1. Explain how noise affects health status. **page 617**
2. List and discuss ways to keep noise at a safe level. **page 618**

Vocabulary Words

noise

sound waves

pitch

amplitude

decibel (dB)

noise pollution

general adaptation syndrome (GAS)

acoustic trauma

temporary threshold shift (TTS)

sound frequency

noise-induced permanent threshold shift

tinnitus

How Noise Affects Health Status

The sounds people hear are produced by sound waves. **Sound waves** are vibrations or movements of air. When someone beats a drum, the drum vibrates and moves the air around and creates sound waves that reach people's ears. Different types of sound waves produce sounds at a different pitch. **Pitch** is the highness or lowness of sound. Some sounds have a high pitch, such as a whistle. Other sounds have a low pitch, such as a motor vehicle engine. Sounds have different amplitudes. **Amplitude** is the loudness of a sound. A **decibel (dB)** is a unit used to measure the loudness of sounds. Sounds that measure more than 70 dBs pollute the environment.

Noise pollution is a loud or constant noise that causes hearing loss, stress, fatigue, irritability, and tension. It is a stressor that can affect health status. The body responds to noise pollution as a threat and goes through the general adaptation syndrome (GAS). The **general adaptation syndrome (GAS)** is a series of body changes that result from stress. Prolonged exposure to noise pollution can cause ulcers, headaches, and high blood pressure. Noise pollution also can cause accidents by preventing people from hearing warnings and interfering with ability to concentrate and perform. It also can cause sleeplessness, increase irritability, and provoke violent reactions. Prolonged noise pollution can cause hearing loss.

According to OSHA, daily exposure of eight hours or more to noise levels averaging over 85 dBs will result in hearing loss. Noise below 85 decibels also can damage hearing, but it will take longer. Noises above 120 dBs can cause immediate and permanent hearing damage. An **acoustic trauma** is an immediate and permanent loss of hearing caused by a short, intense sound.

Exposure to loud noises may cause people's ears to ring or feel full. This ringing sensation or full feeling is a symptom of temporary threshold shift. **Temporary threshold shift (TTS)** is the temporary hearing loss of certain frequencies and amplifications. A **sound frequency** is the number of sound waves produced per minute.

Noise-induced permanent threshold shift is a permanent loss of the ability to hear certain frequencies and amplifications. Hearing becomes muffled and tinnitus may develop. **Tinnitus** (TEYE·nuh·tuhs) is a ringing, buzzing, or hissing sensation in the ears that can reach levels equivalent to 70 dBs. Tinnitus can affect concentration, be a source of great frustration, and interfere with ability to sleep, hold a conversation, and learn.

Noises That Can Cause Permanent Hearing Loss After Eight Hours		Noises That Can Cause Immediate and Permanent Hearing Loss	
Sound	dBs	Sound	dBs
Vacuum	85	Jackhammer (3 ft away)	120
Power lawnmower	85	Earphones on loud	125
City traffic	90	Rock music (maximum)	130
Motorcycle	90	Rivet gun	130
Garbage truck	100	Jet engine (100 ft away)	135
Chain saw	100	Air raid siren	140
Car horn	110	Gun shot	140
Boom stereo in car	115	Rocket launch site	180

Adapted from Association of Hearing Aid Audiologists

How to Keep Noise at a Safe Level

Everyone should be aware which sounds are and are not safe so they can keep noise at a safe level. Many teens listen to music through earphones. Through the earphones, the sounds to which they are listening often exceed safety limits and can cause permanent hearing loss. Rock concerts and personal sound systems also can cause hearing loss. For example, kicker stereos can reach 145 dBs, which is louder than a jet engine.

Recognizing Clues That a Sound Is Too Loud

A sound is unsafe if:

1. You must raise your voice to be heard
2. You cannot hear someone less than two feet (60 centimeters) away
3. You experience pain or ringing in your ears
4. You feel unsteady, dizzy, or nauseated in the presence of the sound or when the sound stops
5. Sounds are muffled when the sound stops
6. Other people can hear your headset or earphones when you wear them

Eight Ways to Avoid Noise Pollution

1. **Keep the volume of radios, compact disc players, stereos, and TVs at safe levels.** Reduce the sound level if it is too loud. Set the volume so that you can carry on a normal conversation.

2. **Avoid listening to music through headphones or headsets at unsafe levels.** Headphones and headsets cover your ears. They produce sounds that immediately reach the ears and can cause hearing loss.

3. **Wear protective earplugs when operating loud machinery or using power tools.** You can purchase earplugs made from foam, rubber, silicone, and wax in most drugstores. Earplugs used to protect hearing are not the same as earplugs designed for swimming.

4. **Wear protective earplugs when attending concerts.** Many music performers wear earplugs to protect their hearing when they perform.

5. **Use your fingers to protect your ears if you do not have earplugs.** You can press your fingers against your ears to temporarily protect them from sounds that are too loud.

6. **Distance yourself from loud sounds if you cannot avoid exposure and do not have earplugs.** Sit at a safe distance from performers and speakers when attending a concert. Objects between you and the sound help reduce the intensity. Conversation only adds to noise levels and can cause stress.

7. **Be considerate of others.** Be aware of the sounds you produce and the effects they can have on others, including on pets. Many people will not tolerate noise. This could lead to legal warnings or penalties. For example, people might call the police if someone is having a party and making too much noise.

8. **Avoid drinking alcohol.** Drinking alcohol intensifies the impact of noise.

Lesson 84

Review

Vocabulary Words

Write a separate sentence using each of the vocabulary words listed on page 616.

Objectives

1. What are ways that noise affects health status? **Objective 1**

2. What is noise pollution? **Objective 1**

3. What are ten causes of noise pollution? **Objective 1**

4. What are six clues that a sound is too loud? **Objective 2**

5. What are eight ways to avoid noise pollution? **Objective 2**

Responsible Decision-Making

Your friends invite you to a concert. Your parents or guardian insist that you wear earplugs. You take the earplugs to the concert. However, you are nervous about using them because you think your friends will make fun of you. Write a response to this situation.

1. Describe the situation that requires you to make a decision.

2. List possible decisions you might make.

3. Name two responsible adults with whom you might discuss your decisions.

4. Evaluate the possible consequences of your decisions. Determine if each decision will lead to actions that:
   • promote health,
   • protect safety,
   • follow laws,
   • show respect for yourself and others,
   • follow the guidelines of your parents and of other responsible adults,
   • demonstrate good character.

5. Decide which decision is most responsible and appropriate.

6. Tell two results you expect if you make this decision.

 ### Effective Communication

Design a poster that shows the decibel levels of sounds in your environment. Include a graphic or picture to illustrate each sound you show. Obtain permission to display the poster in a place where other teens will see it.

 ### Self-Directed Learning

Keep a journal for two days. List noises to which you are exposed. Describe how you felt each time you were exposed to a noise. Consider ways you can protect yourself from noise pollution.

 ### Critical Thinking

Your friend always blasts the radio when you ride in his/her car. (S)he tries to talk over the music and never turns it down. When you get out of the car, your ears are ringing. What might you say to your friend to convince him/her to turn down the volume?

 ### Responsible Citizenship

Evaluate your sound-producing habits. Do you produce sounds that disturb or annoy others? What are these sounds? List actions you can take to improve your sound-producing habits.

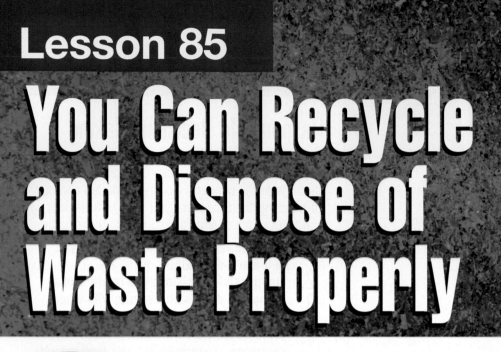

Lesson 85

You Can Recycle and Dispose of Waste Properly

Life Skill **I will precycle, recycle, and dispose of waste properly.**

Do you and your family members use paper products almost every-day? How much food gets thrown away in your house? Consider this— each person in the United States throws away an average of four pounds (1.8 kilograms) of solid waste every day. **Solid waste** is discarded solid materials, such as paper, metals, plastics, glass, leather, wood, rubber, textiles, food, and yard waste. Most solid waste is dumped in landfills. A **landfill** is a place where waste is dumped in layers and buried. This lesson focuses on the issue of waste. Some waste can be precycled or recycled. You will learn ways to precycle and recycle. You also will learn ways to dispose of waste properly.

The Lesson Outline

How to Precycle and Recycle

How to Dispose of Waste

Objectives

1. List and discuss ten tips for precycling. **page 621**
2. List six materials that are commonly recycled. **page 621**
3. List and discuss four ways to dispose of waste. **page 622**

Vocabulary Words

solid waste

landfill

precycling

recycling

sanitary landfill

secure landfill

leachate

incinerator

bio-hazardous waste

medical waste

compost

composting

humus

mulching mower

deep-injection well

hazardous waste

How to
Precycle and Recycle

Solid waste is a problem that affects many parts of the environment. It pollutes the air, water, and soil. The landfills where solid wastes are dumped take up space and can contaminate water supplies and pollute the air.

How To Precycle

Some solid wastes can be precycled. **Precycling** is a process of reducing waste. It includes purchasing products in packages or containers that have been or can be broken down and used again, purchasing products that have little packaging, and repairing existing products rather than throwing them out and buying new ones.

Ten Tips for Precycling

1. Do not purchase paper items not made from paper that has been broken down and used more than once.

2. Do not purchase beverages not in returnable or refillable containers or containers made of materials that can be broken down and used more than once.

3. Do not use disposable diapers made of plastic, paper, or some other throw away material.

4. Do not use just one side of a sheet of paper.

5. Do not use paper napkins or paper towels to dry the hands.

6. Do not use plastic wrap or aluminum foil.

7. Avoid purchasing food items in single-serving containers.

8. Do not purchase nonbiodegradable products.

9. Do not buy items that have a lot of packaging.

10. Do not use plastic or paper bags.

How to Recycle

Some solid wastes can be recycled. **Recycling** is the process of re-forming or breaking down a waste product so that it can be used again. Recycling can help reduce the amount of solid waste in landfills and the pollution caused by wastes that are nonbiodegradable. Nonbiodegradable waste cannot be broken down by natural processes and can last for hundreds of years. Plastics, aluminum cans, and glass are nonbiodegradable wastes. Waste that is biodegradable can be broken down by living organisms such as foods and certain paper products. Recycling is not always appropriate. However, when it is, it can help conserve natural resources because it reduces the need for raw materials. Recycling involves collecting reusable material, processing and marketing it, and reusing it for a new product. Many communities have recycling programs or centers. Recycling can help reduce the amount of raw materials, energy, and water used and cut down the amount of air pollution created by normal processing.

Six Commonly Recycled Materials

- Paper
- Glass
- Used petroleum products
- Yard trimmings
- Plastics
- Aluminum and other metals

What Is In Our Trash?

National averages show that our trash is:

- 38 percent paper products
- 18 percent yard waste
- 8 percent metals
- 8 percent plastics
- 7 percent glass
- 7 percent food waste
- 14 percent other (leather, wood, textiles, rubber)

Municipal and Industrial Solid Waste Division, EPA Office of Solid Waste Management, Washington, D.C.

How to
Dispose of Waste

Individuals, families, industries, businesses, and farms all produce a huge amount of waste. This waste can be disposed of in several different ways.

Ways to Dispose of Waste

1. Landfills

There are two types of landfills. A **sanitary landfill** is a waste disposal land site where solid waste is spread in thin layers, compacted, and covered with a fresh layer of dirt daily. The dirt contains bacteria to help break down the organic material in the garbage. A **secure landfill** is a landfill that has protective liners to reduce or prevent leachate from escaping through water runoff. **Leachate** (LEECH·ayte) is the liquid that drains from a landfill. Hazardous wastes and nonbiodegradable materials should not be sent to a landfill.

2. Incineration

An **incinerator** is a furnace in which solid waste is burned and energy is recovered in the process. Incinerators reduce the volume of solid waste but can release pollutants into the atmosphere. Some incinerators use the heat produced by burning to create steam that provides electricity. Most bio-hazardous waste, or medical waste, is incinerated. **Bio-hazardous waste**, or **medical waste**, is infectious waste from medical facilities. It includes syringes, needles, tubes, blood vials, and other items that can contain tissues and body fluids from a person or animal.

3. Composting

Compost (KAHM·post) is a mixture of decayed organic material generally used to fertilize and condition the soil. **Composting** is the breakdown by bacteria of plant remains to humus. **Humus** (HYOO·mus) is a soil conditioner. In some communities, yard waste is separated from other kinds of waste and transported to compost landfills. Many individuals have their own compost piles. Food wastes such as meat and eggs should not be composted because they will attract flies and rodents. The use of mulching mowers helps reduce yard waste and serves as a natural fertilizer. A **mulching mower** is a lawn mower that cuts the grass into small pieces that can be left on a lawn to decompose naturally.

4. Deep-injection wells

A **deep-injection well** is a well that pumps waste into porous rock far below the level of groundwater. Hazardous wastes may be disposed of in deep-injection wells. **Hazardous waste** is any solid, liquid, or gas in a container that is harmful to humans or animal life. Hazardous waste includes paints, solvents, cleaners, acids, alkalis, pesticides, petroleum products such as gasoline and motor oil, and other toxic chemicals. The disposal of hazardous waste is very important to environmental health. Hazardous waste can leach out of landfills and escape into the environment. Hazard waste cannot be incinerated because it might cause an explosion.

Lesson 85

Review

Vocabulary Words

Write a separate sentence using each of the vocabulary words listed on page 620.

Objectives

1. What are ten tips for precycling? **Objective 1**

2. What are six materials you can recycle? **Objective 2**

3. What is the difference between wastes that are nonbiodegradable and wastes that are biodegradable? **Objective 2**

4. What are four ways to dispose of waste? **Objective 3**

5. What is the difference between a sanitary landfill and a secure landfill? **Objective 3**

Responsible Decision-Making

You go to the beach with your family. As you prepare to swim, you see a syringe lying in the sand. Your sibling already is in the water and calls you to join him/her. Write a response to this situation.

1. Describe the situation that requires you to make a decision.
2. List possible decisions you might make.
3. Name two responsible adults with whom you might discuss your decisions.
4. Evaluate the possible consequences of your decisions. Determine if each decision will lead to actions that:
   - promote health,
   - protect safety,
   - follow laws,
   - show respect for yourself and others,
   - follow the guidelines of your parents and of other responsible adults,
   - demonstrate good character.
5. Decide which decision is most responsible and appropriate.
6. Tell two results you expect if you make this decision.

 Effective Communication

Prepare a 30-second public service announcement (PSA) encouraging people in your community to precycle and recycle. Record your announcement and send the tape to a local radio station.

 Self-Directed Learning

Investigate how your community recycles different materials and disposes of wastes. To locate information, you might contact the recycling center, hazardous waste collection center, or landfill site in your community.

 Critical Thinking

Suppose your sibling paints his/her bedroom. (S)he finishes the job, and there is paint left over. Your sibling is going to pour it down the drain. Why shouldn't (s)he pour the paint down the drain? How should (s)he dispose of the paint?

 Responsible Citizenship

Evaluate your family's precycling and recycling habits and how you dispose of waste. Do you precycle and recycle when appropriate? Do you dispose of solid waste properly? What changes might you make to precycle, recycle, and dispose of waste more efficiently?

You Can Conserve Energy and Natural Resources

Life Skill ▶ **I will help conserve energy and natural resources.**

Energy and natural resources are an important part of the environment. A **natural resource** is anything obtained from the natural environment to meet people's needs. To protect the environment, natural resources must be conserved. **Conservation** is the saving of resources. Your actions can have an impact on resources. This lesson teaches you about the different types of energy and natural resources that exist in the environment. You will learn how to conserve natural resources and energy.

The Lesson Outline

What to Know About Energy and Natural Resources

How to Conserve Energy and Natural Resources

Objectives

1. List and describe sources of energy. **page 625**
2. List 20 ways to conserve energy. **page 626**
3. List ten ways to conserve water. **page 626**

Vocabulary Words

natural resource

conservation

energy

law of conservation of energy

fossil fuel

coal

petroleum

crude oil

oil refinery

natural gas

nuclear energy

uranium

nuclear reactor

hydroelectric power

turbine

solar energy

biomass

bagasse

gasohol

geothermal energy

wind energy

hydrogen power

What to Know About Energy and Natural Resources

Energy is the ability to do work. The **law of conservation of energy** is a scientific theory that says that energy cannot be created or destroyed but can be changed in form. For example, plants use light energy to combine water and carbon dioxide to form sugar. The sugar in plants provides energy for animals and people. Plants are a natural resource that people use for food. There are a variety of resources that are sources of energy.

Fossil Fuels

A **fossil fuel** is a fuel that is formed from plant or animal remains as a result of pressure over many years.

- **Coal** is a black or brown solid that contains stored energy formed from decayed plant. It is the most abundant fossil fuel in the United States.

- **Petroleum**, or **crude oil**, is a black liquid energy source that is trapped in rock beneath Earth's surface. It is removed by drilling wells and pumping the oil through pipelines to tankers or oil refineries. An **oil refinery** is a processing plant that produces gasoline, heating oil, diesel oil, or asphalt from petroleum. Oil also is used to produce fertilizers, pesticides, plastics, synthetic materials, paint, and medical products. After coal, oil is the cheapest fuel.

- **Natural gas** is an energy source that is found underground above deposits of oil. Methane, propane, and butane are types of natural gas. Natural gas is the cleanest burning fossil fuel.

Other Sources of Energy

There are other sources of energy besides fossil fuels.

- **Nuclear energy** is energy produced by splitting atoms of uranium into smaller parts. **Uranium** is a radioactive substance that is mined. It is used to power nuclear reactors and produces a large amount of electrical power. A **nuclear reactor** is a device that splits atoms to produce steam. The steam is used to generate electricity. Nuclear energy is one of the more expensive sources of energy.

- **Hydroelectric power** is electricity generated from flowing or falling water. Dams are built to store water and direct its flow through turbines. A **turbine** is an engine that rotates. Hydroelectric power is an inexpensive source of energy.

- **Solar energy** is the energy of the sun. Solar energy can be converted into electrical energy or heat. Currently the costs of solar energy systems are high. However, solar energy could prove to be an almost unlimited source of power.

- **Biomass** is organic plant matter produced by solar energy. It includes wood, sewage, agricultural wastes, and algae. All of these can be used as sources of energy when they are burned. Bagasse is a biomass source of energy. **Bagasse** is a fibrous waste produced during the processing of sugar cane. Gasohol also is a biomass. **Gasohol** is a blend of grain alcohol and gasoline that is used as a fuel source.

- **Geothermal energy** is heat transferred from underground sources of steam or hot water. It can be used to heat homes, produce electricity, and power industrial plants.

- **Wind energy** is energy from wind. Wind turbines change wind energy to electricity.

- **Hydrogen power** is energy produced by passing electrical current through water to burn the hydrogen. Hydrogen yields a high amount of energy.

How to Conserve Energy and Natural Resources

Most people take energy for granted. They do not always realize how much energy they use. They do not always know how much they waste. They can conserve energy by developing habits that use less energy and by using energy-saving devices.

Twenty Ways to Conserve Energy Supplied by Natural Resources

1. Turn off lights when leaving a room.
2. Use fluorescent lights except for reading.
3. Use lamps when reading.
4. Use light bulbs with a low wattage except when reading.
5. Turn off electrical appliances such as TVs, stereos, and radios when not in use.
6. Use manual instead of electrical appliances.
7. Use rechargeable instead of disposable batteries.
8. Use fans instead of air conditioning.
9. Plant fast-growing trees near a home to keep it cooler.
10. Wear an additional layer of warm clothing in cold weather instead of turning up the heat.
11. Install weather stripping around windows and seal air leaks around doors to prevent heat loss.
12. Turn down the thermostat at night and when away from home.
13. Conserve the amount of hot water used for showers or baths.
14. Dry clothes in warm weather on a clothesline.
15. Purchase energy-efficient products for the home.
16. Try to use a motor vehicle that gets 30 miles (48 kilometers) or more per gallon of gas.
17. Carpool or use public transportation.
18. Ride a bike to save fuel whenever possible.
19. Walk instead of driving a motor vehicle whenever possible.
20. Service the furnace once a year and replace filters frequently.

Ten Ways to Conserve Water

Water is necessary for all forms of life to survive. Ten ways people can conserve water are:

1. Install a low-flow shower head to reduce the amount of water used in showering
2. Take shorter showers
3. Take a shower instead of a bath
4. Check faucets and pipes for leaks
5. Run a washing machine only for a full load of clothes
6. Do not allow water to run while washing and rinsing dishes
7. Run a dishwasher only for a full load
8. Water the lawn only at the coolest time of the day and do not let the water run for long periods of time
9. Plant trees in a yard because they store water and release it into the ground
10. Keep drinking water in the refrigerator instead of allowing tap water to run until it is cool enough to drink

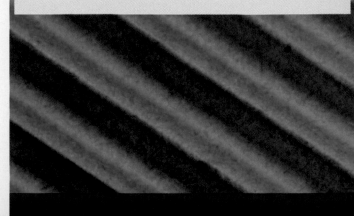

Lesson 86

Review

Vocabulary Words

Write a separate sentence using each of the vocabulary words listed on page 624.

Objectives

1. What are ten sources of energy?
   Objective 1
2. What are fossil fuels? **Objective 1**
3. What are two examples of biomass?
   Objective 1
4. What are ten ways to conserve energy?
   Objective 2
5. What are ten ways to conserve water?
   Objective 3

Responsible Decision-Making

Suppose you usually drive to school alone. Two of your neighbors have cars as well, and suggest that you ride to school together. They say that you can take turns driving. Write a response to this situation.

1. Describe the situation that requires you to make a decision.
2. List possible decisions you might make.
3. Name two responsible adults with whom you might discuss your decisions.
4. Evaluate the possible consequences of your decisions. Determine if each decision will lead to actions that:
   - promote health,
   - protect safety,
   - follow laws,
   - show respect for yourself and others,
   - follow the guidelines of your parents and of other responsible adults,
   - demonstrate good character.
5. Decide which decision is most responsible and appropriate.
6. Tell two results you expect if you make this decision.

 Effective Communication

Make a sign to remind yourself and other family members to turn off the lights and turn down the thermostat when you leave. Hang the sign in a place where family members will see it.

 Self-Directed Learning

Obtain permission from a parent or guardian to visit a power plant in your community. You might visit an oil refinery, a hydroelectric power plant, a nuclear power plant, or a geothermal power plant. Write a short essay describing the power plant.

 Critical Thinking

Suppose you had to live without electricity, petroleum, and natural gas. How would your life be different than it is right now?

 Responsible Citizenship

Work with several friends or classmates to create a puppet show about the importance of conserving energy and natural resources. Ask your teacher or an elementary school principal for permission to present the show to an elementary class.

You Can Help Protect the Natural Environment

Life Skill **I will protect the natural environment.**

The **environment** is everything around a person. The **natural environment** is everything around a person that is not made by people. The natural environment includes plants, animals, insects, mountains, oceans, and the sky. The natural environment influences quality of life. **Quality of life** is the degree to which a person lives life to the fullest capacity. This lesson will help you identify places in which to enjoy the natural environment. You will learn how the natural environment can affect health status. You also will learn ways to improve the natural environment.

The Lesson Outline

What to Know About the Natural Environment

How to Protect the Natural Environment

Objectives

1. Explain how the natural environment affects health status. **page 629**
2. List ten ways to protect the natural environment. **page 630**

Vocabulary Words

environment
natural environment
quality of life
nature preserve
wildlife sanctuary
national parks
state parks
community park
nature trail
recreational trail
beach
zoo
garden
conservatory
leisure time
habitat

What to Know About the
Natural Environment

Think about nature and the natural environment. Picture a forest, an ocean, a mountain, the sky, a park, a field. Just thinking about nature and the natural environment can give a sense of awe and appreciation. People have created places in which to enjoy and appreciate nature. Some communities have parks and nature preserves. Thousands of people visit national parks in areas other than their own. Review the Ten Places Created to Help You Appreciate the Natural Environment. These places provide people with the opportunity to enjoy the natural environment and improve their quality of life.

Ten Places Created to Help You Appreciate the Natural Environment

1. **Nature preserves** A **nature preserve** is an area restricted for the protection of the natural environment.

2. **Wildlife sanctuaries** A **wildlife sanctuary** is a place reserved for the protection of plants and animals.

3. **National and state parks** **National parks** and **state parks** are government-maintained areas of land open to the public.

4. **Community parks** A **community park** is an area of land kept for natural scenery and recreation.

5. **Nature trails** A **nature trail** is a path through a natural environment.

6. **Recreational trails** A **recreational trail** is a path designed for recreational activities, such as walking, jogging, in-line skating, biking, and hiking.

7. **Beaches** A **beach** is the shore of a body of water covered by sand, gravel, or rock.

8. **Zoos** A **zoo** is a park in which animals are cared for and shown to the public.

9. **Garden** A **garden** is an area where trees, flowers, and other plants are grown and landscaping is maintained.

10. **Conservatory** A **conservatory** is a greenhouse in which plants are grown and displayed to the public.

How the Natural Environment Improves Health Status

The natural environment provides:

1. A quiet place to spend time by yourself. This can contribute to your well-being. It gives you time to collect your thoughts.

2. A place for you to spend time with family members and friends. You might spend time with your family members or friends at the zoo, in a park, or at the beach.

3. A place in which you can participate in physical activities. You might enjoy outdoor physical activities, such as hiking, in-line skating, swimming, and playing basketball.

4. A place in which you can enjoy leisure time. **Leisure time** is time free from work or duties. During their leisure time, some teens collect leaves, observe the stars, watch birds, and participate in physical activities.

5. A place in which you can relieve stress. Most people feel more relaxed after walking through a park, spending time at a zoo or at a nature preserve, or visiting a conservatory.

How to Protect the Natural Environment

People need to take responsibility for preserving the natural environment. They need to take actions to protect the natural environment. There are ten actions to take to help protect the natural environment.

1. **Follow all rules.** Many places created to help people enjoy the natural environment post rules to follow. Rules might involve staying in certain areas, keeping pets on a leash, and following safety guidelines.

2. **Do not leave belongings behind.** Whatever you take into a natural area should go with you when you leave the area.

3. **Do not litter or leave other objects.** Bring garbage bags to collect trash and other wastes.

4. **Do not destroy the environment.** Leave as little trace as possible of having been in a natural environment. Do not damage trees or plants. Do not carve initials in trees. Do not write graffiti on rocks, trees, bridges, trail signs, or buildings.

5. **Do not take things out of the natural environment.** Leave everything in its place so that you do not harm the natural habitat. A **habitat** is a place where an animal or plant normally lives. Do not pick flowers. Do not break branches off trees. Do not take animals or other objects from the natural environment.

6. **Do not feed wild animals.** Feeding wild animals makes them dependent on humans for food. They do not learn to feed themselves. Many animals starve to death after people leave the area.

7. **Stay on trails.** Trails are designed to protect people from possible dangers and to protect the natural environment. Walk in single file rather than side-by-side when hiking with two or more people to make sure everyone stays on the trail.

8. **Keep fires small and make sure they are extinguished before leaving.** Follow park rules for building fires. Make sure that fires are completely out before eaving the area.

9. **Be considerate of others when in the natural environment.** Do not make loud noises, such as screaming or playing loud music. Do not "hog" equipment and facilities. Walk or ride on the appropriate side of trails.

10. **Do not drink out of lakes and streams or consume wild plants.** Many lakes and streams are polluted with microorganisms and other pollutants that harm health. Many wild plants are poisonous and can cause illness or death.

Lesson 87

Review

Vocabulary Words

Write a separate sentence using each of the vocabulary words listed on page 628.

Objectives

1. What are ten places that have been created to help people enjoy the natural environment? **Objective 1**

2. What are five ways the natural environment helps improve health status? **Objective 1**

3. What effect can the natural environment have on stress? **Objective 1**

4. What are ten ways to protect the natural environment? **Objective 2**

5. What is a habitat? **Objective 2**

Responsible Decision-Making

You are visiting a park with a person you are dating. You see wildflowers not far away from where you are walking. Your date says that (s)he would like some of the wildflowers. You have to leave the trail to pick the flowers. Write a response to this situation.

1. Describe the situation that requires you to make a decision.
2. List possible decisions you might make.
3. Name two responsible adults with whom you might discuss your decisions.
4. Evaluate the possible consequences of your decisions. Determine if each decision will lead to actions that:
   • promote health,
   • protect safety,
   • follow laws,
   • show respect for yourself and others,
   • follow the guidelines of your parents and of other responsible adults,
   • demonstrate good character.
5. Decide which decision is most responsible and appropriate.
6. Tell two results you expect if you make this decision.

 Effective Communication

Select a natural environment in which to spend a few hours. You might spend time in a community park or a nature reserve. Describe your visit in a creative manner. You might write a poem or story or draw a picture that describes your experience.

 Self-Directed Learning

Do research to find the names, locations, and hours open to the public of five places that have been created in your state to help people appreciate the local environment. Share the information with family members.

 Critical Thinking

Teens who live in large cities may not have many in places in their community where they can enjoy the natural environment. What are five things these teens can do to enjoy the natural environment?

 Responsible Citizenship

Select from Ten Places Created to Help You Appreciate the Natural Environment a place that you have in your community. Write a list of ten actions you can take to help protect and improve this place. Obtain permission from a parent or guardian to take one of the actions on your list.

Lesson 88

You Can Improve the Visual Environment

Life Skill **I will help improve my visual environment.**

The environment is everything around a person. The **visual environment** is everything a person sees regularly. Your visual environment includes what you see when you wake up in the morning, when you look out the window of your home, and when you walk or ride to school. This lesson will help you evaluate the quality of your visual environment. You will learn ways a positive visual environment improves health status. You also will learn ways to improve your visual environment.

The Lesson Outline

What to Know About the Visual Environment
How to Improve the Visual Environment

Objectives

1. Contrast a positive and negative visual environment. **page 633**
2. List and describe five ways a positive visual environment improves health status. **page 633**
3. List and discuss eight ways to improve the visual environment. **page 634**

Vocabulary Words

visual environment
graffiti
visual pollution
terrarium

What to Know About the
Visual Environment

Do you live in a positive visual environment? A positive visual environment exists when the environment is visually appealing. Suppose you are outdoors. You look around and see buildings that are well cared for and a community park with flowers. This is a positive visual environment. Then suppose you are outdoors in another place. You look around and see buildings with broken windows, peeling paint, and graffiti. **Graffiti** is writing or drawings on a public surface. This is a negative visual environment. A negative visual environment contains visual pollution. **Visual pollution** is sights that are unattractive. Visual pollution includes litter, graffiti, and badly cared-for buildings.

Visual pollution also includes materials that are displayed in inappropriate places. For example, billboards advertising alcohol and tobacco products used to be found near schools and playgrounds. Federal law now prohibits alcohol and tobacco companies from putting billboards within a certain distance from schools. A blinking neon sign hanging in a bedroom window also is visual pollution. Areas that are visually polluted seem to invite more visual pollution. For example, people are more likely to dump garbage and throw litter in places that already are polluted. They assume that if an area is polluted, one more piece of litter will not make any difference.

Your visual environment is more than what is outdoors. It includes your indoor surroundings as well. A positive indoor visual environment might be a room that is free of clutter and litter and that is freshly painted. Visual pollution in an indoor environment might include clutter and trash.

Five Ways a Positive Visual Environment Affects Health Status

1. **A positive visual environment improves mood.** The sight of an attractive painting or a sunrise can be energizing. The sight of a beautiful sunset can inspire a sense of awe.

2. **A positive visual environment improves motivation.** The sight of a clean desk and a neat room can help people feel motivated. People are better able to focus and concentrate when they are not distracted by visual pollution.

3. **A positive visual environment helps relieve stress.** Certain sights can be calming. People who are stressed may find looking out the window at a pleasant scene relaxes them.

4. **A positive visual environment contributes to quality of life.** Communities in which there is visual pollution, such as graffiti and litter, often are at high risk for crime and violence. The value of property is lower. People may not have pride in the community. Improving the visual environment is linked to a decrease in crime and violence, an increase in property value, and an increase in community pride.

5. **A positive visual environment can improve social health.** You share the visual environment with others. In fact, you are a part of other people's visual environment. The way you appear and the way you care for your visual environment can affect those around you. Making sure that you are well-groomed and have a clean and healthful appearance can improve social health. It shows others that you care for yourself and have self-respect. Others will find you more attractive.

How to Improve the Visual Environment

Look around your visual environment. It is likely that you will see things that could be improved. The following are ways to improve the visual environment.

1. **Pick up clutter.** Organize your belongings so they are stored neatly. Keep an area free of clutter in which to work on projects.

2. **Clean up litter.** Throw litter in the trash. Keep trash cans available to decrease the likelihood that other people will litter.

3. **Put pictures in your visual environment.** Cover bare or cracked walls with pictures. Pictures can add warmth and provide something at which to look.

4. **Put plants in your visual environment.** Consider adding a plant, an aquarium, or a terrarium to your home. A **terrarium** is a transparent container that holds plants or small animals. Plants add color and can improve the atmosphere.

5. **Improve the view outside your window.** Hang a bird feeder or clean up litter.

6. **Change the colors in your visual environment.** Colors can impact mood. Bright red, yellow, and orange have an energizing effect. Blues and greens have a relaxing effect.

7. **Organize a clean-up campaign.** Many organizations and community groups sponsor clean-up campaigns in the community in which teens can participate. Other efforts include cleaning up abandoned buildings, picking up litter in parks, and planting trees and flowers.

8. **Write to community leaders about visual pollution in your community.** Write letters to officials explaining your concerns about such visual pollution as abandoned buildings and graffiti.

Activity

A View from a Window

Life Skill: I will help improve my visual environment.

Materials: posterboard, colored markers or pens

Directions: Follow the steps below to create a visual environment that appeals to you. On a piece of posterboard, design a window out of which you can see a positive visual environment.

 Draw a frame to represent a window.

Imagine a positive visual environment. Consider the visual environment you would most like to see every day as you look out of a window at school or at home.

 Draw a picture of this environment on the posterboard. Your poster should appear as if you were looking out a window.

 Discuss the effect that environment has on you. Display the window on the classroom wall. Explain to classmates why you find the environment you designed so appealing.

Lesson 88

Review

Vocabulary Words

Write a separate sentence using each of the vocabulary words listed on page 632.

Objectives

1. What are examples of a positive visual environment? **Objective 1**

2. What are examples of a negative visual environment? **Objective 1**

3. What is visual pollution? **Objective 1**

4. What are five ways a positive visual environment affects health status? **Objective 2**

5. What are eight ways to improve the visual environment? **Objective 3**

Responsible Decision-Making

Some of your classmates paint graffiti. They say it is art. They claim they want to improve the visual environment. They encourage you to join them. Write a response to this situation.

1. Describe the situation that requires you to make a decision.

2. List possible decisions you might make.

3. Name two responsible adults with whom you might discuss your decisions.

4. Evaluate the possible consequences of your decisions. Determine if each decision will lead to actions that:
   • promote health,
   • protect safety,
   • follow laws,
   • show respect for yourself and others,
   • follow the guidelines of your parents and of other responsible adults,
   • demonstrate good character.

5. Decide which decision is most responsible and appropriate.

6. Tell two results you expect if you make this decision.

 Effective Communication

You share a bedroom with a younger sibling. Neither of you has been too concerned about keeping the room neat. Now you recognize the benefits of a positive visual environment. You want to start keeping the room neat. What might you say to your sibling to encourage him/her to help keep the room neat?

 Self-Directed Learning

Find and read a book or magazine article on how color influences mood and behavior. Write a one-page summary of the contents. Include a paragraph describing how three different colors influence your mood.

 Critical Thinking

Some teens live in homes in which there is a negative visual environment. What actions might these teens take to improve their visual environment?

 Responsible Citizenship

Identify a way to improve the visual environment in your community. Obtain permission from a parent or guardian and your teacher to implement your plan. Consider asking classmates to help. If possible, take before and after pictures of the project.

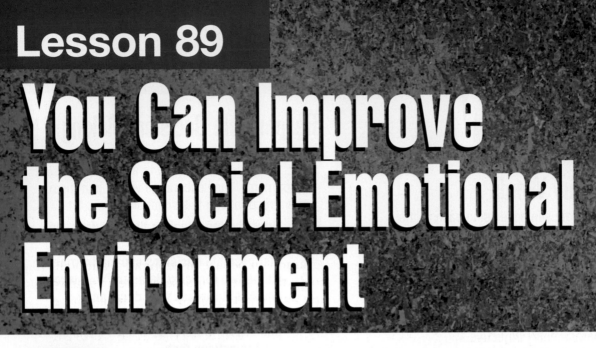

Lesson 89

You Can Improve the Social-Emotional Environment

Life Skill **I will take actions to improve my social-emotional environment.**

The environment is everything around a person. The **social-emotional environment** is the quality of the contacts a person has with the people with whom (s)he interacts. Your interactions with members of your family influence your social-emotional environment. Your interactions with peers and adults in the community also have an influence. This lesson will help you evaluate the quality of your social-emotional environment. You will learn ways a positive social-emotional environment improves health status. You also will learn ways to improve the social-emotional environment.

The Lesson Outline

What to Know About the Social-Emotional Environment

How to Improve the Social-Emotional Environment

Objectives

1. Contrast a positive and negative social-emotional environment. **page 637**

2. List ten ways a positive social-emotional environment improves health status. **page 637**

3. List and discuss seven ways to improve the social-emotional environment. **page 638**

Vocabulary Words

social-emotional environment

social-emotional booster

social-emotional pollutant

alienation

What to Know About the
Social-Emotional Environment

Do you live in a positive social-emotional environment? A positive social-emotional environment exists when you receive plenty of social-emotional boosters. A **social-emotional booster** is an interpersonal contact that helps a person feel encouragement and support, choose responsible behavior, and recognize options. Suppose people around you encourage you to take calculated risks. Suppose they praise you when you do something well. Suppose they recognize and appreciate that you are special and unique and compliment you when you use self-discipline and choose responsible behavior. Suppose they point out to you that you have options or choices. When people do these things, you feel connected and cared about. You have the support you need to take calculated risks. When you are tempted to do something wrong, you quickly turn back. You do not feel totally depressed or down over circumstances in your life. You recognize that there are options even for the most difficult circumstances.

Now suppose you live in a negative social-emotional environment. A negative social-emotional environment exists when you experience too many social-emotional pollutants. A **social-emotional pollutant** is an interpersonal contact that closes options or may cause a person to feel discouraged and alone or to choose wrong behavior. Suppose people around you are disrespectful, put you down, or gossip about you. Suppose people around you try to manipulate and control you. Suppose people around you abuse you in some way. Suppose people around you behave in wrong ways and want you to do the same. Suppose people around you do not want you to improve your circumstances. They tell you that you cannot change the way things are. Actions such as these create a negative social-emotional environment.

If you live in a negative social-emotional environment, you must take actions. If you do not, you can feel discouraged, unsupported, lonely, and alienated. **Alienation** is the feeling of being separate from others. The next part of this lesson gives suggestions for improving the social-emotional environment.

Ten Ways a Positive Social-Emotional Environment Improves Health Status

- Improves self-respect
- Provides support for responsible behavior
- Provides the support and encouragement needed to take calculated risks
- Allows you to correct mistakes, forgive yourself, and move on
- Helps you to be resilient
- Helps you to be optimistic
- Reduces stress
- Helps to prevent and relieve depression
- Helps prevent feelings of loneliness and alienation
- Reduces the risk of psychosomatic diseases

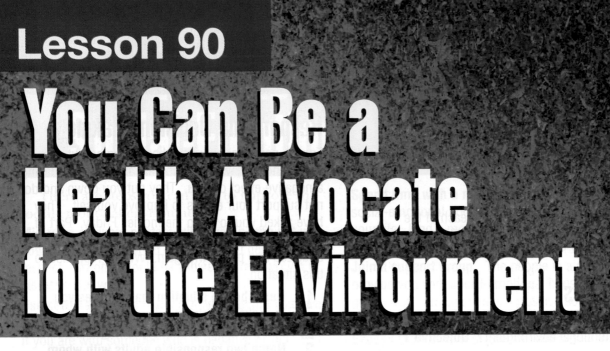

Lesson 90

You Can Be a Health Advocate for the Environment

Life Skill I will be a health advocate for the environment.

Are you satisfied with the environment in which you live? Or do you think that some things could or should be changed to improve the quality of life? You can help make others aware of the changes you consider important by participating in health advocacy. **Health advocacy** is taking responsibility to improve the quality of life. Health advocacy for the environment includes taking responsibility for the environment and encouraging others to do the same. This lesson focuses on health advocacy for the environment. You will learn how to promote health by promoting a healthy environment.

Vocabulary Words

health advocacy
health advocate
health advocate for the environment

The Lesson Outline

What to Know About Health Advocacy for the Environment

How to Be a Health Advocate for the Environment

Objectives

1. Discuss four actions taken by health advocates for the environment. **page 641**
2. List and describe six ways to be a health advocate for the environment. **page 642**

What to Know About Health Advocacy for the Environment

A **health advocate** is a person who promotes health. A **health advocate for the environment** is a person who promotes a healthful environment. Health advocates for the environment take actions to improve the quality of the environment. They avoid actions that may threaten the environment. Health advocates for the environment work together with other people to promote environmental health. They encourage others to join them in taking responsibility for the environment. They have successfully influenced the passage of laws that protect the environment.

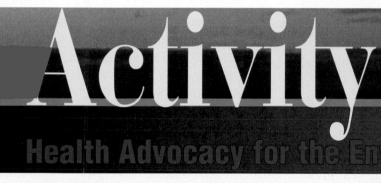

Activity

Health Advocacy for the Environment

Life Skill: I will be a health advocate for the environment.

Materials: paper, pen or pencil

Directions: Complete the steps in this activity to become a health advocate for the environment.

 1. **Identify action items from lists such as the following in this unit:**

- Twenty Actions You Can Take to Keep the Air Clean (page 608)
- Fifteen Ways to Help Keep the Water Safe (page 614)
- Twenty Ways to Conserve Energy Supplied by Natural Resources (page 626)
- Ten Ways to Conserve Water (page 626)
- How to Improve the Visual Environment (page 634)
- How to Improve the Social-Emotional Environment (page 638)
- How to Be a Health Advocate for the Environment (page 642)

 2. **Divide into groups according to your teacher's instructions.** Each group will take responsibility for one list.

3. **Classmates work in groups to make a creative presentation for their class and other classes.** The presentation should illustrate or demonstrate the actions identified in the group's assigned list in a way that will encourage members of the audience to help preserve or improve the environment.

How to Be a Health Advocate for the Environment

You can be a health advocate for the environment. You also can be a role model to others when you take responsibility for the environment. There are a variety of ways to become an effective health advocate for the environment.

1. **Take responsibility for your own actions regarding the environment.** Do not allow circumstances or peer pressure to cause you to forget or avoid your responsibility for a healthy environment. For example, do not throw crumpled fast-food bags out the window of a motor vehicle and contribute to roadside litter because the other teens with you want to get rid of them before they return the family car. Instead, take advantage of the opportunity to be both a health advocate for the environment and a role model for your friends.

2. **Stay informed about environmental issues that affect your community, the nation, and the world.** New discoveries are made every day. New technology brings about change rapidly. Keep current on the changes and how they affect environmental issues. Read about environmental issues in newspapers and magazines, and learn about factors that may harm the quality of your environment. Recognize that scientists and environmental groups have differing opinions about environmental issues. Make sure the information you read or hear and the source from which it comes are reliable.

3. **Take actions to promote the environment.** Review the lessons in this unit for actions you can take to promote the environment. Look for ways you can protect and improve the environment, such as conserving water and energy, recycling, building a compost pile, planting trees, and maintaining an environment free from litter.

4. **Encourage others to protect the environment.** Share the information you have learned in this unit with family members and friends. Invite others to join your efforts to protect the environment.

5. **Volunteer to work on environmental improvement projects in your community.** Identify environmental organizations or groups involved in improving your community. Obtain permission from a parent or guardian to volunteer to help these organizations or groups.

6. **Organize environmental improvement projects.** Being a health advocate for the environment involves taking responsibility. Suppose you see a need for improvement in an area of the environment, such as air or water pollution. Don't wait for someone else to organize an environmental improvement project. Choose a way to improve your environment and take action.

Lesson 90

Review

Vocabulary Words

Write a separate sentence using each of the vocabulary words listed on page 640.

Objectives

1. What is a health advocate for the environment? **Objective 1**

2. What are four actions taken by health advocates for the environment? **Objective 1**

3. What are six ways to be a health advocate for the environment? **Objective 2**

4. How can you stay informed about environmental issues? **Objective 2**

5. What can you do if you see a need for improvement in the environment? **Objective 2**

Responsible Decision-Making

You want to join the school environmental club. Your friends want you to join another club that is "more fun." Your friends say that this club has the popular students as its members and the environmental club does not. Write a response to this situation.

1. Describe the situation that requires you to make a decision.
2. List possible decisions you might make.
3. Name two responsible adults with whom you might discuss your decisions.
4. Evaluate the possible consequences of your decisions. Determine if each decision will lead to actions that:
   • promote health,
   • protect safety,
   • follow laws,
   • show respect for yourself and others,
   • follow the guidelines of your parents and of other responsible adults,
   • demonstrate good character.
5. Decide which decision is most responsible and appropriate.
6. Tell two results you expect if you make this decision.

Effective Communication

Choose an environmental issue that affects your community. Write a letter to a community official in which you voice your concern about the issue.

Self-Directed Learning

Write a letter to an environmental agency, group, or organization. Request information that explains the purpose of the organization.

Critical Thinking

Many people believe that they cannot make a difference in the quality of the environment. What arguments might you offer to convince these people that they can make a difference?

Responsible Citizenship

Teens can make a difference in the environment. List three actions you can take right now to help improve the environment. Ask your parents or guardian for permission to take these actions.

Review Questions

Prepare for the unit test. Review your answers for each Lesson Review in this unit. Then write answers to each of the following questions:

1. What is the difference between a developed country and a developing country? **Lesson 81**

2. How might the thinning of the ozone layer affect health? **Lesson 81**

3. How can you stay informed about environmental issues? **Lesson 81**

4. How might health status be affected if cilia are destroyed by air pollutants? **Lesson 82**

5. How might breathing secondhand smoke affect health status? **Lesson 82**

6. What are the signs of sick building syndrome (SBS)? **Lesson 82**

7. How might you know if water from the faucet were unsafe to drink? **Lesson 83**

8. What is the difference between hard water and soft water? **Lesson 83**

9. How does bottled water compare to tap water as far as safety for drinking? **Lesson 83**

10. What are three noises that can cause immediate and permanent hearing loss? **Lesson 84**

11. How might you protect your ears if you attend a loud concert? **Lesson 84**

12. How might noise pollution increase the risk of having an accident? **Lesson 84**

13. What is the difference between precycling and recycling? **Lesson 85**

14. What are three examples of commonly recycled materials? **Lesson 85**

15. Why might composting make a lawn greener? **Lesson 85**

16. What is the most abundant fossil fuel in this country? **Lesson 86**

17. How many miles per gallon should an energy-efficient motor vehicle get? **Lesson 86**

18. How might you set your thermostat to conserve energy? **Lesson 86**

19. What is the difference between a conservatory and a wildlife sanctuary? **Lesson 87**

20. Why should you avoid feeding wild animals unless there is a sign that permits you to do so? **Lesson 87**

21. Why should you take drinking water with you to a park rather than drinking out of a lake or stream? **Lesson 87**

22. What is the difference between a positive and negative visual environment? **Lesson 88**

23. How might you improve the visual environment in your home or apartment? **Lesson 88**

24. How might you improve the visual environment from a window? **Lesson 88**

25. Why do most people need social-emotional boosters? **Lesson 89**

26. What might you do if a friend constantly puts you down? **Lesson 89**

27. What might a teen do who does not get social-emotional boosters from significant adults? **Lesson 89**

28. What are the characteristics of a health advocate for the environment? **Lesson 90**

29. How can you stay informed about environmental issues that affect your community, nation, and world? **Lesson 90**

30. What are six ways you can be a health advocate for the environment? **Lesson 90**

Vocabulary Words

Number a sheet of paper from 1–10. Select the correct vocabulary word and write it next to the corresponding number. DO NOT WRITE IN THIS BOOK.

developing country	air pollution
landfill	sound waves
natural gas	health advocacy
natural environment	alienation
graffiti	water pollution

1. _____ is a contamination of the air that causes negative effects on life and health. **Lesson 82**

2. The _____ is everything around a person that is not made by people. **Lesson 87**

3. _____ are vibrations or movements of air. **Lesson 84**

4. A _____ is a country that is working to achieve an acceptable standard of health conditions. **Lesson 81**

5. A _____ is a place where waste is dumped in layers and buried. **Lesson 85**

6. _____ is writing or drawing on a public surface. **Lesson 88**

7. _____ is the feeling of being separate from others. **Lesson 89**

8. _____ is an energy source that is found underground above deposits of oil. **Lesson 86**

9. _____ is contamination of water that causes negative effects on life and health. **Lesson 83**

10. _____ is taking responsibility to improve the quality of life. **Lesson 90**

Health Literacy

Effective Communication

Write a 30-second public service announcement explaining the dangers of noise pollution. Explain how noise pollution can cause temporary and permanent hearing loss. Discuss ways to recognize that a sound is too loud and to avoid noise pollution. Record your announcement. Ask your parents or guardian for permission to send it to a local radio station.

Self-Directed Learning

Locate a book on one of the environmental issues discussed in this Unit. Look through the book. Write a one-page summary about the contents. Explain why the particular environmental issue is important to the environment.

Critical Thinking

Why is it important that everyone keep informed about and help protect the environment?

Responsible Citizenship

As a responsible citizen you should try to improve your environment. Make a list of actions you can take to improve your environment. Obtain permission from your parents or guardian to implement one of your plans.

Responsible Decision-Making

Suppose you go out to lunch with a classmate. You get your lunch to go at a fast-food restaurant. When you are finished eating, your friend tells you to throw the trash out the window of the motor vehicle. (S)he says that no one will ever know and that someone will pick it up eventually. Write a response to this situation.

1. Describe the situation that requires you to make a decision.
2. List possible decisions you might make.
3. Name two responsible adults with whom you might discuss your decisions.
4. Evaluate the possible consequences of your decisions. Determine if each decision will lead to actions that:
   - promote health,
   - protect safety,
   - follow laws,
   - show respect for yourself and others,
   - follow the guidelines of your parents and of other responsible adults,
   - demonstrate good character.
5. Decide which decision is most responsible and appropriate.
6. Tell two results you expect if you make this decision.

Health Behavior Inventory of Life Skills

Number from 1 to 10 on a sheet of paper. Read each life skill carefully. Write YES or NO next to the same number on your paper. Each YES response indicates a life skill you practice to promote your health status. Each NO response indicates a life skill you do not practice. Plan to begin practicing these life skills.

1. I will stay informed about environmental issues.
2. I will help keep the air clean.
3. I will help keep the water safe.
4. I will help keep noise at a safe level.
5. I will precycle, recycle, and dispose of waste properly.
6. I will help conserve energy and natural resources.
7. I will protect the natural environment.
8. I will help improve my visual environment.
9. I will take actions to improve my social-emotional environment.
10. I will be a health advocate for the environment.

Multicultural Health

Different countries have different environmental issues. What are five important environmental issues in your country? Research another country. What are five important environmental issues in that country? What are five global environmental issues?

Family Involvement

Make an information sheet on ways to keep the water safe. Include a brief explanation of how water pollution can affect health status. Share the information sheet with your family. Discuss ways you and other family members can improve your behavior to help keep the water safe. For example, your family might decide to use phosphate-free detergents and biodegradable soaps and shampoos.

Health Behavior Contract

Copy and complete the following health behavior contract. Evaluate your progress.
Share the results with your family.

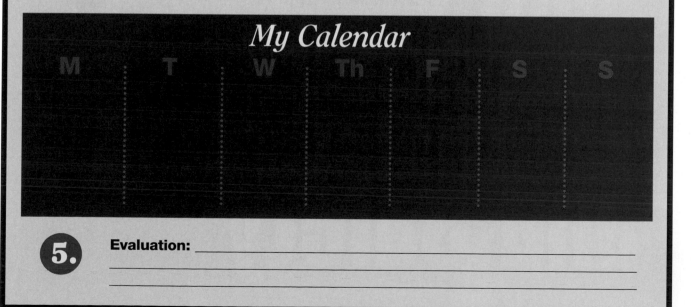

Health Behavior Contract

1. Name_____Date_____

2. **Life Skill:** I will help keep the air clean.

3. **Effects on Health Status:** Air pollution harms health status in different ways. Air pollution can interfere with the action of cilia in the respiratory system. This can increase the likelihood of respiratory diseases and infections such as asthma, emphysema, bronchitis, and lung cancer. Air pollution also contributes to heart disease, eye and throat irritation, and a weakened immune system. By helping to keep the air clean, I will reduce the likelihood that air pollution affects my health status.

4. **Plan and Method to Record Progress:** I will review the list of Twenty Actions You Can Take to Keep the Air Clean. When I take one of these actions, I will write the activity in the space provided for the day of the week. I will list ways I benefited from taking these action in the evaluation.

My Calendar

M	T	W	Th	F	S	S

5. Evaluation: _____
_____

Unit 10

Injury Prevention and Safety

Lesson 91

You Can Reduce the Risk of Unintentional Injuries

I will follow safety guidelines to reduce the risk of unintentional injuries.

Lesson 92

You Can Be Safe During Severe Weather and Natural Disasters

I will follow safety guidelines for severe weather and natural disasters.

Lesson 93

You Can Reduce the Risk of Motor Vehicle Injuries

I will follow guidelines for motor vehicle safety.

Lesson 94

You Can Reduce the Risk of Violence

I will practice protective factors to reduce the risk of violence.

Lesson 95

You Can Respect Authority and Obey Laws

I will respect authority and obey laws.

Lesson 96

You Can Protect Yourself from People Who Might Harm You

I will practice self-protection strategies.

Lesson 97

You Can Stay Away from Gangs

I will stay away from gangs.

Lesson 98

You Can Reduce the Risk of Being Injured by a Weapon

I will not carry a weapon.

Lesson 99

You Can Participate in Victim Recovery If You Have Been Harmed by Violence

I will participate in victim recovery if I am harmed by violence.

Lesson 100

You Can Be Ready to Give First Aid

I will be skilled in first aid procedures.

Lesson 91

You Can Reduce the Risk of Unintentional Injuries

Life Skill I will follow safety guidelines to reduce the risk of unintentional injuries.

An **unintentional injury** is an injury caused by an accident. Unintentional injuries are the leading cause of death for teens. Some causes of unintentional injuries are motor vehicle accidents, fires, burns, falls, drownings, and poisoning. Lesson 93 will include safety guidelines to reduce the risk of unintentional injuries from motor vehicle accidents. This lesson will include ways to reduce the risk of unintentional injuries in the home, community, and workplace. You will learn how to prevent poisoning, falls, fires and suffocation. You also will learn how to prevent drownings and bicycle accidents. This lesson also covers laws and safety guidelines that protect you if you get a part-time job.

The Lesson Outline

What to Know About Unintentional Injuries in the Home

What to Know About Unintentional Injuries in the Community

Objectives

1. Outline ways to reduce the risk of unintentional injuries in the home. **pages 651–652**

2. Outline ways to reduce the risk of unintentional injuries in the community. **page 653**

3. Discuss ways to reduce the risk of unintentional injuries in the workplace. **page 654**

Vocabulary Words

unintentional injury

poisoning

carbon monoxide

smoke detector

heat detector

suffocation

strangulation

Occupational Safety and Health Act

repetitive strain injury (RSI)

What to Know About Unintentional Injuries in the Home

Many accidents that result in unintentional injury and death occur in the home. The home is the most dangerous place for young children and older people.

How to Reduce the Risk of Unintentional Injuries from Poisoning

Poisoning has recently surpassed falling to become the leading cause of death in the home. **Poisoning** is a harmful chemical reaction from a substance that enters the body. It includes reactions to drugs. Other substances that may be poisonous when swallowed are household cleaners, polish, ammonia, nail polish remover, antifreeze, insecticides, rat poison, and certain plants. Taking very high doses of vitamin and mineral supplements also may result in poisoning. Most cases of poisoning in a home are the result of young children swallowing household products and OTC drugs.

Certain substances cause poisoning when inhaled, such as auto exhaust, airplane glue, gasoline, and carbon monoxide. **Carbon monoxide** is an odorless, tasteless gas. It is emitted from motor vehicles, stoves, heaters, lawnmowers, and chimneys.

Lesson 100 will include more information about first aid for poisoning.

Ways to Reduce the Risk of Poisoning

- Use childproof containers on potential poisons and keep them out of the reach of children.
- Place warning stickers on any potential poisons.
- Place childproof latches on the doors of all cabinets in which harmful substances are kept.
- Do not keep a motor vehicle or lawnmower running in a closed garage.
- Do not use outdoor grills indoors.
- Check chimneys regularly for blockage.

How to Reduce the Risk of Injuries Due to Falls

Falls are a leading cause of injury and death in the home. Half of all falls are caused by hazards such as poor lighting, loose carpets, trailing wires, and unsteady stair rails. Most spinal cord injuries are the result of falls. Young children are at particular risk because their sense of balance is not fully developed. Teens injured due to falls often have taken unnecessary risks and may have ignored safety precautions or been showing off. Teens have been injured and killed from falls off rooftops, bridges, mountains, and windows in high buildings.

Ways to Reduce the Risk of Falls

- Do not take risks in high places, such as going too close to a drop-off or hanging out a window.
- Use a sturdy ladder when climbing to reach an object. Keep your body in the center of the step to avoid losing balance. Face the ladder when climbing down.
- Place an infant or young child in a playpen, crib, or safety seat when (s)he must be out of your sight.
- Use appropriate child safety devices to block stairways and windows.
- Do not run in the home.
- Be cautious if wearing shoes with slippery bottoms or high heels.

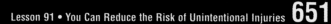

How to Reduce the Risk of Injuries Due to Fires

Most deaths and injuries related to fires occur in the home. Most home fires are caused by improper use and disposal of cigarettes, cigarette lighters, and matches. All homes should be equipped with a fire extinguisher, a heat detector, and at least one smoke detector on each floor. A **smoke detector** is an alarm that sounds when smoke is detected. A **heat detector** is a device that sounds an alarm when the room temperature rises above a certain level. A fire escape plan should be set up in advance that includes at least two different ways to escape from each room and designates a place outside the home to meet. Take the following actions should a fire occur.

1. Alert everyone if a fire begins.
2. Place a cloth, wet if possible, over the face.
3. Crawl out of the home on hands and knees to stay below the smoke line.
4. Feel doors for heat before opening. Do not open doors that are warm or hot. Open cool doors slowly.
5. Stuff rugs, blankets, or clothes around door cracks to stop smoke from entering if you cannot leave a room. Call out a window for help.
6. Call 9-1-1 or the fire department after you have escaped.
7. Meet family members at the designated meeting place.
8. Do not go back into a burning building.
9. Tell fire officials if people or animals are inside the building.

Ways to Reduce the Risk of Fires

- Have a no smoking policy in the home.
- Keep all matches, cigarette lighters, and flames out of children's reach.
- Do not overload electrical outlets or run cords under rugs.
- Do not leave items such as irons or electric hair styling products plugged in for long periods of time.
- Check food cooking on a stove often.

How to Reduce the Risk of Injuries Due to Suffocation

Suffocation is a condition in which there is lack of oxygen due to an obstruction to passage of air into the lungs. Suffocation due to choking is the leading cause of death among infants. Young children may choke by placing objects in their mouths, such as small toys, coins, or food.

Suffocation also may be due to strangulation. **Strangulation** is choking to death due to pressure on the throat. Teens have accidentally strangled on material tied around the neck, such as a scarf, that caught on another object, such as a car door. Children have strangled on cords from window coverings, strings on toys, ropes tied into lassoes, and pieces of clothing.

Ways to Reduce the Risk of Suffocation

- Keep small objects out of the reach of children.
- Do not allow children to play with plastic bags or toys that are not appropriate for their age.
- Check sleeping infants and children to be sure breathing is not blocked by a pillow, blanket, or stuffed toy.
- Cut food into small pieces that are easy to swallow.
- Do not tie a rope or cord around the neck, even as a joke.

What to Know About
Unintentional Injuries in the Community

Teens often are injured in the community. They may be injured because they disregard safety guidelines. Peers may influence them to be daring. They may be stressed or overtired and careless or less alert. They risk injury when they ride a bicycle and can be at risk for drowning when near bodies of water. Teens also may be injured in the workplace.

How to Reduce the Risk of Injuries Due to Drownings

Drowning is the third leading cause of accidental death. Drownings most often occur when people are swimming or playing in water. Many people who drown are strong swimmers who become tired or are pulled under by the current. Drownings also can result from boating accidents. Alcohol is a major factor in teen-related drownings and most boating accidents. Many drownings occur in swimming pools and whirlpools. Many young children are injured and killed by drowning in bathtubs, toilets, and sinks.

Ways to Reduce the Risk of Drownings

- Learn to swim.
- Never swim or use a hot tub alone.
- Wear a personal flotation device (life jacket) when boating or participating in water sports.
- Swim only in areas designated safe to swim and in sight of a lifeguard.
- Stay out of the water in threatening weather such as thunderstorms.
- Do not swim in unlighted areas.
- Leave the water if you have cramps or are tired.
- Enforce an alcohol-free policy for all people around pools and water.
- Never boat with others who speed or do not follow safety guidelines.

How to Reduce the Risk of Injury Due to Bicycling

Most deaths and serious injuries due to bicycling involve head injuries. The most serious injuries occur when bikes collide with motor vehicles.

Ways to Reduce the Risk of Injuries from Bicycling Accidents

- Wear a bicycle helmet.
- Obey traffic rules followed by motor vehicle drivers.
- Ride on the right, with the flow of traffic.
- Check that the bicycle and all safety equipment, such as brakes, lights, and reflectors, are in good condition.
- Wear clothing that will not get caught in the bicycle.
- Wear reflective clothing at night.
- Wear shoes at all times.
- Watch for the sudden opening of motor vehicle doors.
- Walk the bicycle across busy streets.
- Do not ride double.
- Beware of unsafe road conditions, such as ice and potholes.

- Have training before boating or participating in water sports.
- Do not overload a boat or personal watercraft such as a jet ski.
- Do not leave a child alone near swimming pools, bathtubs, or bodies of water.
- Check the depth of water before entering.
- Install a fence and childproof latches around swimming pools.
- Do not walk on untested ice.

Q&A
Ways to Reduce the Risk of Injury in the Workplace

Q: What type of injuries occur in the workplace?

A: The workplace is second only to the home as the most frequent site of unintentional injuries. Common work-place injuries to teens involve driving a motor vehicle or heavy equipment such as tractors and using power tools. Machine-related accidents, electrocution, and homicide also account for many deaths in the workplace.

Q: I will be working in construction over summer vacation. What will my employer do to protect my health and safety?

A: According to law, your employer must meet safety guidelines for healthful working conditions. The **Occupational Safety and Health Act** is a series of minimum safety and health standards that all employers must meet. Recognized health hazards must be eliminated. Employees must receive a regular review of safety regulations. New employees must be trained on equipment and made aware of hazards.

Q: My younger sibling is looking for a part-time job. Are there any rules about minors who work?

A: The Fair Labor Standards Act (FLSA) contains child labor laws to protect the health and safety of minors. The act limits the hours minors under age 16 can work and prohibits employing minors under age 18 for certain occupations.

Q: I work at a fast food restaurant after-school. For what kinds of injuries should I watch?

A: Most injuries in the workplace among 16- and 17-year-olds were in food preparation and service jobs. The most common types of injuries in food service were sprains, strains, cuts, bruises, scrapes, heat burns, fractures, and dislocation.

Q: I volunteer at a health organization where I type on a computer. Why might my hands be feeling numb?

A: An increasingly common workplace injury is RSI. **Repetitive strain injury (RSI)** is an injury that occurs from repeated physi-cal movements. RSI damages tendons, nerves, muscles, and other soft body tissues. Using computer devices, such as keyboards and mice, often contributes to the injury. Symptoms include tingling; tightness; pain, and stiffness in the hands, wrists, fingers, arms, and elbows; weak-ness in hands; and a need to massage hands, wrists, and elbows. To prevent RSI when typing, sit straight and relax your hands and wrists. Keep the com-puter screen at eye level and position the keyboard so hands and wrists are straight. Take a 15-minute break at least every two hours.

Lesson 91

Review

Vocabulary Words

Write a separate sentence using each of the vocabulary words listed on page 650.

Objectives

1. What are ways to reduce the risk of poisoning? Falls? Fires? Suffocation? **Objective 1**

2. What are ways to reduce the risk of drownings? Bicycle accidents? **Objective 2**

3. What are the most common injuries in teens who are working? **Objective 3**

4. How does the Occupational Safety and Health Act protect people in the workplace? **Objective 3**

5. What are the working guidelines for minors in the Fair Labor Standards Act (FLSA)? **Objective 3**

Responsible Decision-Making

You are going mountain biking with some friends. when you all meet, you notice that they are not wearing safety helmets. They say they are not going to wear their helmets and tell you not to wear yours. Write a response to this situation.

1. Describe the situation that requires you to make a decision.
2. List possible decisions you might make.
3. Name two responsible adults with whom you might discuss your decisions.
4. Evaluate the possible consequences of your decisions. Determine if each decision will lead to actions that:
   • promote health,
   • protect safety,
   • follow laws,
   • show respect for yourself and others,
   • follow the guidelines of your parents and of other responsible adults,
   • demonstrate good character.
5. Decide which decision is most responsible and appropriate.
6. Tell two results you expect if you make this decision.

Effective Communication

Select one category of unintentional injuries that may occur in the home. Write a public service announcement (PSA) about ways to reduce the risk of these injuries. Obtain permission from a parent or guardian to submit your PSA to a local radio station.

Self-Directed Learning

Obtain permission from a parent or guardian. Call the local Poison Control Center. Obtain a list of items that are potential poisons. Place a warning sticker or sign on any of these items you may have in your home.

Critical Thinking

Falls are a leading cause of death in elderly people. Why might elderly people be at high risk of injury and death from falling?

Responsible Citizenship

Design a poster that provides information about safety guidelines in the workplace. Your poster should include information from the Occupational Safety and Health Act (OSHA) or Fair Labor Standards Act (FLSA). Obtain permission from a local business or factory to hang your poster where employees will see it.

Lesson 92

You Can Be Safe During Severe Weather and Natural Disasters

Life Skill I will follow safety guidelines for severe weather and natural disasters.

The **weather** is the condition of the atmosphere at a particular time and place. A **natural disaster** is an event caused by nature that results in damage or loss. You may live in a high-risk area for a particular weather condition or natural disaster. Your travels may take you to an area where severe weather or natural disasters are common. This lesson tells you how to be prepared for severe weather or natural disasters. You will learn five steps your family can take to be ready. This lesson also includes safety guidelines to follow should severe weather or a natural disaster occur. You will learn what to do if there is a landslide, flood, earthquake, tornado, hurricane, wildland fire, electrical storm, or winter storm.

The Lesson Outline

How to Prepare for Severe Weather and Natural Disasters

What to Know About Safety Guidelines for Severe Weather and Natural Disasters

Objectives

1. List five ways to prepare for severe weather and natural disasters. **page 657**

2. Discuss ways to stay safe during a landslide, flood, earthquake, tornado, hurricane, wildland fire, electrical storm, and winter storm. **pages 657–660**

Vocabulary Words

weather

natural disaster

landslide

flood

flash flood

earthquake

tornado

tornado watch

tornado warning

hurricane

wildland fire

electrical storm

severe thunderstorm watch

severe thunderstorm warning

winter storm

How to Prepare for Severe Weather and Natural Disasters

> Prepare yourself and your family for a severe weather emergency or natural disaster by taking the following actions.

1. Contact your local emergency management office or chapter of the American Red Cross for a copy of their emergency plans.

2. Know the warning signals for your community, such as sirens or announcements.

3. Develop an emergency communication plan. Have a plan for getting together in case family members are in separate locations. Identify one contact person in your area and one contact person out of town. Make sure all family members know the name and phone number of these two people.

4. Teach all family members how and when to turn off gas, electricity, and water.

5. Prepare an emergency supply kit that includes:

   - Flashlight
   - Extra batteries
   - Battery-operated radio
   - First aid kit
   - Emergency food and water
   - Non-electric can opener
   - Cash and credit cards
   - Sturdy shoes

What to Know About Safety Guidelines for Severe Weather and Natural Disasters

What to Know About Safety Guidelines for Landslides

A **landslide** is a rapid movement of a mass of earth or rock. If there is a risk of landslides, take the following actions.

- Listen to the radio or watch TV for the latest developments.
- Evacuate immediately if instructed to do so.
- Look for landslide warning signs such as doors or windows cracking; new cracks in walls or foundations; cracks widening on the ground or pavement; water breaking through ground surface in new locations; fences, utility poles, or trees tilting or moving; and a faint rumbling sound increasing in volume.

What to Do During a Landslide

If you are indoors:

1. Stay inside.
2. Take cover under a desk, table, or other piece of sturdy furniture.

If you are outdoors:

1. Try to get out of the path of the landslide.
2. Run to the nearest high ground in a direction away from the path.
3. Run to the nearest shelter, such as a building or group of trees, if debris is approaching.
4. Curl into a tight ball and protect your head if escape is not possible.

What to Know About Safety Guidelines for Floods

A **flood** is a rising and overflowing of a body of water on to normally dry land. A **flash flood** is a flood that occurs suddenly. Flash floods are the number one weather-related cause of death in the United States. If there is a risk of floods, take the following actions.

- Listen to the radio or watch TV for the latest developments.
- Fill bathtubs, sinks, and jugs with clean water in case water becomes contaminated.
- Bring outdoor belongings indoors, if time permits.
- Move valuable household possessions to the upper floors or to safe ground.
- Be prepared to evacuate.
- Turn off utilities at the main switch and turn off the main gas valve if instructed to do so.
- Evacuate immediately if instructed to do so.

What to Do During a Flood

If you are indoors:

1. Turn on a radio or TV for the latest emergency information.
2. Keep your emergency supply kit handy.

If you are outdoors:

1. Climb to higher ground and stay there.
2. Avoid walking through flood waters of more than several inches.

If you are in a motor vehicle:

1. Do not drive through flood waters.
2. Abandon the vehicle if it stalls and climb to higher ground.
3. Do not attempt to move a stalled vehicle.

What to Know About Safety Guidelines for Earthquakes

An **earthquake** is a violent shaking of Earth's surface caused by the shifting of plates that make up Earth's crusts. If there is a risk of earthquakes, take the following actions.

- Keep the emergency supply kit close by.
- Identify safe places in the room, such as against an inside wall or a piece of heavy furniture.
- Evacuate immediately if instructed to do so.

What to Do During an Earthquake

If you are indoors:

1. Take cover under a piece of heavy furniture or against an inside wall and hold on tightly.
2. Stay inside.
3. Do not try to leave a building.
4. Be prepared for aftershocks.

If you are outdoors:

1. Move into the open, away from buildings, street lights, and utility wires.
2. Get off a bridge as soon as possible.
3. Be prepared for aftershocks.

What to Know About Safety Guidelines for Tornadoes

A **tornado** is a violent, rapidly spinning windstorm that has a funnel-shaped cloud. A **tornado watch** is a warning issued when weather conditions are such that tornadoes are likely to develop. A **tornado warning** is a warning issued when a tornado has been sighted or indicated by radar. If there is a risk of tornadoes, take the following actions.

- Gather family members together. Be prepared to move to the safest place.
- Listen to the radio or watch TV for the latest developments.
- Keep the emergency supply kit available.
- Evacuate immediately if instructed to do so.

What to Do During a Tornado

If you are indoors:

1. Go at once to the basement, storm cellar, lowest level of the building, or an inner hallway or small inner room without windows.
2. Stay away from windows and corners.
3. Get under a piece of sturdy furniture such as a table and hold on to it.
4. Protect your head and neck.
5. Get out and find shelter elsewhere if you are in a mobile home.

If you are outdoors:

1. Seek shelter indoors.
2. Lie in a ditch or low-lying area or crouch near a building.
3. Use your arms to protect your head and neck.

If you are in a motor vehicle:

1. Do not try to out-drive a tornado.
2. Get out of the vehicle immediately.
3. Seek shelter indoors.
4. Lie in a ditch or low-lying area or crouch near a building.
5. Use your arms to protect your head and neck.

What to Know About Safety Guidelines for Hurricanes

A **hurricane** is a tropical storm with heavy rains and winds in excess of 74 miles (118.4 kilometers) per hour. If there is a risk of hurricanes, take the following actions.

- Listen to the radio or watch TV for the latest developments.
- Bring outdoor objects indoors.
- Secure buildings by closing and boarding up windows.
- Turn the refrigerator and freezer to the coolest settings and open them only when necessary.
- Fill bathtubs, sinks, and jugs with clean water in case water becomes contaminated.
- Store valuables and personal papers in a waterproof container on the highest level of the building.

What to Do During a Hurricane

If you are indoors:

1. Secure your home by unplugging appliances and turning off the electricity and the main water valve.
2. Evacuate immediately if instructed to do so.
3. Stay inside, away from windows.
4. Keep a supply of flashlights and extra batteries handy.
5. Avoid open flames, such as candles, as a source of light.
6. Turn off major appliances to reduce power.
7. Avoid mobile homes.

What to Know About Safety Guidelines for Wildland Fires

A **wildland fire** is a fire that occurs in the wilderness. If there is a risk of wildland fires, take the following actions.

- Listen to the radio or watch TV for the latest developments.
- Take down flammable drapes and curtains and close all blinds and window coverings.
- Close gas valves and turn off pilot lights.
- Turn on a light in each room for visibility in heavy smoke.
- Place valuables that would not be damaged by water in a pool or pond.
- Leave sprinklers on roofs and on anything that might be damaged if adequate water is available.
- Evacuate immediately if asked to do so.

What to Do During a Wildland Fire

1. Do not attempt to outrun the fire if you are trapped.
2. Crouch in a body of water if possible.
3. Cover your head and upper body with wet clothing.
4. Seek shelter in a cleared area or bed of rocks if water is not available.
5. Breathe the air close to the ground through a wet cloth.

What to Know About Electrical Storms

An **electrical storm** is a storm that has lightning and thunder. A **severe thunderstorm watch** is a warning that is issued when the weather conditions are such that a severe thunderstorm is likely to develop. A **severe thunderstorm warning** is a warning that is issued when a severe thunderstorm has been sighted or indicated by radar. If there is a risk of electrical storms, take the following actions.

- Review the safety guidelines for tornadoes and flash floods, which may accompany thunderstorms.
- Listen to a battery-operated radio for the latest weather developments.
- Turn off the TV.
- Bring outdoor objects indoors.
- Close and board up windows.

What to Do During an Electrical Storm

If you are indoors:

1. Do not handle any electrical equipment or telephones.
2. Avoid bathtubs, water faucets, and sinks.
3. Avoid open doors, and windows and all electrical equipment.

If you are outdoors:

1. Go inside a building or motor vehicle, if possible.
2. Go to an open space and squat low to the ground, if you must stay outside.
3. Stand in the woods in an area protected by a low clump of trees.
4. Avoid tall structures such as towers, fences, and telephone or power lines.
5. Avoid golf clubs, tractors, fishing rods, bicycles, and camping equipment.
6. Stay away from bodies of water.
7. Crouch forward with your feet together and your hands on your knees if you feel your hair stand on end, which indicates that lightning is about to strike.
8. Do not lie flat on the ground.

If you are in a motor vehicle:

1. Pull safely to the shoulder of the road away from any trees.
2. Stay in the car and turn on the emergency flashers until rain subsides.
3. Avoid flooded roadways.

What to Know About Safety Guidelines for Winter Storms

A **winter storm** is a storm in the form of freezing rain, sleet, ice, heavy snow, or blizzards. If there is a risk of winter storms, take the following actions.

- Listen to the radio or watch TV for the latest developments.
- Make preparations in case you are isolated and without electricity.

What to Do During a Winter Storm

If you are indoors:

1. Remain indoors until the storm has passed.
2. Close all windows and doors.

If you are outdoors or in a motor vehicle:

1. Seek shelter immediately.
2. Travel only if necessary.
3. Pack winter storm supplies in your motor vehicle—sand, shovel, rope, scraper, flares, heavy blanket, warm clothing—in case of evacuation.

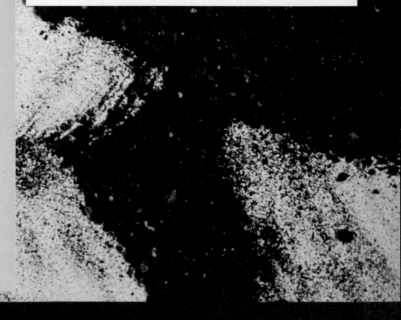

Lesson 92

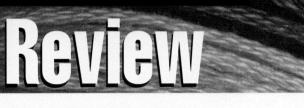

Vocabulary Words

Write a separate sentence using each of the vocabulary words listed on page 656.

Objectives

1. What are five ways to prepare for severe weather and natural disasters? **Objective 1**

2. What should be kept in an emergency supply kit? **Objective 1**

3. What are ways to stay safe during a landslide? Flood? Earthquake? Tornado? Hurricane? **Objective 2**

4. What are ways to stay safe during wildland fires? **Objective 2**

5. What are ways to stay safe during an electrical storm? Winter storm? **Objective 2**

Responsible Decision-Making

Your younger sibling is watching a TV program. A warning comes across the screen announcing a severe thunderstorm warning in the area. You tell your sibling the safety guidelines for electrical storms include turning off the TV. (S)he does not want to stop watching the program. Write a response to this situation.

1. Describe the situation that requires you to make a decision.
2. List possible decisions you might make.
3. Name two responsible adults with whom you might discuss your decisions.
4. Evaluate the possible consequences of your decisions. Determine if each decision will lead to actions that:
   • promote health,
   • protect safety,
   • follow laws,
   • show respect for yourself and others,
   • follow the guidelines of your parents and of other responsible adults,
   • demonstrate good character.
5. Decide which decision is most responsible and appropriate.
6. Tell two results you expect if you make this decision.

 Effective Communication

Select one of the severe weather conditions or natural disasters that might affect your community. Write a public service announcement (PSA) identifying the safety guidelines for your choice. Obtain permission from a parent or guardian to submit your PSA to a local radio station.

 Self-Directed Learning

Electrical storms are a fairly common occurrence. Find out the causes of this kind of storm and what signs weather professionals look for to forecast them.

 Critical Thinking

Suppose you are in a car on the way home from visiting a friend when a bulletin comes on the radio that there is a tornado warning. What should you do?

 Responsible Citizenship

Select a country other than the one in which you live, and identify the severe weather conditions and natural disasters that occur. Draw a map of the country with symbols to designate the regions at risk for different weather conditions and natural disasters.

Lesson 93

You Can Reduce the Risk of Motor Vehicle Injuries

Life Skill **I will follow guidelines for motor vehicle safety.**

Have you recently obtained your driver's license? Will you be getting your license soon? Having a driver's license is a privilege and responsibility. A driver's license gives you "legs" and allows you new freedoms. At the same time, it adds to your responsibilities. You must drive safely to protect yourself and the passengers in your motor vehicle from accidents. Motor vehicle accidents are the leading cause of unintentional injuries and deaths for teens. If you drive the family motor vehicle, you must protect family property and insurance coverage. This lesson discusses ways to reduce the risk of unintentional injuries from motor vehicle accidents and violence. You will learn ways to protect yourself as a driver and as a passenger.

The Lesson Outline

What to Know About Motor Vehicle Accidents

What to Know About Violence Involving Motor Vehicles

Objectives

1. Explain the responsibilities of a driver including obtaining a valid license, being a defensive driver, and avoiding high-risk driving and traffic violations. **pages 663–664**

2. Discuss the importance of air bags, safety belts, and child safety restraint systems. **page 664**

3. List 20 guidelines for motor vehicle safety. **page 665**

4. Discuss ways a person can reduce the risk of injury from road rage. **page 666**

5. List 25 ways to protect against violence involving motor vehicles. **page 666**

Vocabulary Words

learner's permit

graduated license

defensive driver

high-risk driving

traffic violation

air bag

safety belt

child safety restraint

road rage

carjacking

What to Know About Motor Vehicle Accidents

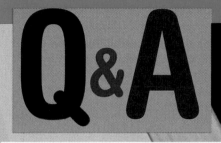

Q: My birthday is almost here, and I will be old enough to drive. How can I obtain a valid driver's license?

A: Before you obtain a driver's license, you must pass a written test and a driving test. Many teens take a driver education course to gain the knowledge and skills needed to pass these tests. The courses are required in several states and are offered by schools, community organizations, and private companies. Check on state laws and opportunities to learn driving skills. You may have to get a learner's permit or a graduated license first. A **learner's permit** is an authorization to drive when supervised by a licensed driver of a certain age. A **graduated license** is a conditional license given to new drivers. People with a graduated license have restricted driving privileges, such as being allowed to drive only during the day. The likelihood of accidents in the first year of driving is high. One in five 16-year-old male drivers and one in ten 16-year-old female drivers have an accident during the first year of driving.

Q: I live in an area where signs are posted for animal crossings. Are there ways to avoid hitting deer?

A: Be a defensive driver. Guard against the unforeseen actions of animals. Motorists most often hit animals at dusk and at dawn. Control your speed so you can stop suddenly if needed. If you see an animal in the road, honk your horn but do not flash your lights.

Q: My family's insurance agent has stressed the importance of being a defensive driver. What does this mean?

A: A **defensive driver** is a driver who guards against the unsafe actions of other drivers. Defensive driving is one way to reduce the risk of accidents. It includes taking the following actions.

- Observe traffic laws and speed limits.
- Make sure the intersection is clear when the light turns green.
- Never tailgate.
- Stay alert.
- Avoid distractions such as loud music or talking on a cellular phone while driving.
- Listen to traffic reports and adjust plans accordingly.
- Check that all parts of a motor vehicle are working properly.

Q: My classmate says (s)he can take any turn as well as a race driver. Should I ride with him/her?

A: No. **High-risk driving** is dangerous driving that can result in accidents. It includes behaviors such as speeding, trying to beat red lights or a train, racing other drivers, jumping hills, drinking and driving, doing "doughnuts" or "fishtails," and hanging out of motor vehicles. Do not ride in a motor vehicle with a driver who chooses high-risk driving. If you already are in the vehicle, ask the driver to stop or get out and call another person for a ride.

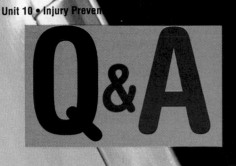

Q: My friend says (s)he can drink up to two drinks without it affecting his/her driving and that drinking and driving is OK if (s)he sticks to these limits. Is this true?

A: No. It is against the law for your friend to drink if (s)he is under the age of 21. Drinking alcohol is the leading cause of motor vehicle accidents in teens. Teens interviewed after motor vehicle accidents involving drinking admitted that they thought they were safe drivers. Alcohol impairs judgment, reaction time, and motor skills. Drinking is a leading cause of high-risk driving.

Q: The parent or guardian of the child for whom I childsit drives me home. Last time, I suspected that (s)he had been drinking. What should I do if this happens again?

A: Even if an adult who has been drinking insists (s)he is OK, call your parents or guardian for a ride. Call a taxi or other responsible adult if they cannot be reached.

Q: My friend got a speeding ticket and is worried about the consequences. What can (s)he expect?

A: A **traffic violation** is any violation of the current traffic code. After a certain amount of traffic violations, a license can be revoked, or taken away for a period of time. Motor vehicle insurance rates will increase. A person may have to attend additional driver education classes. Serious violations, such as speeding, driving without a license, and driving under the influence of alcohol or other drugs, may result in imprisonment, a criminal record, fines, and the risk of injuring or killing oneself and others.

Q: My motor vehicle has an air bag. Do I need to wear a safety belt?

A: Yes. An **air bag** is a cushion in motor vehicles that inflates upon impact. Air bags cushion people from being thrown into the wheel, dashboard, and windshield. A **safety belt** is a seat belt and shoulder strap. Air bags are not a substitute for safety belts. Air bags often are effective in protecting people involved in frontal crashes but offer little or no protection in side, rear, and roll-over crashes. Safety belts should be worn by the driver and all passengers at all times. The lap belt should be snug and low across the hips and pelvis and the shoulder belt snug and across the chest and collarbone.

Q: I will be driving my younger siblings to daycare. What actions can I take so they are safe?

A: The National Highway Traffic Safety Administration recommends that all children under the age of 12 should ride in the back seat of a motor vehicle. This protects them from injury due to airbags and puts them farthest away from most impacts. All infants and small children must be placed in a child safety restraint placed in the back seat of a motor vehicle. A **child safety restraint** is a seat designed for a small child that is secured in the back seat of a motor vehicle. Motor vehicle safety seats for small infants face the rear. Seats for older infants face the front. Older children up to 60 pounds (27 kilograms) may need special motor vehicle booster seats. Always read the seat directions for proper use.

Activity

A Contract for Motor Vehicle Safety

Life Skill: I will follow guidelines for motor vehicle safety.

Materials: paper, pen or pencil

Directions: Your family motor vehicle belongs to your parents or guardian. You must protect your family's property and insurance coverage and earn your family's trust when driving. Use the steps below to make a Contract for Motor Vehicle Safety. DO NOT WRITE IN THIS BOOK.

 Make a copy or copy on a separate sheet of paper a Contract for Motor Vehicle Safety.

 Review the Contract for Motor Vehicle Safety. Add additional guidelines to the contract.

 Ask your parents or guardian to review with you the Contract for Motor Vehicle Safety and to add other guidelines.

 Sign and date the contract and ask your parents or guardian to sign and date it.

Contract for Motor Vehicle Safety

I recognize that driving a motor vehicle is a privilege that has been granted to me. I understand that I must obey all traffic laws and drive in a safe manner. I will follow each of the 20 safety guidelines in this contract. I understand that my driving privileges will be taken away if I break this contract.

1. I will obtain permission from my parents or guardian before driving any motor vehicle.
2. I will obey all traffic laws, including speed limits.
3. I will wear a safety belt when I am in a motor vehicle.
4. I will follow curfews and community guidelines.
5. I will not allow more passengers in my motor vehicle than there are safety belts.
6. I will not allow passengers in my motor vehicle who do not demonstrate good character.
7. I will not drink alcohol or use drugs.
8. I will not drive if I have taken OTC or prescription drugs that warn against operating a motor vehicle.
9. I will not be a passenger in a motor vehicle with anyone I know or suspect has been drinking or using drugs.
10. I will not be a passenger in a motor vehicle whose driver does not have a valid driver's license.

11. I will not allow peers to pressure me to practice unsafe driving habits.
12. I will avoid driving in severe weather, such as snowstorms and thunderstorms.
13. I will not drive in situations in which I do not feel safe, such as in heavy traffic.
14. I will not drive if I am tired.
15. I will recognize that other drivers may not be operating a motor vehicle safely and will drive defensively.
16. I will not participate in behavior that may be distracting when driving.
17. I will keep music and voices at a reasonable volume so I can hear sirens and other traffic sounds.
18. I will not allow another person to drive my motor vehicle without permission of my parent or guardian.
19. I will carry my license and registration with me when I am driving a motor vehicle.
20. I will keep a copy of my insurance coverage in the dashboard of my motor vehicle.
    Other conditions for the contract include:_____

_____

Signed,_____

(teen)   (date)

_____

(parents or guardian)   (date)

What to Know About Violence Involving Motor Vehicles

Teens need to protect themselves from violence while driving or riding in motor vehicles. Some people pretend to be helpful and assault people who have motor vehicle trouble. Others hitchhike and rob or injure people who stop and give them a ride. Some motorists become violent toward other motorists. **Road rage** is violent and aggressive actions of drivers and passengers in motor vehicles toward other drivers. Examples include making obscene hand gestures or remarks, throwing objects at or bumping other vehicles, keying vehicles, following another driver, and physically threatening another driver. People who have road rages injure others by fighting, hitting them with a vehicle, or using weapons such as firearms.

Events cited as provoking drivers and passengers to participate in road rages include slow driving, loud music, refusing to allow another motorist to pass or cutting him/her off, taking a parking space, tailgating, and failing to signal. The American Automobile Association (AAA) Foundation for Traffic Safety recommends that to prevent provoking other drivers and passengers you avoid eye contact with an aggressive driver, stay calm and do not react to a person trying to provoke you, keep a safe distance from people driving unpredictably, and report incidences of road rage to the police or 9-1-1.

Carjacking is motor vehicle theft that occurs by force or threat of force while the driver and/or passengers are still in the motor vehicle. Protect yourself by following the 25 strategies listed below.

1. Always park in a safe and well-lighted area where there are other people and vehicles.
2. Lock your motor vehicle at all times and keep your keys with you.
3. Have someone walk you to your motor vehicle.
4. Check the front and back seats before getting into a motor vehicle.
5. Never leave infants or small children in an unattended motor vehicle.
6. Never leave the keys in the ignition or the engine running.
7. Keep valuables out of sight.
8. Keep the fuel tank full. Fill it only during daytime.
9. Keep your motor vehicle in good condition to prevent breakdowns.
10. Try to drive in safe, well-lighted areas.
11. Have a car phone to use in case of emergency.
12. Keep a "Send help" sign in your vehicle to display if your vehicle breaks down.
13. Keep a flashlight and road flares in your trunk.
14. Stay in your motor vehicle, keep your doors locked and windows rolled up, and honk your horn at a police motor vehicle when your motor vehicle breaks down.
15. Do not get out of the motor vehicle if someone other than a police officer stops and offers help. Do not roll down the window and ask the person to call the police.
16. Drive to a nearby phone and call 9-1-1 if you see someone in need of help.
17. Never hitchhike or pick up a hitchhiker.
18. Do not drive home if you think you are being followed. Go to a store, police station, or well-lighted area where there are other people. Call the police.
19. Be cautious of anyone approaching your motor vehicle when it is stopped.
20. Keep the doors locked and windows rolled up.
21. Keep a sunroof closed and do not drive a convertible with the top down.
22. Keep your motor vehicle in gear when at a stoplight or stop sign. Allow enough distance between your motor vehicle and the one ahead to drive away.
23. Do not resist if an armed person demands your vehicle or your keys.
24. Do not give your keys to other people.
25. Get a latch inside for your trunk so that you can escape if forced inside.

Lesson 93

Review

Vocabulary Words

Write a separate sentence using each of the vocabulary words listed on page 662.

Objectives

1. What steps can be take to obtain a valid driver's license? Be a defensive driver? Avoid high-risk driving? Avoid traffic violations? **Objective 1**

2. Why are air bags recommended? Safety belts? Child safety restraint systems? **Objective 2**

3. What are 20 guidelines for motor vehicle safety? **Objective 3**

4. How can a person reduce the risk of injury caused by road rage? **Objective 4**

5. What are 25 self-protection strategies to keep safe from motor vehicle violence? **Objective 5**

Responsible Decision-Making

Your classmate has a new sports motor vehicle. (S)he asks you if you want to go for a ride and see how fast the vehicle can go. Write a response to this situation.

1. **Describe the situation that requires you to make a decision.**

2. **List possible decisions you might make.**

3. **Name two responsible adults with whom you might discuss your decisions.**

4. **Evaluate the possible consequences of your decisions. Determine if each decision will lead to actions that:**
   - **promote health,**
   - **protect safety,**
   - **follow laws,**
   - **show respect for yourself and others,**
   - **follow the guidelines of your parents and of other responsible adults,**
   - **demonstrate good character.**

5. **Decide which decision is most responsible and appropriate.**

6. **Tell two results you expect if you make this decision.**

Effective Communication

Your classmate gets very angry when other drivers cut him/her off. (S)he makes obscene hand gestures at the other drivers. What might you say to your classmate about the risks of this behavior?

Self-Directed Learning

Obtain permission from a parent or guardian. Call or visit the local department or agency of motor vehicles. Obtain information on licensing laws in your state. Write a one-page essay about your findings. Include information about the legal driving age, whether or not a learner's permit or graduating license is required, and what tests are required to obtain a license.

Critical Thinking

How might peer pressure increase the risk of motor vehicle accidents? How might a teen respond to this peer pressure?

Responsible Citizenship

Make an additional copy of the Contract for Motor Vehicle Safety and share it with a sibling or other teen. Suggest that this person sign the contract and share it with a parent or guardian.

You Can Reduce the Risk of Violence

Life Skill I will practice protective factors to reduce the risk of violence.

Violence has become too commonplace in society. Acts of violence are seen on television and videotapes, and music lyrics often describe violent behaviors. Being exposed to violence again and again may result in getting used to it and being unable to recognize what is and is not violent. In fact, it might lead to being unable to tell the difference between what is right and what is wrong. This lesson will explain how to reduce the risk of violence. You will learn about different types of violent behavior. You will learn risk factors and protective factors for violence. You also will learn why assertive behavior helps reduce the risk of violence.

The Lesson Outline

What to Know About Violence

What to Know About Risk Factors for Violence

What to Know About Protective Factors for Violence

How Assertive Behavior Reduces the Risk of Violence

Objectives

1. List and discuss nine types of violence. **pages 669–670**
2. Identify 20 risk factors that increase the likelihood that a person will become a perpetrator or victim of violence. **page 671**
3. Identify 20 protective factors that reduce the likelihood that a person will become a perpetrator or victim of violence. **page 672**
4. Explain how passive, aggressive, and assertive behavior influence the risk of being a perpetrator or victim of violence. **page 673**

Vocabulary Words

violence

nonviolence

perpetrator of violence

victim of violence

bullying

bully

fighting

assault

homicide

murder

suicide

sexual harassment

rape

child abuse

domestic violence

parent abuse

desensitization

risk factor

protective factor

resiliency

passive behavior

aggressive behavior

assertive behavior

What to Know About
Violence

Violence is the use of physical force to injure, damage, or destroy oneself, others, or property. **Nonviolence** is the avoidance of the threatened or actual use of physical force to injure, damage, or destroy oneself, others, or property.

A **perpetrator of violence** is a person who commits a violent act. A **victim of violence** is a person who has been harmed by violence. There are different kinds of violence.

Bullying

Bullying is an attempt by a person to hurt or frighten people who are perceived to be smaller or weaker. A **bully** is a person who hurts or frightens people who are perceived to be smaller or weaker. Most teens have been bullied at one time or another. In fact, three-fourths of high school students say they have been bullied. Bullying someone is violent behavior and wrong.

Fighting

Fighting is taking part in a physical struggle. About 40 percent of high school students say they have been involved in at least one fight per year. Eight percent of high school students say they have been in a fight in the last 30 days in which someone needed medical treatment for an injury. Males are more likely than females to get into fights. Fighting is risky. Many teens are injured. In most cases where a teen has been murdered, the violence began with a fight.

Assault

Assault is a physical attack or threat of attack. There are more assault injuries to teens than there are to people of any other age group. In some cases, assault occurs because a person wants to harm another person. In other cases, assault occurs as a result of another type of crime. For example, a teen might push down another teen to take a jacket or other item. One out of four people who have been assaulted require emergency medical treatment.

Homicide

Homicide is the accidental or purposeful killing of another person. **Murder** is a homicide that is purposeful. Homicide or murder is death from injuries that resulted when one person harmed another. Most homicides follow arguments and fights between people who know each other. Homicide is one of the top ten leading causes of death. It is the second leading cause of death in teens.

Suicide

Suicide is the intentional taking of one's own life. It is a deadly and final solution to temporary problems. Teens who commit suicide usually have experienced depression, anger, hopelessness, alcohol and other harmful drug use, family problems, and relationship problems for which they might have received help. Suicide is the third leading cause of death among teens. Teen females are three times more likely than males to commit suicide. Lesson 10 contains more information on suicide and suicide prevention strategies.

Sexual Harassment

Sexual harassment is unwanted sexual behavior that ranges from making sexual comments to forcing another person into unwanted sex acts. Sexual harassment sometimes occurs in schools. Title IX, a federal law, makes it clear that sexual harassment should never occur in a school.

Rape

Rape is the threatened or actual use of physical force to get someone to have sex without giving consent. An important part of this definition are the words "without consent." There are laws to interpret what "without consent" means. If a person does not agree willingly to sex, there is no consent and sex is considered rape. The law states that people under a certain age and people who do not have certain mental abilities are considered unable to give consent. The law considers these people unable to give consent even if they agree to have sex. A person who has sex with someone described as not able to give consent is guilty of committing rape.

Child Abuse

Child abuse is the harmful treatment of a minor. Child abuse may involve physical abuse, emotional abuse, sexual abuse, or neglect. The most common type of child abuse is neglect. This is followed by physical abuse and emotional abuse. A family member is the perpetrator 85 to 90 percent of the time. In most cases, the family member who harms a teen was abused as a child. Teens who are abused often are abusive when they are older and become parents. More than 80 percent of people in prison report that they were abused during their childhood. Children and teens have a right to be protected and kept safe by the important adults in their life. No one has the right to abuse them.

Domestic Violence

Domestic violence is violence that occurs within a family. Child abuse is one type of domestic violence. There are other types of domestic violence. One marriage partner may abuse or harm the other. This person may physically beat a partner. Or, this person might emotionally harm a partner by repeatedly making cruel and critical comments. This person also might force a partner to have sex without consent. Domestic violence also includes violence between other family members, such as brothers, sisters, stepbrothers, and stepsisters. **Parent abuse** is the harmful treatment of a parent. It is estimated that one-half of all families have experienced some type of domestic violence. Half of all married couples say that violence has occurred at least once during their marriage. Females are more likely to be killed by their husband or partner or by their former husband or partner than by anyone else.

WARNING:
TV Programs, Videos, Music, and Reading Materials That Contain Violence Are Dangerous to Health

Desensitization is the effect of reacting less and less to the exposure of something. You can become desensitized to violence if you see, hear, and read about violence again and again. You may ignore signs of violent behavior in others. You may behave in violent ways and think it is no big deal.

What to Know About
Risk Factors for Violence

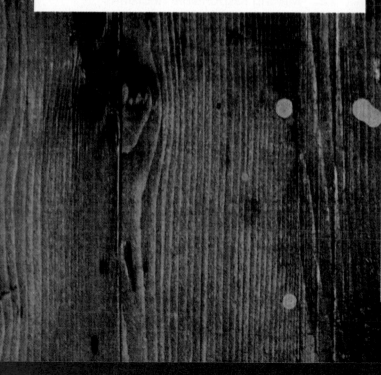

A **risk factor** is something that increases the likelihood of a negative outcome. Read the list Twenty Risk Factors That Increase the Likelihood That You Will Be a Perpetrator or Victim of Violence. You may find that some factors describe your behavior or the characteristics of the environment in which you live. If so, you have some risk factors for violence. You may be more at risk for behaving in violent ways and for being harmed.

Risk factors refer only to the statistical probability that something negative will happen. This does not mean that you will actually behave in violent ways or be harmed by others. You have varying degrees of control over the different risk factors. For example, you do not have control over the family in which you are raised or whether you are born rich or poor. However, you do have control over whether or not you carry a weapon to school. Knowing about risk factors is an important step in protecting yourself and others from violence.

Twenty Risk Factors That Increase the Likelihood That You Will Be a Perpetrator or Victim of Violence

1. Failing to recognize violent behavior
2. Lacking self-respect
3. Being raised in a dysfunctional family
4. Living in an adverse environment
5. Lacking social skills
6. Being unable to manage anger
7. Being unable to manage stress
8. Not participating in physical and recreational activities
9. Having suicidal tendencies
10. Resolving conflict in harmful ways
11. Practicing discriminatory behavior
12. Lacking responsible decision-making skills
13. Being unable to resist negative peer pressure
14. Using alcohol and other harmful drugs
15. Carrying a weapon
16. Belonging to a gang
17. Challenging authority and breaking laws
18. Failing to take precautions to protect yourself
19. Avoiding recovery if you have been a victim of violence
20. Repeating violence if you have been a juvenile offender

What to Know About
Protective Factors for Violence

A **protective factor** is something that increases the likelihood of a positive outcome. Read the list Twenty Protective Factors That Reduce the Likelihood That You Will Be a Perpetrator or Victim of Violence. You may find some protective factors that describe your behavior or characteristics of the environment in which you live. If so, you have some protection from violence. You are more likely to behave in nonviolent ways and be harmed by others.

Protective factors refer only to the statistical probability that your health, safety, and well-being will be protected. There is a chance that something beyond your control will affect your health, safety, and/or well-being in negative ways. For example, you might be a victim of random violence such as a drive-by shooting. However, the more protective factors that apply to you, the more likely you are to be protected from violence. Having protective factors in your life helps promote resiliency. **Resiliency** is the ability to adjust, recover, bounce back, and learn from difficult times.

Twenty Protective Factors That Reduce the Likelihood That You Will Be a Perpetrator or Victim of Violence

1. Recognizing violent behavior
2. Having self-respect
3. Being raised in a healthful family
4. Living in a nurturing environment
5. Having social skills
6. Being able to manage anger
7. Being able to manage stress
8. Participating in physical and recreational activities
9. Practicing suicide prevention strategies
10. Being able to resolve conflict
11. Avoiding discriminatory behavior
12. Making responsible decisions
13. Being able to resist negative peer pressure
14. Avoiding the use of alcohol and other harmful drugs
15. Staying away from weapons
16. Staying away from gangs
17. Showing respect for authority and obeying laws
18. Practicing self-protection strategies
19. Participating in recovery if you have been a victim of violence
20. Changing your behavior if you have been a juvenile offender in the past

How Assertive Behavior Reduces the Risk of Violence

Your behavior can influence the likelihood that you will be a perpetrator or victim of violence.

Passive behavior is the holding back of ideas, feelings, and decisions. People who have passive behavior find conflict very unsettling. As a result, they back off when there is a disagreement. They keep their anger to themselves. Bottled-up anger will continue to grow when it is not expressed. People with passive behavior may explode and lash out. They are at risk for being perpetrators of violence. People with passive behavior also are at risk for being victims of violence. This is because they do not stand up for themselves or expect others to treat them with respect. If they are harmed by others, they may keep it a secret in order to avoid conflict.

Assertive behavior is the honest expression of ideas, feelings, and decisions without worrying or feeling threatened. People who are assertive respect others and expect others to respect them. They are not controlling, forceful, or intimidating. They do not keep anger bottled up inside. They communicate in healthful ways and are able to resolve conflict without fighting. As a result, they are not at risk for being perpetrators of violence. People with assertive behavior also are less likely to be victims of violence. They expect to be treated with respect. They do not allow others to take advantage of them. They do not keep it a secret if they suspect wrong behavior.

Aggressive behavior is the use of words or actions that are disrespectful toward others. People who are aggressive are controlling. They are at risk for being perpetrators of violence. They may use force or intimidation to convince others to do what they want them to do. People who are aggressive also are at risk for being victims of violence. Their actions may provoke others into retaliation or into defending themselves. As a result, they are harmed by others.

You Can Respect Authority and Obey Laws

Life Skill I will respect authority and obey laws.

All societies are governed by laws that are regulated by people in positions of authority. A **law** is a rule of conduct or action recognized to be binding and is enforced by a controlling authority. **Authority** is the power and right to apply laws and rules. Laws usually represent the beliefs of a majority of people in a community, state, or nation. Every citizen has the responsibility to know and obey existing laws. This lesson will explain how you develop a moral code. You will learn that when you respect authority and obey laws, you protect yourself and others from injury. This lesson also will explain why some teens challenge authority and break laws. You will learn the consequences associated with being a juvenile offender.

The Lesson Outline

How to Develop a Moral Code

Why Some Teens Challenge Authority and Break Laws

What to Know About Juvenile Offenders

Objectives

1. Explain how a person develops a moral code. **page 677**
2. Explain why some teens challenge authority and break laws. **page 678**
3. Discuss the consequences juvenile offenders may experience. **pages 679–680**
4. Identify ways juvenile offenders can change their behavior to show respect for authority and obey laws. **page 680**

Vocabulary Words

law

authority

moral code

conscience

role conformity

social reciprocity

mentor

juvenile offender

delinquent behavior

status offenses

rehabilitation of juvenile offenders

probation

restitution

juvenile detention

prison

diversion

boot camp

parole

How to Develop a Moral Code

Laws are designed to protect the rights of people in a community, state, or nation. Many laws protect the health and safety of people. They may prevent violence and injury. You would think that everyone would want to obey laws. However, people have their own moral codes. A **moral code** is a set of rules a person uses to control behavior. People develop a moral code in three stages.

Stage 1: Will I get into trouble?

The first stage of moral development occurs in early childhood. During childhood, people decide what is right and wrong based upon whether they think they will be rewarded or punished for what they do. They decide what they will do by asking the question, "Will I get into trouble?" They do not completely understand the reasons why their parents, guardian, and other caregivers punish or reward certain actions. However, they want to please their parents, guardian, and other caregivers. They also want to avoid punishment.

Between the ages of five and seven, people begin to develop a conscience. A **conscience** is an inner sense of right and wrong that prompts responsible behavior and causes feelings of guilt following wrong behavior. The moral code learned early in life forms the basis of people's conscience. Their conscience makes them feel obligated to do what is right. Wrong actions make them feel guilty.

Stage 2: What will people think of me if I behave this way?

People reach the second stage of moral development between the ages of 10 and 13. This stage is referred to as role conformity. **Role conformity** is the desire to behave in ways that other people approve. People decide what they will do by asking, "What will people think of me if I behave this way?" They are most concerned with behaving in ways that are expected by the people with whom they feel close. At this age, people understand what behavior is expected and which behavior is right and which is wrong.

Stage 3: Is my behavior responsible?

During the third stage of moral development, people commit to a set of principles that guide their behavior. In this book, you have learned The Responsible Decision-Making Model. This model provides six criteria for deciding if behavior is responsible. These criteria can be used as a set of principles to help determine right behavior from wrong behavior. If you must decide if a behavior is right or wrong, ask if your behavior:

- promotes health,
- protects safety,
- follows laws,
- shows respect for you and others,
- follows the guidelines of your parents and of other responsible adults,
- demonstrates good character.

If the answer to all of the above is "yes," you can have a clear conscience. If the answer to any of the above is "no," you must reconsider your behavior. Your behavior does not guarantee that your rights and the rights of others will be protected. Having respect for the rights of others is a necessary quality that helps prevent injury and violence. It is necessary to develop the ability to care how others feel when treated in certain ways and to care about other people. **Social reciprocity** is the act of people treating others as they themselves wish to be treated. Many people in our society live by a moral code that says, "I will treat others as I expect to be treated."

Why Some Teens Challenge Authority and Break Laws

Teens who have a solid moral code respect authority and obey laws. What about teens who challenge authority and break laws? Why might they choose behaviors that put themselves and others at risk for injury? Why might they be involved in actions that promote violence.

Consider the three stages of moral development. In the first stage, right and wrong are learned based upon the behavior that was rewarded or punished. Parents, guardians, and other caregivers made choices about rewards and punishments. If they were very clear as to what was expected, a person had guidelines for his/her behavior. If they always followed through and gave consequences for wrong behavior, a person learned that wrong behavior would have negative outcomes.

Some teens are raised in families in which they did not have clear expectations for their behavior. Their parents, guardian, or other caregivers may not have disciplined them for wrong behavior. Or, they may have been disciplined in an inappropriate way, such as with physical abuse. As a result, they did not develop a conscience and do not feel obligated to do what is right. When they behave in wrong ways, they do not feel guilty. These teens need mentors to help them examine the difference between right behaviors and wrong behaviors. A **mentor** is a responsible person who guides another person. When troubled teens have a mentor, they have someone to whom they are accountable for right actions.

Consider the second stage of moral development. In the second stage, people are motivated to behave in ways that other people approve. This stage of moral development occurs between the ages of 10 and 13. Peer groups have a tremendous influence at these ages. Suppose members of a person's peer group respected authority and obeyed laws. Then that person would behave in the same way. However, some teens hang out with the wrong crowd. They may hang out with peers who get into trouble or they may hang out with gang members. Then these teens behave the same way. To change their behavior, troubled teens must break away from peers who behave in wrong ways.

Consider the third stage of moral development. In the third stage, people develop a set of principles to guide their behavior. They treat others as they wish to be treated. Some teens put their rights ahead of the rights of others. They want what they want right now. They do not care about the rights of others or consider the effects of their actions on others. If they harm someone, they do not care. Teens who have no principles to guide their behavior get themselves in trouble. They are dangerous. They may become juvenile offenders. The next part of this lesson examines what you should know about juvenile offenders.

What to Know About
Juvenile Offenders

A **juvenile offender** is a minor who commits a criminal act. Juvenile offenders are involved in delinquent behavior. **Delinquent behavior** is an illegal action committed by a juvenile. Delinquent behavior includes serious crimes, such as homicide, rape, drug trafficking, prostitution, robbery, assault, burglary, auto theft, and arson. Delinquent behavior also includes status offenses. **Status offenses** are types of behavior for which an adult would not be arrested, such as truancy, alcohol use, running away, defying parents or guardians, and breaking curfew.

Many juvenile offenders who are arrested stop committing crimes and do not become repeat offenders. They fear being arrested, put on probation, or sentenced to serve time in a correctional facility. Other juvenile offenders mature and change their behavior. Another group of juvenile offenders responds favorably to rehabilitation. **Rehabilitation of juvenile offenders** is the process of helping juvenile offenders change wrong behavior to responsible behavior. Juvenile offenders may experience the following consequences.

1. **Being placed on probation. Probation** is a sentence in which an offender remains in the community under the supervision of a probation officer for a specific period of time. Probation is the most common sentence that judges use for juvenile offenders. More than two-thirds of juvenile offenders are sentenced to probation. During probation, judges set restrictions and conditions for juvenile offenders. For example, juvenile offenders may be ordered to obey laws, obey parents or a guardian, attend school, avoid contact with other juvenile offenders, take drug tests, and make some form of restitution. **Restitution** is making good for any loss or damage. It is a way to make up for what has been taken, damaged, hurt, or done. It might involve making a payment, returning stolen property, or performing community service.

2. **Spending time in a correctional facility.** Juvenile offenders who engage in illegal behavior or violate the terms of their probation may be sent to a correctional facility. These include detention centers, training schools, ranches, forestry camps, farms, halfway houses, and group homes. **Juvenile detention** is the temporary physical restriction of juveniles in special facilities until the outcome of their legal case is decided. Detention centers are secure custody facilities where juvenile offenders are kept. Detention centers also are known as juvenile halls. Juvenile offenders usually are held in detention centers for a period of several hours to 90 days while they wait for their court hearing. They are held there because they may be a threat to others. Or, their home environment may be unacceptable. Or, they may be in need of physical or mental health treatment.

3. **Spending time in prison.** A **prison** is a building, usually with cells, where convicted criminals stay. Some people feel that the best way to deal with juvenile offenders is to treat them as adults and keep them in prison. These people are concerned about juvenile offenders who repeat crimes. Many states have changed their laws so that teens as young as 14 years old can be tried as adults for any crime. People who are opposed to trying juvenile offenders as adults feel that the results would be negative. They are afraid juvenile offenders will spend time in prison without changing their behavior. They are concerned about the influence adult criminals might have on juvenile offenders. They also are concerned that juvenile offenders will be sexually and physically abused by adult criminals while they are in prison.

4. **Experiencing a diversion approach.** **Diversion** is an approach to rehabilitation that involves sending juvenile offenders somewhere to learn how to obey laws. Juvenile offenders may be sent to social agencies, child welfare departments, mental health agencies, substance abuse clinics, shoplifters' programs, crisis intervention programs, and runaway shelters. Youth Service Bureaus offer services such as drop-in centers, school outreach programs, and crisis intervention programs.

5. **Going to boot camp.** A **boot camp** is a camp that uses rigorous drills, hard physical training, and structure to teach discipline and obedience. At boot camp, juvenile offenders live under very strict rules. They may have to wake up at 5 a.m. and go to bed at 9 p.m. They may not be allowed to watch television, listen to the radio, or swear. Most boot camps include education and therapy efforts. Juvenile offenders often end up in boot camp in exchange for reduced sentences.

6. **Being paroled and being involved in aftercare.** **Parole** is a conditional release from a sentence in a correctional facility. Aftercare is support and supervised services that juvenile offenders receive when they are released and must live and interact in the community. Once out on parole, juvenile offenders are assigned an aftercare officer who makes certain they follow the conditions of parole and stay out of trouble. Juvenile offenders who do not follow the conditions of their parole are returned to correctional facilities.

How Teens Who Have Been Juvenile Offenders Can Change Behavior

- Improve difficult family relationships.
- Spend time with a mentor.
- Ask trusted adults for feedback on their behavior.
- Work to improve self-respect.
- Choose friends who obey laws.
- Make restitution for wrong actions.
- Become involved in school activities.
- Develop job-related skills.
- Volunteer in the community.
- Attend a support group.

Lesson 95

Review

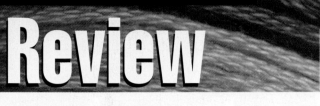

Vocabulary Words

Write a separate sentence using each of the vocabulary words listed on page 676.

Objectives

1. How does a person develop a moral code? **Objective 1**

2. Why do some teens challenge authority and break laws? **Objective 2**

3. What are examples of status offenses for which juvenile offenders can be arrested? **Objective 3**

4. What are six possible consequences of being a juvenile offender? **Objective 3**

5. What are ten ways juvenile offenders can change their behavior to show respect for authority and obey laws? **Objective 4**

Responsible Decision-Making

You are with two friends at a fast food restaurant. Your friends suggest taking all the straws, napkins, and packets of sugar, salt and pepper. Write a response to this situation.

1. **Describe the situation that requires you to make a decision.**

2. **List possible decisions you might make.**

3. **Name two responsible adults with whom you might discuss your decisions.**

4. **Evaluate the possible consequences of your decisions. Determine if each decision will lead to actions that:**
   - promote health,
   - protect safety,
   - follow laws,
   - show respect for yourself and others,
   - follow the guidelines of your parents and of other responsible adults,
   - demonstrate good character.

5. **Decide which decision is most responsible and appropriate.**

6. **Tell two results you expect if you make this decision.**

Effective Communication

Make a list of ten expectations that you have for other people's behavior. For example, you might list, "I expect a person who borrows something from me to return it." Review your list to determine if you have the same expectations of your own behavior.

Self-Directed Learning

Browse the newspaper or magazines or watch television for a story about a person who has committed a violent crime. Consider what has been written or shown about the crime and the person who committed it. Does this person show remorse for his/her actions? What form of restitution do you believe is appropriate for the crime?

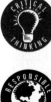

Critical Thinking

Why is it important for you to associate with peers who respect authority and obey laws?

Responsible Citizenship

Write a letter to a person who helps to protect the health and safety of your community. For example, you might write a parole officer, a police officer, prosecuting attorney, or the mayor. Express your gratitude for the job the person is doing.

Lesson 96

You Can Protect Yourself from People Who Might Harm You

Life Skill **I will practice self-protection strategies.**

An **unnecessary risk** is a chance that is not worth taking after the possible outcomes are considered. You can avoid unnecessary risks that jeopardize your personal safety. **Self-protection strategies** are strategies that can be practiced to protect oneself from violence. This lesson includes a discussion of each of the five principles of self-protection. The lesson also identifies self-protection strategies to protect you from violence. You will learn protection strategies to keep you safe at home, in public places, and in social situations. You will learn what to do if you are stalked or sexually harassed.

The Lesson Outline

What to Know About Self-Protection

What to Know About Self-Protection at Home

What to Know About Self-Protection in Public Places

What to Know About Self-Protection in Social Situations

What to Do If You Are Stalked

What to Do If You Are Sexually Harassed

Objectives

1. List and discuss five principles of self-protection. **page 683**
2. List 22 self-protection strategies to practice at home. **page 684**
3. List 22 self-protection strategies to practice in public places. **page 685**
4. List 14 self-protection strategies to follow in social situations. **page 686**
5. List steps to take if a person is stalked or sexually harassed. **pages 687–688**

Vocabulary Words

unnecessary risk

self-protection strategies

random violence

street smart

perpetrator of violence

acquaintance rape

date rape

stalking

restraining order

sexual harassment

What to Know About
Self-Protection

Random violence is violence over which a person has no control. A person may be a cashier in a store and be injured during a robbery. This person is a victim of random violence. Random violence is unsettling because there is nothing victims can do to avoid their fate. But, many acts of violence can be prevented by being aware of danger. This does not mean that you need to live in a state of fear, but you do need to be cautious. Consider the five principles of self-protection.

1. **Trust your feelings about people.** Accept the fact that some people, including people you know, might harm you. These people may have been harmed themselves. Trust yourself if you have a gut level feeling that a person or a group of people may be dangerous. Be on guard when this person or group is around. Avoid the person or group whenever possible.

2. **Tell your parents or guardian if there is a person you believe to be dangerous.** A trusted adult needs to know when you suspect someone who is or has been around you is dangerous. This person may have done nothing wrong—yet. But, for added protection, a trusted adult should know about your feelings. A trusted adult can talk over self-protection with you.

3. **Trust your feelings about situations.** When you sense that a situation might be dangerous, trust your feelings. Get out of the situation as soon as possible. Avoid the situation if you can. If the situation poses an immediate threat, scream to get the attention of others. Never worry about being embarrassed that you might be wrong.

4. **Practice being street smart at all times.** **Street smart** is being aware of possible danger and knowing what to do. Pay attention to people who are around you. Know how close they are to you and what they are doing. Find out where you are going so you do not look lost. Do not walk too close to buildings where someone can jump out and surprise you. Carry yourself with confidence. Practice screaming. Keep one hand and arm free when you carry something. Give up a personal belonging, such as a watch, rather than risk being harmed. Do not carry all your money in one place.

5. **Practice self-protection strategies at all times.** Behave in safe ways at all times. Never let down your guard or take your safety for granted.

What to Know About
Self-Protection at Home

Members of your family must cooperate to keep your home safe from perpetrators. A **perpetrator of violence** is a person who commits a violent act. A perpetrator may enter your home intending to take possessions or to cause harm to you or family members. A perpetrator may enter your home without intent to cause harm, be surprised, and respond by harming someone in your family. You can reduce the risk of being harmed in your home by practicing self-protection strategies.

Self-Protection Strategies for the Home

1. Keep windows and doors locked at all times, even when you are home.

2. Make sure your home has extra-security dead-bolts on all entry doors.

3. Be aware that chain locks are easily ripped off a door.

4. Consider having a home security alarm system installed.

5. Consider getting a dog and placing "Beware of Dog" signs on your property.

6. Do not give out your house key to anyone other than a trusted friend.

7. Do not hide your extra keys outside your home.

8. Consider having a one-way viewer or peephole in your door.

9. Leave one or more lights on at night.

10. Have your mail, newspaper delivery, and other services discontinued when you leave for an extended period of time.

11. Ask a trusted neighbor to check your home and vary the position of the drape when you leave for an extended period of time.

12. Always have your keys ready before going to your door.

13. Do not go inside if there are signs that someone has entered your home. Go to a safe place and call the police.

14. Never let a stranger into your home unless you are sure it is safe to do so.

15. Always give the impression someone else is in the home with you when speaking on the phone or answering the door.

16. Ask to see identification before allowing a repair person to enter your home.

17. Do not open the door, when someone asks to come in and make an emergency phone call. You can always make the call yourself if you want to do so.

18. Report any stranger who does not have identification to the police.

19. Be cautious about giving out information on where you live to people in person, on the phone, or by mail.

20. Do not talk to the person if you receive a crank phone call. Hang up immediately.

21. Report continuous, obscene, or bothersome phone calls to the telephone company and police.

22. Keep a list of emergency phone numbers, such as the number for the police and fire departments, by the phone.

What to Know About
Self-Protection in Public Places

You come from and go to many different places. You walk through the streets in your community. When you finish part-time work, you may walk home or to a car. You may stop at an automatic money machine to get some money from the bank. Whenever you are in public places, other people might harm you. You can reduce the risk of being harmed in public places by practicing self-protection strategies.

Self-Protection Strategies for Public Places

1. Avoid walking alone at night or in high-risk areas.

2. Stay on well-lighted streets and avoid deserted areas, alleys, and staircases when walking alone.

3. Keep your distance if someone in a car stops to ask you for directions. Ignore the person or call out directions to him/her.

4. Never accept a ride from a stranger or someone you do not trust.

5. Never hitchhike.

6. Wear comfortable shoes that allow you to run from trouble.

7. Do not talk to strangers who approach you.

8. Seek help in a nearby store or building with other people. Walk briskly with your head up and move in a confident manner if you think you are being followed.

9. Carry a loud siren, whistle, or buzzer to get attention if you need it.

10. Avoid using bank money machines whenever possible. If you use a money machine, do so during the day.

11. Stay away from areas where there are gangs.

12. Carry a chemical spray such as tear gas to use in case you are attacked.

13. Carry a flashlight at night and use it to light up potentially dangerous areas. It also could be used as a weapon in an emergency.

14. Carry your purse tucked under your elbow and hold it firmly with one hand. (Instead of carrying a purse, consider wearing a waist pack and carrying only what you need.)

15. Avoid using alcohol or other drugs so that you think clearly and make wise decisions about what you should do.

16. Wait only in safe and well-lighted areas for public transportation. After boarding, stay with a group of people or sit near the driver if possible.

17. Do not go into places that are deserted.

18. Yell, scream, or shout loudly for help if someone is bothering you in a public place.

19. Be sure to vary your walking route if you routinely walk to and from school or work.

20. Speed up, cross the street, turn around, run, or do whatever you feel necessary if you feel a person may be following you.

21. Do not turn your back toward a street or a lobby when you are using a public telephone; turn your back toward the telephone.

22. Use pay telephones only when they are in well-lighted places where there are many other people.

What to Know About Self-Protection in Social Situations

You are in many social situations. Sometimes you meet new people. Other times, you socialize with friends and other people you already know. When you socialize, you do not expect to be harmed, especially when you socialize with people you know. However, a perpetrator might be an acquaintance. A perpetrator might be someone with whom you have had a few dates. One type of violence that occurs is acquaintance rape. **Acquaintance rape** is rape in which the rapist is known to the person who is raped. One kind of acquaintance rape is date rape. **Date rape** is rape that occurs in a dating situation. Whenever you socialize, other people are in a position to harm you. You can reduce the risk of being harmed in social situations by practicing self-protection strategies.

Self-Protection Strategies for Social Situations

1. Stay away from places where you will be alone with a person you do not know well or whom you do not trust.

2. Do not go anywhere with a stranger even if you are supposed to meet other people.

3. Trust your gut feelings about other people.

4. Choose to be with other people when you socialize with someone for the first time.

5. Do not use alcohol or other drugs.

6. Set limits for expressing affection and communicate these limits to others.

7. Do not pressure another person to drink alcohol or to express affection beyond limits. Know that a person who has been drinking is accountable for sexual behavior.

8. Avoid behavior that might be interpreted as sexually teasing or seductive.

9. Respect the limits other people have set for expressing affection. Never pressure someone beyond limits.

10. Ask the other person to tell you clear limits when you are confused or feel you are getting mixed messages.

11. Do not assume you and another person want to express affection in the same ways or have the same limits.

12. Use physical force if someone continues sexual behavior after you have set limits.

13. Attend workshops, seminars, or classes to be clear on issues regarding acquaintance rape.

14. Pay attention to warning signs that indicate a person might harm you: disrespectful attitude toward you, dominating attitude, extreme jealousy, unnecessary physical roughness, and/or a history of violent and/or abusive behavior.

What to Do If You Are Stalked

Stalking is obsessing about a person with the intent to threaten or harm that person. Most of the people who harm others are male. Most of the people being stalked are female. Typically, people who stalk others are trying to form a relationship with the person they stalk. They may feel that by stalking they are able to get the other person's attention. Stalking also may begin when a relationship has just ended. The stalker may be upset and want to scare the victim into continuing the relationship. In some cases, a stalker takes further action, and stalking leads to injury or murder. There are steps to take to reduce the risk of being injured if you are stalked.

Steps to Take If You Are Stalked

1. Contact the police department to report the stalking. Consider pressing charges against the person who is stalking you. This may be enough to frighten and stop the person.

2. Keep a record of each case of stalking. Write down the date, time, what was said, and what happened.

3. Save any evidence, including notes and letters that may have been written to you and answering machine tapes with messages left on them.

4. Try to obtain a restraining order. A **restraining order** is an order by a court that forbids a person from doing a particular act.

5. Tell your parents or guardian and school officials what is happening. Tell them everything so they can do all they can to help protect you.

6. Seek appropriate counseling or join a support group for victims of stalking.

What to Do If You Are Sexually Harassed

Sexual harassment is unwanted sexual behavior that ranges from making sexual comments to forcing another person into unwanted sex acts. Examples of sexual harassment include telling sexual jokes, making inappropriate gestures, staring someone up and down, and touching, and grabbing or pinching someone in sexual ways. Males as well as females are sexually harassed. There are steps to take if you are sexually harassed.

Steps to Take If You Are Sexually Harassed

1. Ask the person who is harassing you to stop. Be direct about what behavior is bothering you. Describe the situation and the behavior that made you uncomfortable.

2. Keep a record of what happened. Write down the date and time, describe the situation and behavior, and explain how you handled the situation. Save any notes, letters, or pictures.

3. Check to see if there are guidelines to follow for the specific situation. For example, if the harassment was at school, check school guidelines; if at work, check work guidelines.

4. Report the harassment to the appropriate person in charge. This may be a boss, teacher, or school counselor.

5. Determine if you want to take legal action.

Lesson 96

Review

Vocabulary Words

Write a separate sentence using each of the vocabulary words listed on page 682.

Objectives

1. What are five principles of self-protection? **Objective 1**

2. What are 22 self-protection strategies to practice at home? **Objective 2**

3. What are 22 self-protection strategies to practice in public places? **Objective 3**

4. What are 14 self-protection strategies to practice in social situations? **Objective 4**

5. What are steps to take if a person is stalked? Sexually harassed? **Objective 5**

Responsible Decision-Making

A female friend has a part-time job as a childsitter for a family you know. She asks you to keep a big secret and tells you that the father of the children for whom she sits teases her in a sexual way. She says she is very uncomfortable, but she does not know what to do. She is afraid to tell anyone because he is generous in what he pays for childsitting. Write a response to this situation.

1. Describe the situation that requires your friend to make a decision.

2. List possible decisions your friend might make.

3. Name two responsible adults with whom your friend might discuss her decisions.

4. Evaluate the possible consequences of your friend's decisions. Determine if each decision will lead to actions that:
   - promote health,
   - protect safety,
   - follow laws,
   - show respect for your friend and others,
   - follow the guidelines of your friend's parents and of other responsible adults,
   - demonstrate good character.

5. Decide which decision is most responsible and appropriate for your friend.

6. Tell two results your friend can expect if she makes this decision.

Effective Communication

Tape a 30-second public service announcement (PSA) about how to be street smart. Play your tape for classmates.

Self-Directed Learning

Interview a police officer about crime in your community. Before the interview, prepare ten questions to ask. Take notes on the police officer's responses.

Critical Thinking

Suppose a neighbor makes you feel uneasy. You cannot pinpoint exactly what (s)he does that makes you feel this way. Why is it responsible to tell a trusted adult that you are uneasy when this neighbor is nearby?

Responsible Citizenship

Use five index cards. Write a self-protection strategy for the home on each card. Tape one card to the refrigerator. In a few days, exchange it for another card. Continue until all five cards have been displayed on the refrigerator to remind family members to stay safe.

Lesson 97

You Can Stay Away from Gangs

Life Skill **I will stay away from gangs.**

A **gang** is a group of people involved in violent and illegal activities. Some gangs consist of a few neighborhood teens. Others have thousands of members who cooperate in highly organized illegal activities. Gang violence is an increasing problem. Gangs have moved from big cities to smaller cities, suburbs, and rural areas. This lesson will give you facts about gangs. You will learn how to recognize gang members. You will learn why it is risky to belong to a gang. This lesson also outlines ways you can protect yourself from gangs.

The Lesson Outline

How to Recognize Gangs

Why It Is Risky to Belong to a Gang

How to Protect Yourself from Gangs

Objectives

1. List and discuss eight characteristics of gang members.
    page 691
2. Discuss reasons why it is risky to belong to a gang.
    pages 692–693
3. List ten ways to resist gang membership. **page 694**
4. Explain how a teen who belongs to a gang can leave the gang.
    page 694
5. Discuss reasons why some teens have become anti-gang gang members. **page 694**

Vocabulary Words

gang

hard-core gang member

regular gang member

wanna-be

could-be

prestige crime

jumping-in

anti-gang gang

How to Recognize
Gangs

You may have a mental picture of what gang members are like. There are ways gang members are alike and different. For example, gang members have been raised in families who have different income levels. They may live in big cities, small cities, or rural areas. However, most gang members have some common characteristics of which you should be aware.

1. **Gang members band together as a group.** Gang members hang out only with other gang members. They refer to their groups as "crews" or "posses."

2. **Gang members play specific roles.** Gangs have clear structures. A **hard-core gang member** is a senior gang member who has the most influence. There usually are several hard-core gang members who are leaders and tell others what to do. A **regular gang member** is a gang member who belongs to the gang and obey the hard-core gang members. A **wanna-be** is a child or teen who is not a gang member, but may wear gang clothing and engage in violent or criminal behavior to prove worthy of being a gang member. A **could-be** is a child or teen who is interested in belonging to a gang, perhaps due to a family member or friend. A could-be often is a younger friend and family member of gang members.

3. **Gang members follow specific rules.** Gangs have strict rules for the behavior of gang members. These rules are set by hard-core gang members. The rules may be written down in a code book. There are harsh consequences for gang members who break the rules. The rules may include hanging out only with other gang members and committing certain crimes.

4. **Gang members operate within a territory.** Gang members refer to this territory as their "turf." They may draw graffiti on buildings to let others know it is their turf. They consider members of other gangs to be trespassers if they enter their turf. Gang members may injure and kill people who "trespass" on their turf.

5. **Gang members wear certain colors or types of clothing.** Gang members identify themselves with a certain color or style of dress. They may choose one specific color to wear or one particular item of clothing to wear, such as a scarf or colored shoelaces.

6. **Gang members have their own vocabulary, logos, and signals.** Gang members invent code words to use among themselves. They invent ways to identify themselves as members of the gang, such as hand signals and handshakes. Gangs identify themselves by writing graffiti, or "tagging." Gang logos are used as graffiti as a public statement of turf and of intimidation.

7. **Gang members identify themselves by nicknames.** When people join gangs they are given a nickname, or street name. The nickname is used to disguise the gang member when (s)he is involved in illegal activity.

8. **Gang members often have tattoos.** Gang members get tattoos to identify themselves as members of the gang. They are a sign that a member is pledging to be in the gang for life.

Why It Is Risky to Belong to a Gang

Belonging to a gang is risky. Belonging to a gang often means being with young people who have enemies. Rivalry exists among gangs. Gang rivalry results in fighting, homicide, and other acts of violence. Gang members have sought revenge against rival gang members for insults, "trespassing" on gang turf, and personal disputes. If gang members feel they have been insulted or cheated, they feel their honor is at stake. They must restore their honor by seeking revenge. Revenge might include an assault or a drive-by shooting. Family members of gang members are at risk as well. Gang members often retaliate against the family members of rival gang members. Gang members often carry weapons to protect themselves from rival gangs. They also are involved in illegal weapon sales. Gang members often are involved in illegal drug use and drug trafficking. These activities can lead to violence.

Gang members may commit crimes to gain respect from other gang members. A **prestige crime** is a crime committed to gain status from other gang members. A gang member may assault another gang member, participate in a drive-by shooting, or steal in an effort to establish a tough reputation.

Gang members also participate in violence against their own gang members. Gang members who do not follow orders are beaten.

Teens who want to join a gang must participate in violent behaviors before they are admitted to a gang. These teens must go through an initiation period to prove they are "worthy" of gang membership. During the initiation period, they are subject to any gang member's demand at any time. They must commit violent crimes to prove themselves. Teens who are going through initiation often commit the most serious crimes so that the gang members do not have to do the "dirty work" themselves. Initiation demands may include murder, drug trafficking, weapons dealing, getting tattoos, carving or burning gang symbols into the skin, robbery, beating up other people, participating in a drive-by shooting, and beating up or killing rival gang members. Initiation may involve jumping-in. **Jumping-in** is an initiation rite in which a potential gang member is beaten by gang members. The potential gang member may have to fight all of the gang members either one by one or all at once. This initiation rite may continue for hours or even days. Teens have been severely injured and died from jumping-in. Initiation for females may involve being "sexed-in." This means they are forced to have sex with one or more male gang members. This puts them at risk for infection with HIV and other STDs and unwanted pregnancy.

Sometime teens are used by gang members. They may believe they are being initiated into a gang. Gang members demand they participate in criminal activities. They demand they participate in sexual activities. After these teens have committed the crimes, they are told they are not worthy of being gang members.

Why Teens Join Gangs

Myth: I feel left out and the gang will help me feel like I belong.

Truth: Being a gang member does not give a sense of belonging. Belonging means that teens who are gang members are considered property of the gang. Gang leaders believe they "own" their members and can use them to do whatever they want. Gang members only are accepted and "liked" by gang members if they behave the way gang leaders want them to. Gang members who break a rule or have a different opinion than other gang members may be injured or killed. Gang members always have to watch out for breaking a rule or getting on the wrong side of a gang leader.

Myth: I can escape family problems by being in a gang.

Truth: Many gang members have been raised in dysfunctional families. They have been raised in families in which there is physical abuse, sexual abuse, drug abuse, and neglect. Teens who think about joining a gang may believe they will be escaping the abuse. They believe that unlike their family members, gang members will care for them and pay attention to them. However, these same abusive behaviors continue among gang members. Gangs are even more dysfunctional. Gang leaders abuse gang members. Fighting, drug abuse, and rape are common among gang members.

Myth: I only get money for the things I want by being involved in gang activities.

Truth: Gangs are a big business. Gang members make their money from drug trafficking, stealing, and committing other illegal activities. When large amounts of money and illegal activities are involved, violence follows. Gang members are more likely to get a criminal record from these activities than make money. A person who has a criminal record often has more difficulty finding a job. Gang members are at high risk of dropping out of school. Not having an education increases the risk of poverty.

Myth: I can get protection from gang members.

Truth: Gang members may offer to protect you from others. However, once a teen is a member of a gang the risk of harm and threats from others are greatly increased. Teens are harmed being initiated into gangs. They are constantly at risk of being harmed by rival gang members. Involvement in drug trafficking and criminal activity also increases the risk of being harmed.

How to Protect Yourself from Gangs

Ways to Protect Yourself from Gangs

You know that it is risky to belong to a gang. Practicing using The Model for Using Resistance Skills to stick to resist pressure to join gangs. Tell a parent, guardian, or responsible adult if you are pressured to join a gang. You can avoid gangs by taking the following actions.

1. Stay away from gang members.
2. Avoid gang turf and places where gang activity takes place as much as possible.
3. Be aware of gang colors in your community and in nearby communities.
4. Do not listen to music that supports gang activities.
5. Do not stay out late at night.
6. Do not write graffiti.
7. Spend time with family members and mentors.
8. Obey laws and respect authority.
9. Avoid alcohol and other drug use.
10. Set goals and make plans to reach them.

How a Gang Member Can Leave a Gang

Teens who joined gangs when they were younger often were not aware of what being in a gang involves. Gang members often realize that being in a gang was not what they had hoped. They recognize that it is risky, stressful, and, at times, boring. However, they may be afraid to try to leave the gang. They know that other gang members may harm them or their family members. Some gangs allow members to leave if they survive a severe beating, or "jumping-out." However, many do not survive. Other gangs say they will not allow gang members to leave under any circumstances. However, it is not too late for teens who are in gangs. Help is available. Many teens have successfully left gangs and started lives without gangs, violence, and fear. Law enforcement officers have helped protect many gang members who wanted to leave their gangs. Many communities have gang counselors who help gang members leave gangs. Teens who want to leave a gang may move to another neighborhood, community, or state to be safe. Others return to their neighborhood and avoid gang members. The best way to avoid leaving a gang is not to join one in the first place.

Safety in Numbers

Some teens who live in communities in which there are gangs have formed anti-gang gangs. An **anti-gang gang** is a group of teens who stay together to avoid pressure and protect themselves from gang members. The goal of anti-gang gangs is for teens to continue with daily activities without being pressured or threatened by gang members. Anti-gang gangs walk together as a group to and from school and make arrangements to escort one another to school activities. An adult may accompany them for additional protection. These teens recognize that gang members are less likely to pressure them to join a gang when they are in a group. They do not hang around gang members or participate in gang activities. They do not wear clothing or take other actions to identify themselves as a group. Anti-gang gangs are informal, and any teen who wants to avoid gangs can become involved.

Lesson 97
Review

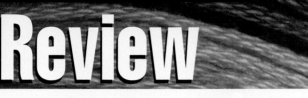

Vocabulary Words

Write a separate sentence using each of the vocabulary words listed on page 690.

Objectives

1. What are eight characteristics of gang members? **Objective 1**

2. Why is it risky to belong to a gang? **Objective 2**

3. What are ten ways to resist gang membership? **Objective 3**

4. How might a teen who belongs to a gang leave the gang? **Objective 4**

5. Why do some teens become anti-gang gang members? **Objective 5**

Responsible Decision-Making

A classmate is pressuring you to join a gang. (S)he says it will give you a sense of belonging and protect you from harm and threats. (S)he tells you that if you try it and don't like it, you can leave. Write a response to this situation.

1. Describe the situation that requires you to make a decision.

2. List possible decisions you might make.

3. Name two responsible adults with whom you might discuss your decisions.

4. Evaluate the possible consequences of your decisions. Determine if each decision will lead to actions that:
   • promote health,
   • protect safety,
   • follow laws,
   • show respect for yourself and others,
   • follow the guidelines of your parents and of other responsible adults,
   • demonstrate good character.

5. Decide which decision is most responsible and appropriate.

6. Tell two results you expect if you make this decision.

 ### Effective Communication

Your younger sibling tells you (s)he made money after school. A gang member paid your sibling to keep an eye out for police officers in the neighborhood for a few minutes. Your sibling tells you (s)he is excited about making money for "doing nothing." What might you tell your sibling?

 ### Self-Directed Learning

Check the library or the Internet for information about anti-gang gangs. Do anti-gang gangs exist in your community? In your neighborhood? In your school? If so, how did they get started?

 ### Critical Thinking

Why is it important to be aware of gang territories in your community? Why is it important to recognize colors and clothing worn by gangs in your community and nearby communities?

 ### Responsible Citizenship

Design a poster titled 50 Things to Do Besides Joining a Gang. Target the poster toward children. Obtain permission from a parent or guardian. Ask a principal of a middle or elementary school for permission to hang the poster where children will see it.

Lesson 98

You Can Reduce the Risk of Being Injured by a Weapon

Life Skill I will not carry a weapon.

Weapons are widely available in society. According to several surveys, one in five high school students has carried a gun, knife, or club to school or someplace else. Teens are more likely to use weapons to solve disagreements today than they were in the past. In many cases, fighting with fists has been replaced by fighting with guns and weapons. This lesson emphasizes the risks associated with carrying a weapon. This lesson also includes ten ways to reduce the risk of being injured by a weapon. You will learn ways to protect yourself if someone you know has a weapon.

Vocabulary Words
weapon
concealed weapon

The Lesson Outline
Why It Is Risky to Carry a Weapon
How to Reduce the Risk of Being Injured by a Weapon

Objectives
1. State the laws regarding the sale of handguns and rifles to teens. **page 697**
2. State the law regarding carrying a concealed weapon. **page 697**
3. List and discuss four reasons why carrying a weapon increases the risk of being injured. **page 697**
4. List and discuss ten ways to reduce the risk of being injured by a weapon. **page 698**

Why It Is Risky to Carry a Weapon

A **weapon** is an instrument or device used for fighting. Guns, knives, razor blades, pipe bombs, brass knuckles, clubs, and stun guns are examples of weapons. Guns are the weapons most likely to be used to harm teens. Most states have laws regarding the possession and use of guns. These laws forbid the sale of handguns to people under the age of 21 and rifles to people under the age of 18. Many states also have strict regulations regarding the sale of ammunition. The law forbids people of any age from carrying a concealed weapon. A **concealed weapon** is a weapon that is hidden partially or fully from view. There also are laws that regulate the way guns may be transported in cars and that prohibit carrying weapons to school.

Why Carrying a Weapon Increases the Risk of Injury

1. **Carrying a weapon increases the risk of injury due to accidents.** Every day, a teen dies or is seriously injured in a gun accident. In most cases, the victim was "fooling around with the gun." (S)he may not have known how to handle the gun or may have been showing off the gun to impress others or gain status. (S)he may have thought the gun was not loaded and wondered what it would be like to pull the trigger. The victim may have been handling a gun that was bought in an illegal manner. Or, (s)he may have been around a person handling a gun for one of the above reasons.

2. **Carrying a weapon increases the risk that it will be used to settle a fight.** Teens who carry a weapon may use the weapon if they get into a fight. If they had not had the weapon, they might have settled their disagreement in a different way. But, when emotions are strong and someone has a weapon, it is easy to use it. Once the weapon has been used, there is no way to take back any injury that has been inflicted. If a teen has a weapon, there also is the possibility that another person will wrestle it away and use it to get even.

3. **Carrying a weapon increases the risk of it being used in a crime.** Teens who commit crimes may intend to use a weapon only to frighten their victim. But they may actually use the weapon if the victim puts up a fight. Once a weapon is used, there is no way to take back any injury that has been inflicted.

4. **Carrying a weapon, particularly a gun, increases the risk of suicide.** Sometimes teens experience hard times. They may feel depressed and not know how to handle their situation. They may be taking drugs. These situations can lead to thoughts of suicide. In most cases, thoughts of suicide pass. However, if a weapon is available, a teen might use it. This action cannot be taken back.

How to Reduce the Risk of Being Injured by a Weapon

There are actions you can take to reduce the risk of being injured by a weapon.

1. **Do not purchase a weapon illegally.** Most states have laws forbidding the sale of guns to people under the age of 18. Suppose you want to purchase a gun for hunting. Ask your parents or guardian for permission. Learn how to use the gun. Keep it in a safe place. Do not carry it with you at inappropriate times.

2. **Do not carry a concealed weapon.** Carrying a concealed weapon without a permit is against the law for a person of any age. Always follow laws because they protect you and others.

3. **Do not carry a weapon to school.** Remember, you are forbidden to carry a weapon to school. You need to graduate from high school and do not want to be suspended. Keep your school safe.

4. **Encourage others to avoid buying, carrying, or concealing a weapon.** Be a positive influence. The fewer weapons there are in your community, the safer you and others will be.

5. **Do not pretend you are going to use a weapon.** Pretending can be misinterpreted. This behavior may threaten others into violence. For example, suppose you point your finger in your pocket to pretend you have a gun. Another person may respond with violence for self-protection.

6. **Avoid being around people who buy, carry, conceal, or use weapons.** You want to stay safe, and you cannot be certain what will happen if another person has a weapon. If you are around people who sell weapons to teens, they are criminals. They might be involved in other crimes, such as drug trafficking. Stay away from these people.

7. **Do not argue with someone who has a weapon.** Keep your distance. Try not to provoke or argue with this person. Remember, weapons often are used to inflict injury when someone becomes emotional. Remain calm.

8. **Avoid being in situations in which there will be weapons.** You may know that other teens will carry a weapon to a specific event. If so, stay away from the event.

9. **Leave a weapon untouched if you find it.** The weapon may have been used in a crime. If so, it may have fingerprints on it that would help solve the crime. The exact location of the weapon may be important.

10. **Tell a responsible adult if you find a weapon.** Someone needs to know the location of the weapon. A responsible adult, such as a parent, guardian, teacher, or law enforcement officer, can make arrangements, remove the weapon, and put it in a safe place.

Lesson 98

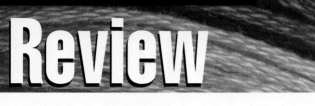

Review

Vocabulary Words

Write a separate sentence using each of the vocabulary words listed on page 696.

Objectives

1. What are the laws regarding the sale of handguns and rifles to teens? **Objective 1**

2. What is the law regarding carrying a concealed weapon? **Objective 2**

3. What are four reasons why carrying a weapon increases the risk of injury? **Objective 3**

4. What are ten ways to reduce the risk of being injured by a weapon? **Objective 4**

5. Why should a person avoid arguing with someone who has a weapon? **Objective 4**

Responsible Decision-Making

You and a friend are driving through a fast food restaurant. You spot a man putting a knife into the trash bin behind the restaurant. Your friend says, "Let's get out of here and pretend we didn't see anything." Write a response to this situation.

1. Describe the situation that requires you to make a decision.
2. List possible decisions you might make.
3. Name two responsible adults with whom you might discuss your decisions.
4. Evaluate the possible consequences of your decisions. Determine if each decision will lead to actions that:
   - promote health,
   - protect safety,
   - follow laws,
   - show respect for yourself and others,
   - follow the guidelines of your parents and of other responsible adults,
   - demonstrate good character.
5. Decide which decision is most responsible and appropriate.
6. Tell two results you expect if you make this decision.

Effective Communication

Write a rap or a poem about why it is risky to carry a weapon. Ask your teacher for permission to perform the rap or poem in class.

Self-Directed Learning

Check the library or the Internet for statistics about injuries or deaths caused by weapons during the last year. Chart the information to share with classmates.

Critical Thinking

Why might a teen want to carry a weapon? What reasons might you give the teen for not carrying the weapon?

Responsible Citizenship

Do research at the library or call a local law enforcement agency. Find out the laws in your state regarding the sale of handguns and rifles and ammunition. Make a poster to illustrate the laws. Ask a school official for permission to display the poster in a prominent place in your school.

You Can Participate in Victim Recovery If You Have Been Harmed by Violence

Life Skill I will participate in victim recovery if I am harmed by violence.

A **victim of violence** is a person who has been harmed by violence. Victims of violence may suffer physical injuries. They may lose money or property. They may be hurt emotionally. The emotional hurt that follows violence often is deeper and lasts longer than the physical injuries. Time does not heal all wounds. This lesson discusses victim recovery. You will learn how victims respond to being harmed. You will learn reasons why victims need help to fully recover. You also will learn what victim recovery includes and how victims can become survivors of violence.

The Lesson Outline

What to Know About Victims of Violence

What to Know About Victim Recovery

Objectives

1. Discuss the symptoms experienced by victims of violence. **page 701**
2. Explain post traumatic stress disorder. **page 701**
3. Give two examples of secondary victimizations. **page 701**
4. Outline five aspects of victim recovery. **page 702**
5. List and discuss five reasons why victims of violence need to participate in victim recovery. **page 702**

Vocabulary Words

victim of violence

post-traumatic stress disorder (PTSD)

secondary victimization

perpetrator of violence

victim recovery

survivor of violence

empowered

resilient

self-protection strategies

What to Know About
Victims of Violence

Victims of violence may experience different reactions in the period after being harmed. They may be highly emotional, feel depressed, and cry often. At first, they may avoid talking and being with others. They may neglect everyday tasks and have difficulty concentrating. They may have difficulty sleeping or have nightmares and flashbacks. They usually are very angry and afraid. They may try to numb their feelings with alcohol or other drugs.

Victims of violence do not respond in the same ways. Their response may be influenced by the way they usually act or by the kind of violence they experienced. For example, teens who have been victims of burglary may be afraid when home alone. Teens who have been victims of sexual abuse may have difficulties relating to people of the opposite sex. Teens who have experienced the murder of a relative may fear the loss of other people about whom they care deeply.

Some victims are able to recover from physical injuries and emotional hurt without help. However, most do not recover quickly or easily. Often victims experience pain for many years. **Post-traumatic stress disorder (PTSD)** is a condition in which a person relives a stressful experience again and again. PTSD is common in people who have experienced violence. The signs of PTSD include difficulty falling asleep or staying asleep, being irritable, and having trouble concentrating. When something reminds these people of what happened, they respond with much emotion.

Victims often experience additional pain or problems after violence. **Secondary victimization** is hurtful treatment experienced by victims after they experience violence. There are at least two kinds of secondary victimization. The first occurs if a victim must face the perpetrator. The **perpetrator of violence** is a person who commits a violent act. Many victims must attend the trial of the perpetrator. The trial may be delayed several times, and they may have to answer painful questions. The second kind of victimization involves being blamed for what happened. Family members and friends may try to find fault with the victim's behavior. If they can find fault, they convince themselves that this type of violence will never happen to them. Secondary victimization usually is not intentional. Family members and friends do not want the victim to suffer further. People act in these ways because violence causes emotion.

What to Know About
Victim Recovery

Victim recovery is a person's return to physical and emotional health after being harmed by violence. Victim recovery may include:

- treatment for physical injuries,
- treatment for emotional pain,
- support from family and friends,
- repayment for money or property losses,
- education in self-protection skills.

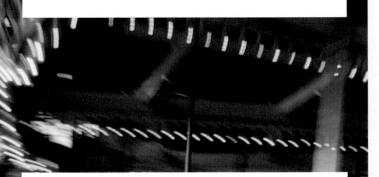

The purpose of recovery programs is to help victims survive the pain, heal, and move forward with self-confidence. A **survivor of violence** is a person who has been harmed by violence, participated in recovery, and feels empowered. To be **empowered** is to be energized because a person has some control over his/her decisions and behavior. Survivors of violence are resilient. To be **resilient** is to be able to adjust, recover, bounce back, and learn from difficult times.

Five Reasons Why Victims of Violence Need to Participate in Victim Recovery

1. **Victims of violence may need a complete medical examination if they have experienced physical injuries.** They may need blood tests to determine if they have become infected with any STDs including HIV.

2. **Victims of violence may need help with trust issues.** To have close relationships, teens must feel safe. Teens who have been victims of violence may not trust others again without help.

3. **Victims of violence may lack self-respect and allow others to harm them.** They may have been abused often. As a result, they may not believe they deserve respect. Without help, they may continue to allow others to treat them with disrespect.

4. **Victims of violence may need to learn better ways to protect themselves. Self-protection strategies** are strategies that can be practiced to protect oneself from violence. For example, a teen may drink too much and then be in a risk situation in which (s)he is harmed. Suppose (s)he continues to drink and be in risk situations. The result might be further violence.

5. **Victims who do not fully recover are at risk for behaving in violent ways.** This is especially true if violence occurred in the family. Victims who were abused by parents or a guardian may grow up and be parents themselves someday. They learned how to parent from their parents or guardian. Without outside help, they may parent in the same ways and abuse their children.

Lesson 99
Review

Vocabulary Words

Write a separate sentence using each of the vocabulary words listed on page 700.

Objectives

1. What are the symptoms experienced by victims of violence? **Objective 1**

2. What are the symptoms of post traumatic stress disorder? **Objective 2**

3. What are two examples of secondary victimization? **Objective 3**

4. What are five aspects of victim recovery? **Objective 4**

5. What are five reasons why victims of violence need to participate in victim recovery? **Objective 5**

Responsible Decision-Making

A classmate confides that his stepfather physically abuses him when his mother is not at home. He has kept the abuse a secret from his mother. He plans to avoid being alone with his stepfather. He says he will handle the situation this way because he will leave after high school. Write a response to this situation.

1. Describe the situation that requires your classmate to make a decision.
2. List possible decisions your classmate might make.
3. Name two responsible adults with whom your classmate might discuss his/her decisions.
4. Evaluate the possible consequences of your classmate's decisions. Determine if each decision will lead to actions that:
   • promote health,
   • protect safety,
   • follow laws,
   • show respect for your classmate and others,
   • follow the guidelines of your classmates's parents and of other responsible adults,
   • demonstrate good character.
5. Decide which decision is most responsible and appropriate for your classmate.
6. Tell two results your classmate can expect if (s)he makes this decision.

Effective Communication

Ask three people to respond to the terms victim of violence and survivor of violence. Do not share the definitions with the three people. How do their responses to the two terms differ? Why is choice of words important?

Self-Directed Learning

Use the card catalog at the library to find a book, tape, or video about a survivor of violence who was resilient. Share with a classmate or family member what you learned from the book, tape, or video about violence, victimization, and resiliency.

Critical Thinking

Suppose a classmate has been raped. (S)he did not know the perpetrator and was not in a risk situation. Other students in your school begin to find fault with your classmate. Why might these students respond to the violent rape of a classmate by blaming him/her?

Responsible Citizenship

Identify local organizations, agencies, groups, and health care facilities that deal with victim recovery. Make a pamphlet that identifies what services each offers. Ask your parents or guardian for permission to send the list to the local newspaper and request that it be published.

You Can Be Ready to Give First Aid

Life Skill **I will be skilled in first aid procedures.**

An **emergency** is a serious situation that occurs without warning and calls for quick action. An emergency exists whenever a person is injured or experiences sudden illness. The person needs immediate care. **First aid** is the immediate and temporary care given to a person who has been injured or suddenly becomes ill. This lesson includes A Guide to First Aid Procedures. The guide includes explains how to make an emergency telephone call, follow universal precautions, obtain consent to give first aid, and adminster first aid procedures. When you know first aid procedures, you can respond quickly to an emergency. You will not panic if someone is injured or ill.

The Lesson Outline

The table of contents for A Guide to First Aid Procedures appears on the next page.

Objectives

1. Explain the correct procedure for making an emergency telephone call. **page 707**
2. Explain how to obtain consent (actual and implied). **page 708**
3. Explain how to follow universal precautions when giving first aid. **pages 709**
4. Discuss steps to take when checking a victim. **pages 710–711**
5. Explain first aid procedures for choking; rescue breathing; CPR; heart attack; stroke; bleeding; shock; poisoning; burns; injuries to muscles, bones, and joints; sudden illnesses; heat-related illnesses; cold-temperature-related illnesses. **pages 712–749**

Vocabulary Words

The vocabulary words are listed in the activity on page 750.

A Guide to First Aid Procedures

What to Know About
First Aid Kits

It is important to keep first aid kits where they might be needed. Keep a first aid kit at home and in the family car. Carry a first aid kit when you participate in outdoor activities, such as camping and hiking. Ask where first aid kits are kept when you are away from home. You can purchase a first aid kit from a drugstore or the local chapter of the American Red Cross.

You also can purchase items and put together a first aid kit yourself. Keep items needed to follow universal precautions in your first aid kit. Universal precautions are discussed later. Add special medicines you or family members need. Check the first aid kit often. Some of the items have expiration dates and will need to be replaced. Be certain flashlight batteries work.

cold pack

activated charcoal

syrup of ipecac

plastic bags

triangular bandage

antiseptic ointment

disposable gloves

gauze pads and roller gauze

adhesive tape

hand cleaner

adhesive bandages

small flashlight and extra batteries

scissors and tweezers

blanket

What to Know About
Emergency Telephone Calls

Be prepared to make an emergency telephone call. Learn the telephone numbers to call in your community. Check out the telephone numbers to call when you travel to another community. In many communities, calling 9-1-1 will reach assistance for fire, police, and medical emergencies. The local phone book will tell whether a community has a 9-1-1 emergency assistance telephone number. Dial the operator (the number 0) if you do not know the correct number to call.

An emergency dispatcher will answer the telephone when you call 9-1-1. An **emergency dispatcher** is a person who decides who to contact when there is a call for help. The call may be directed to the police, fire station, poison control center, rescue squad, or emergency medical team.

No Prank Calls

Never make prank calls to your local emergency telephone number.

More than 35 percent of all calls made to 9-1-1 are for nonemergencies. The emergency dispatcher must take time to answer the telephone and evaluate each call. Unnecessary calls and prank calls can take time away from real emergency calls. These calls may slow down help to people who really need it.

How to Make an Emergency Telephone Call

1. Remain calm and speak clearly.

2. Describe the exact location of the emergency. Give the address and ways for emergency personnel to find the location. Naming the closest intersection or a landmark is helpful.

3. Give your name, what happened, the number of people involved, the condition of the injured people, and the help that has been given.

4. Give the telephone number of the telephone you are using. This makes it possible for someone to call you back if you get disconnected or more information is needed.

5. Listen carefully if you are told how to care for the victim. Write down directions if necessary. Give directions to other people who are caring for the victim.

6. Do not hang up the telephone until you are told to do so.

7. Return to the victim. Provide care if appropriate. Stay with the victim until help arrives.

What to Know About
Consent to Give First Aid

> You must have consent to give first aid. Consent means permission. There are two types of consent.

Actual Consent

Actual consent is oral or written permission to give first aid from a mentally competent adult. Tell the victim who you are, what you plan to do, and the first aid training that you have had. If the person gives you permission, this is actual consent. Do not give first aid to a conscious adult who does not give you permission.

A parent or guardian must give actual consent if the victim is a child or is not mentally competent. A supervising adult with legal permission from parents to care for an infant or child also can give actual consent. Do not give first aid to a conscious infant or child when a parent or guardian says "no." Do not give first aid to a conscious infant or child when a supervising adult with legal permission to care for an infant or child says "no."

Implied Consent

Implied consent is permission to give first aid to:

- a mentally competent adult victim who is unconscious;
- an adult victim who is not mentally competent, when no adult who can grant actual consent is present;
- an infant or child when no adult who can grant actual consent is present.

Good Samaritan Laws

Good Samaritan laws are laws that protect people who give first aid in good faith and without gross negligence or misconduct. Many states have Good Samaritan laws to protect people who give first aid. Lawsuits usually do not occur if a person giving first aid has the skills to do so. Lawsuits do occur when a minor injury is made worse because of the first aid given. Good Samaritan laws cannot provide complete legal protection. Anyone giving first aid should be properly trained and apply the correct procedures and skills.

Perform only the first aid skills you have been trained to give. Do not perform skills beyond your knowledge such as those you may see on a television show.

What to Know About
Universal Precautions

You must protect your health when giving first aid to another person. A victim's body fluids might contain harmful pathogens. For example, blood and certain other body fluids might contain HIV or HBV. HIV is found in blood, semen, vaginal secretions, and urine. A person who is infected with HIV will develop AIDS. HBV also is found in blood. A person who is infected with HBV will develop hepatitis B. You can help a victim and not risk infection with these pathogens.

Universal precautions are steps taken to prevent the spread of disease by treating all human blood and certain body fluids as if they contained HIV, HBV, and other pathogens. Follow universal precautions in any situation in which you might have contact with blood and certain other body fluids.

FOLLOW UNIVERSAL PRECAUTIONS
- Wear Disposable Latex Gloves
- Always Use a Face Mask

1. Wear disposable latex gloves. Latex gloves are made of a special rubber through which pathogens cannot pass. Your hands and fingers may have tiny cuts or openings you cannot see. Pathogens in a victim's blood or certain other body fluids may enter your bloodstream through these tiny cuts or openings. Wearing latex gloves protects you from contact with the victim's blood. Do not wear the same gloves more than once. Do not wear the same gloves to give first aid to another victim.

2. Wash your hands with waterless antiseptic hand cleanser after removing gloves. This provides extra protection.

3. Use a face mask or shield with a one-way valve when performing first aid for breathing emergencies. You may have tiny cuts or openings in your lips or mouth. There may be blood in the saliva or vomit in the victim's mouth. The victim may be bleeding from the mouth or nose. The face mask protects you from the victim's blood. Follow the instructions provided with the face mask. Do not use the face mask to give first aid to more than one victim without sterilizing it.

4. Take other precautions to avoid contact with the victim's blood. Cover any cuts, scrapes, or rashes on your body with a plastic wrap or sterile dressing. Avoid touching objects that have had contact with the victim's blood.

5. Do not eat or drink anything while giving first aid. Wash hands after giving first aid and before eating or drinking. This will prevent pathogens from entering your body.

6. Do not touch your mouth, eyes, or nose while caring for a victim.

What to Know About
Checking a Victim

A **victim assessment** is a check of the injured or medically ill person to determine if:

- the victim has an open airway,
- the victim is breathing,
- the victim's heart is beating,
- the victim is severely bleeding,
- the victim has other injuries.

FOLLOW UNIVERSAL PRECAUTIONS
- Wear Disposable Latex Gloves
- Always Use a Face Mask

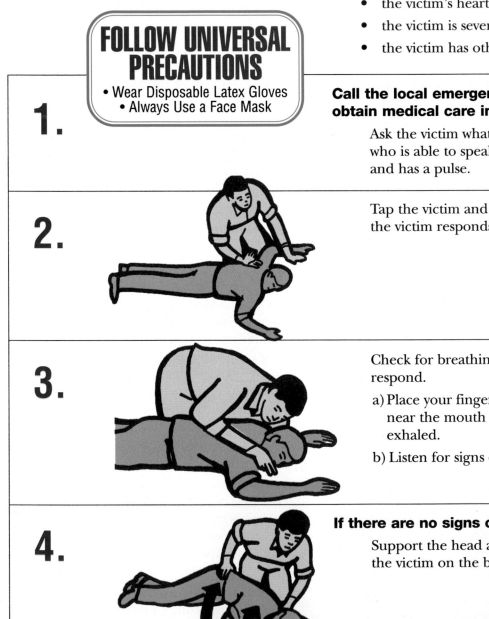

1. **Call the local emergency number and obtain medical care immediately.**

Ask the victim what happened. A victim who is able to speak to you is breathing and has a pulse.

2. Tap the victim and shout loudly to see if the victim responds.

3. Check for breathing if the victim does not respond.

a) Place your finger under the nose or near the mouth to feel for air being exhaled.

b) Listen for signs of breathing.

4. **If there are no signs of breathing...**

Support the head and neck and position the victim on the back.

5.

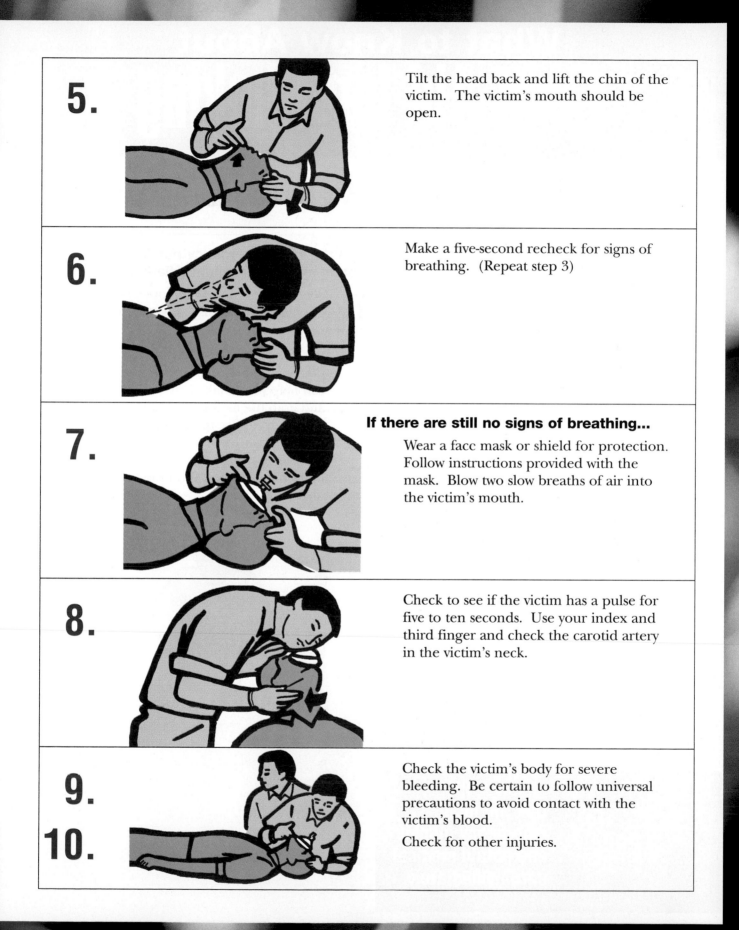

Tilt the head back and lift the chin of the victim. The victim's mouth should be open.

6.

Make a five-second recheck for signs of breathing. (Repeat step 3)

7.

If there are still no signs of breathing...

Wear a facc mask or shield for protection. Follow instructions provided with the mask. Blow two slow breaths of air into the victim's mouth.

8.

Check to see if the victim has a pulse for five to ten seconds. Use your index and third finger and check the carotid artery in the victim's neck.

9.

10.

Check the victim's body for severe bleeding. Be certain to follow universal precautions to avoid contact with the victim's blood.

Check for other injuries.

What to Know About
First Aid for Choking

Choking is an emergency in which the airway is blocked. A piece of food or other small object may block the airway. A conscious victim will cough to try to dislodge it. If a victim can talk, the victim is getting enough air. Encourage the victim to continue trying to cough up the object. Call for help if the victim cannot cough up the object.

A victim may not get enough air to talk or cough. Or, the cough may be very weak. This tells you that the airway is completely blocked. The victim may indicate that (s)he is not breathing. The **universal distress signal** is a warning that a person has difficulty breathing and is shown by clutching at the throat with one or both hands.

The airway must be opened quickly when someone is choking. **Abdominal thrusts** are a series of thrusts to the abdomen that force air from the lungs to dislodge an object. The method of giving abdominal thrusts is different for adults, children, and infants.

What to Do If You Are Choking

Call the local emergency number and obtain medical care immediately.

1. Get the attention of someone around you. Use the universal distress signal if you are unable to speak.

2. Give yourself abdominal thrusts if no one can help you. Make a fist with one hand and grab the fist with your other hand. Give yourself five quick abdominal thrusts. Apply pressure inward and push up toward your diaphragm in one smooth movement. Repeat until the object is dislodged.

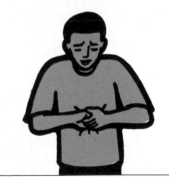

Call the local emergency number and obtain medical care immediately.

What to Do If an Adult or Older Child Is Conscious and Choking

1.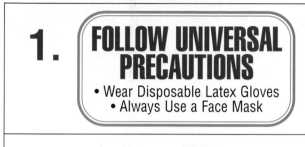

Call the local emergency number and obtain medical care immediately.

Ask the victim if (s)he is choking. Do not do anything if the victim can speak or cough easily. Encourage the victim to continue coughing to dislodge the object.

2.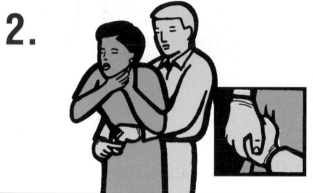

If the victim cannot speak, breathe, or cough...

Stand behind the victim and wrap your hand around the victim's waist. Make a fist with one hand. Place the thumb side of the fist into the victim's abdomen above the navel and below the rib cage. Grab your fist with the other hand.

3.

Give five quick abdominal thrusts. Apply pressure inward and push up toward the victim's diaphragm in one smooth movement. Repeat the cycle of five abdominal thrusts until the object is dislodged.

The victim may need rescue breathing after the object is dislodged. Stay with the victim and watch for breathing difficulties.

What to Do If an Adult or Older Child Is Not Conscious and Is Choking

1.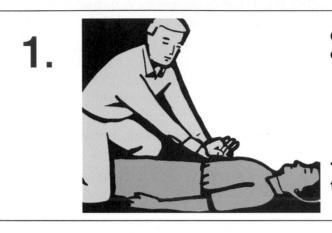

Call the local emergency number and obtain medical care immediately.

Roll the victim on his/her back. Place the heel of your hand just above the navel. Point your fingers toward the victim's head and give five quick abdominal thrusts.

The victim may need rescue breathing if the object is not dislodged.

What to Do If an Infant or Young Child Is Choking

1.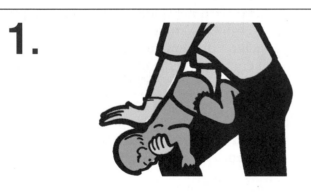

If the victim cannot cough, cry, or breathe...

Place the victim face down on your forearm or upper leg. Support the victim's head by placing your hand around the lower jaw and chest. Use the heel of your other hand and give five quick blows to the victim's back between the shoulder blades.

2.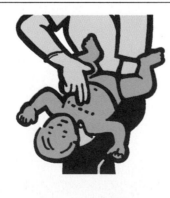

Place the victim face up on your upper leg. Make certain that the victim's head is lower than the trunk. Press two or three fingers in the center of the breastbone (just below an imaginary line between the nipples). Give five quick chest thrusts. Repeat back blows and chest thrusts until the object is dislodged.

The victim may need rescue breathing after the object is dislodged. Stay with the victim and watch for breathing difficulties.

What to Know About
Rescue Breathing

A victim will become unconscious without oxygen after a period of time. The heart will stop beating and blood will stop circulating to body organs. The different body systems will fail and the victim will die. **Rescue breathing** is a way of breathing air into an unconscious victim who is not breathing, but has a pulse. Rescue breathing gives a victim the oxygen needed to stay alive.

How to Use a Face Mask

A face mask or shield should be worn for rescue breathing. Place it between your mouth and nose and the victim's mouth and nose. This helps prevent you from having contact with the victim's body fluids.

Follow the instruction provided with the face mask or shield. The instructions might include:

Adults and Children

1. Apply the rim of the mask between the victim's lower lip and chin, thus pulling back the lower lip to keep the mouth open under the mask. Position the end marked "nose" over the victim's nose.

2. Seal the mask. Open the airway and blow slowly.

3. Remove your mouth. Allow the victim to exhale. Continue until the chest rises.

   (If the victim vomits, remove the mask and clear the victim's airway. Reapply the mask.)

Infants

Follow procedures except reverse the mask so the end marked "nose" is under the chin.

How to Give Rescue Breathing to Adults and Older Children

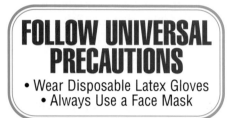

FOLLOW UNIVERSAL PRECAUTIONS
• Wear Disposable Latex Gloves
• Always Use a Face Mask

1.

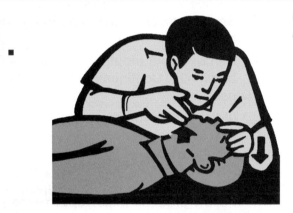

Call the local emergency number and obtain medical care immediately.

Roll the victim on his/her back. Tilt the victim's head back in the following way. Place one hand under the victim's chin and lift up while pressing down on the victim's forehead with your other hand. Pinch the victim's nostrils shut.

2.

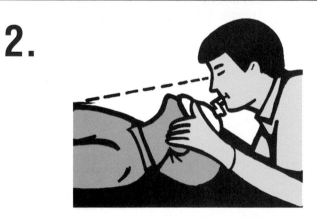

Wear a face mask or shield for protection. Follow instructions provided with mask. Apply mask. Open airway. Give two slow breaths. Watch to see if the victim's chest slowly rises.

3.

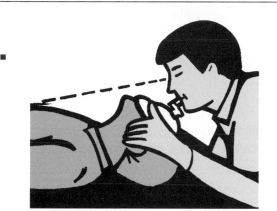

Check to see if the victim has a pulse. Use your index and third finger and find the carotid artery in the neck. The carotid artery is the large artery where the pulse can be felt.

4.

If the pulse is present, but the victim is still not breathing...

Give one slow breath about every five seconds. Remove your mouth after each breath so the victim can exhale.

5.

Recheck pulse and breathing every minute. Continue rescue breathing as long as the victim is not breathing, but has a pulse.

If the victim does not have a pulse, the heart is not beating. CPR is needed. CPR is illustrated in the next section.

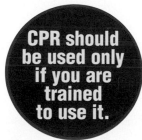

CPR should be used only if you are trained to use it.

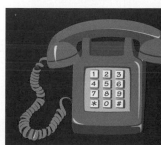

Call the local emergency number and obtain medical care immediately.

How to Give Rescue Breathing to Infants and Young Children

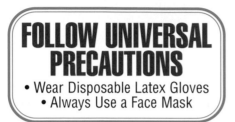

FOLLOW UNIVERSAL PRECAUTIONS
• Wear Disposable Latex Gloves
• Always Use a Face Mask

1.

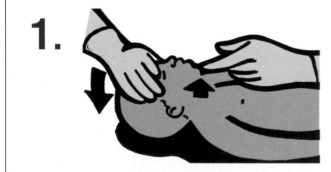

Call the local emergency number and obtain medical care immediately.

Roll the victim on his/her back. Tilt the victim's head back slightly.

2.

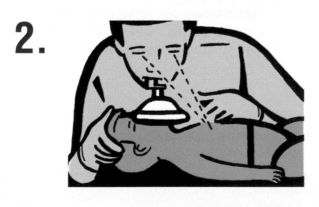

Wear a face mask or shield for protection. Follow instructions provided with mask. Apply mask. Open airway. Give two slow breaths. Watch to see if the victim's chest slowly rises. Remove your mouth to allow the victim to exhale.

3. Check to see if the victim has a pulse. Use your index and third finger and check the brachial artery on the inside of the upper arm.

4. **If the pulse is present, but the victim is still not breathing...**

Give one slow breath about every three seconds. Remove your mouth after each breath so the victim can exhale.

5. Recheck pulse and breathing every minute. Continue rescue breathing as long as the victim is not breathing, but has a pulse.

If the victim does not have a pulse, the heart is not beating. CPR is needed. CPR is illustrated in the next section.

CPR should be used only if you are trained to use it.

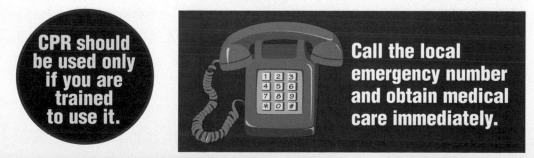

Call the local emergency number and obtain medical care immediately.

What to Know About
Cardiopulmonary Resuscitation (CPR)

Cardiopulmonary resuscitation (CPR) is a first aid technique that is used to restore heartbeat and breathing. CPR should be used only if you are trained to use it. Contact your local chapter of the American Red Cross to find out when CPR training classes are held.

CPR

CPR should be used only if you are trained to use it.

FOLLOW UNIVERSAL PRECAUTIONS
• Wear Disposable Latex Gloves
• Always Use a Face Mask

The ABCs of CPR help you determine the need for CPR.

A-Airway   Open the victim's airway.

B-Breathing   Perform rescue breathing if breathing has stopped.

C-Circulation   Perform CPR if a pulse is absent.

How to Give CPR to Adults and Older Children

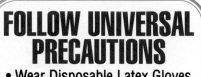

FOLLOW UNIVERSAL PRECAUTIONS
- Wear Disposable Latex Gloves
- Always Use a Face Mask

CPR should be used only if you are trained to use it.

1.

Make a victim assessment.

Call the local emergency number and obtain medical care immediately.

A person who is trained in CPR should:

Roll the victim on his/her back. Find the lower part of the breastbone and measure up the width of two fingers from that point. Place the heel of your other hand on the sternum next to the fingers. Place the other hand on top of the first hand.

2.

Position shoulders over hands to exert pressure straight down. Compress the chest 15 times (at a rate of 80 compressions per minute). Exert enough pressure to depress the breastbone one and one-half to two inches. Each compression forces blood from the heart to other parts of the body.

3.

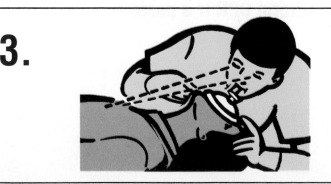

Wear a face mask or shield for protection. Follow instructions provided with mask. Apply mask. Open airway. Give two slow breaths. Watch to see if the victim's chest slowly rises. Remove the mouth to allow the victim to exhale.

4.

Do three more sets of 15 compressions and two slow breaths.

5.

Make a five-second check to see if the victim has a pulse and is breathing.

6.

If the victim does not have a pulse...

Continue sets of 15 compressions and two slow breaths.

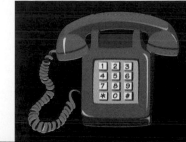

Call the local emergency number and obtain medical care immediately.

How to Give CPR to Children

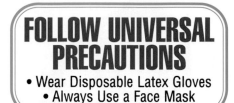

FOLLOW UNIVERSAL PRECAUTIONS
• Wear Disposable Latex Gloves
• Always Use a Face Mask

CPR should be used only if you are trained to use it.

1.

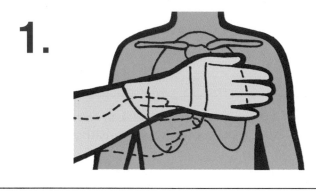

Make a victim assessment.

Call the local emergency number and obtain medical care immediately.

A person who is trained in CPR should:

Roll the victim on his/her back. Place the heel of your hand on the center of the breastbone.

2.

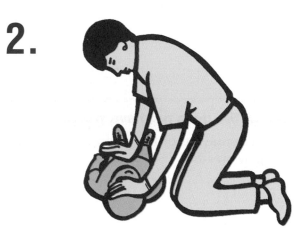

Position shoulders over the hand to exert pressure straight down. Compress the chest five times (at a rate of 60 compressions per minute).

3.

Wear a face mask or shield for protection. Follow instructions provided with mask. Apply mask. Open airway. Give one slow breath. Watch to see if the victim's chest slowly rises. Remove the mouth to allow the victim to exhale.

4.

Repeat sets of five compressions and one slow breath for about one minute. (12 sets)

5.

Make a five-second check to see if the victim has a pulse and is breathing.

6.

If the victim does not have a pulse...

Continue sets of five compressions and one slow breath. Recheck pulse and breathing every few minutes.

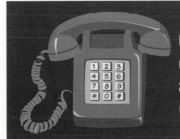

Call the local emergency number and obtain medical care immediately.

How to Give CPR to Infants

FOLLOW UNIVERSAL PRECAUTIONS
• Wear Disposable Latex Gloves
• Always Use a Face Mask

CPR should be used only if you are trained to use it.

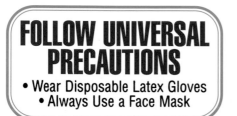

1.

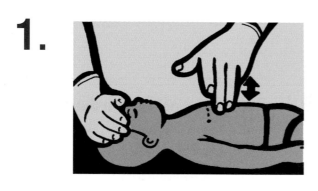

Make a victim assessment.

Call the local emergency number and obtain medical care immediately.

A person who is trained in CPR should:

Roll the victim on his/her back. Place the third and fourth finger on the center of the breastbone. Compress the chest five times.

2.

Wear a face mask or shield for protection. Follow instructions provided with mask. Apply mask. Open airway. Give one slow breath. Watch to see if the victim's chest slowly rises. Remove the mouth to allow the victim to exhale.

3. Repeat sets of five compressions and one slow breath for about one minute. (12 sets)

4. Check to see if the victim has a pulse and is breathing.

5. **If the victim does not have a pulse...**

Continue sets of five compressions and one slow breath. Recheck for pulse and breathing every few minutes.

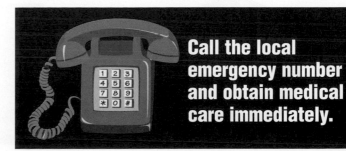

Call the local emergency number and obtain medical care immediately.

What to Know About
First Aid for Heart Attack

A **heart attack** is the death of cardiac muscle caused by a lack of blood flow to the heart. The blocked blood vessel prevents blood from getting to the heart tissue. Without blood, the heart tissue does not receive oxygen. This usually causes pain in the center of the chest, beneath the breastbone. **Cardiac arrest** is the death of the heart muscle. Prompt action must be taken for warning signs of heart attack to prevent cardiac arrest.

First aid for heart attack involves these steps:

Call the local emergency number and obtain medical care immediately.

1. Have the victim stop activity and rest in a comfortable position.

2. Ask the victim about his/her condition. Does the victim have a history of heart disease? Is the victim taking any medication?

3. Comfort the victim until help arrives.

4. Observe the victim for changes in condition.

If cardiac arrest occurs, the victim is not breathing and has no pulse...

A person who is trained in CPR should:

5. Perform CPR and rescue breathing.

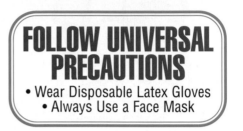

FOLLOW UNIVERSAL PRECAUTIONS
- Wear Disposable Latex Gloves
- Always Use a Face Mask

The warnings signs of heart attack include:

- Persistent pain or pressure in the center of the chest that is not relieved by resting or changing position
- Pain that spreads from the center of the chest to the shoulder, arm, neck, jaw, or back
- Dizziness
- Sweating
- Fainting
- Difficulty breathing
- Shortness of breath
- Pale or bluish skin color
- Moist face
- Irregular pulse

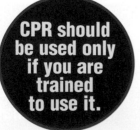

CPR should be used only if you are trained to use it.

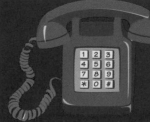

Call the local emergency number and obtain medical care immediately.

What to Know About
First Aid for Stroke

A **stroke** is a condition caused by a blocked or broken blood vessel in the brain. A stroke can occur when a clot moves through the bloodstream and lodges in the brain. A clot can form inside one of the arteries in the brain or a blood vessel in the brain can burst. A head injury or tumor may cause an artery to burst. Blood cannot get to all parts of the brain and some tissue dies.

The damage that occurs depends on the part of the brain that is affected. A victim may suffer a loss of vision or slurred speech. Body parts can become paralyzed. Sometimes blood cannot flow to parts of the brain that control heart rate or breathing and death results. Prompt action must be taken for signs of stroke to prevent disability and death.

First aid for stroke involves these steps:

Call the local emergency number and obtain medical care immediately.

1. Keep the victim lying down with the head and shoulders raised to relieve the force of blood on the brain.

2. Check the airway. Keep the victim's air passage open.

3. Position the victim on his/her side if there is fluid or vomit in the mouth.

4. Do not give the victim anything to drink.

5. Comfort the victim until help arrives.

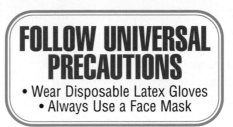

FOLLOW UNIVERSAL PRECAUTIONS
• Wear Disposable Latex Gloves
• Always Use a Face Mask

The warning signs of stroke include:

- Slowed breathing rate
- Unequal size of pupils in the eyes
- Slurred speech
- Paralysis on one side of the body
- Blurred vision
- Severe headache

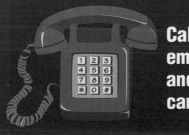

Call the local emergency number and obtain medical care immediately.

What to Know About
First Aid for Bleeding

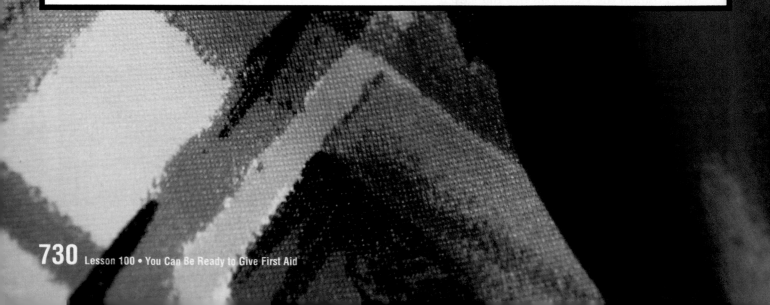

A **wound** is an injury to the body's soft tissues. A **closed wound** is an injury to the soft tissues under the skin. An **open wound** is an injury in which the skin's surface is broken. There are many types of wounds.

Bruise. A **bruise** is a wound in which damage to soft tissues and blood vessels causes bleeding under the skin. The tissues change color and swell. A bruise may appear red and change to blue or purple. Large bruises may indicate serious damage to deeper body tissues.

Incision. An **incision** is a cut caused by a sharp-edged object, such as a knife, razor, scissors, or broken glass. Bleeding from an incision may be heavy. There may be damage to large blood vessels, nerves, and deep soft body tissues if the cut is deep.

Laceration. A **laceration** is a cut that causes a jagged or irregular tearing of the skin. Bleeding can be heavy. There is the risk of infection because foreign matter is forced through the skin.

Abrasion. An **abrasion**, or scrape, is a wound caused by rubbing or scraping away of the skin. There is the risk of infection as dirt and other matter can become ground into the wound. An abrasion may be painful if the scraping away of the skin exposes nerve endings.

Avulsion. An **avulsion** is a wound in which the skin or other body tissue is separated or completely torn away. This injury may result in a piece of skin hanging as a flap. It may result in a body part, such as a finger, being completely torn from the body. Bleeding is heavy if deeper tissues are damaged.

Puncture. A **puncture** is a wound produced when a pointed instrument pierces the skin. A needle, nail, piece of glass, knife, or gunshot can cause a puncture wound. Puncture wounds do not usually bleed much unless a major blood vessel is damaged. The risk of infection from a puncture wound is high. A tetanus shot may be given if the victim has not had one recently.

How to Prevent Infection

A wound must be kept clean to prevent infection. An **infection** is a condition in which pathogens enter the body and multiply. Wash minor wounds with soap and water. Do not wash more serious wounds that require medical care. Closely watch the wounded area for signs of infection. There may be swelling and redness. The wounded area may become warm, throb with pain, or discharge pus. Red streaks may develop by the wound and move toward the heart.

There are steps to take when signs of infection occur.

1. Keep the area clean and soak it with warm water.
2. Apply an antibiotic ointment.
3. Elevate the infected area above the level of the heart.
4. Seek medical attention.

FOLLOW UNIVERSAL PRECAUTIONS
• Wear Disposable Latex Gloves
• Always Use a Face Mask

An Ounce of Prevention— The Tetanus Shot?

If you have ever stepped on a nail or been bitten by an animal, your physician may have given you a tetanus shot. Some wounds, especially puncture wounds, put you at risk for infection with tetanus. **Tetanus** or **lockjaw** is a bacteria that grows in the body and produces a strong poison that affects the nervous system and muscles. A DPT is an immunization given in childhood to protect against tetanus, diphtheria, and pertussis (whooping cough). A booster shot is needed every five to ten years after the childhood series. A booster shot also is needed when a wound is caused by a dirty object, such as a rusty nail.

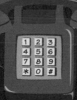

Call the local emergency number and obtain medical care immediately.

How to Control Bleeding

The first priority in any wound is to stop severe bleeding and prevent germs from entering the wound. A person with a wound may bleed to death in a matter of minutes.

1.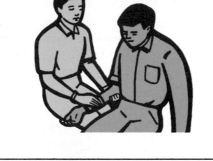

Call the local emergency number and obtain medical care immediately.

Cover the wound with a clean cloth or sterile dressing and apply direct pressure with your hand. Add more cloth if the blood soaks through, but do not remove the first piece of cloth. Do not remove any foreign objects that are lodged deep in the wound.

2.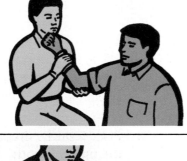

Elevate the wounded body part above the level of the heart. This helps reduce blood flow to the area.

3.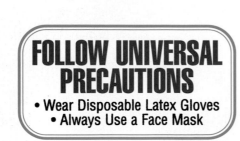

Cover the cloth or sterile dressing with a roller bandage.

4.

FOLLOW UNIVERSAL PRECAUTIONS
• Wear Disposable Latex Gloves
• Always Use a Face Mask

If bleeding does not stop...

Continue to apply direct pressure to the wound. Locate the closest pressure point. The pressure point technique compresses the main artery that supplies blood to the affected body part. This technique stops circulation within the limb. It is important to remember that if the use of pressure points is necessary, it should be used with direct pressure and elevation. Using pressure points to stop bleeding is not a substitute for direct pressure.

How to Stop a Nosebleed

A **nosebleed** is a loss of blood from the mucous membranes that line the nose. Many teens have nosebleeds. Most nosebleeds are caused by a blow to the nose or cracked mucous membranes in the nose. Nosebleeds are usually easy to control.

1. Have the victim sit with his/her head slightly forward and pinch the nostrils firmly together. Sitting slightly forward helps the blood flow toward the external opening of the nose instead of backward down the throat.

2. The nostrils should be pinched firmly together for about five minutes before releasing. The victim should breathe through the mouth and spit out any blood in the mouth.

3. An ice pack may be applied to the bridge of the nose.

4. Repeat this procedure for another ten minutes if the bleeding does not stop.

5. Get prompt medical help if bleeding continues or if you suspect serious injury.

FOLLOW UNIVERSAL PRECAUTIONS
- Wear Disposable Latex Gloves
- Always Use a Face Mask

What to Do When a Tooth Is Knocked Out

A **knocked-out tooth** is a tooth that has been knocked out of its socket. There are various recommendations on how to respond to this emergency.

1. Place a sterile dressing in the space left by the missing tooth. Have the victim bite down to hold the dressing in place.

2. Place the tooth in a cup of cold milk, or in water if milk is not available. Do not touch the root of the tooth.

3. The victim should see a dentist immediately. The sooner the tooth is placed back inside the socket, the better the chance it can be saved.

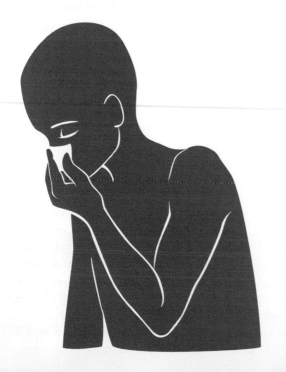

What to Know About
First Aid for Shock

Any serious injury or illness can lead to shock. **Shock** is a dangerous reduction in blood flow to the body tissues. The body organs fail to function properly when they do not receive oxygen. Shock can lead to collapse, coma, and death if untreated. Signs of shock include rapid, shallow breathing; cold, clammy skin; rapid, weak pulse; dizziness; weakness; and fainting.

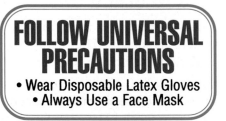

FOLLOW UNIVERSAL PRECAUTIONS
• Wear Disposable Latex Gloves
• Always Use a Face Mask

CPR should be used only if you are trained to use it.

First aid for shock involves the following steps:

Call the local emergency number and obtain medical care immediately.

1. Have the victim lie down. Elevate the legs about 8 to 12 inches above the level of the heart unless you suspect head, neck, or back injuries or broken bones in the hips or legs. Leave the victim lying flat if you are unsure of the victim's injuries.

2. Improve the victim's circulation.

   A Airway   Keep the victim's airway open.

   B Breathing   Perform rescue breathing if necessary. Remember to use a face mask or shield.

   C Circulation If you have completed CPR training, perform CPR if the victim has no pulse.

3. Control for external bleeding. Wear latex gloves.

4. Help the victim maintain normal body temperature. Cover the victim with a blanket if (s)he is cold.

5. Do not give the victim anything to eat or drink.

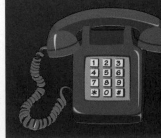

Call the local emergency number and obtain medical care immediately.

What to Know About
First Aid for Poisoning

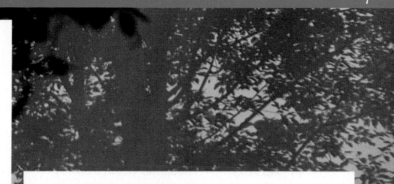

A **poison** is a substance that causes injury, illness, or death if it enters the body. Poisoning can occur when a person:

- **swallows a poison,**
- **breathes a poison,**
- **has poison on the skin that is absorbed into the body.**

Most cases of poisoning occur when small children swallow medicines or products, such as cleaning solutions or pesticides. Some people are poisoned by certain foods, such as shellfish or mushrooms. Some substances cause poisoning in larger amounts. For example, a person can be poisoned by taking too many pills or by drinking too much alcohol too quickly. Combinations of drugs, such as alcohol and sleeping pills, can cause poisoning.

Poisoning also can occur from breathing the fumes of household products, such as glue, paints, and cleaners. Certain gases cause poisoning. For example, a well-known tennis athlete died from carbon monoxide poisoning. Chlorine that is added to swimming pools is dangerous to breathe. Fumes from certain drugs, such as crack cocaine, also can cause poisoning.

Some poisons get on the skin and are absorbed into the body. Products, such as pesticides and fertilizers, can cause poisoning if they get on the skin. People using these products should wear gloves and clothing to prevent poisoning. They also should wear a mask to keep from breathing in fumes from these products. Poisons from plants, such as poison ivy and poison oak, can get on the skin. They are absorbed into the body and cause a reaction.

Poisoning can occur when a needle is used to inject drugs into the body. Bites or stings from insects, spiders, bees, snakes, and marine life can cause poisoning.

The signs of poisoning include difficulty breathing, nausea, vomiting, chest and abdominal pain, sweating, and seizures. Skin rashes and burns on the lips or tongue also may indicate poisoning.

What to Do for Poisoning

Steps to be taken when you suspect someone has been poisoned:

Call the local emergency number and obtain medical care immediately.

1. Be cautious. Protect your health and safety. Do not risk injury.

2. Move the victim to a safe location if necessary.

3. Treat the victim for life-threatening emergencies.

A	**Airway**	Keep the victim's airway open.
B	**Breathing**	Perform rescue breathing if necessary. Remember to use a face mask or shield.
C	**Circulation**	If you have completed CPR training, perform CPR if the victim has no pulse.

4. Gather information about the cause of poisoning. Determine the type of poison. Ask the victim what the type of poison might be. Be on the lookout for empty bottles and containers or needles. Recognize fumes and odors that may be the cause. Be alert to the environment. Are there bees, snakes, or poisonous plants in the area? Try to determine how much poison has been taken and when.

The Poison Control Center will tell you whether or not to induce vomiting in the victim. Victims who have swallowed acid substances, bleach or gasoline products should not vomit. These substances can burn the esophagus, mouth, and throat if the victim vomits. A victim with seizures or who is unconscious or semiconscious may be advised not to vomit. You may be advised to dilute the poison by having the victim drink water or milk.

Syrup of Ipecac is a liquid used to induce vomiting in victims who have swallowed certain poisons. It can be bought at local drugstores. Victims between the ages of one to 12 are given one tablespoon of the syrup followed by two glasses of water. Victims over age 12 are given two tablespoons of the syrup followed by two glasses of water. The victim usually vomits within 20 minutes after taking the syrup.

The victim may be advised to take activated charcoal after vomiting. Activated charcoal is a product used to absorb poisons that have been swallowed. It is sold in both liquid and powder forms at drugstores. It counteracts the effects of the poison that remains after a person has vomited.

FOLLOW UNIVERSAL PRECAUTIONS
- Wear Disposable Latex Gloves
- Always Use a Face Mask

CPR should be used only if you are trained to use it.

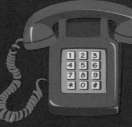

Call the local emergency number and obtain medical care immediately.

What to Do If You Touch a Poisonous Plant

Touching poisonous plants, such as poison ivy, poison sumac, or poison oak, can result in skin redness, swelling, and itching. If you touch a poisonous plant:

1. Wash the affected body parts with soap and water immediately.

2. Remove any clothing that may have some of the poison on it.

3. Use over-the-counter drugs to relieve the reactions that result.

4. Call a physician if the reactions are severe.

What to Do for Snakebites

Poisoning can occur from being bitten by a poisonous snake, such as a coral snake or a pit viper. Examples of pit vipers are rattlesnakes, copperheads, and water moccasins. Symptoms of a bite from a poisonous snake include pain at the site of the wound, rapid pulse, dimmed vision, vomiting, and shortness of breath. The victim may experience shock and become unconscious.

Call the local emergency number and obtain medical care immediately.

1. Treat for shock.

2. Keep the victim still. This will reduce the speed with which the poison can travel through the body.

3. Keep the bitten area below the level of the heart.

4. Get the victim of a snakebite prompt medical care.

Call the local emergency number and obtain medical care immediately.

What to Do for Beestings

Stings from bees are one of the most common insect-related problems. Beestings can create a serious health problem for people who are allergic. These people should carry medication to prevent a serious allergic reaction. They also should wear a Medic Alert tag.

Most people do not have an allergic response to beestings. The bee will leave its stinger in the skin when it stings.

Call the local emergency number and obtain medical care immediately.

1. Remove the stinger. Do not try to remove the stinger with a tweezer. The tweezer will force the bee's venom into the body. Flick the stinger away with a nail file, fingernail, credit card, or a similar object. Hornets, wasps, and yellow jackets do not leave stingers in the skin.

2. Place something cold over the area to relieve the pain.

What to Do for Spider Bites

Being bitten by a black widow spider can be deadly. A bite from this spider will produce a dull, numbing pain. Headache, muscular weakness, vomiting, and sweating may occur.

Call the local emergency number and obtain medical care immediately.

1. Wash the bitten area with soap and water.

2. Apply ice to relieve the pain.

3. Get prompt medical help. An antivenum may be given. An antivenum is a medicine that reduces the effects of the poison.

A bite from the brown recluse spider also is dangerous. A bite from this spider produces an open ulcer. Chills, nausea, and vomiting may follow.

1. Wash the affected part with soap and water.

2. Get prompt medical help.

FOLLOW UNIVERSAL PRECAUTIONS
• Wear Disposable Latex Gloves
• Always Use a Face Mask

Call the local emergency number and obtain medical care immediately.

What to Do for Marine Animal Stings

Stings from marine animals, such as the sting ray, sea urchin, spiny fish, jellyfish, sea anemone, or man-of-war can cause serious allergic reactions. Breathing difficulties, heart problems, and paralysis may result. A victim should be removed from the water as soon as possible.

Call the local emergency number and obtain medical care immediately.

Stings from a sting ray, sea urchin, or spiny fish:

1. Remove the sting ray, sea urchin, or spiny fish.

2. Flush the area where the sting is with water.

3. Do not move the injured part.

4. Soak the injured area with hot water for 30 minutes to relieve pain.

5. Clean the wounded area and apply a bandage.

6. Seek medical attention. A tetanus shot may be required.

Stings from a jellyfish, sea anemone, or man-of-war:

1. Remove the victim from the water as soon as possible.

2. Soak the area with vinegar as soon as possible. Vinegar offsets the effects of the toxin from the sting. Rubbing alcohol or baking soda can be used if vinegar is not available.

3. Do not rub the wound. Rubbing spreads the toxin and increases pain.

FOLLOW UNIVERSAL PRECAUTIONS
• Wear Disposable Latex Gloves
• Always Use a Face Mask

Prompt medical attention is needed for a victim who:
• does not know what stung him/her,
• has had a previous allergic reaction to a sting,
• has been stung on the face or neck,
• has difficulty breathing.

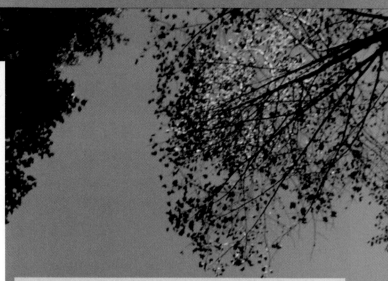

What to Do for Tick Bites

A tick is an insect that attaches itself to any warm-blooded animal. It feeds on the blood of the animal. There is great concern about diseases spread by ticks. Two such diseases are Lyme disease and Rocky Mountain spotted fever. **Lyme disease** is a bacterial disease transmitted through a tick. The ticks that spread Lyme disease are those on field mice and deer. The ticks are very small. The bacteria that cause Lyme disease are transmitted through the bite of an infected tick. A rash starts and spreads to be about seven inches across. The center of the rash is light red and the outer ridges are darker red and raised. A victim may have fever, headaches, and weakness. Prompt medical attention is needed. Antibiotics are used for treatment.

Rocky Mountain spotted fever is a potentially life-threatening disease carried by a tick. Cases of this disease are not confined to the Rocky Mountain region. Symptoms include high fever, weakness, rash, leg pains, and coma. Prompt medical attention is needed. Antibiotics are used for treatment.

How to Remove a Tick

A tick should always be removed from the body.

1. Grasp the tick with tweezers as close to the skin as possible.

2. Use a glove or plastic wrap to protect your fingers if you do not have tweezers.

3. Pull the tick slowly away from the skin.

4. Wash the area with soap and water. Also, wash your hands with soap and water.

5. Apply an antibiotic ointment or antiseptic to the area to prevent infection.

6. Observe the area for signs of infection.

7. Obtain medical help if the tick cannot be removed or if part of it remains under the skin. Medical help also is needed if signs of Lyme disease or Rocky Mountain spotted fever develop.

Do not put nail polish or petroleum jelly on a tick bite to suffocate the tick. Do not try to kill the tick by burning it with a match. These are not appropriate first aid procedures.

What to Know About
First Aid for Burns

A **burn** is an injury caused by heat, electricity, chemicals, or radiation. The seriousness of a burn depends on:

- the cause of the burn,
- the length of time the victim was exposed to the source of the burn,
- the location of the burn on the body,
- the depth of the burn,
- the size of the burn,
- the victim's age and health condition.

Burns are usually described as first-degree burns, second-degree burns, or third-degree burns. These descriptions help explain the seriousness of the burn.

FOLLOW UNIVERSAL PRECAUTIONS
- Wear Disposable Latex Gloves
- Always Use a Face Mask

What to Do for First-Degree Burns

A **first-degree burn** is a burn which affects the top layer of skin. Most sunburns are first-degree burns. The skin becomes red and dry and the area may swell. The area is painful to touch. First-degree burns usually heal in six days without permanent scarring.

First aid for a first-degree burn:

1. Stop the burning. Get the victim out of the sun. Put out flames that are burning clothes or skin.

2. Cool the burned area with water as soon as possible. Soak the area with tap water, a garden hose, or have the victim get into the bath or shower. Use sheets or towels soaked in cold water to cool a burn on the face or other areas that cannot be soaked. Keep adding cool water.

3. Wear latex gloves. Loosely bandage the area with a dry, sterile dressing.

4. Place cotton or gauze between burned fingers and toes.

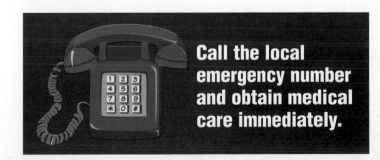

Call the local emergency number and obtain medical care immediately.

What to Do for Second-Degree Burns

A **second-degree burn** is a burn that involves the top layers of the skin. The skin becomes red. Blisters form and may open and discharge a clear fluid. The skin appears wet and mottled. Second-degree burns usually heal in two to four weeks. Slight scarring may occur.

First aid for a second-degree burn:

Call the local emergency number and obtain medical care immediately.

1. Stop the burning. Remove the victim from the source of the burn.

2. Cool the burned area with cool water or cold cloths. Keep the cover loose. This helps prevent infection and reduces pain. Do not break blisters or remove tissue.

4. Elevate the burned area above heart level.

5. Cover the victim with clean, dry sheets if burns cover large parts of the body. Treat for shock.

FOLLOW UNIVERSAL PRECAUTIONS
- Wear Disposable Latex Gloves
- Always Use a Face Mask

What to Do for Third-Degree Burns

A **third-degree burn** is a burn that involves all layers of the skin and some underlying tissues. A third-degree burn may affect fat tissue, muscle tissue, bones, and nerves. The skin becomes darker and appears charred. The underlying tissues may appear white. A third-degree burn is painless if nerve endings are destroyed. It also can be very painful. Third-degree burns may take months or years to treat. Permanent scarring often occurs. Some victims require skin grafting and plastic surgery.

First aid for a third-degree burn:

Call the local emergency number and obtain medical care immediately.

1. Treat the victim for shock.

2. Check immediately if the victim is breathing. Give rescue breathing if necessary. Do not open blisters or remove pieces of tissue. Do not apply cold.

3. Cover the burned area with a dry, sterile dressing; clean cloth; or sheet.

What to Do for Electrical Burns

An **electrical burn** is a burn that occurs when electricity travels through the body. The cause may be lightning or contact with faulty electrical equipment or a power line. The seriousness of an electrical burn depends on the strength of the electrical current. It also depends on the path the current takes through the body. An electrical burn can be very deep. There may be a wound where the electrical current enters and where it leaves the body.

First aid for an electrical burn:

Call the local emergency number and obtain medical care immediately.

1. Do not go near the victim until the source of electricity is turned off.

2. Get prompt medical attention.

3. Treat the victim for shock.

4. Do not move the victim.

5. Cover the burn with a dry, sterile dressing. Do not use cool water or compresses as the victim may be in shock.

What to Do for Chemical Burns

A **chemical burn** is a burn that occurs when chemicals in a laboratory or in products get on the skin or into the eyes or body. The burn continues as long as there is contact with the chemical.

First aid for a chemical burn:

Call the local emergency number and obtain medical care immediately.

1. Remove the source of the chemical. Have the victim remove any clothing with the chemical on it.

2. Flush the skin or eyes with cool, low-pressure running water. If the chemical is dry or solid, brush it off with a cloth before flushing with water. Take special precautions if one eye is involved. Have the victim turn the head and run the water from the nose away from the eye. This keeps water with the chemical in it from running into the other eye.

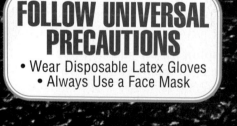

FOLLOW UNIVERSAL PRECAUTIONS
• Wear Disposable Latex Gloves
• Always Use a Face Mask

What to Know About
First Aid for Injuries to Muscles, Bones, and Joints

There are 206 bones in the body and more than 600 muscles. A joint is the point at which two bones meet. Ligaments are the fibers that connect bones together. Tendons are tough tissue fibers that connect muscles to bones. Injuries involving muscles, bones, and joints are common in teens. The most common injuries are fractures, dislocations, sprains, and strains.

A **splint** is material or a device used to protect and immobilize a body part. A splint should only be used when you need to move a victim without emergency help and need to keep an injured body part still. A splint should only be used if it can be used without hurting the victim. A folded blanket, towel, sheet, or bandage might be used as a soft splint. Rolled-up newspapers or boards may be used as a rigid splint. Emergency medical personnel may use a board as a splint.

First aid when using a splint:

Call the local emergency number and obtain medical care immediately.

1. Attempt to splint the injury in the position you find it.

2. A splint for an injured bone must include the joints above and below the fracture.

3. A splint for an injured joint must include the bones above and below the injured joint.

4. Check for circulation so that the splint is not too tight.

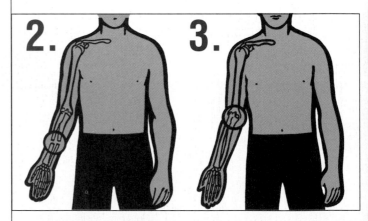

What to Do for Fractures

A **fracture** is a break or a crack in a bone. An **open fracture** is a fracture in which there is a break in the skin. A **closed fracture** is a fracture in which there is no break in the skin. A fracture can be very serious if a break in a bone damages an artery or interferes with breathing. The signs of a fracture include pain, swelling, loss of movement, and deformity. Signs of a fracture of the skull include bleeding from the head or ears, drowsiness and headache.

First aid for fractures:

Call the local emergency number and obtain medical care immediately.

1. Treat for bleeding and shock.

2. Keep the injured part from moving. Use a splint when appropriate. Keep a victim with a head injury still.

3. Apply ice to the break or crack to prevent swelling.

4. Follow universal precautions. Control bleeding.

5. Get prompt medical help.

What to Do for Dislocations

A **dislocation** is the movement of a bone from its joint. Dislocations often are accompanied by stretched ligaments. The signs of a dislocation are pain, swelling upon movement, loss of movement, and deformity.

First aid for a dislocation:

Call the local emergency number and obtain medical care immediately.

1. Splint above and below the dislocated joint.
2. Apply cold compresses.

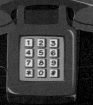

Call the local emergency number and obtain medical care immediately.

FOLLOW UNIVERSAL PRECAUTIONS
- Wear Disposable Latex Gloves
- Always Use a Face Mask

What to Do for Sprains

A **sprain** is an injury to the ligaments, tendons, and soft tissue around a joint caused by undue stretching. The signs of a sprain include pain that increases with movement or weight bearing, tenderness, and swelling.

First aid for sprains:

1. Follow the RICE treatment.
2. Get prompt medical help if a fracture is suspected.

What to Do for Strains

A **strain** is an overstretching of muscles and/or tendons. One of the most common strains involves the muscles of the back. Signs of strain include pain, swelling, stiffness, and firmness to the area.

First aid for strains:

1. Follow the RICE treatment.
2. Get prompt medical help for a severe strain.

How to Use the RICE Treatment

Rest: Rest the injured part for 24 to 72 hours. Longer rest is required for severe injuries. Do not exercise the injured area until there is complete healing.

Ice: Apply cold water, a cold compress, or ice pack for 20 minutes as soon as possible after the injury occurs. Apply several times a day for one to three days. Wrap ice in a cloth before placing on the skin. Applying cold water reduces pain, swelling, inflammation, and tissue damage.

Compression: Wrap the injury with an elastic bandage to limit swelling. The compression should not be too tight so as to restrict blood flow. Remove the wrap periodically and check.

Elevation: Raise the injured body part above the level of the heart to reduce swelling and drain blood and fluid from the area.

What to Know About
First Aid for Sudden Illnesses

Sudden illness is an illness that occurs without warning signals of what is actually happening. It is difficult to determine if the situation is an emergency. Signs of sudden illness may include dizziness and confusion, weakness, changes in skin color, nausea, vomiting, and diarrhea. Seizures, paralysis, slurred speech, difficulty seeing, and severe pain may also indicate sudden illness.

First aid for sudden illness:

Call the local emergency number and obtain medical care immediately.

1. Give first aid for life-threatening conditions.
2. Keep the victim calm.
3. Cover the victim with a blanket if (s)he is chilled.
4. Do not give an unconscious victim anything to eat or drink.
5. Get prompt medical attention.

FOLLOW UNIVERSAL PRECAUTIONS
- Wear Disposable Latex Gloves
- Always Use a Face Mask

What to Do for Fainting

6. If the victim has fainted: Put the victim on his/her back. Elevate the victim's legs 8 to 12 inches above the level of the heart. (Do not elevate the legs if you suspect a head or back injury.) Loosen tight clothing. Do not splash water on the victim, slap the victim's face, or use smelling salts.

What to Do for Vomiting

7. If the victim is vomiting: Turn the victim on his/her side.

What to Do for Seizures

8. If the victim has a seizure: Place something under the victim's head to cushion the head from injury. Remove objects that might injure the victim. Loosen the clothing around the victim's neck. Do not restrain the victim. Do not place anything in the victim's mouth or between the teeth. Look for a Medic Alert tag.

What to Know About
First Aid for Heat-Related Illnesses

Heat-related illnesses are conditions that result from exposure to temperatures higher than normal. Heat cramps, heat exhaustion, and heat stroke are the most common heat-related illnesses.

What to Do for Heat Cramps

Heat cramps are painful muscle spasms in the legs and arms due to excessive fluid loss through sweating.

First aid for heat cramps:

1. Have the victim rest in a cool, shaded area.
2. Give the victim cool water to drink.
3. Stretch the muscle gently.

What to Do for Heat Exhaustion

Heat exhaustion is extreme tiredness due to the body's inability to regulate its temperature. Heat exhaustion can be life-threatening. A victim of heat exhaustion will have a body temperature that is below normal. Other signs of heat exhaustion include cool, moist, pale, or red skin; nausea; headache; dizziness; fast pulse, and weakness.

First aid for heat exhaustion:

Call the local emergency number and obtain medical care immediately.

1. Have the victim rest in a cool place.
2. Have the victim lie down and elevate the feet.
3. Give the victim cool water to drink.
4. Observe the victim for signs of heat stroke.

What to Do for Heat Stroke (Sunstroke)

Heat stroke is an overheating of the body that is life-threatening. Sweating ceases so that the body cannot regulate its temperature. The victim has a high body temperature and rapid pulse and respiration rate. The skin becomes hot and dry. A victim feels weak, dizzy, and has a headache. A victim may be unconscious.

First aid for heat stroke:

Call the local emergency number and obtain medical care immediately.

1. Have the victim rest in a cool place.
2. Remove heavy clothing.
3. Wrap the victim in cool, wet towels or sheets.
4. Place ice packs near the neck, armpits, and groin.
5. Continue cooling the victim until a body temperature of 102°F (38.9°C) is reached.
6. Treat life-threatening emergencies.

FOLLOW UNIVERSAL PRECAUTIONS
• Wear Disposable Latex Gloves
• Always Use a Face Mask

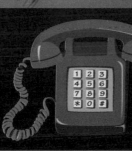

Call the local emergency number and obtain medical care immediately.

What to Know About
First Aid for Cold-Temperature-Related Illnesses

Cold-temperature-related illnesses are conditions that result from exposure to low temperatures. The most common cold-temperature-related emergencies are frostbite and hypothermia.

FOLLOW UNIVERSAL PRECAUTIONS
- Wear Disposable Latex Gloves
- Always Use a Face Mask

What to Do for Frostbite

Frostbite is the freezing of body parts, often the tissues of the extremities. Frostbite may involve the fingers, toes, ears, and nose. People exposed to subfreezing temperatures or snow are at risk for developing frostbite. Signs of frostbite include numbness in the affected area, waxy appearance of skin, and skin discolored and cold to touch.

First aid for frostbite:

Call the local emergency number and obtain medical care immediately.

1. Do not attempt rewarming if a medical facility is nearby. Take the following steps if medical help is not available.

2. Remove any clothing or jewelry that interferes with circulation.

3. Handle the affected area gently.

4. Soak the affected body part in water that has a temperature between 100°F (37.8°C) and 105°F (40.6°C). Test the water by having someone who has not been exposed to the cold place the hand in the water. Water that is too warm for the hand is too warm to use for the victim. Warming usually takes 25 to 40 minutes, until the tissues are soft.

5. Apply warm, moist cloths to warm the ears, nose, or face.

6. Do not rub the affected body part.

7. Do not allow a victim to walk on frostbitten toes or feet, even after rewarming.

8. Slightly elevate the affected part.

9. Place dry, sterile gauze between the toes and fingers to absorb moisture and avoid having them stick.

What to Do for Hypothermia

Hypothermia is a reduction of the body temperature so that it is lower than normal. Hypothermia results from overexposure to cool temperatures, cold water, moisture, and wind. The temperature can be as high as 50°F (11.7°C) and a person can suffer from hypothermia.

Most cases of hypothermia are mild. The victim will shiver and feel cold. The pulse rate slows down and becomes irregular as the body temperature drops. Eventually, a victim can become unconscious. A victim can die if hypothermia is not treated.

First aid for hypothermia:

Call the local emergency number and obtain medical care immediately.

1. Get the victim into a warm environment.

2. Handle the victim gently.

3. Remove any wet clothing, and replace it with dry clothing.

4. Place something warm above and below the victim, such as blankets.

5. Cover the victim's head.

For mild hypothermia (body temperature above 90°F [32.2°C]):

6. Warm the victim. Use an electric blanket or tub of water with a temperature no greater than 105°F (40.6°C). Keep the victim's legs and arms out of the water. Do not have the victim's arms or legs covered by the electric blanket.

7. Place hot packs on the victim's head, neck, chest, and groin. Be careful not to burn the victim.

For profound hypothermia (body temperature below 90°F [32.2°C]):

8. Do not rewarm a victim who can be transported to a medical facility within 12 hours.

9. Calm the victim.

10. Move the victim as little as possible.

11. Do not give CPR to the victim unless there is no pulse. Continue CPR until the victim is transported to a medical facility.

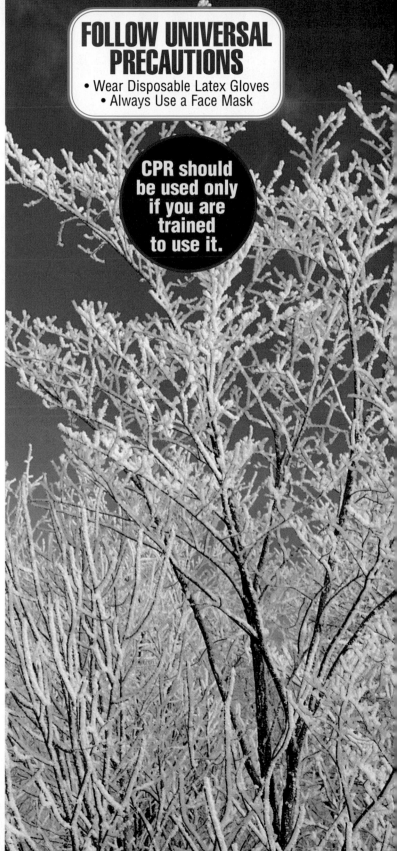

FOLLOW UNIVERSAL PRECAUTIONS
- Wear Disposable Latex Gloves
- Always Use a Face Mask

CPR should be used only if you are trained to use it.

Activity

Ready for Emergencies

Life Skill: I will be skilled in first aid procedures.

Materials: 54 index cards, tape, pencil or marker

Directions: This activity helps you review how to make an emergency telephone call, follow universal precautions, obtain consent to give first aid, and administer first aid procedures. Your teacher will write each one of the vocabulary words listed below on a separate index card. The cards should be shuffled and placed with the words facing down. Your classmates should form a line in front of the teacher. Each classmate will come forward and turn so that his/her back is facing the teacher. The teacher will tape an index card to the back of each classmate. No one will know what word or words are on the card taped to his/her back. Each classmate is to guess the word(s) by approaching other classmates, using the following rules.

 Walk up to a classmate and turn your back to the classmate so that (s)he can read what is written on the card taped to your back.

 Ask the classmate a question that can be answered by "yes" or "no." For example, you might ask, "Is this a cold-temperature-related illness?"

 When you guess what word(s) are on the index card taped on your back, take the card off.

 Take turns with classmates providing information about the word(s) on your index card. For example, if you had "laceration" on your card, you would describe what a laceration is and the first aid procedures for this injury.

emergency	heart attack	lockjaw	open fracture
first aid	cardiac arrest	nosebleed	closed fracture
emergency dispatcher	stroke	knocked-out tooth	dislocation
actual consent	wound	shock	sprain
implied consent	closed wound	poison	strain
Good Samaritan laws	open wound	Lyme disease	sudden illness
universal precautions	bruise	burn	heat-related illnesses
victim assessment	incision	first-degree burn	heat cramps
choking	laceration	second-degree burn	heat exhaustion
universal distress signal	abrasion	third-degree burn	heat stroke
abdominal thrusts	avulsion	electrical burn	cold-temperature-related illnesses
rescue breathing	puncture	chemical burn	frostbite
cardiopulmonary resuscitation (CPR)	infection	splint	hypothermia
	tetanus	fracture	

Lesson 100

Review

Vocabulary Words

Write a separate sentence using 15 of the vocabulary words listed on page 750.

Objectives

1. What is the correct procedure for making an emergency telephone call? **Objective 1**

2. How would you obtain actual consent to give first aid? **Objective 2**

3. What universal precautions must be followed when giving first aid? **Objective 3**

4. What are steps to take when checking a victim? **Objective 4**

5. What are first aid procedures for: Rescue breathing? CPR? Heart attack? Stroke? Bleeding? Shock? Poisoning? Burns? Injuries to muscles, bones, and joints? Heat-related illnesses? Cold-temperature-related illnesses? **Objective 5**

Responsible Decision-Making

Your friends are bored and looking for some excitement. One friend suggests making a prank call to 9-1-1. This friend says you could prank a teacher at your school. You could make up a story about his/her house being on fire. Then you could hide and watch the fire trucks arrive. Your friends laugh when they imagine how embarrassed your teacher will be. Write a response to this situation.

1. Describe the situation that requires you to make a decision.

2. List possible decisions you might make.

3. Name two responsible adults with whom you might discuss your decisions.

4. Evaluate the possible consequences of your decisions. Determine if each decision will lead to actions that:
   - promote health,
   - protect safety,
   - follow laws,
   - show respect for yourself and others,
   - follow the guidelines of your parents and of other responsible adults,
   - demonstrate good character.

5. Decide which decision is most responsible and appropriate.

6. Tell two results you expect if you make this decision.

 Effective Communication

Prepare a three-minute story for an evening newscast in which you discuss the importance of following universal precautions when giving first aid.

 Self-Directed Learning

Make a list of telephone numbers that may be needed for emergencies, such as the Poison Control Center, your physician, fire, police, etc. Place these numbers by the telephones in your home.

 Critical Thinking

A friend falls down the stairs at your house and is bleeding. You grab your family's first aid kit. Should you wear the latex gloves in the first aid kit to give first aid?

 Responsible Citizenship

Have a family discussion about the importance of being prepared for an emergency. Discuss places where a first aid kit might be kept. Tell family members what should be kept in a first aid kit.

Unit 10
Unit Review

Review Questions

Prepare for the unit test. Review your answers for each Lesson Review in this unit. Then write answers to each of the following questions:

1. What are five ways to reduce the risk of drownings? **Lesson 91**

2. What are the most common injuries among teens who work in fast-food restaurants? **Lesson 91**

3. What are the symptoms of repetitive strain injury (RSI)? **Lesson 91**

4. What is the difference between a severe thunderstorm watch and a severe thunderstorm warning? **Lesson 92**

5. What actions would you take if you heard the siren for a tornado warning? **Lesson 92**

6. What are warning signs that a landslide might occur? **Lesson 92**

7. What should you do if the driver in the motor vehicle next to you begins to show road rage? **Lesson 93**

8. Why should you wear a safety belt if a motor vehicle has air bags? **Lesson 93**

9. Why should infants be placed in a child safety restraint in the back seat of a motor vehicle? **Lesson 93**

10. What can happen if you see, hear, and read about violence again and again? **Lesson 94**

11. What are five risk behaviors for violence? **Lesson 94**

12. Why might a person with passive behavior become a perpetrator of violence? **Lesson 94**

13. How do people develop a moral code? **Lesson 95**

14. What are examples of delinquent behavior for which you could be punished? **Lesson 95**

15. What happens when a teen is put on probation because of delinquent behavior? **Lesson 95**

16. What are five ways you can be street smart? **Lesson 96**

17. What should you do if you are sexually harassed? **Lesson 96**

18. What are five self-protections strategies for social situations? **Lesson 96**

19. How would you recognize a gang member? **Lesson 97**

20. Why should you stay away from gangs? **Lesson 97**

21. What are some reasons teens join gangs? **Lesson 97**

22. What does it mean when someone is convicted for carrying a concealed weapon? **Lesson 98**

23. What are the laws regarding the purchase of handguns by teens? **Lesson 98**

24. What are five reasons why carrying a weapon is risky? **Lesson 98**

25. Why may victims of violence need a complete medical examination? **Lesson 99**

26. Why do some people blame victims of violence for what happened even when they were not at fault? **Lesson 99**

27. What is the purpose of recovery programs for victims of violence? **Lesson 99**

28. What would you do if you were alone and choking? **Lesson 100**

29. What would you do if you had a severe nosebleed? **Lesson 100**

30. What would you do if you were stung by a bee? **Lesson 100**

Vocabulary Words

Number a sheet of paper from 1–10. Select the correct vocabulary word and write it next to the corresponding number. DO NOT WRITE IN THIS BOOK.

safety belt	unintentional injury
weapon	emergency
empowered	poison
probation	resiliency
random violence	landslide

1. A _____ is a rapid movement of a mass of earth or rock. **Lesson 92**

2. A _____ is a group of people involved in violent and illegal activities. **Lesson 97**

3. An _____ is an injury caused by an accident. **Lesson 91**

4. A _____ is a seat belt and shoulder strap. **Lesson 93**

5. _____ is a sentence in which an offender remains in the community under the supervision of a probation officer for a specific period of time. **Lesson 95**

6. _____ is violence over which a person has no control. **Lesson 96**

7. A _____ is an instrument or device used for fighting. **Lesson 98**

8. An _____ is a serious situation that occurs without warning and calls for quick action. **Lesson 100**

9. _____ is the ability to adjust, recover, bounce back, and learn from difficult times. **Lesson 94**

10. To be _____ is to be energized because a person has some control over his/her decisions and behavior. **Lesson 99**

Health Literacy

Effective Communication

Write a 60-second public safety announcement (PSN) that explains ways to reduce the risk of unintentional injuries from motor vehicle accidents. Include information about obtaining a valid driver's license, defensive driving, high-risk driving, drinking and driving, speeding tickets, air bags and safety belts, and child restraint systems.

Self-Directed Learning

Status offenses are types of behavior for which an adult would not be arrested. Contact a community law enforcement agency, such as the local police department, and find out the status offenses for juveniles in your community and the consequences of the offenses. Share this information with a classmate.

Critical Thinking

Suppose your friend was the victim of a violent crime. Your friend is having difficulty recovering from the incident. What could you do to help your friend in his/her recovery?

Responsible Citizenship

In this lesson, you learned that seeing, hearing, and reading about violence desensitizes your response to violence. Make a list of TV programs, videos, music, and reading materials that do not contain violence. Share this list with your family members. Suggest that you stop watching, listening to, and reading about violence.

Responsible Decision-Making

You go to your friend's house after school. Your friend's parents are not home. Your friend takes you into his/her parents' bedroom and pulls out a pistol. (S)he suggests that you set up a target and practice shooting the pistol. Write a response to this situation.

1. **Describe the situation that requires you to make a decision.**
2. **List possible decisions you might make.**
3. **Name two responsible adults with whom you might discuss your decisions.**
4. **Evaluate the possible consequences of your decisions. Determine if each decision will lead to actions that:**
   - **promote health,**
   - **protect safety,**
   - **follow laws,**
   - **show respect for yourself and others,**
   - **follow the guidelines of your parents and of other responsible adults,**
   - **demonstrate good character.**
5. **Decide which decision is most responsible and appropriate.**
6. **Tell two results you expect if you make this decision.**

Health Behavior Inventory of Life Skills

Number from 1 to 10 on a sheet of paper. Read each life skill carefully. Write YES or NO next to the same number on your paper. Each YES response indicates a life skill you practice to promote your health status. Each NO response indicates a life skill you do not practice. Plan to begin practicing these life skills.

1. **I will follow safety guidelines to reduce the risk of unintentional injuries.**
2. **I will follow safety guidelines for severe weather and natural disasters.**
3. **I will follow guidelines for motor vehicle safety.**
4. **I will practice protective factors to reduce the risk of violence.**
5. **I will respect authority and obey laws.**
6. **I will practice self-protection strategies.**
7. **I will stay away from gangs.**
8. **I will not carry a weapon.**
9. **I will participate in victim recovery if I am harmed by violence.**
10. **I will be skilled in first aid procedures.**

Multicultural Health

Identify another country in which gangs are a problem. The problem might be an increase in gang violence. Write an essay describing the problem this country is having with gangs and what is being done to resolve the problem.

Family Involvement

Review A Guide to First Aid Procedures with family members. With which first aid procedures are family members familiar? With which are they not familiar? What are ways your family can improve knowledge of first aid procedures?

Health Behavior Contract

Copy and complete the following health behavior contract. Evaluate your progress.
Share the results with your family.

Health Behavior Contract

1. Name_____ Date_____

2. **Life Skill:** I will follow safety guidelines to reduce the risk of unintentional injuries.

3. **Effects on Health Status:** Unintentional injuries are the leading cause of death for teens. Following safety guidelines to reduce the risk of unintentional injuries will protect my health status. It will help me reduce the risk of unintentional injuries in the home, community, and workplace. It will help me reduce the risk of motor vehicle accidents, bicycle accidents, fires, burns, falls, drownings, poisoning, and suffocation. It will help me protect myself if I have a part-time job.

4. **Plan and Method to Record Progress:** I will follow guidelines to reduce the risk of unintentional injuries in the home, community, and workplace. When I use one of these guidelines, I will write the guideline in the space provided for the day of the week. I will list ways that I benefited from following guidelines to reduce the risk of unintentional injuries.

My Calendar

M	T	W	Th	F	S	S

5. **Evaluation:** _____
_____
_____

Glossary

Sound	As in	Symbol	Example
ă	c<u>a</u>t, t<u>a</u>p	a	metatasis (muh·TAS·tuh·suhs)
ā	m<u>a</u>y, s<u>a</u>me	ay	beta-endorphins (BAY·tuh·en·DOR·finz)
a	w<u>ea</u>r, d<u>a</u>re	ehr	pituitary (pi·TOO·i·tehr·ee)
ä	f<u>a</u>ther, t<u>o</u>p	ah	audiologist (awh·dee·AH·luh·jist)
ar	c<u>ar</u>, p<u>ar</u>k	ar	giardiasis (jee·ar·dee·AH·sis)
ch	<u>ch</u>ip, tou<u>ch</u>	ch	botulism (BAH·chuh·li·zuhm)
ĕ	b<u>e</u>t, t<u>e</u>st	e	diuretic (dy·yuh·REH·tik)
ē	p<u>ea</u>, n<u>ee</u>d	ee	amenorrhea (ah·me·nuh·REE·uh)
er	p<u>er</u>k, h<u>ur</u>t	er	chancre (SHAN·ker)
g	<u>g</u>o, bi<u>g</u>	g	smegma (SMEG·muh)
ï	t<u>i</u>p, l<u>i</u>ve	i	epididymis (e·puh·DI·duh·mus)
ī	s<u>i</u>de, b<u>y</u>	y, eye	diabetes (dy·uh·BEE·teez)
j	<u>j</u>ob, e<u>dg</u>e	j	gingivitis (jin·juh·VY·tuhs)
k	coo<u>k</u>, a<u>ch</u>e	k	trachea (TRAY·kee·uh)
ō	b<u>o</u>ne, kn<u>ow</u>	oh	alveoli (al·vee·OH·ly)
ô	m<u>o</u>re, p<u>ou</u>r	or	norepinephrine (NOR·ep·uh·nef·rin)
ȯ	s<u>aw</u>, <u>a</u>ll	aw	gallbladder (GAWL·bla·der)
oi	c<u>oi</u>n, t<u>oy</u>	oy	thyroid (THY·roid)
ou	<u>ou</u>t, n<u>ow</u>	ow	Cowper's (KOW·purz)
s	<u>s</u>ee, le<u>ss</u>	s	seminiferous (se·muh·NI·fuh·ruhs)
sh	<u>sh</u>e, mi<u>ss</u>ion	sh	dehydration (dee·HY·dray·shuhn)
ŭ	c<u>u</u>p, d<u>u</u>g	uh	antioxident (an·ty·AHKS·uh·dent)
u	w<u>oo</u>d, p<u>u</u>ll	u	pulmonary (PUL·muh·nehr·ee)
ü	r<u>u</u>le, <u>u</u>nion	oo	eutrophication (yoo·TROH·fik·a·shun)
w	<u>w</u>e, a<u>w</u>ay	w	wound (WOOND)
y	<u>y</u>ou, <u>y</u>ard	yu	celiac sprue (SEE·lee·ak sproo)
z	<u>z</u>one, rai<u>s</u>e	z	resiliency (ri·ZIL·yuhn·see)
zh	vi<u>s</u>ion, mea<u>s</u>ure	zh	malocclusion (ma·luh·KLOO·zhuhn)
ə	<u>a</u>round, m<u>u</u>g	uh	chlamydia (kluh·MID·ee·uh)

A

abandonment: removing oneself from those whose care is one's responsibility.

abdominal thrusts: a series of thrusts to the abdomen that force air from the lungs to dislodge an object.

abrasion: a wound caused by rubbing or scraping away of the skin.

abstinence: voluntarily choosing not to do something.

abstinence from sex: voluntarily choosing not to be sexually active.

abuse: the harmful treatment of another person.

abuser: a person who is abusive.

acid rain: rain or another form of precipitation that has a high acid content.

acne: a skin disorder in which pores in the skin are clogged with oil.

acoustic nerve: the nerve that connects the inner ear to the brain.

acoustic trauma: an immediate and permanent loss of hearing caused by a short, intense sound.

acquaintance rape: rape in which the rapist is known to the person who is raped.

Acquired Immunodeficiency Syndrome (AIDS): a condition that results in a breakdown of the body's ability to fight infection.

action plan: a detailed description of the steps a person will take to reach a goal.

active immunity: resistance to disease due to the presence of antibodies.

active listening: a way of responding to show that a person hears and understands.

actual consent: oral or written permission to give first aid from a mentally competent adult.

acyclovir (ay·SEE·kloh·vir)**:** an antiviral drug approved for the treatment of herpes simplex infections.

addiction: a compelling need to take a drug or engage in a specific behavior.

adipose (AD·eh·POHZ) **tissue:** fat that accumulates around internal organs, within muscle, and under the skin.

adolescence: the period of growth between childhood and adulthood.

adrenal glands: endocrine glands that secrete several hormones, including adrenaline.

adrenaline: a hormone that prepares the body to react during times of stress or in an emergency.

adverse environment: an environment that interferes with a person's growth, development, and success.

advertisement (ad): a paid announcement about a product or service.

advertising: a form of selling products and services.

aerobic exercise: one in which large amounts of oxygen are required continually for an extended period of time.

affection: a fond or tender feeling that a person has toward another person.

affective disorder: a disorder involving moods that are extreme.

afterbirth: the placenta that is expelled after delivery.

age: to grow older.

aggressive behavior: the use of words or actions that are disrespectful toward others.

agility: the ability to rapidly change the position of the body.

AIDS dementia complex: a loss of brain function caused by HIV infection.

air bag: a cushion in motor vehicles that inflates upon impact.

air pollution: a contamination of the air that causes negative effects on life and health.

Al-Anon: a recovery program for people who have friends or family members with alcoholism.

alarm stage: the first stage of the GAS in which the body gets ready for quick action.

Al-Ateen: a recovery program for teens who have a family member or friend with alcoholism.

emergency room: a facility within a hospital where emergency services are provided without an appointment.

emotion: a specific feeling.

emotional abuse: "putting down" another person and making the person feel worthless.

empathy: the ability to share in another person's emotions or feelings.

emphysema: a condition in which the alveoli lose most of their ability to function.

empowered: to be energized because a person has some control over his/her decisions and behavior.

enabler: a person who supports the harmful behavior of others.

endocrine system: consists of glands that control many of the body's activities by producing hormones.

energy: the ability to do work.

enmeshment: a condition in which a person becomes obsessed with the needs of another person and no longer can recognize his/her own needs.

enriched food: a food in which nutrients lost during processing are added back into the food.

entertainment: something that is designed to hold the interest of people.

environment: everything around a person.

Environmental Protection Agency (EPA): a federal regulatory agency responsible for reducing and controlling environmental pollution.

environmental tobacco smoke: exhaled smoke and sidestream smoke.

enzyme: a protein that regulates chemical reactions.

ephedrine: a stimulant that is found naturally in the ephedra plant.

epidermis: the outer layer of skin cells.

epididymis (e·puh·DI·duh·mus)**:** a comma-shaped structure along the upper rear surface of the testes where sperm mature.

epiglottis: a flap that covers the entrance to the trachea when a person swallows foods or beverages.

epilepsy: a disorder in which abnormal electrical activity in the brain causes a temporary loss of control of the mind and body.

erection: a process that occurs when the penis swells with blood and elongates.

esophagus: a tube connecting the mouth to the stomach.

essential amino acids: the nine amino acids the body cannot produce.

essential body fat: the amount of body fat needed for optimal health.

estrogen: a hormone produced by the ovaries that stimulates the development of female secondary sex characteristics and affects the menstrual cycle.

estrogen replacement therapy (ERT): synthetic estrogen given as a drug to reduce the symptoms of menopause and to help prevent osteoporosis.

ethnic restaurant: a restaurant that serves food that is customary for people of a specific culture.

eugenol: a chemical that numbs the back of the throat and reduces the ability to cough.

eulogy: a formal speech praising someone who has recently died.

Eustachian tube: the tube that connects the middle ear and the back of the nose.

eutrophication (yoo·TROH·fik·a·shun)**:** the build-up of nutrients in water that causes an overgrowth of plants which use up oxygen.

exclusion: a service for which a health insurance plan will not pay.

exercise: planned, structured, and repetitive bodily movement done to improve or maintain one or more components of physical fitness.

exercise addiction: the compelling need to exercise.

exercise-induced asthma (EIA): a condition in which a person has difficulty breathing during or shortly after strenuous physical activity.

exhaustion stage: the third stage of the GAS in which wear and tear on the body increases the risk of injury, illness, and premature death.

expenses: amounts of money needed to purchase or do something.

extended care facility: a facility that provides nursing, personal, and residential care.

extended family members: members of a family in addition to parents, brothers, and sisters.

extinction: the death of all members of a species of animal or plant.

F

fad diet: a quick weight loss strategy that is popular for a short time.

Fallopian tube: a four-inch (ten-centimeter)-long tube that connects an ovary to the uterus.

false image appeal: an advertising technique that tries to convince a person that (s)he will have a certain image if (s)he purchases a specific product or service.

family: a group of people who are related by blood, adoption, or marriage.

family health history: information about the health of a person's blood relatives.

family relationships: the connections a person has with family members, including extended family members.

family value: a standard that is held and copied by members of a family.

fan: a person who watches and supports sports without actively participating in them.

fast food: food that can be served quickly.

fat: a nutrient that provides energy and helps the body store and use vitamins.

fat ketosis (kee·TOH·sis): a condition in which excessive ketones are released into the blood.

fat-soluble vitamin: a vitamin that dissolves in fat and can be stored in the body.

faulty thinking: a thought process in which a person ignores or denies facts or believes false information.

Federal Bureau of Investigation (FBI): a federal government agency that is responsible for federal criminal offenses, including investigation of health fraud such as insurance scams.

Federal Trade Commission (FTC): a federal government agency that enforces consumer protection laws and monitors trade practices and the advertising of foods, drugs, and cosmetics.

female reproductive system: consists of organs in the female body that are involved in producing offspring.

fermentation: a process in which yeast, sugar, and water are combined to produce alcohol and carbon dioxide.

fertilization: the union of an ovum and a sperm.

fetal alcohol syndrome (FAS): the presence of severe birth defects in babies born to mothers who drink alcohol during pregnancy.

fiber: the part of grains and plant foods that cannot be digested.

fighting: taking part in a physical struggle.

filling: the material that a dentist uses to repair a cavity in a tooth.

first aid: the immediate and temporary care given to a person who has been injured or suddenly becomes ill.

first-degree burn: a burn which affects the top layer of skin.

fitness skills: skills that can be used in sports and physical activities.

FITT formula: a formula in which each letter represents a factor for determining how to obtain fitness benefits from physical activity: F-Frequency, I-Intensity, T-Time, and T-Type.

five stages of grief: psychological stages of grieving that include denial, anger, bargaining, depression, and acceptance.

fixer: a person who tries to fix other people's problems.

flash flood: a flood that occurs suddenly.

flashback: a sudden hallucination a person has long after having used a drug.

flexibility: the ability to bend and move the joints through the full range of motion.

flood: a rising and overflowing of a body of water on to normally dry land.

flu: a highly contagious viral infection of the respiratory tract.

flunitrazepam (floo·nuh·TRAZ·i·pam): an odorless, colorless sedative drug.

fluoride: a mineral that strengthens the enamel of teeth.

food additives: substances intentionally added to food.

food allergy: an abnormal response to food that is triggered by the immune system.

Food and Drug Administration (FDA): a federal government agency that monitors the safety of cosmetics and food and the safety and effectiveness of new drugs, medical devices, and prescription and OTC drugs.

food group: a category of foods that contain similar nutrients.

Food Guide Pyramid: a guide that tells how many servings from each food group are recommended each day.

food intolerance: an abnormal response to food that is not caused by immune system.

food label: a panel of nutrition information required on all processed foods regulated by the Food and Drug Administration (FDA).

food-borne illness: an illness caused by consuming foods or beverages that have been contaminated with pathogens.

formal intervention: an action by people, such as family members, who want a person to get treatment.

formaldehyde: a colorless gas with a strong odor.

fortified food: a food in which nutrients not usually found in the food are added.

fossil fuel: a fuel that is formed from plant or animal remains as a result of pressure over many years.

foster care: an arrangement in which another unrelated adult assumes temporary responsibility for a child.

fracture: a break or a crack in a bone.

free weight: a barbell or dumbbell.

freestanding emergency center: a facility that is not part of a hospital that provides emergency care.

fresh water: water that is not contaminated or salty.

friendship: a special relationship with someone a person likes.

frostbite: the freezing of body parts, often the tissues of the extremities.

fungi: single- or multi-celled parasitic organisms.

G

gallbladder: an organ that stores bile.

gambling addiction: the compelling need to bet money or something else.

gang: a group of people involved in violent and illegal activities.

garden: an area where trees, flowers, and other plants are grown and landscaping is maintained.

gasohol: a blend of grain alcohol and gasoline that is used as a fuel source.

gastroenteritis (gas·tro·en·tuh·RI·tuhz): a food-borne illness in which the bacterium *Campylobacter jejuni* contaminates animal products, especially chicken.

gateway drug: a drug whose use increases the likelihood that a person will use other harmful drugs.

gene: a unit of hereditary material.

general adaptation syndrome (GAS): a series of body changes that result from stress.

generational cycle of teen pregnancy: occurs when a teen whose mother was a teen parent becomes pregnant.

generic-name drug: a drug that contains the same active ingredients as a brand-name drug.

genetic counseling: a process in which a trained professional interprets medical information concerning genetics to prospective parents.

genetic predisposition: the inheritance of genes that increase the likelihood of developing a condition.

genital herpes: an STD caused by the herpes simplex virus (HSV) that produces cold sores or fever blisters in the genital area and mouth.

genital warts: an STD caused by certain types of the human papilloma virus (HPV) that produces wart-like growth on the genitals.

geothermal energy: heat transferred from underground sources of steam or hot water.

gerontologist: a person who specializes in the study of aging.

gerontology: the study of aging.

gestational diabetes: diabetes that occurs in some females during pregnancy.

giardia lamblia: a parasite that lives in the intestines of humans and other mammals and causes giardiasis.

giardiasis (jee·ar·dee·AH·sis)**:** a stomach and intestinal infection that causes abdominal cramps, nausea, gas, and diarrhea.

gingivitis (jin·juh·VY·tuhs)**:** a condition in which the gums are red, swollen, and tender and bleed easily.

gland: a group of cells or an organ that secretes hormones.

glaucoma: a condition in which the pressure of the fluid in the eye is high and may damage the optic nerve.

glittering generality appeal: an advertising technique that includes a claim that is exaggerated to appeal to an emotion.

global environmental issues: environmental concerns that can affect the quality of life of people everywhere.

global learner: a person who learns best by combining visual, auditory, and kinesthetic ways of learning.

global warming: an increase in Earth's temperature.

glucose: a simple sugar that is the main source of energy for the body.

goal: a desired achievement toward which a person works.

gonorrhea: a highly contagious STD caused by the gonococcus bacterium *Niesseria gonorrhoeae*.

Good Samaritan laws: laws that protect people who give first aid in good faith and without gross negligence or misconduct.

government hospital: a hospital that is run by the federal, state, or local government for the benefit of a specific population.

graduated license: a conditional license given to new drivers.

graffiti: writing or drawing on a public surface.

grand mal: a major seizure in which a person may have convulsions.

grandparents' rights: the visitation rights with grandchildren courts have awarded grandparents when their son's or daughter's marriage ends.

greenhouse effect: a process by which water vapor and gases in the atmosphere absorb and reflect infrared rays and warm Earth's surface.

grief: intense emotional suffering caused by a loss, disaster, or misfortune.

grooming: keeping the body clean and having a neat appearance.

Group A carcinogen: a substance that causes cancer in humans.

gynecologist: a physician who specializes in female reproductive health.

H

habitat: a place where an animal or plant normally lives.

hair: a threadlike structure consisting of dead cells filled with keratin.

hair follicle: a pit on the surface of the skin that contains nutrients a hair needs to grow.

hairspray: a spray that stiffens hair to keep it in place.

halfway house: a live-in facility that helps a person who is drug-dependent gradually adjust to living independently in the community.

hallucination: an imagined sight, sound, or feeling.

hallucinogens: a group of drugs that interfere with senses and cause hallucinations.

hand-eye coordination: the use of the hands together with the eyes during movement.

hangnail: a strip of skin torn from the side or base of a fingernail.

hangover: an aftereffect of using alcohol and other drugs.

hard-core gang member: a senior gang member who has the most influence.

harmful relationship: a relationship that harms self-respect, interferes with productivity and health, and includes violence and/or drug misuse and abuse.

hashish: a drug that is made from marijuana.

hashish oil: the liquid resin from the cannabis plant.

hate crime: a crime motivated by prejudice.

hay fever: a common term for seasonal respiratory allergies.

hazardous waste: any solid, liquid, or gas in a container that is harmful to humans or animal life.

hazing activity: an activity in which a person is forced to participate in a dangerous or demeaning act to become a member of a club or group.

health advocacy: taking responsibility to improve the quality of life.

health advocate: a person who promotes health.

health advocate for the environment: a person who promotes a healthful environment.

health behavior contract: a written plan to develop the habit of practicing a life skill.

health behavior inventory: a checklist a person completes to learn if (s)he is practicing life skills for health.

health care: the professional medical and dental help that promotes a person's health.

health career: a profession or occupation in the health field for which one trains.

health care facility: a place where people receive health care.

health care practitioner: an independent health care provider who is licensed to practice on a specific area of the body.

health care provider: a trained professional who provides people with health care.

health care system: a system that includes health care providers, health care facilities, and payment for health care.

health center: a facility that provides routine health care to a special population.

health department clinic: a facility in most state and local health departments that keeps records and performs services.

health fraud: the advertising, promotion, and sale of products and services that have not been scientifically proven safe and/or effective.

health history: a record of a person's health habits, past health conditions, and medical care, allergies and drug sensitivities, and health facts about family members.

health insurance: financial protection that provides benefits for sickness or injury.

health knowledge: the information and understanding a person has about health.

health literate person: a person skilled in effective communication, self-directed learning, critical thinking (problem solving), and responsible citizenship.

health maintenance organization (HMO): a business that organizes health care services for its members.

health status: the condition of a person's body, mind, emotions, and relationships.

healthful behavior: an action a person chooses that promotes health; prevents injury, illness, and premature death; and improves the quality of the environment.

healthful body composition: a high ratio of lean tissue to fat tissue in the body.

healthful friendship: a balanced relationship that promotes mutual respect and healthful behavior.

healthful relationship: a relationship that promotes self-respect, encourages productivity and health, and is free of violence and/or drug misuse and abuse.

healthful situation: a circumstance that promotes health; prevents injury, illness, and premature death; and improves the quality of the environment.

health-related fitness: the ability of the heart, lungs, muscles, and joints to function at optimal capacity.

healthy helper syndrome: a state in which a person feels increased energy, relaxation, and improved mood as a result of giving service to others.

hearing aid: an electronic device worn in or near the ear that improves hearing.

heart: a four-chambered muscle that pumps blood throughout the body.

heart attack: the death of cardiac muscle caused by a lack of blood flow to the heart.

heart rate: the number of times the heart contracts each minute.

heart-healthy diet: a low-fat diet rich in fruits, vegetables, whole grains, nonfat and low-fat milk products, lean meats, poultry, and fish.

heat cramps: painful muscle spasms in the legs and arms due to excessive fluid loss through sweating.

heat detector: a device that sounds an alarm when the room temperature rises above a certain level.

heat exhaustion: extreme tiredness due to the body's inability to regulate its temperature.

heat stroke: an overheating of the body that is life-threatening.

heat-related illnesses: conditions that result from exposure to temperatures higher than normal.

helminth: a parasitic worm.

helper T cell: a white blood cell that signals B cells to produce antibodies.

hemoglobin: an iron-rich protein that helps transport oxygen and carbon dioxide in the blood.

hemophilia: an inherited condition in which blood does not clot normally.

heredity: the passing of characteristics from biological parents to their children.

heroin: an illegal narcotic derived from morphine.

herpes simplex virus type 1 (HSV-1): a virus that causes cold sores or fever blisters in the mouth or on the lips.

herpes simplex virus type 2 (HSV-2): a virus that causes genital sores but also may cause sores in the mouth.

hidden anger: anger that is not recognized and is expressed in an inappropriate way.

high blood pressure: a blood pressure of 140/90 mm Hg or greater for an extended time.

high density lipoproteins (HDLs): substances in the blood that carry cholesterol to the liver for breakdown and excretion.

high-risk driving: dangerous driving that can result in accidents.

HIV negative: a term used to describe a person who does not have antibodies for HIV present in his/her blood.

HIV positive: a term used to describe a person who has antibodies for HIV present in his/her blood.

HIV wasting syndrome: a substantial loss in body weight that is accompanied by high fevers, sweating, and diarrhea.

home health care: care provided within a patient's home.

home HIV test: an HIV test that allows a person to take a blood sample at home, place drops of blood on a test card, mail the card to a lab, and call a toll-free number to get results.

homemaker: a person who manages a home.

homicide: the accidental or purposeful killing of another person.

honest talk: the straightforward sharing of feelings.

hormone: a chemical messenger that is released directly into the bloodstream.

hospice: a facility for people who are dying and their families.

hospital: a health care facility where people can receive medical care, diagnosis, and treatment on an inpatient or outpatient basis.

hospitalization insurance: insurance that pays the cost of a hospital stay.

hostility syndrome: a physical state in which the body is in the fight-or-flight state at all times.

huffing: inhaling fumes to get high.

human immunodeficiency virus (HIV): a pathogen that destroys infection-fighting T cells in the body.

humor appeal: an advertising technique that contains a catchy slogan, jingle, or cartoon that gets attention.

humus (HYOO·mus)**:** a soil conditioner.

hunger: the physiological need for food.

hurricane: a tropical storm with heavy rains and winds in excess of 74 miles (118.4 kilometers) per hour.

hydroelectric power: electricity generated from flowing or falling water.

773

hydrogen power: energy produced by passing electrical current through water to burn the hydrogen.

hymen: a thin membrane that stretches across the opening of the vagina.

hyperactive: to not be able to sit or stand still.

hyperopia (or farsightedness): a refractive error in which close objects appear blurred and distant objects are seen clearly.

hyperthyroidism: a condition in which the thyroid gland is overactive.

hypnotic: a drug that produces drowsiness and sleep.

hypoglycemia (hy·po·gly·SEE·mee·uh): a condition in which the pancreas produces too much insulin, causing the blood sugar level to be low.

hypothermia: a reduction in the body temperature so that it is lower than normal.

I

ice: a smokable form of pure methamphetamine.

ideal family: a family that has all the skills needed for loving, responsible relationships.

illegal drug use: the use of a controlled drug without a prescription.

I-message: a statement that contains a specific behavior or event, the effect of the behavior or event on a person, and the emotions that result.

immune system: removes harmful organisms from the blood and combats pathogens.

immunity: the body's resistance to disease-causing agents.

immunization: a substance that contains dead or weakened pathogens that is introduced into the body to give more immunity.

immunotherapy: a process in which the immune system is stimulated to fight cancer cells.

implied consent: permission to give first aid to: a mentally competent adult victim who is unconscious; an adult victim who is not mentally competent, when no adult who can grant actual consent is present; an infant or child when no adult who can grant actual consent is present.

inactive decision-making style: a habit in which a person fails to make choices, and this failure determines the outcome.

incest: having sexual intercourse with a family member.

incinerator: a furnace in which solid waste is burned and energy is recovered in the process.

incision: a cut caused by a sharp-edged object, such as a knife, razor, scissors, or broken glass.

income: money received.

incomplete protein: a protein from plant sources that does not contain all of the essential amino acids.

independent: to be able to rely on oneself.

indication for use: a symptom or condition for which the OTC drug should be used.

infection: a condition in which pathogens enter the body and multiply.

infectious disease: an illness caused by pathogens that can be spread from one living thing to another.

influenza: a highly contagious viral infection of the respiratory tract.

infomercial: a TV program meant to sell products or services.

ingredients listing: the list of the ingredients in a food.

ingrown toenail: a toenail that grows into the skin.

inguinal hernia: a hernia in which some of the intestine pushes through the inguinal canal into the scrotum.

inhalants: chemicals that affect mood and behavior when inhaled.

injecting drug user: a person who injects illegal drugs into the body with syringes, needles, and other injection equipment.

injection drug use: drug use that involves injecting drugs into the body.

inpatient care: treatment that requires a person to stay overnight at a facility.

insomnia: the prolonged inability to fall asleep, stay asleep, or get back to sleep once a person is awakened during the night.

instant gratification: choosing an immediate reward regardless of potential harmful effects.

insulin: a hormone that regulates the blood sugar level.

insulin-dependent diabetes mellitus (IDDM): a type of diabetes in which the body produces little or no insulin.

insurance policy: the legal document issued to the policyholder that outlines the terms of the insurance.

integumentary (in·TEH·gyuh·ment·tuh·ree) **system:** covers and protects the body and consists of skin, glands associated with the skin, hair, and nails.

interdependence: a condition in which two people depend upon one another, yet each has a separate identity.

interest: additional money that is paid for the use of a larger sum of money.

intergroup conflict: a conflict that occurs between two or more groups of people.

Internet: an on-line telecommunications system that connects computer networks from around the world.

interpersonal conflict: a conflict that occurs between two or more people.

intimacy: a deep and meaningful kind of sharing between two people.

intragroup conflict: a conflict that occurs between people that identify themselves as belonging to the same group.

intrapersonal conflict: a conflict that occurs within a person.

invisible fat: fat that cannot be seen when looking at the food.

involuntary muscle: a muscle that functions without a person's control.

isokinetic exercise: an exercise using special machines that provide weight resistance through the full range of motion.

isometric exercise: one in which a muscle is tightened for about five to eight seconds and there is no body movement.

isoniazid (eye·soh·NEE·uh·sud): a drug that prevents tuberculosis in people in close contact with infected people.

isotonic exercise: one in which a muscle or muscles move a moderate amount of weight eight to 15 times.

J

jaundice: yellowing of the skin and whites of the eyes.

joint: the point where two bones meet.

joint custody: an arrangement in which both partners keep legal custody of a child or children.

jumping-in: an initiation rite in which a potential gang member is beaten by gang members.

juvenile detention: the temporary physical restriction of juveniles in special facilities until the outcome of their legal case is decided.

juvenile offender: a minor who commits a criminal act.

K

Kaposi's sarcoma (KS): a type of cancer that affects people who are infected with HIV.

keratin: a tough protein that makes up nails and hair.

kidney: an organ that filters the blood and excretes waste products and excess water in the form of urine.

kinesthetic learner: a person who learns best by acting out something, touching an object, or repeating a motion.

knocked-out tooth: a tooth that has been knocked out of its socket.

L

labia majora: the heavy folds of skin that surround the opening of the vagina.

labia minora: two smaller folds of skin located within the labia majora.

labor: the process of childbirth.

laceration: a cut that causes a jagged or irregular tearing of the skin.

lactase deficiency (LAK·tays dee·FEE·shuhn·see): a condition in which lactase, an enzyme that breaks down the milk sugar present in the cells of the small intestine, is missing.

lacto-ovo-vegetarian diet: a diet that excludes fish, poultry, and red meat.

lacto-vegetarian diet: a diet that excludes eggs, fish, poultry and meat.

mental disorder: a mental or emotional condition that makes it difficult for a person to live in a normal way.

mental health clinic: a facility that provides services for people who have mental disorders.

mentor: a responsible person who guides another person.

mescaline: an illegal hallucinogen made from the peyote cactus.

metabolism (muh·TAB·uh·liz·uhm): the rate at which food is converted into energy in body cells.

metastasis (muh·TAS·tuh·suhs): the spread of cancer.

methamphetamine: a group of stimulant drugs that fall within the amphetamine family.

methcathinone: a stimulant that has effects similar to those of methamphetamine.

methylphenidate: a stimulant that is used to treat Attention Deficit Hyperactivity Disorder.

migraine headache: severe head pain that is caused by dilation of blood vessels in the brain.

mind-body connection: the close relationship between mental and physical responses.

mineral: a nutrient that regulates many chemical reactions in the body.

miscarriage: the natural ending of a pregnancy before a baby is developed enough to survive on its own.

mites: tiny, eight-legged animals that resemble spiders.

mixed message: a message that gives out two different meanings.

Model for Using Resistance Skills, The: a list of suggested ways to resist negative peer pressure.

modem: an electronic device that allows computers to send, receive, and retrieve information over telephone lines.

moderate amount of physical activity: roughly equivalent to physical activity that uses approximately 150 calories of energy per day, or 1000 calories per week.

moderation: placing limits to avoid excess.

monogamous marriage: a marriage in which partners have sex only with each other.

mons veneris: the fatty tissue that covers the front of the pubic bone and serves as a protective cushion for the internal reproductive organs.

moral code: a set of rules a person uses to control behavior.

morphine: a narcotic found naturally in opium that is used to control pain.

motor neurons: carry responding impulses to muscles and glands from the brain and spinal cord.

motor vehicle emissions: substances released into the atmosphere by motor vehicles with gasoline engines.

mousse: a foam that keeps hair in place.

mucous membrane: a type of tissue that lines body cavities and secretes mucus.

mucus: a thick secretion that moistens, lubricates, and protects mucous membranes.

mulching mower: a lawn mower that cuts the grass into small pieces that can be left on the lawn to decompose naturally.

multiple sclerosis (MS): a disease in which the protective covering of nerve fibers in the brain and spinal cord are destroyed.

murder: a homicide that is purposeful.

muscular dystrophy: a genetic disease in which the muscles progressively deteriorate.

muscular endurance: the ability of the muscle to continue to perform without fatigue.

muscular strength: the maximum amount of force a muscle can produce in a single effort.

muscular system: consists of muscles that provide motion and maintain posture.

musculoskeletal injury: an injury to muscles and joints.

myocardial infarction (my·oh·KAR·dee·uhl in·FARK·shun) **(MI):** the medical term for heart attack.

myopia (or nearsightedness): a refractive error in which distant objects appear blurred and close objects are seen clearly.

N

narcolepsy: a chronic sleep disorder in which a people are excessively sleepy even after adequate nighttime sleep.

narcotics: a group of drugs that slow down the central nervous system and relieve pain.

National Collegiate Athletic Association (NCAA): the organization that regulates athletics at the college level and sets eligibility requirements.

National Council Against Health Fraud (NCAHF): an organization that provides legal counsel and assistance to victims of health fraud.

National Health Information Center (NHIC): an agency that refers consumers to organizations that can provide health-related information.

National Institute for Occupational Safety (NIOSH): a federal regulatory agency that conducts research on health hazards in the workplace.

national parks: government- maintained areas of land open to the public.

natural disaster: an event caused by nature that results in damage or loss.

natural environment: everything around a person that is not made by people.

natural gas: an energy source that is found underground above deposits of oil.

natural resource: anything obtained from the natural environment to meet our needs.

nature preserve: an area restricted for the protection of the natural environment.

nature trail: a path through a natural environment.

negative peer pressure: influence from peers to behave in a way that is not responsible.

negative self-esteem: a person's belief that (s)he is not worthy and does not deserve respect.

neglect: failure to provide proper care and guidance.

nervous system: carries messages to and from the brain and spinal cord and all other parts of the body.

neuron: a nerve cell that is the structural and functional unit of the nervous system.

nicotine: a stimulant drug found in tobacco products, including cigarettes and chewing tobacco.

nicotine addiction: the compelling need for nicotine.

nicotine chewing gum: chewing gum that releases nicotine when chewed.

nicotine patch: a patch worn on the skin of the upper body or arms that releases nicotine into the bloodstream at a slow rate.

nicotine withdrawal syndrome: the body's reaction to quitting tobacco products.

nitrogen oxides: nitrogen-containing chemicals that irritate the respiratory system and appear as a yellow-brown haze in the atmosphere.

nitroglycerin: a drug that widens the coronary arteries allowing more oxygen to get to cardiac muscle.

nits: tiny white lice eggs that attach to body hair.

noise: a sound that produces discomfort or annoyance.

noise pollution: a loud or constant noise that causes hearing loss, stress, fatigue, irritability, and tension.

noise-induced permanent threshold shift: a permanent loss of the ability to hear certain frequencies and amplifications.

non-insulin-dependent diabetes mellitus (NIDDM) (dy·uh·BEE·teez me·luh·tuhs)**:** a type of diabetes in which the body produces insulin but it cannot be used by cells.

nonrapid eye movement (NREM) sleep: the period of sleep in which the eyes are relaxed.

nonverbal behavior: the use of actions to express emotions and thoughts.

nonviolence: the avoidance of the threatened or actual use of physical force to injure, damage, or destroy oneself, others, or property.

norepinephrine (NOR·ep·uh·nef·rin)**:** a substance that helps transmit brain messages along certain nerves.

nosebleed: a loss of blood from the mucous membranes that line the nose.

nuclear energy: energy produced by splitting atoms of uranium into smaller parts.

nuclear reactor: a device that splits atoms to produce steam.

nutrient: a substance in food that helps with body processes, helps with growth and repair of cells, and provides energy.

nutrition: the study of what people eat and of eating habits and how these affect health status.

physical fitness plan: a written plan of physical activities to develop each of the components of fitness and a schedule for doing them.

physical intimacy: the sharing of physical affection.

physical punishment: a disciplinary technique in which an act is used to teach a child not to repeat undesirable behavior.

physician: an independent health care provider who is licensed to practice medicine.

pitch: the highness or lowness of sound.

pituitary (pi·TOO·i·tehr·ree) **gland:** an endocrine gland that produces hormones that control growth and other glands.

placenta: rich in blood vessels and anchors the embryo to the uterus.

plagiarism (PLAY·juh·riz·uhm): copying and passing off the ideas or words of another person or persons as one's own.

plaque: hardened deposits.

plasma: the liquid component of blood that carries blood cells and dissolved materials.

platelet: a particle that helps the blood clot.

player agent: a person who represents athletes in contract negotiations with professional teams and with companies who want endorsements.

pneumocystis carinii pneumonia (PCP): a form of pneumonia that may affect people infected with AIDS.

pneumonia: an infection in the lungs caused by bacteria, viruses, or other pathogens.

podiatrist: a doctor of podiatric medicine (DPM) who specializes in problems of the feet.

poison: a substance that causes injury, illness, or death if it enters the body.

poisoning: a harmful chemical reaction from a substance that enters the body.

pollen: a yellowish powder made in flowers and grass.

pollutants: harmful substances in the environment.

pollution: any change in air, water, soil, noise level, or temperature that has a negative effect on life and health.

pollution standard index: a measure of air quality based on the sum of the levels of five different pollutants.

positive peer pressure: influence from peers to behave in a responsible way.

positive self-esteem: a person's belief that (s)he is worthy and deserves respect.

postpartum period: the span of time that begins after the baby is born.

post-traumatic stress disorder (PTSD): a condition in which a person relives a stressful experience again and again.

poverty: a condition in which a person does not have sufficient resources to eat and live healthfully.

power: the ability to combine strength and speed.

precycling: a process of reducing waste.

preexisting condition: a health problem that person had before being covered by the insurance.

preferred provider: a health care provider who appears on a list that has been approved by the health insurance provider.

preferred provider organization (PPO): a health insurance plan that has a contract with a group of health care providers who agree to provide health care services at a reduced rate.

prejudice: suspicion, intolerance, or irrational hatred directed at an individual or group of people.

premature birth: the birth of a baby before it is fully developed; less than 38 weeks from time of conception.

premature death: death before a person reaches his/her predicted life expectancy.

premature heart attack: a heart attack that occurs before age 55 in males and age 65 in females.

premenstrual syndrome (PMS): a combination of physical and emotional symptoms that affect a female a week to ten days prior to menstruation.

premium: a specific amount of money that will guarantee that an insurance company will help pay for health services.

prenatal care: the care that is given to the mother-to-be and baby before birth.

presbyopia (prez·bee·OH·pee·uh): a refractive error caused by weakening of eye muscles and hardening of the cornea.

prescription: a written order from a physician or other licensed health professional.

prescription drug: a medicine that can be obtained only with a written order from a licensed health professional.

prestige crime: a crime committed to gain status from other gang members.

preventive discipline: training in which a parent explains correct behavior and the consequences of wrong behavior.

primary care: general health care.

primary syphilis: the first stage of syphilis.

principle of cool-down: states that a workout should end with five to ten minutes of reduced exercise to help the heart rate, breathing rate, body temperature, and circulation return to the nonexercising state.

principle of fitness reversibility: states that fitness benefits are lost when training stops.

principle of overload: states that a workout must include exercise beyond what a person usually does to gain additional fitness benefits.

principle of progression: states that the amount and intensity of exercise during workouts must be increased gradually.

principle of specificity: states that a workout should include a specific type of exercise to obtain the desired fitness benefits.

principle of warm-up: states that a workout should begin with three to five minutes of easy exercise to increase blood flow, raise the temperature in muscles, and stretch muscles.

prison: a building, usually with cells, where convicted criminals stay.

private hospital: a hospital that is owned by private individuals and operates as a profit-making business.

proactive decision-making style: a habit in which a person describes the situation that requires a decision, identifies and evaluates possible decisions, and makes a decision and takes responsibility for the consequences.

probation: a sentence in which an offender remains in the community under the supervision of a probation officer for a specific period of time.

procrastinate: to postpone something until a future time.

products: material goods, such as food, medicine, and clothing, that are made for consumers to purchase.

progesterone: a hormone that changes the lining of the uterus.

progress appeal: an advertising technique that emphasizes that a product or service is "new and improved."

projection: blaming others for actions or events for which they are not responsible.

promiscuous: to engage in sexual intercourse with many people.

promise breaker: a person who is not reliable.

proof: a measure of the amount of alcohol in a beverage.

prostate gland: a gland that produces a fluid that helps keep sperm alive.

prostitution: sexual activity for pay.

protective factor: something that increases the likelihood of a positive outcome.

protein: a nutrient that is needed for growth; to build, repair, and maintain body tissues; to regulate body processes; and to supply energy.

protein loading: an eating strategy in which extra protein is eaten to increase muscle size.

protozoa: tiny, single-celled organisms that produce toxins that cause disease.

PSI: a measure of air quality based on the sum of the levels of five different pollutants.

psilocybin: an illegal hallucinogen made from a specific type of mushroom.

psychological dependence: a strong desire to continue using a drug for emotional reasons.

psychological intimacy: the sharing of needs, emotions, weaknesses, and strengths.

psychosomatic disease: a physical disorder caused or aggravated by emotional responses.

puberty: the stage of growth and development when both the male and female body become capable of producing offspring.

pubic lice: infestation of the pubic hair by pubic or crab lice that survive by feeding on human blood.

pulmonary artery: a blood vessel that carries blood from the heart to the lungs to pick up oxygen and release carbon dioxide.

pulp: the living tissue within a tooth.

pulse: the surge of blood that results from the contractions of the heart.

puncture: a wound produced when a pointed instrument pierces the skin.

purge: to rid the body of food by vomiting or by using laxatives and diuretics.

Q

quack: a person or company who is involved in health fraud.

quality of life: the degree to which a person lives life to the fullest capacity.

R

radiation therapy: treatment of cancer with high-energy radiation to kill or damage cancer cells.

radon: an odorless, colorless radioactive gas that is released by rocks and soil.

rain forest: a hot, wet forested area that contains many species of trees, plants, and animals.

random event: an event over which a person has little or no control.

random violence: violence over which a person has no control.

rape: the threatened or actual use of physical force to get someone to have sex without giving consent.

rape survivor: a person who has been raped.

rape trauma syndrome: a condition in which a rape survivor experiences emotional responses and physical symptoms over a period of time.

rapid eye movement (REM) sleep: the period of sleep characterized by rapid eye movements behind closed eyelids.

razor: a device with a sharp blade used for shaving hair.

reaction time: the time it takes a person to move after (s)he hears, sees, feels, or touches a stimulus.

reactive decision-making style: a habit in which a person allows others to make his/her decisions.

recall: an order to take a product off the market due to safety concerns.

recovery program: a group that supports members as they change behavior to be responsible and healthful.

recreational trail: a path designed for recreational activities, such as walking, jogging, in-line skating, biking, and hiking.

recruitment: contact by a coach or representative of a college athletic department about enrolling and playing sports at a college.

rectum: a short tube at the end of the large intestine that stores wastes temporarily.

recycling: the process of re-forming or breaking down a waste product so that it can be used again.

red blood cell: a blood cell that transports oxygen to body cells and removes carbon dioxide from body cells.

redshirt year: a year in which an athlete practices with the team without competing to keep an extra year of eligibility.

reference materials: publications that contain facts and information and are used for consultation.

reflex action: an involuntary action in which a message is sent to the spinal cord, is interpreted, and is responded to immediately.

refractive error: a variation in the shape of the eyeball that affects the way images are focused on the retina and blurs vision.

regular gang member: a gang member who belongs to the gang and obey the hard-core gang members.

regular physical activity: physical activity that is performed on most days of the week.

regulatory agency: an agency that enforces laws to protect the general public.

rehabilitation of juvenile offenders: the process of helping juvenile offenders change wrong behavior to responsible behavior.

rejection: the feeling of being unwelcome or unwanted.

relapse: a return to a previous behavior or condition.

relationship: a connection a person has with another person.

relationship addiction: the compelling need to be connected to another person.

relaxer: a product that helps take curl out of hair.

remarriage: a marriage in which a previously married person marries again.

repetitions: the number of times an exercise is performed in one set.

repetitions maximum: the maximum amount of resistance that can be moved a specified number of times.

repetitive strain injury (RSI): an injury that occurs from repeated physical movements.

request for medical nonintervention: a person's refusal of specific life support systems when there is no reasonable expectation of recovering or regaining a meaningful life.

rescue breathing: a way of breathing air into an unconscious victim who is not breathing, but has a pulse.

resiliency (ri·ZIL·yuhn·see): the ability to adjust, recover, bounce back, and learn from difficult times.

resilient: to be able to adjust, recover, bounce back, and learn from difficult times.

resistance exercise: an exercise in which a force acts against muscles.

resistance skills: skills that help a person say "no" to an action or to leave a situation.

resistance stage: the second stage of the GAS in which the body attempts to regain internal balance.

respect: high regard for someone or something.

respiratory system: provides body cells with oxygen and removes carbon dioxide that cells produce as waste.

responsible decision: a choice that leads to actions that promote health, protect safety, follow laws, show respect for self and others, follow the guidelines of parents and other responsible adults, and demonstrate good character.

Responsible Decision-Making Model, The: a series of steps to follow to assure that the decisions a person makes result in actions that promote health, protect safety, follow laws, show respect for self and others, follow the guidelines of parents and of other responsible adults, and demonstrate good character.

responsible drug use: the correct use of legal drugs to promote health and well-being.

rest: a period of relaxation.

restitution: making good for any loss or damage.

restraining order: an order by a court that forbids a person from doing a particular act.

retainer: a plastic device with wires that keep the teeth from moving back to their original places.

retina: the inner lining of the eyeball.

reward appeal: an advertising technique that offers a special prize, gift, or coupon when a product or service is purchased.

Reye's syndrome: a disease that causes swelling of the brain and deterioration of liver function.

rheumatic fever: an auto-immune action in the heart that can cause fever, weakness, and damage to the valves in the heart.

rheumatic heart disease: permanent heart damage that results from rheumatic fever.

rheumatoid arthritis: a condition in which joints become deformed and may lose function.

rhinovirus: a virus that infects the nose.

RICE treatment: a technique for treating musculoskeletal injuries that involves rest, compression, and elevation.

rickettsia (ri·KET·see·uh): pathogens that grow inside living cells and resemble bacteria.

ringworm: a skin condition that causes small, red, ring-shaped marks on the skin.

risk: a chance that a person takes that has an unknown outcome.

risk behavior: an action a person chooses that threatens health; can cause injury, illness, and premature death; and destroys the environment.

risk factor: something that increases the likelihood of a negative outcome.

risk situation: a circumstance that threatens health; can cause injury, illness, and premature death; and destroys the environment.

tampon: a small tube of cotton placed inside the vagina to absorb the menstrual flow.

tar: a sticky, thick fluid that is formed when tobacco is burned.

target heart rate: a heart rate of 75 percent of maximum heart rate.

teaching hospital: a hospital that is associated with a medical school and/or school of nursing.

television addiction: the compelling need to watch television.

temporary threshold shift (TTS): the temporary hearing loss of certain frequencies and amplifications.

tendon: tough tissue fiber that attaches muscles to bones.

terminal illness: an illness that will result in death.

terrarium: a transparent container that holds plants or small animals.

tertiary syphilis: the final stage of syphilis in which spirochetes damage body organs.

testes: male reproductive glands that produce sperm cells and testosterone.

testicular self-examination: a screening procedure for testicular cancer in which a male checks his testes for lumps or tenderness.

testimonial appeal: an advertising technique that uses a spokesperson who names the benefits of a specific product or service.

testosterone (te·STAH·tuh·rohn): a hormone that produces male secondary sex characteristics.

tetanus: a bacteria that grows in the body and produces a strong poison that affects the nervous system and muscles.

texturizing hair cream: a product that puts curl in a male's hair.

THC: a drug found in the cannabis plant that produces psychoactive effects.

therapeutical equivalence: when two drugs are chemically the same and produce the same medical effects.

thermal inversion: a condition that occurs when a layer of warm air forms above a layer of cool air.

thermal pollution: a harmful condition caused by the addition of heated water to a water supply.

third-degree burn: a burn that involves all layers of the skin and underlying tissues.

thrill-seeking addiction: the compelling need to take unnecessary risks.

thrush: a fungal infection of the mucous membranes of the tongue and mouth.

thymus gland: a gland that causes white blood cells to become T cells.

thyroid gland: an endocrine gland that produces thyroxin.

thyroxin: a hormone that controls metabolism and calcium balance in the body.

time management: organizing time to accomplish priorities.

time management plan: a plan that shows how a person will spend time.

time out: a calming-down period of time.

tinnitus (TEYE·nuh·tuhs): a ringing, buzzing, or hissing sensation in the ears that can reach levels equivalent to 70 dBs.

tissue: a group of similar cells that work together.

tobacco: a plant that contains nicotine.

tobacco cessation program: a program to help a person stop smoking or using smokeless tobacco.

tolerance: a condition in which the body becomes used to a substance.

topical fluoride: a fluoride product that is applied directly to the teeth.

tornado: a violent, rapidly spinning windstorm that has a funnel-shaped cloud.

tornado warning: a warning issued when a tornado has been sighted or indicated by radar.

tornado watch: a warning issued when weather conditions are such that tornadoes are likely to develop.

toxemia of pregnancy: a disorder of pregnancy characterized by high blood pressure, tissue swelling, and protein in the urine.

toxic shock syndrome (TSS): a severe illness resulting from infection with toxin-producing strains of *Staphylococcus*.

toxin: a substance that is poisonous.

trachea (TRAY·kee·uh): a tube through which air moves to the lungs.

tracking disorder: a learning disability in which a person has difficulty following a series of words or images.

traditional marriage: an emotional, spiritual, and legal commitment a man and woman make to one another.

traffic violation: any violation of the current traffic code.

training ceiling: the upper limit of overload required to obtain fitness benefits without risking injury or illness.

training principles: guidelines to follow to obtain maximum fitness benefits and reduce the risk of injuries and illnesses.

training threshold: the minimum amount of overload required to obtain fitness benefits.

training zone: the range of overload required to obtain fitness benefits.

trichomoniasis (trik·oh·moh·NY·uh·sis): an STD caused by the single-celled protozoan *Trichomonas vaginalis.*

trihalomethanes: harmful chemicals that are produced when chlorine attacks pollutants in water.

tryptophan: an amino acid that helps promote relaxation.

tubal pregnancy: occurs when a fertilized egg implants in a Fallopian tube instead of in the uterus.

tuberculin skin test: the injection of a protein substance under the skin in the forearm.

tuberculosis: a bacterial infection of the lungs.

tumor: an abnormal growth of tissue.

turbine: an engine that rotates.

tutor: a person who works with individual students to help them with schoolwork.

Twelve Step Program: a program which helps people recover from their past and gain wholeness.

Type I diabetes: a type of diabetes in which the body produces little or no insulin.

Type II diabetes: a type of diabetes in which the body produces insulin but it cannot be used by cells.

U

ulcer: an open sore on the skin or on a mucous membrane.

ultrasound: a procedure in which high-frequency sound waves are used to provide an image of the developing baby.

ultraviolet (UV) radiation: a type of radiation that comes from the sun and also is emitted by sunlamps and tanning booths.

umbilical cord: a ropelike structure that connects the embryo to the placenta.

underweight: a body weight that is 10 percent or more below desirable body weight.

unintentional injury: an injury caused by an accident.

United States Department of Agriculture (USDA): a federal government agency that enforces standards to ensure the safe processing of food and oversees the distribution of food information to the public.

United States Postal Service (USPS): a federal government agency that offers postal services and protects the public when products and services are sold through the mail.

universal distress signal: a warning that a person has difficulty breathing and is shown by clutching at the throat with one or both hands.

universal precautions: steps taken to prevent the spread of disease by treating all human blood and certain body fluids as if they contained HIV, HBV, and other pathogens.

unnecessary risk: a chance that is not worth taking after the possible outcomes are considered.

unsaturated fat: a type of fat obtained from plant products and fish.

uranium: a radioactive substance that is mined.

ureter (YU·ruh·ter): a narrow tube that connects the kidneys to the urinary bladder.

urethra (yu·REE·thruh): a narrow tube extending from the urinary bladder to the outside of the body through which urine passes out of the body.

urgent care center: a facility that is not part of a hospital that provides emergency care.

urinary bladder: a muscular sac that stores urine.

urinary system: removes liquid wastes from the body and maintains the body's water balance.

urine: a pale yellow liquid composed of water, salts, and other waste products.

uterus: a muscular organ that receives and supports the fertilized egg during pregnancy and contracts during childbirth to help with delivery.

V

vaccine: a substance that contains dead or weakened pathogens that is introduced into the body to give more immunity.

vagina: a muscular tube that connects the uterus to the outside of the body.

value: a standard or belief.

vas deferens: two long, thin tubes that act as a passageway for sperm and a place for sperm storage.

V-chip: a small electronic device that allows television programs to be blocked.

vegan diet: a diet that excludes foods of animal origin.

vegetarian diet: a diet in which vegetables are the foundation and meat, fish, and poultry are restricted or eliminated.

vein: a blood vessel that returns blood to the heart.

vena cava: one of two large veins that returns blood rich in carbon dioxide to the right atrium.

ventricle: one of the lower two chambers of the heart.

victim assessment: a check of the injured or medically ill person to determine if: the victim has an open airway, the victim is breathing, the victim's heart is beating, the victim is severely bleeding, the victim has other injuries.

victim of violence: a person who has been harmed by violence.

victim recovery: a person's return to physical and emotional health after being harmed by violence.

video: a tape of video images and sound that is recorded and played using a videocassette recorder and a TV.

villi: small folds in the lining of the small intestine.

violence: the use of physical force to injure, damage, or destroy oneself, others, or property.

viral hepatitis: a viral infection of the liver.

virus: the smallest known pathogen.

visible fat: fat that can be seen when looking at food.

visitation rights: guidelines set for the visitation of children by the parent who does not have custody.

visual acuity: sharpness of vision.

visual environment: everything a person sees regularly.

visual learner: a person who learns best by seeing or creating images and pictures.

visual pollution: sights that are unattractive.

vitamin: a nutrient that helps the body use carbohydrates, proteins, and fats.

voluntary hospital: a hospital that is owned by a community or organization and does not operate for profit.

voluntary muscle: a muscle a person can control.

volunteer: a person who provides a service without pay.

volunteer burnout: a loss of enthusiasm about volunteering that results from feeling overwhelmed.

volunteer center: an organization that matches people with volunteer jobs.

W

walk-in surgery center: a facility where surgery is performed on an outpatient basis.

wanna-be: a child or teen who is not a gang member, but may wear gang clothing and engage in violent or criminal behavior to prove worthy of being a gang member.

warm-up: a period of three to five minutes of easy physical activity to prepare the muscles to do more work.

wart: a contagious growth that forms on the top layer of the skin.

water: a nutrient that is involved with all body processes, makes up the basic part of the blood, helps with waste removal, regulates body temperature, and cushions the spinal cord and joints.

water pollution: contamination of water that causes negative effects on life and health.

water runoff: water that runs off the land into a body of water.

water-soluble vitamin: a vitamin that dissolves in water and cannot be stored by the body in significant amounts.

weapon: an instrument or device used for fighting.

weather: the condition of the atmosphere at a particular time and place.

web site: a specific location where information is found.

weight machine: an apparatus that provides resistance to a muscle or group of muscles.

weight management: a diet and exercise plan to maintain a desirable weight and body composition.

weight training: a conditioning program in which free weights or weight machines provide resistance for muscles.

wellness: the quality of life that results from a person's health status.

Wellness Scale, The: a scale that shows the ranges in quality of life.

Western blot: a blood test used to check for antibodies for HIV and to confirm an ELISA test.

wheal: a round skin lump that indicates sensitivity to a particular allergen.

white blood cell: a blood cell that attacks, surrounds, and destroys pathogens that enter the body, and prevents them from causing infection.

wildland fire: a fire that occurs in the wilderness.

wildlife sanctuary: a place reserved for the protection of plants and animals.

wind energy: energy from wind.

winter storm: a storm in the form of freezing rain, sleet, ice, heavy snow, or blizzards.

wisdom: good judgment and intelligence in knowing what is responsible and appropriate.

withdrawal symptoms: unpleasant reactions that occur when a person who is physically dependent on a drug no longer takes it.

workaholism: the compelling need to work to fill an emptiness.

work ethic: an attitude of discipline, motivation, and commitment toward tasks.

World Wide Web (WWW): a graphic system on the Internet made up of a huge connection of documents.

wound: an injury to the body's soft tissues.

wrong decision: a choice that leads to actions that harm health, are unsafe, are illegal, show disrespect for self and others, disregard the guidelines of parents and of other responsible adults, and lack good character.

Y

you-message: a statement that blames or shames another person.

Z

zoo: a park in which animals are cared for and shown to the public.